FIRST AID FOR THE® INTERNAL MEDICINE BOARDS

TAO T. LE, MD
Senior Fellow, Division of Allergy and Clinical Immunology
Department of Medicine
Johns Hopkins University
Baltimore, Maryland

PETER CHIN-HONG, MD
Assistant Professor, Division of Infectious Diseases
Department of Medicine
University of California at San Francisco
San Francisco, California

THOMAS E. BAUDENDISTEL, MD, FACP
Associate Director Internal Medicine Residency
Department of Medicine
California Pacific Medical Center
San Francisco, California

LEWIS RUBINSON, MD, PHD
Senior Fellow, Division of Pulmonary and Critical Care Medicine
Johns Hopkins University
Fellow, Center for Biosecurity
University of Pittsburgh Medical Center
Pittsburgh, Pennsylvania

McGraw Hill

Boston Burr Ridge, IL Dubuque, IA Madison, WI New York San Francisco St. Louis
Bangkok Bogotá Caracas Kuala Lumpur Lisbon London Madrid Mexico City
Milan Montreal New Delhi Santiago Seoul Singapore Sydney Taipei Toronto

The McGraw-Hill Companies

First Aid for the® Internal Medicine Boards
International Edition 2006

Exclusive rights by McGraw-Hill Education (Asia), for manufacture and export. This book cannot be re-exported from the country to which it is sold by McGraw-Hill. The International Edition is not available in North America.

10 09 08 07 06 05 04 03 02 01
20 09 08 07 06
CTF SLP

ISBN 007-142166-1

NOTICE

Medicine is an ever-changing science. As new research and clinical experience broaden our knowledge, changes in treatment and drug therapy are required. The authors and the publisher of this work have checked with sources believed to be reliable in their efforts to provide information that is complete and generally in accord with the standards accepted at the time of publication. However, in view of the possibility of human error or changes in medical sciences, neither the authors nor the publisher nor any other party who has been involved in the preparation or publication of this work warrants that the information contained herein is in every respect accurate or complete, and they disclaim all responsibility for any errors or omissions or for the results obtained from use of the information contained in this work. Readers are encouraged to confirm the information contained herein with other sources. For example and in particular, readers are advised to check the product information sheet included in the package of each drug they plan to administer to be certain that the information contained in this work is accurate and that changes have not been made in the recommended dose or in the contraindications for administration. This recommendation is of particular importance in connection with new or infrequently used drugs.

When ordering this title, use ISBN 007-123996-0

Printed in Singapore

DEDICATION

To the contributors to this and future editions, who took time to share their knowledge, insight, and humor for the benefit of residents and clinicians.

and

To our families, friends, and loved ones, who endured and assisted in the task of assembling this guide.

CONTENTS

AUTHORS

DIANA M. ANTONIUCCI, MD
Clinical Instructor, Division of Endocrinology and Metabolism
Department of Medicine
University of California at San Francisco

AMIN N. AZZAM, MD
Research Fellow
Department of Psychiatry
University of California at San Francisco

SCOTT W. BIGGINS, MD
Fellow, Division of Gastroenterology
Department of Medicine
University of California at San Francisco

THOMAS CHEN, MD, PHD
Staff Physician
Department of Hematology and Oncology
San Francisco VA Medical Center

JOSH COHEN, MD
Fellow, Division of Cardiology
Department of Medicine
University of California at San Francisco

PARAM DEDHIA, MD
Instructor, Department of Medicine
Assistant Program Director, Geriatric Educational Center
Johns Hopkins University

KAREN EARLE, MD
Clinical Instructor, Division of Endocrinology and Metabolism
Diabetes Center
Department of Medicine
University of California at San Francisco

JOSÉ EGUÍA, MD
Assistant Professor, Division of Infectious Diseases
Department of Medicine
University of California at San Francisco

JOEY ENGLISH, MD, PHD
Clinical Instructor
Department of Neurology
University of California at San Francisco

JONATHAN GRAF, MD
Assistant Professor, Division of Rheumatology
Department of Medicine
University of California at San Francisco

CINDY LAI, MD
Assistant Clinical Professor, Division of General Internal Medicine
Department of Medicine
University of California at San Francisco

SERGE LINDNER, MD
Fellow, Division of Geriatrics
Department of Medicine
University of California at San Francisco

CHRISTIAN MERLO, MD, MPH
Clinical Instructor, Division of Pulmonary and Critical Care Medicine
Department of Medicine
Johns Hopkins University

ALAN C. PAO, MD
Fellow, Division of Nephrology
Department of Medicine
University of California at San Francisco

MICHAEL RAFII, MD, PHD
Chief Resident
Department of Neurology
Johns Hopkins University

MARC RIEDL, MD
Clinical Instructor, Division of Clinical Immunology and Allergy
Department of Medicine
University of California at Los Angeles

JONATHAN E. ROSENBERG, MD
Clinical Instructor, Division of Hematology and Oncology
Department of Medicine
University of California at San Francisco

SANJIV SHAH, MD
Fellow, Division of Cardiology
Department of Medicine
University of California at San Francisco

LINDA W. SHIUE, MD
Assistant Clinical Professor
Department of Medicine
University of California at San Francisco and
Palo Alto Medical Foundation

ROBERT TROWBRIDGE, MD
Assistant Professor
Department of Medicine
University of Vermont School of Medicine
Maine Hospitalist Service
Maine Medical Center

SIEGRID YU, MD
Chief Resident
Department of Dermatology
University of California at San Francisco

SENIOR REVIEWERS

ADRIAN M. CASILLAS, MD
Associate Professor, Division of Clinical Immunology and Allergy
Department of Medicine
David Geffen School of Medicine
University of California at Los Angeles

HUGO QUINNY CHENG, MD
Associate Clinical Professor, Division of General Internal Medicine
Department of Medicine
University of California at San Francisco

CHARLES DALEY, MD
Professor and Chief, Division of Mycobacterial and Respiratory Infections
Department of Medicine
National Jewish Medical and Research Center

G. DAVID ELKIN, MD
Associate Professor
Department of Psychiatry
University of California at San Francisco

JOHN W. ENGSTROM, MD
Professor and Vice-Chair
Department of Neurology
Director, Neurology Residency Program
University of California at San Francisco

ELYSE FOSTER , MD
Professor of Clinical Medicine, Division of Cardiology
Department of Medicine
University of California at San Francisco

KENNETH H. FYE, MD
Clinical Professor, Division of Rheumatology
Department of Medicine
University of California at San Francisco

KAREN HAUER, MD
Associate Professor of Clinical Medicine
Director of Internal Medicine Clerkships
Department of Medicine
University of California at San Francisco

ROBERT M. JASMER, MD
Assistant Professor, Division of Pulmonary and Critical Care Medicine
Department of Medicine
Co-Director, Pulmonary and Critical Care Medicine Fellowship Program
University of California at San Francisco

C. BREE JOHNSTON, MD, MPH
Associate Professor, Division of Geriatrics
Department of Medicine
San Francisco VA Medical Center
University of California at San Francisco

R. JEFFREY KOHLWES, MD, MPH
Director, PRIME Residency Program
Department of Medicine
San Francisco VA Medical Center
University of California at San Francisco

UMESH MASHARANI, MB, BS, MRCP
Professor, Division of Endocrinology and Metabolism
Department of Medicine
University of California at San Francisco

TOBY A. MAURER, MD
Associate Professor and Chief
Department of Dermatology
San Francisco General Hospital
University of California at San Francisco

ANDREW D. MICHAELS, MD, FACC, FAHA
Assistant Professor, Division of Cardiology
Department of Medicine
University of California at San Francisco

WILLIS H. NAVARRO, MD
Assistant Clinical Professor, Division of Hematology and Oncology
Department of Medicine
University of California at San Francisco

RUDOLPH A. RODRIGUEZ, MD
Associate Professor, Division of Nephrology
Department of Medicine
University of California at San Francisco

HOPE S. RUGO, MD
Clinical Professor, Division of Hematology and Oncology
Department of Medicine
University of California at San Francisco

NEIL STOLLMAN, MD
Associate Professor, Division of Gastroenterology
Department of Medicine
University of California at San Francisco

NORAH TERRAULT, MD, MPH
Assistant Professor, Division of Gastroenterology
Department of Medicine
University of California at San Francisco

JUDITH WALSH, MD, MPH
Associate Professor, Division of General Internal Medicine
Department of Medicine
University of California at San Francisco

LISA G. WINSTON, MD
Assistant Professor, Division of Infectious Diseases
Department of Medicine
University of California at San Francisco

PREFACE

With *First Aid for the® Internal Medicine Boards,* we hope to provide residents and clinicians with the most useful and up-to-date preparation guide for the American Board of Internal Medicine (ABIM) certification and recertification exams. This new addition to the *First Aid* series represents an outstanding effort by a talented group of authors and includes the following:

- A practical exam preparation guide with resident-tested test-taking and study strategies
- Concise summaries of thousands of board-testable topics
- Hundreds of high-yield tables, diagrams, and illustrations
- Key facts in the margins highlighting "must know" information for the boards
- Mnemonics throughout, making learning memorable and fun

We invite you to share your thoughts and ideas to help us improve *First Aid for the® Internal Medicine Boards.* See How to Contribute, p. xv.

Baltimore Tao Le
San Francisco Peter Chin-Hong
San Francisco Thomas E. Baudendistel
Baltimore Lewis Rubinson

ACKNOWLEDGMENTS

This has been a collaborative project from the start. We gratefully acknowledge the thoughtful comments, corrections, and advice of the residents, international medical graduates, and faculty who have supported the authors in the development of *First Aid for the® Internal Medicine Boards.*

For input into the design of this book and for help in coordinating faculty reviewers, we first want to thank Cynthia Fenton. For reviewing content manuscript, we would like to thank Alex Walley and Elizabeth Turner.

For additional feedback, we also thank Leila Alpers, Nader Banki, Kirsten Bibbins-Domingo, Charles Chiu, Janet Diaz, Martin Garcia, Liz Goldman, Chris Hall, James Hamrick, Dave Hemsey, Jo Ix, Lenny Katz, Brent Kinder, Stacey Jolly, Kiran Khush, Bernie Lo, Rick Loftus, Dana McClintock, Deepu Nair, Robert Ross, Hilary Seligman, Michael Shiloh, Neil Trivedi, Abhilash Vaishnav, Eduard Vasilevskis, Doug White and Rachel Zemans.

For support and encouragement throughout the process, we are grateful to Thao Pham, Linda Shiue, Lisa Kinoshita, Kai Baudendistel, and Selina Bush.

Thanks to our publisher, McGraw-Hill, for the valuable assistance of their staff. For enthusiasm, support, and commitment to this challenging project, thanks to our editor, Catherine Johnson. For outstanding editorial work, we thank Andrea Fellows. A special thanks to Rainbow Graphics for remarkable production work.

Baltimore Tao Le
San Francisco Peter Chin-Hong
San Francisco Thomas E. Baudendistel
Baltimore Lewis Rubinson

HOW TO CONTRIBUTE

To continue to produce a high-yield review source for the ABIM exam, you are invited to submit any suggestions or corrections. We also offer **paid internships** in medical education and publishing ranging from three months to one year (see next page for details). Please send us your suggestions for

- Study and test-taking strategies for the ABIM
- New facts, mnemonics, diagrams, and illustrations
- Low-yield topics to remove

For each entry incorporated into the next edition, you will receive a $10 gift certificate, as well as personal acknowledgment in the next edition. Diagrams, tables, partial entries, updates, corrections, and study hints are also appreciated, and significant contributions will be compensated at the discretion of the authors. Also let us know about material in this edition that you feel is low yield and should be deleted.

The preferred way to submit entries, suggestions, or corrections is via electronic mail. Please include name, address, institutional affiliation, phone number, and e-mail address (if different from the address of origin). If there are multiple entries, please consolidate into a single e-mail or file attachment. Please send submissions to:

firstaidteam@yahoo.com

Otherwise, please send entries, neatly written or typed or on disk (Microsoft Word), to:

First Aid for the Internal Medicine Boards
P.O. Box 27
Woodstock, MD 21163-9982
Attention: Contributions

NOTE TO CONTRIBUTORS

All entries become property of the authors and are subject to editing and reviewing. Please verify all data and spellings carefully. In the event that similar or duplicate entries are received, only the first entry received will be used. Include a reference to a standard textbook to facilitate verification of the fact. Please follow the style, punctuation, and format of this edition if possible.

INTERNSHIP OPPORTUNITIES

The author team is pleased to offer part-time and full-time paid internships in medical education and publishing to motivated physicians. Internships may range from three months (e.g., a summer) up to a full year. Participants will have an opportunity to author, edit, and earn academic credit on a wide variety of projects, including the popular *First Aid* series. Writing/editing experience, familiarity with Microsoft Word, and Internet access are desired. For more information, e-mail a résumé or a short description of your experience along with a cover letter to **firstaidteam@yahoo.com**.

Introduction: Guide to the ABIM

INTRODUCTION

For house officers, the ABIM is the culmination of three years of hard work. For practicing physicians, it becomes part of their maintenance of certificate. However, the certification and recertification process does not simply represent yet another set of exams in a series of expensive tests. To your patients, it means that you have the level of clinical knowledge and competency required to provide good clinical care. In fact, according to a poll conducted for the ABIM, about 72% of adult patients are aware of their physicians' board-certification status.

The majority of your patients will be aware of your certification status.

In this chapter we talk more about the ABIM and provide you with proven approaches to conquering the exam. For a detailed description of the ABIM, visit **www.abim.org** or refer the *Certification Examination in Internal Medicine Information Booklet*, which can also be found on the ABIM Web site.

ABIM—THE BASICS

How Do I Register to Take the Exam?

You can register for the exam online by going to "On-Line Services" at www.abim.org. The registration fee is currently about $1000. If you miss the application deadline, a $300 nonrefundable late fee is tacked on. Check the ABIM Web site for the latest registration deadlines, fees, and policies.

Register early to avoid an extra $300 late fee.

What if I Need to Cancel the Exam or Change Test Centers?

The ABIM currently provides partial refunds if a written cancellation is received before certain deadlines. You can also change your test center with a written request for a specific deadline. Check the ABIM Web site for the latest information on its refund and cancellation policy as well as procedures. Expect these policies to change significantly when the ABIM implements the computer-based testing (CBT) format in 2006.

How Is the ABIM Test Structured?

The ABIM is currently a two-day paper-based test administered at test centers around the country. The exam is divided into four three-hour blocks during those two days. Each block has 90 questions for a total of 360 questions. One or more of the booklets will contain a "glossy" section of color images that you will need to refer to in order to answer some of the questions. During the time allotted for each block, you can answer test questions in any order as well as review responses and change answers. Examinees cannot go back and change answers from previous blocks.

The ABIM will migrate the certification exam to a CBT format (remember your USMLEs?) by **August 2006** (see Figure 1). Therefore, the structure of the exam is likely to change drastically. The new CBT exam will be administered by Pearson VUE, a division of Pearson Education, at about 200 centers throughout the United States. Please check the ABIM Web site for Web demos, updates, and details about the new format.

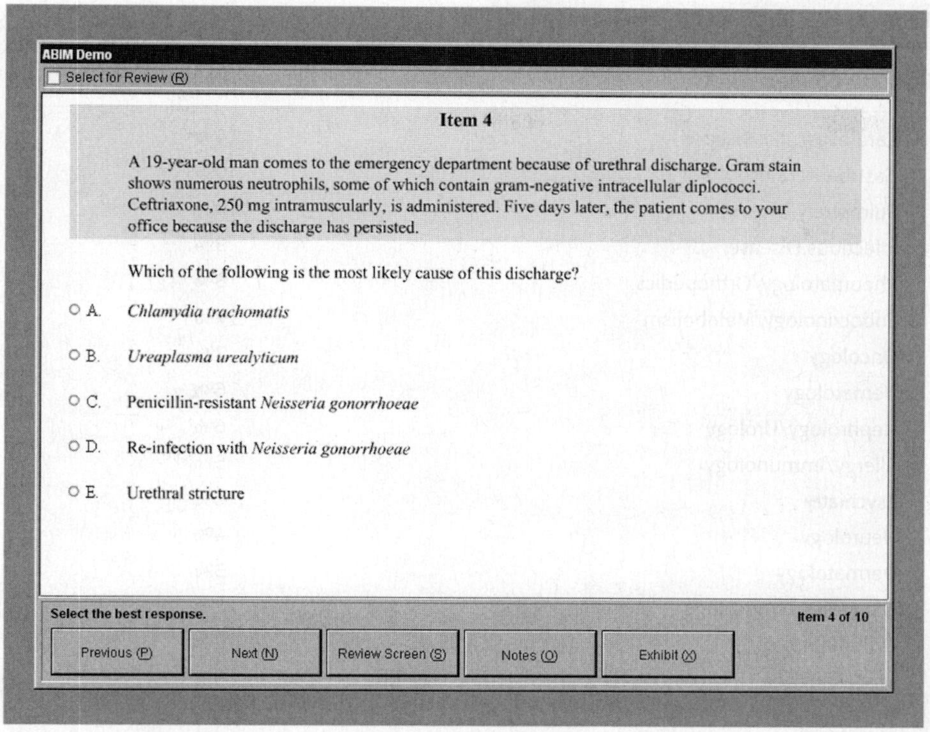

FIGURE 1. ABIM CBT format for 2006.

What Types of Questions Are Asked?

All questions are **single-best-answer** types only. You will be presented with a scenario and a question followed by four to six options. Virtually all questions on the ABIM are vignette based. A substantial amount of extraneous information may be given, or a clinical scenario may be followed by a question that could be answered without actually requiring that you read the case. Some questions require interpretation of photomicrographs, radiology studies, photographs of physical findings, and the like. It is your job to determine which information is superfluous and which is pertinent to the case at hand.

Virtually all questions are case based.

Question content is based on a content "blueprint" developed by the ABIM (see Table 1). This blueprint may change from year to year, so check the ABIM Web site for the latest. About 75% of the **primary content** focuses on traditional subspecialties such as cardiology and gastroenterology. The remaining **25%** pertains to certain outpatient or related specialties and subspecialties such as allergy/immunology, dermatology, and psychiatry. There are also **cross-content** questions that may integrate information from multiple primary content areas.

TABLE 1. ABIM Certification Blueprint

Primary Content Areas	Relative Proportions
Cardiovascular Disease	14%
Gastroenterology	10%
Pulmonary Disease	10%
Infectious Disease	9%
Rheumatology/Orthopedics	8%
Endocrinology/Metabolism	7%
Oncology	7%
Hematology	6%
Nephrology/Urology	6%
Allergy/Immunology	5%
Psychiatry	4%
Neurology	4%
Dermatology	3%
Obstetrics/Gynecology	2%
Ophthalmology	2%
Miscellaneous	3%
Total	100%
Cross-Content Areas	**Relative Proportions**
Critical Care Medicine	10%
Geriatric Medicine	10%
Prevention	6%
Women's Health	6%
Clinical Epidemiology	3%
Ethics	3%
Nutrition	3%
Palliative/End-of-Life Care	3%
Adolescent Medicine	2%
Occupational Medicine	2%
Substance Abuse	2%

Source: www.abim.org, 2005.

How Are the Scores Reported?

The passing scores are set before the exam administration, so your passing is not influenced by the relative performance of others taking the test with you. Scoring and reporting of test results may take up to **three months.** In addition, your pass/fail status will be available to you on the ABIM Web site through the "On-Line Services" within a day of the results being mailed to you. Note that you need to register to access this feature.

Your score report will give you a "pass/fail" decision, the overall number of questions you answered correctly with a corresponding percentile, and the number of questions you answered correctly with a corresponding percentile for the primary and cross-content subject areas noted in the blueprint. Each year, be-

TABLE 2. First-Time Test Taker Performance

Year	Number Taking	Percentage Passed
2004	7056	92%
2003	6751	92%
2002	7074	87%
2001	6802	88%
2000	7048	86%

Source: www.abim.org, 2005.

tween **20 and 40 questions** on the exam do not count toward your final score. Again, these may be "experimental" questions or questions that are later disqualified. Historically, between **85% and 90%** of first-time examinees pass on the first attempt (see Table 2). About 90% of examinees who are recertifying pass on the first attempt, and about 97% are ultimately successful with multiple attempts. There is no limit on the number of retakes if an examinee fails.

THE RECERTIFCATION EXAM

The recertification exam is given every year in November. It consists of **three modules** lasting two hours each. Each module has 60 questions, for a total of **180 questions.** You get two minutes per question. In contrast to the initial certification exam, the recertification exam is currently administered as a CBT at a Pearson VUE testing site. Performance on the recertification exam is similar to that of the certification exam; however, pass rates have been trending downward over the last few years (see Table 3).

Check the ABIM Web site for the latest passing requirements.

TEST PREPARATION ADVICE

The good news about the ABIM is that it tends to focus on the diagnosis and management of diseases and conditions that you have likely seen as a resident and that you should expect to see as an internal medicine specialist. Assuming that you have performed well as a resident, *First Aid* and a good source of practice questions may be all you need. However, consider using *First Aid* as a **guide** and using multiple resources, including a standard textbook, journal review articles, MKSAP, or a concise electronic text such as *UpToDate,* as part

TABLE 3. Recertification Performance

Year	Percent Passed
2001	92%
2002	92%
2003	85%

of your studies. Original research articles are low yield, and very new research (i.e., research done less than one to two years before the exam) will not be tested. In addition, there are a number of high-quality board review courses offered around the country. Board review courses are very expensive but can help those who need some focus and discipline.

The ABIM tends to focus on the horses, not the zebras.

Ideally, you should start your preparation early in your **last year of residency,** especially if you are starting a demanding job or fellowship right after residency. Cramming in the period between end of residency and the exam is **not advisable.**

Use a combination of First Aid, *textbooks, journal reviews, and practice questions.*

As you study, concentrate on the **nuances of management,** especially for difficult or complicated cases. For **common diseases,** learn both common and **uncommon presentations;** for **uncommon diseases,** focus on the **classic presentations** and manifestations. Draw on the experiences of your residency training to anchor some of your learning. When you take the exam, you will realize that you've seen most of the clinical scenarios in your three years of wards, clinics, morning report, case conferences, or grand rounds.

Other High-Yield Areas

Focus on topic areas that are typically not emphasized during residency training but are board favorites. These include the following:

- Topics in outpatient specialties (e.g., allergy, dermatology, ENT, ophthalmology)
- Formulas that are needed for quick recall (e.g., alveolar gas, anion gap, creatinine clearance)
- Basic biostatistics (e.g., sensitivity, specificity, positive predictive value, negative predictive value)
- Adverse effects of drugs

TEST-TAKING ADVICE

By this point in your life, you have probably gained more test-taking expertise than you care to admit. Nevertheless, here are a few tips to keep in mind when taking the exam:

- For long vignette questions, read the question stem and scan the options; **then** go back and read the case. You may get your answer without having to read through the whole case.
- There's no penalty for guessing, so you should **never** leave a question blank.
- Good pacing is key. You need to leave adequate time to get to all the questions. Even though you have two minutes per question on average, you should aim for a pace of 90 to 100 seconds per question. If you don't know the answer within a short period, make an educated guess and move on.
- It's okay to **second guess** yourself. Research shows that our "second hunches" tend to be better than our first guesses.
- Don't panic with "impossible" questions. They may be **experimental questions** that won't count. Again, take your best guess and move on.
- Note the age and race of the patient in each clinical scenario. When ethnicity is given, it is often relevant. Know these well, especially for more common diagnoses.

Never, ever leave a question blank! There's no penalty for guessing.

- Questions often describe clinical findings instead of naming eponyms (e.g., they cite "tender, erythematous bumps in the pads of the finger" instead of "Osler's node").

TESTING AND LICENSING AGENCIES

American Board of Internal Medicine
510 Walnut Street, Suite 1700
Philadelphia, PA 19106-3699
215-446-3500 or 800-441-2246
Fax: 215-446-3633
www.abim.org

Educational Commission for Foreign Medical Graduates (ECFMG)
3624 Market Street
Philadelphia, PA 19104-2685
215-386-5900
Fax: 215-386-9196
www.ecfmg.org

Federation of State Medical Boards (FSMB)
P.O. Box 619850
Dallas, TX 75261-9850
817-868-4000
Fax: 817-868-4098
www.fsmb.org

CHAPTER 1

Allergy and Immunology

Marc Riedl, MD

DIAGNOSTIC TESTING IN ALLERGY

Allergy Skin Testing

- Confirmatory test for the presence of **allergen-specific IgE antibody.**
- **Puncture skin testing:** Adequate for most purposes. A drop of allergen extract is placed on the skin surface, and epidermal puncture is performed with a specialized needle.
- **Intradermal skin testing:** Used for venom and penicillin testing; 0.02 mL of allergen is injected intracutaneously using a 26- to 27-gauge needle.
- All skin testing should use positive (histamine) and negative (saline) controls.
- Skin-testing **wheal-and-flare reactions** are measured 15–20 minutes after placement.

Laboratory Allergy Testing

- Radioallergosorbent (**RAST**) serologic testing is performed to confirm the presence of **allergen-specific IgE antibody.**
- Results are comparable to skin testing for pollen- and food-specific IgE.
- Useful when skin testing is either not available or not possible owing to skin conditions or interfering medications (e.g., antihistamine use).
- RAST testing alone is generally **not** adequate for **venom or drug allergy** testing.

Delayed-Type Hypersensitivity Skin Testing

- An effective screening test for functional **cell-mediated immunity.**
- Involves **intradermal injection of 0.1 mL of purified antigen.** The standard panel includes ***Candida*, mumps, tetanus toxoid,** and **PPD.**
- The injection site is examined for **induration 48 hours** after injection.
- Approximately 95% of normal subjects will respond to one of the abovementioned antigens.
- The absence of a response suggests deficient cell-mediated immunity or anergy.

Allergen Patch Testing

- The appropriate diagnostic test for **allergic contact dermatitis.**
- Suspected substances are applied to the skin with adhesive test strips for 48 hours.
- The skin site is examined 48 and 72 hours after application for evidence of erythema, edema, and vesiculation (reproduction of contact dermatitis).

GELL AND COOMBS CLASSIFICATION OF IMMUNOLOGIC REACTIONS

The traditional framework used to describe immune-mediated reactions; not inclusive of all complex immune processes.

Type I: Immediate Reactions (IgE Mediated)

- Specific antigen exposure causes **cross-linking of IgE on mast cell/basophil surfaces,** leading to the release of histamine, leukotrienes, prostaglandins, and **tryptase.**
- Mediator release causes symptoms of **urticaria, rhinitis, wheezing, diar-**

rhea, vomiting, hypotension, and **anaphylaxis,** usually within **minutes** of antigen exposure.
- **Late-phase** type I reactions may cause **recurrent symptoms 4–8 hours** after exposure.

Type II: Cytotoxic Reactions

- Mediated by **antibodies,** primarily IgG and IgM, **directed at cell surface or tissue antigens.**
- Antigens may be native, foreign, or haptens (small foreign particles attached to larger native molecules).
- Antibodies **destroy cells** by **opsonization** (coating for phagocytosis), **complement-mediated lysis,** or **antibody-dependent cellular cytotoxicity.**
- Clinical examples include penicillin-induced autoimmune **hemolytic anemia** and certain forms of **autoimmune thyroiditis.**

Type III: Immune Complex Reactions

- Exposure to antigen in genetically predisposed individuals causes **antigen-antibody complex** formation.
- Antigen-antibody complexes **activate complement and neutrophil** infiltration.
- Results in tissue inflammation, most commonly affecting the **skin, kidneys, joints,** and **lymphoreticular system.**
- Clinically presents with symptoms of **"serum sickness" 10–14 days after exposure;** most frequently caused by **β-lactam antibiotics** or nonhuman antiserum (antithymocyte globulin, antivenoms).

Gell-Coombs classification system–

ACID

Anaphylactic–type I
Cytotoxic–type II
Immune complex–type III
Delayed hypersensitivity–type IV

Type IV: Delayed Hypersensitivity Reactions (T-Cell Mediated)

- Exposure to antigen causes direct activation of **sensitized T cells,** usually CD4+ cells.
- T-cell activation causes tissue **inflammation 48–96 hours after exposure.**
- The most common clinical reaction is **allergic contact dermatitis** such as that resulting from **poison ivy.**

ASTHMA

A **chronic inflammatory disorder** of the airway resulting in **airway hyperresponsiveness, airflow limitation,** and **respiratory symptoms.** Often begins in childhood, but may have adult onset. **Atopy** is a strong identifiable **risk factor** for the development of asthma. Subtypes include exercise-induced, occupational, aspirin-sensitive, and cough-variant asthma.

Symptoms

Symptoms include **dyspnea** (at rest or with exertion), **cough, wheezing,** mucus hypersecretion, chest tightness, and nocturnal awakenings with respiratory symptoms. Symptoms may have identifiable **triggers** (e.g., exercise, exposure to cat dander, NSAIDs, exposure to cold).

Exam

- **Acute exacerbations: Expiratory wheezing,** prolonged expiratory phase, increased respiratory rate.

- **Severe exacerbations: Pulsus paradoxus,** cyanosis, lethargy, use of accessory muscles of respiration, silent chest (absence of wheezing due to lack of air movement).
- **Chronic asthma without exacerbation:** Minimal to no wheezing. Signs of allergic rhinosinusitis (boggy nasal mucosa, posterior oropharynx cobblestoning, suborbital edema) are commonly found. **Exam may be normal** between exacerbations.

DIFFERENTIAL

- **Upper airway obstruction:** Foreign body, tracheal compression, tracheal stenosis, vocal cord dysfunction.
- **Other lung disease:** Emphysema, chronic bronchitis, cystic fibrosis, allergic bronchopulmonary aspergillosis, Churg-Strauss syndrome, chronic eosinophilic pneumonia, obstructive sleep apnea, restrictive lung disease, pulmonary embolism.
- **Cardiovascular disease**: CHF, ischemic heart disease.
- **Respiratory infection:** Bacterial or viral pneumonia, bronchiectasis, sinusitis.

DIAGNOSIS

Diagnosed by the history and objective evidence of **obstructive lung disease.**

- **PFTs:** Show a **decreased FEV_1/FVC ratio** with **reversible obstruction** (> 12% increase in FEV_1 after bronchodilator) and **normal diffusing capacity.**
- **Methacholine challenge:** Useful if baseline lung function is normal but clinical symptoms are suggestive of asthma. A positive methacholine challenge test is not diagnostic of asthma, but a negative test indicates that asthma is unlikely **(high sensitivity, lower specificity).**

TREATMENT

Acute exacerbations are treated as follows:

- **Initial treatment: Inhaled rapid-acting β_2-agonists** (albuterol), one dose q 20 minutes × 1 hour; **O_2** to keep saturation > 90%.
  - **Good response:** With a peak expiratory flow (PEF) > 80% of predicted or personal best after albuterol, continue albuterol q 3–4 h and institute appropriate chronic therapy (see below).
  - **Incomplete response:** With a PEF 60–80% of predicted or personal best, consider systemic corticosteroids; continue inhaled albuterol q 60 minutes × 1–3 hours if continued improvement is seen.
  - **Poor response or severe episode:** With a PEF < 60% of predicted or personal best, give systemic corticosteroids and consider systemic epinephrine (preferably IM), IV theophylline, and/or IV magnesium.
- Patients with improved symptoms, a PEF > 70%, and O_2 saturation > 90% for 60 minutes after the last treatment may be discharged home with appropriate outpatient therapy and follow-up. Oral corticosteroids are appropriate in most cases.
- Patients with **incomplete responses** after the initial two hours of treatment (persistent moderate symptoms, PEF < 70%, O_2 saturation < 90%) should be admitted for **inpatient therapy** and monitoring with inhaled **albuterol, O_2,** and **systemic corticosteroids.**
- Patients with a **poor response** to initial therapy (severe symptoms, lethargy, confusion, PEF < 30%, P_{O_2} < 60, P_{CO_2} > 45) should be admitted to the **ICU** for treatment with **inhaled albuterol, O_2, IV corticosteroids,** and **possible intubation** and mechanical ventilation.

Chronic asthma therapy is based on asthma severity as defined by the National Asthma Education and Prevention Program (NAEPP) guidelines. The treatment regimen should be **reviewed every 1–6 months,** with changes made depending on symptoms and clinical course.

- All asthma patients should use **2–4 puffs** of a **short-acting bronchodilator as needed for symptoms. Use of a short-acting bronchodilator ≥ 2 times per week** may indicate the need for increased control therapy.
- **Mild intermittent asthma (symptoms ≤ 2 days per week and ≤ 2 nights per month; PEF ≥ 80%): No daily medication** is needed.
- **Mild persistent asthma (symptoms > 2 days/week but < 1 time per day or > 2 nights per month; PEF ≥ 80%):**
  - **Low-dose inhaled corticosteroids** are preferred.
  - Other medications include leukotriene modifiers, theophylline, and cromolyn.
- **Moderate persistent asthma (daily symptoms or > 1 night per week and PEF 60–80%):**
  - **Low- to medium-dose inhaled corticosteroids** and **long-acting inhaled β_2-agonists** are preferred.
  - Alternative therapy involves inhaled corticosteroids and leukotriene modifiers or theophylline.
- **Severe persistent asthma (continuous symptoms; PEF < 60%):**
  - **High-dose inhaled corticosteroids and long-acting inhaled β_2-agonists.**
  - **Oral corticosteroids** at a dosage of up to 60 mg QD may be necessary.

Additional treatment considerations include the following:

- Recognize the exacerbating effects of **environmental factors** such as allergens, air pollution, smoking, and weather (cold and humidity).
- Use potential **exacerbating medications with caution** (aspirin, NSAIDs, β-blockers).
- Always consider **medication compliance and technique** as possible complicating factors in poorly controlled asthma.
- Treatment of **coexisting conditions (rhinitis, sinusitis, GERD)** may improve asthma.

Asthma symptoms that occur more than twice weekly generally indicate the need for inhaled corticosteroid therapy.

COMPLICATIONS

- Hypoxemia, respiratory failure, pneumothorax or pneumomediastinum.
- Frequent hospitalization and previous intubation are warning signs of potentially fatal asthma.
- A subset of patients with chronic asthma develop **airway remodeling,** leading to accelerated, irreversible loss of lung function.

ALLERGIC RHINITIS

The most **common cause** of chronic rhinitis. Allergic factors are present in 75% of rhinitis cases. May be **seasonal or perennial;** incidence is greatest in adolescence and decreases with advancing age. Usually persistent, with occasional spontaneous remission.

SYMPTOMS

- Sneezing, nasal itching, rhinorrhea, nasal congestion, sore throat, throat clearing, itching of the throat and palate.
- Sleep disturbance; association with obstructive sleep apnea.

- Concomitant conjunctivitis with ocular itching, lacrimation, and puffiness.

EXAM

Patients present with swollen nasal turbinates with pale or bluish mucosa, clear nasal discharge, clear to white secretions along the posterior wall of the oropharynx, infraorbital darkening, conjunctival erythema, and lacrimation.

DIFFERENTIAL

- **Nonallergic rhinitis:** Vasomotor or gustatory rhinitis.
- **Rhinitis medicamentosa:** Overuse of vasoconstricting nasal sprays, leading to rebound nasal congestion and associated symptoms.
- **Hormonal rhinitis:** Associated with pregnancy, use of OCPs, and hypothyroidism.
- **Drug-induced rhinitis:** Common causes include β-blockers, α-blockers, and cocaine.
- **Atrophic rhinitis:** Develops in elderly patients with atrophy of the nasal mucosa.
- **Infectious rhinosinusitis:** Acute viral syndromes lasting 7–10 days; bacterial sinusitis.
- **Nasal obstruction due to a structural abnormality:** Septal deviation, nasal polyposis, nasal tumor, foreign body.

DIAGNOSIS

Based on history and **positive skin testing** to common aeroallergens (e.g., grass/tree/weed pollen, house dust mites, cockroaches, dog and cat dander, mold).

TREATMENT

- **Allergen avoidance measures:** Most effective for house dust mites (involves use of allergen-impermeable bed and pillow casings and washing of bedding in hot water). Indoor pollen exposure can be reduced by keeping windows closed and using air conditioners.
- **Antihistamines:** Reduce sneezing, rhinorrhea, and pruritus. Less effective for nasal congestion; most effective if used regularly. Not effective for nonallergic rhinitis. Nonsedating antihistamines are preferable.
- **Oral decongestants:** Effectively reduce nasal congestion in allergic and nonallergic rhinitis. May cause insomnia and exacerbate hypertension or arrhythmia.
- **Intranasal steroids:** The most effective medication for allergic and nonallergic rhinitis. No significant systemic side effects; most beneficial when used regularly.
- **Allergen immunotherapy:** Indicated as an alternative or adjunct to medications. The only effective therapy that has been demonstrated to modify the long-term course of the disease.

Intranasal steroids are the most effective treatment for allergic rhinitis.

COMPLICATIONS

Chronic sinusitis and otitis; exacerbation of asthma.

HYPERSENSITIVITY PNEUMONITIS

A complex immune-mediated lung disease resulting from repeated inhalational exposure to a wide variety of **organic dusts** (see Table 1-1). Presents in acute, subacute, and chronic forms.

TABLE 1-1. Selected Causes of Hypersensitivity Pneumonitis

DISEASE	ANTIGEN	SOURCE
Farmer's lung	*Micropolyspora faeni, Thermoactinomyces vulgaris.*	Moldy hay.
"Humidifier lung"	Thermophilic actinomycetes.	Contaminated humidifiers, heating systems, or air conditioners.
Bird-fancier's lung ("pigeon breeder's disease")	Avian proteins.	Bird serum and excreta.
Bagassosis	*Thermoactinomyces sacchari* and *T. vulgaris.*	Moldy sugar-cane fiber (bagasse).
Sequoiosis	*Graphium, Aureobasidium,* and other fungi.	Moldy redwood sawdust.
Maple bark stripper's disease	*Cryptostroma (Coniosporium) corticale.*	Rotting maple tree logs or bark.
Mushroom picker's disease	Same as farmer's lung.	Moldy compost.
Suberosis	*Penicillium frequentans.*	Moldy cork dust.
Detergent worker's lung	*Bacillus subtilis* enzyme.	Enzyme additives.

Reproduced, with permission, from Tierney LM et al. *Current Medical Diagnosis & Treatment 2005,* 44th ed. New York: McGraw-Hill, 2005: 293.

SYMPTOMS

- **Acute:** Nonproductive cough, shortness of breath, fever, diaphoresis, myalgias occurring 6–12 hours after intense antigen exposure.
- **Chronic:** Insidious onset of dyspnea, productive cough, fatigue, anorexia, weight loss.

EXAM

- **Acute:** Patients are ill-appearing with fever, respiratory distress, and dry rales (wheezing is **not** a prominent symptom). Exam may be normal in asymptomatic patients between episodes of acute hypersensitivity pneumonitis.
- **Chronic:** Dry rales, decreased breath sounds, digital clubbing.

DIFFERENTIAL

- **Acute:**
  - **Pneumonia:** Bacterial, viral, or atypical.
  - **Toxic fume bronchiolitis:** Sulfur dioxide, ammonia, chlorine.
  - **Organic dust toxic syndrome:** Inhalation of dusts contaminated with bacteria and fungi.
- **Subacute or chronic:** Chronic bronchitis, idiopathic pulmonary fibrosis, chronic eosinophilic pneumonia, collagen vascular disease, sarcoidosis, primary pulmonary histiocytosis, alveolar proteinosis.

DIAGNOSIS

- PFTs:
  - **Acute: Restrictive pattern** with decreased FVC and FEV_1. **Decreased DL_{CO}** is common.
  - **Chronic:** Combined obstructive and restrictive pattern.
- **Radiographic:**
  - **Acute:** CXR shows transient patchy, peripheral, bilateral interstitial infiltrates. CT typically shows ground-glass opacifications and diffuse consolidation (see Figure 1-1).
  - **Subacute:** CXR shows nodular, patchy infiltrates and fibrosis; CT shows centrilobular nodules with areas of ground-glass opacity.
  - **Chronic:** CXR shows fibrotic changes with honeycombing and areas of emphysema; CT shows honeycombing, fibrosis, traction bronchiectasis, ground-glass opacities, and small nodules.
- **Lab tests:**
  - **Acute:** Elevated WBC count; elevated ESR.
  - **Acute or chronic: High titers of precipitating IgG** against the offending antigen (indicates exposure, not necessarily disease). Double-gel immunodiffusion is preferred, as ELISA may be too sensitive.
- **Bronchoalveolar lavage:** Lymphocytosis with predominance of CD8+ T cells.
- **Lung biopsy:** Interstitial and alveolar noncaseating granulomas; "foamy" macrophages; predominance of lymphocytes.
- **Inhalational challenge:** Not required or recommended for diagnosis; helpful when data are lacking or diagnosis is unclear. Performed only with careful medical monitoring.

TREATMENT

- Avoidance of offending antigen.
- Oral corticosteroids at a dosage of 40–80 mg QD with tapering after clinical improvement.

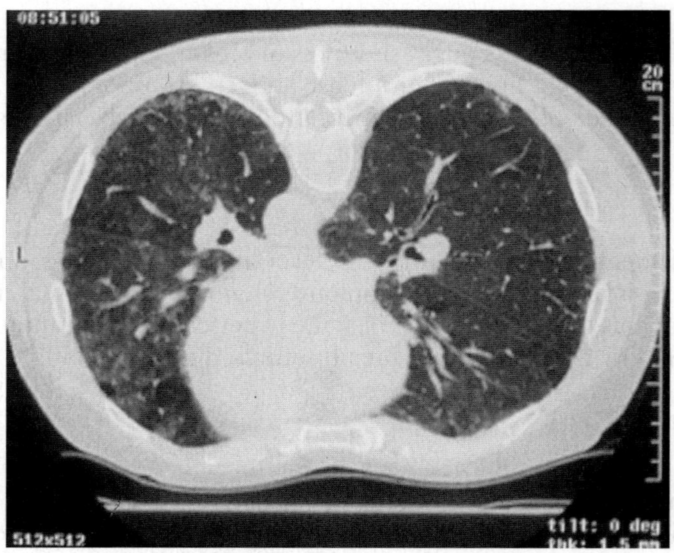

FIGURE 1-1. CT scan of acute hypersensitivity pneumonitis demonstrating scattered regions of ground-glass and nodular infiltrates.

(Courtesy of JS Wilson. Reproduced, with permission, from Kasper DL et al [eds]. *Harrison's Principles of Internal Medicine,* 16th ed. New York: McGraw-Hill, 2005:1518.)

Complications

- Irreversible loss of lung function.
- Death is uncommon but has been reported.

ALLERGIC BRONCHOPULMONARY ASPERGILLOSIS (ABPA)

An immunologic reaction to antigens of *Aspergillus* present in the bronchial tree.

Symptoms

Asthma (may be cough variant or exercise induced); expectoration of golden brown mucous plugs; fever with acute flare.

Exam

Wheezing, rales, or bronchial breath sounds; digital clubbing and cyanosis (late-stage disease).

Differential

Asthma without ABPA, pneumonia (bacterial, viral, fungal, acid-fast bacilli), Churg-Strauss syndrome, eosinophilic pneumonias, CF.

Diagnosis

- **Essential criteria** for ABPA-S (seropositive) are as follows:
  - Presence of **asthma.**
  - Positive immediate **skin tests to *Aspergillus*.**
  - Elevated total serum **IgE (> 1000 ng/mL).**
  - Elevated serum ***Aspergillus*-specific IgE and/or IgG.**
- Other features include the following:
  - The above plus central bronchiectasis = ABPA-CB (with central bronchiectasis).
  - Precipitating antibodies to *Aspergillus*.
  - Peripheral blood eosinophilia (> 1000/mm^3).
  - CXR showing infiltrates (transient or fixed).
  - Sputum culture that is positive for *Aspergillus* or that contains *Aspergillus* hyphae.

ABPA should be considered in any patient with poorly controlled asthma, particularly in the presence of CXR infiltrates.

Treatment

- **Prednisone;** itraconazole as an adjunctive medication.
- Chronic inhaled corticosteroids to control asthma.

Complications

Corticosteroid-dependent asthma, irreversible loss of pulmonary function, chronic bronchitis, pulmonary fibrosis, death due to respiratory failure or cor pulmonale.

ALLERGIC FUNGAL SINUSITIS

An immunologic reaction to fungal aeroallergens (*Aspergillus, Bipolaris, Curvularia, Alternaria, Fusarium*) that causes chronic, refractory sinus disease.

SYMPTOMS

Sinus congestion and obstruction that are refractory to antibiotics; thick mucoid **secretions** (**"peanut butter"** appearance); nasal polyposis; proptosis; asthma.

EXAM

Presents with thickening of the sinus mucosa, allergic mucin on rhinoscopy, and nasal polyps.

DIFFERENTIAL

- **Chronic rhinosinusitis:** Bacterial, allergic (nonfungal).
- Nasal polyposis without allergic fungal sinusitis.
- **Invasive fungal disease:** Seen in immunocompromised individuals (HIV, diabetes).
- Mycetoma (fungus ball).

DIAGNOSIS

- **Diagnostic criteria** include the following:
  - Chronic sinusitis for > 6 months.
  - **Allergic mucin:** Contains many eosinophils and fungal hyphae.
  - **Sinus CT:** Opacification of the sinus (often unilateral) with **hyperattenuated,** expansile material.
  - Absence of invasive fungal disease.
- **Other supportive findings:** Peripheral blood eosinophilia and immediate skin tests positive to fungus.

TREATMENT

- **Surgical** removal of allergic mucin.
- **Prednisone** 0.5–1.0 mg/kg for weeks with slow tapering.
- Intranasal corticosteroids; nasal irrigation.

COMPLICATIONS

Bony erosions from expansion of allergic mucin; surgical complications; high recurrence rate despite therapy.

URTICARIA AND ANGIOEDEMA

Localized edema in the skin or mucous membranes. Individual wheals (hives) typically last < 24 hours. Presents in acute (< 6 weeks of symptoms) and chronic (> 6 weeks) forms.

When used regularly at adequate doses, antihistamines successfully treat most cases of urticaria.

SYMPTOMS

Pruritic hives and painful soft tissue swelling on the lips, oral mucosa, periorbital area, hands, and feet. Individual skin lesions resolve in < 24 hours without residual scarring. Angioedema may take longer to fully resolve.

EXAM

Erythematous, blanching skin wheals; soft tissue swelling as described above. No scarring or pigmentary changes can be seen at previously affected sites. Exam may be normal between symptomatic flares.

DIFFERENTIAL

- **IgE-mediated allergic reaction:** Food, medication, insect stings.
- **Non-IgE reactions:** Aspirin, narcotics, radiocontrast media.
- **Physical urticaria:** Pressure, vibratory, solar, cholinergic, local heat and cold.
- **Autoimmunity:** Vasculitis, associated thyroiditis.
- **Infections:** Mononucleosis, viral hepatitis, fungal and parasitic disease.
- **Idiopathic:** Accounts for the majority of chronic urticaria cases.
- **Isolated angioedema:** Consider hereditary angioedema or acquired angioedema (associated with vasculitis and neoplasms).
- **Other:** Dermatographism; cutaneous mastocytosis.

DIAGNOSIS

- Clinical history suggests diagnostic testing.
- Provocative testing for physical urticarias.
- ESR, ANA, skin biopsy (if necessary to exclude vasculitis), antithyroid antibodies if autoimmunity is suspected.
- CBC, viral hepatitis panel, stool O&P if history is suggestive of infection.
- If angioedema alone, obtain C1 inhibitor assay to exclude hereditary angioedema; determine C1q level to exclude acquired angioedema.

The vast majority of chronic urticaria cases are idiopathic. Extensive laboratory evaluation in the absence of systemic symptoms or unusual features is generally not beneficial.

TREATMENT

- Avoid inciting exposure or treat the underlying condition if it is identified.
- **Antihistamines:** Regular use of nonsedating H_1 antagonists is preferred. Sedating H_1 antagonists may also be used QHS; H_2 antagonists may be helpful adjunctive medication.
- Ephedrine (OTC) is helpful for acute flares.
- Leukotriene modifiers are beneficial in some cases.
- Oral corticosteroids for severe, refractory cases.
- Epinephrine for life-threatening laryngeal edema.
- Danazol or stanozolol for chronic treatment of hereditary angioedema.

COMPLICATIONS

Laryngeal edema.

ATOPIC DERMATITIS

A chronic inflammatory skin disease that is often associated with a personal or family **history of atopy.** Usually begins in childhood.

SYMPTOMS

Characterized by intense **pruritus** and an erythematous papular rash typically occurring in the flexural areas of the elbows, knees, ankles, and neck. Pruritus precedes the rash (**"an itch that rashes").** Chronic atopic dermatitis manifests as thickened nonerythematous plaques of skin (lichenification).

EXAM

Presents with an erythematous papular rash in **flexural areas** as well as with excoriations, serous exudate, lichenification (if chronic), and other findings of atopic disease (boggy nasal mucosa, conjunctival erythema, expiratory wheezing).

Differential

- **Other dermatitis:** Seborrheic, irritant, contact, psoriasis.
- **Neoplasia:** Cutaneous T-cell lymphoma.
- **Infectious:** Scabies, candidiasis, tinea versicolor.
- **Hyper-IgE syndrome:** Usually diagnosed in childhood.

Diagnosis

Diagnosis is readily made through the history and physical. Consider skin biopsy to rule out cutaneous T-cell lymphoma in new-onset eczema in an adult.

Treatment

- **Skin hydration:** Lotions, emollients.
- **Topical corticosteroids.**
- **Antihistamines** to reduce pruritus.
- Avoid skin irritants (e.g., abrasive clothing, temperature extremes, harsh soaps).
- Avoid allergic triggers if identified (food, aeroallergens; more common in children).
- Treat bacterial, fungal, and viral **superinfection** as necessary.
- Topical **tacrolimus/pimecrolimus** and oral corticosteroids for severe disease.

Complications

- **Chronic skin changes:** Scarring, hyperpigmentation.
- **Cutaneous infection:** Bacterial (primarily *S. aureus*), viral (primarily HSV); risk of eczema vaccinatum with smallpox vaccine.

ALLERGIC CONTACT DERMATITIS

A lymphocyte-mediated delayed hypersensitivity reaction causing a skin rash on an antigen-exposed area.

Symptoms

Characterized by a **pruritic** rash that typically appears 5–21 days after the initial exposure or 12–96 hours after reexposure in sensitized individuals. The typical pattern is **erythema** leading to **papules** and then **vesicles.** The rash precedes pruritus and appears in the distribution of antigen exposure (see Figure 1-2).

Exam

- **Acute stage:** Skin erythema, papules, vesicles.
- **Subacute or chronic stage:** Crusting, scaling, lichenification, and thickening of skin.

Differential

Atopic dermatitis, seborrheic dermatitis, irritant dermatitis (antigen-nonspecific irritation, usually due to chemicals or detergents), psoriasis.

Diagnosis

- **Location of the rash:** Suggests the cause—feet (shoes), neck/ears (jewelry), face (cosmetics/hair products).
- **Allergy patch testing:** See above.

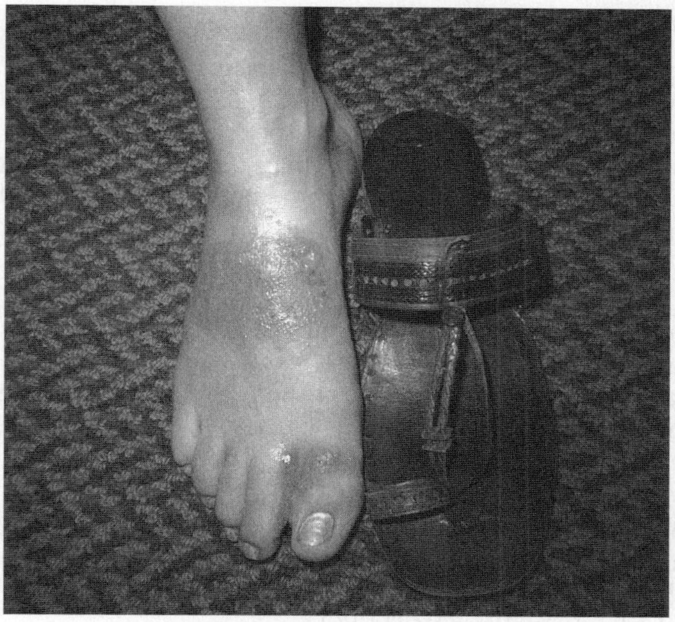

FIGURE 1-2. Contact dermatitis.

Erythematous papules, vesicles, and serous weeping localized to areas of contact with the offending agent are characteristic. (Reproduced, with permission, from Hurwitz RM. *Pathology of the Skin: Atlas of Clinical-Pathological Correlation.* Stamford, CT: Appleton & Lange, 1991:3.) (Also see Color Insert.)

TREATMENT

Antigen avoidance, topical corticosteroids, antihistamines for pruritus, oral prednisone in severe or extensive cases.

COMPLICATIONS

Secondary infection from scratching affected skin.

ANAPHYLAXIS

A systemic type I (IgE-mediated) hypersensitivity reaction that is often life-threatening. Requires **previous exposure** (known or unknown) for sensitization. Risk factors include parenteral antigen exposure and repeated interrupted antigen exposure. Common causes are **foods** (especially peanuts and shellfish), **drugs** (especially penicillin), **latex, stinging insects,** and **blood products.**

SYMPTOMS

Symptoms include skin erythema, pruritus, urticaria, angioedema, laryngeal edema, wheezing, chest tightness, cramping abdominal pain, nausea, vomiting, diarrhea, diaphoresis, dizziness, a sense of "impending doom," hypotension, syncope, and shock. Most frequently appear **seconds to minutes after exposure,** but may be delayed several hours for ingested agents.

EXAM

Urticaria, angioedema, flushing, wheezing, stridor, diaphoresis, hypotension, tachycardia.

DIFFERENTIAL

- **Other types of shock:** Cardiogenic, endotoxic, hemorrhagic.
- **Cardiovascular disease:** Arrhythmia, MI.
- **Scombroid:** Histamine poisoning from spoiled fish.
- **Anaphylactoid reaction:** Nonspecific mast cell activation (**not** IgE).
- **Other:** Carcinoid syndrome, pheochromocytoma, severe cold urticaria, vasovagal reaction, systemic mastocytosis, panic attack.

DIAGNOSIS

- Elevated **serum tryptase** drawn 30 minutes to three hours after onset can help confirm the diagnosis.
- **Presence of allergen-specific IgE antibody** by skin or RAST testing (best performed one month after event).

TREATMENT

The treatment of anaphylaxis consists of the prompt administration of epinephrine. Mortality is strongly associated with delays in epinephrine administration.

- **Epinephrine** 1:1000 0.3 mL IM: Repeat every 15 minutes as needed.
- **Maintain airway:** O_2, inhaled bronchodilators, intubation if necessary.
- Rapid IV fluids if hypotensive.
- **Diphenhydramine** 50 mg IV/IM/PO.
- **Corticosteroids** (prednisone 60 mg or equivalent) IV/IM/PO: Reduces late-phase recurrence of symptoms 4–8 hours later.
- Vasopressor medications in the presence of persistent hypotension.
- IV epinephrine 1:10,000 0.3 mL only in terminal patients.
- Consider **glucagon and/or atropine for patients on β-blockers** whose symptoms are refractory to therapy.
- Monitor patients for 8–12 hours after reaction.
- Ensure that patients have access to injectable epinephrine and antihistamines on discharge.

COMPLICATIONS

Respiratory obstruction, cardiovascular collapse, death.

ANAPHYLACTOID REACTIONS

Clinically indistinguishable from anaphylactic reactions, but caused by nonspecific mast cell activation **(not IgE mediated).** May occur with first exposure to medication. Common causes include radiocontrast media, vancomycin, amphotericin, opiates, and general anesthetics (induction agents and muscle relaxants).

DIAGNOSIS

- Elevated **serum tryptase** drawn 30 minutes to three hours after onset helps confirm mast cell release.
- **Absence of allergen-specific IgE** antibody to suspected antigens by skin or RAST testing (best performed one month after event).

TREATMENT

- Same as that for anaphylaxis.
- **Vancomycin:** Slow infusion rate.
- **Radiocontrast media:** Use low-osmolality forms.
- Anaphylactoid reactions are **generally preventable with pretreatment** using corticosteroids and antihistamines. Pretreatment is recommended for patients with a history of reactions to radiocontrast media.

FOOD ALLERGY

True (IgE-mediated) food allergy in adults is most commonly caused by **peanuts, crustaceans, tree nuts,** and **fish.** Sensitivities to these foods tend to be lifelong. Multiple food allergies are rare in adults. Anaphylactic signs and symptoms occur **minutes to two hours after ingestion.**

DIFFERENTIAL

- Nonallergic food intolerance (lactase deficiency, celiac disease, symptoms due to vasoactive amines).
- Food poisoning, including scombroid.
- Anaphylaxis due to other causes.
- Eosinophilic gastroenteritis.

DIAGNOSIS

- Anaphylaxis may be confirmed with **elevated serum tryptase** if the test is conducted 30 minutes to three hours after the reaction.
- **Positive allergy skin or RAST tests** to food antigen.
- Double-blind placebo-controlled food challenge if diagnosis is unclear.

TREATMENT

- Treat anaphylaxis in an acute setting (see above).
- Eliminate implicated food from diet.
- Ensure patient access to injectable epinephrine.

STINGING INSECT ALLERGY

Allergic reactions occur to three major stinging insect families: **vespids** (yellow jackets, hornets, wasps), **apids** (honeybees and bumblebees), and **fire ants.** Reactions are classified into **local** (symptoms at the sting site) and **systemic** (anaphylactic).

SYMPTOMS/EXAM

- **Local reaction:** Swelling and erythema; pain at the sting site lasting several hours.
- **Large local reaction:** Extensive swelling and erythema at the sting site lasting up to one week; nausea and malaise.
- **Systemic reaction:** Anaphylactic symptoms occurring within 15 minutes of sting.

DIFFERENTIAL

- **Toxic venom reaction:** Results from large venom burden delivery by **multiple simultaneous stings.** The pharmacologic properties of venom may cause hypotension and shock.
- Anaphylaxis due to other causes.

DIAGNOSIS

- Systemic reactions may be confirmed by **elevated serum tryptase** if drawn 30 minutes to three hours after reaction.
- Any systemic reaction should be confirmed with **venom-specific IgE by allergy skin or RAST testing** owing to the risk of recurrence with repeat sting. Testing should be performed several weeks after the reaction owing to mast cell depletion.

Any adult who reacts systemically to an insect sting, regardless of reaction severity, should be evaluated for venom immunotherapy.

TREATMENT

- **Large local:** Antihistamines, analgesics, short prednisone course for severe or disabling local reactions.
- **Systemic:** Treatment is the same as that for anaphylaxis (see above).
- **Venom immunotherapy** is recommended for patients with a history of systemic reaction and positive venom-specific IgE tests. Immunotherapy is 98% effective in preventing systemic allergic reactions on re-sting.
- Insect avoidance.
- Ensure patient access to antihistamines and injectable epinephrine.

DRUG ALLERGY

Only a small portion of adverse drug reactions are drug hypersensitivity reactions (immune mediated), of which a small subset represents true drug allergy (IgE mediated).

The vast majority of adverse drug reactions are due to predictable drug effects and are not true drug allergy.

SYMPTOMS

Immunologic drug reactions may present with a wide range of symptoms. Common symptoms include urticaria, angioedema, morbilliform rash, blistering mucocutaneous lesions, cough, dyspnea, wheezing, anaphylaxis, arthralgias, fever, and lymphadenopathy.

EXAM

- **Dermatologic findings:** Urticaria, angioedema, morbilliform rash, purpura, petechiae, exfoliative dermatitis, bullous skin lesions.
- **Other:** Wheezing, lymphadenopathy, jaundice, fever.

DIFFERENTIAL

- **Nonimmunologic adverse drug reaction:** Dose-related toxicity, pharmacologic side effects, drug-drug interactions.
- **Pseudoallergic reaction:** Direct mast cell release (opiates, vancomycin, radiocontrast media).
- Nondrug causes of presenting symptoms

Diagnostic drug allergy skin testing is standardized and predictive only for penicillin.

DIAGNOSIS

- Based on clinical judgment using the general **criteria** outlined in Table 1-2.
- Available **diagnostic testing supportive** of an immunologic mechanism to explain the drug reaction. See Table 1-3 for useful tests.
- The drug challenge procedure is the definitive diagnostic test but should be performed only by an experienced clinician if an absolute indication exists for the drug.

TREATMENT

- **Discontinuation of drug:** In most instances, symptoms promptly resolve if the diagnosis is correct.
- If the drug is absolutely indicated, refer the patient for **graded challenge/desensitization.**
- **Symptomatic treatment for specific symptoms:** Antihistamines, topical corticosteroids, bronchodilators; oral corticosteroids in severe cases.

TABLE 1-2. General Diagnostic Criteria for Drug Hypersensitivity Reactions

- The patient's symptoms are consistent with an immunologic drug reaction.
- The patient was administered a drug known to cause the symptoms.
- The temporal sequence of drug administration and the appearance of symptoms are consistent with a drug reaction.
- Other causes of the symptoms are effectively excluded.
- Laboratory data are supportive of an immunologic mechanism to explain the drug reaction. (Not present or available in all cases.)

- **Patient education:** Educate patients with regard to the risk of future reaction, drug avoidance, and cross-reactive medications.

COMPLICATIONS

- **Fatal drug hypersensitivity:** Anaphylaxis, toxic epidermal necrolysis.
- **"Multiple drug allergy syndrome":** Lack of patient/physician understanding of adverse drug reactions leads to multiple medication avoidance and restrictive, ineffective medical therapy.

TABLE 1-3. Diagnostic Testing and Therapy for Drug Hypersensitivity

Immunologic Reaction	Clinical Manifestations	Laboratory Tests	Therapeutic Considerations
Type I	Anaphylaxis, angioedema, urticaria, bronchospasm.	Skin testing, RAST testing, serum tryptase.	Discontinue drug; epinephrine, antihistamines, systemic corticosteroids, bronchodilators; inpatient monitoring if severe.
Type II	Hemolytic anemia, thrombocytopenia, neutropenia.	Direct/indirect Coombs' test.	Discontinue drug; consider systemic corticosteroids; transfusion in severe cases.
Type III	Serum sickness, vasculitis, glomerulonephritis.	Immune complexes, ESR, complement studies, ANA/ANCA, C-reactive protein, tissue biopsy for immunofluorescence studies.	Discontinue drug; NSAIDs, antihistamines; systemic corticosteroids or plasmapheresis if severe.
Type IV	Allergic contact dermatitis, maculopapular drug rash.[a]	Patch testing, lymphocyte proliferation assay.[b]	Discontinue drug; topical corticosteroids, antihistamines; systemic corticosteroids if severe.

[a] Suspected type IV reaction; mechanism not fully elucidated.

[b] Investigational test.

MASTOCYTOSIS

A disease characterized by **excessive numbers of mast cells** in the skin, internal organs, and bone marrow. Caused by a somatic **kit gene mutation.** Has variable severity ranging from the isolated cutaneous form to indolent systemic disease to aggressive lymphoma-like disease or mast cell leukemia.

Symptoms

Pruritus, flushing, urticaria, diarrhea, nausea, vomiting, abdominal pain, headache, hypotension, anaphylaxis.

Exam

Presents with **urticaria pigmentosa** (a pigmented macular skin rash that urticates with stroking) as well as with lymphadenopathy, hepatomegaly, and splenomegaly.

Differential

- **Anaphylaxis:** Drugs, foods, venoms, exercise induced, idiopathic.
- **Flushing syndromes:** Scombroid, carcinoid, VIPoma, pheochromocytoma.
- **Shock:** Cardiogenic, hemorrhagic, endotoxic.
- **Angioedema:** Hereditary or acquired.
- **Other:** Panic attack.

Diagnosis

- Diagnosed by the presence of one major plus one minor or three minor criteria.
- **Major criteria:** Characteristic multifocal dense **infiltrates of mast cells on bone marrow** biopsy.
- **Minor criteria:**
    - Spindle-shaped morphology of mast cells on **tissue biopsy.**
    - Detection of the **c-kit mutation.**
    - **Flow cytometry** of bone marrow mast cells coexpressing CD117, CD2, and CD25.
    - **Serum tryptase** level > 20 ng/mL.

Treatment

- H_1 and H_2 antagonists.
- Epinephrine for episodes of anaphylaxis.
- Topical steroids for skin lesions.
- Oral corticosteroids for advanced disease.
- Bone marrow transplantation for patients with aggressive disease or associated hematologic disorders.

PRIMARY IMMUNODEFICIENCY IN ADULTS

Adult primary immunodeficiencies (non-HIV) generally present in the second or third decade of life with **recurrent respiratory infections** due to antibody deficiency (hypogammaglobulinemia). Conditions include **common variable immunodeficiency** (CVID), **selective IgA deficiency,** IgG subclass deficiency, and selective antibody deficiency with normal immunoglobulins (SADNI).

SYMPTOMS

Frequent **respiratory tract infections** (sinusitis, otitis, pneumonia); a need for IV or prolonged oral antibiotic courses to clear infections; **chronic GI symptoms** such as diarrhea, cramping abdominal pain, or malabsorption.

EXAM

Nasal congestion and discharge; respiratory wheezing or rales; digital clubbing secondary to chronic lung disease; lymphadenopathy; splenomegaly.

DIFFERENTIAL

- CVID.
- **Selective IgA deficiency:** Most common, with an incidence of 1:500; generally asymptomatic.
- **IgG subclass deficiency:** Generally asymptomatic.
- SADNI.
- Hypogammaglobulinemia due to loss (GI, renal).
- Hypogammaglobulinemia due to medications (immunosuppressants, anticonvulsants).
- HIV, CF, allergic respiratory disease.

DIAGNOSIS

- **History** of recurrent infection.
- **Antibody deficiency** by laboratory testing:
  - **CVID: Low IgG (< 500),** usually with low IgA and/or IgM.
  - **Selective IgA deficiency: Absence of IgA (< 7) with normal IgG** and IgM.
  - **IgG subclass deficiency:** Low levels of one or more IgG subclasses (IgG1, IgG2, IgG3, IgG4). Clinical significance is unclear.
  - **SADNI:** Normal immunoglobulin levels with failure to produce protective antibody levels against specific immunizations (most commonly *Pneumococcus*).
- **Exclusion of other causes** of hypogammaglobulinemia (antibody loss due to protein-losing enteropathy or nephropathy, medication, lymphopenia).

TREATMENT

- **CVID:**
  - **IVIG** 300 mg/kg monthly.
  - Aggressive treatment of infection.
  - Monitor lung function; pulmonary hygiene for bronchiectasis.
- **Selective IgA deficiency:**
  - **Antibiotic therapy and/or prophylaxis** as necessary.
  - **IVIG is contraindicated** owing to possible anti-IgA IgE antibody.
  - Patients should receive only **washed blood products** owing to the **risk of anaphylaxis** with exposure to IgA.
- **IgG subclass deficiency and SADNI:**
  - Antibiotic therapy as needed.
  - IVIG is reserved for rare patients with significant infection despite preventive antibiotics.

COMPLICATIONS

- **CVID**: Variable T-cell deficiency, GI **malignancy** (gastric cancer, small bowel lymphoma), **bronchiectasis, lymphoproliferative** disease, noncaseating granulomas of internal organs, **autoimmune disease.**
- **Selective IgA deficiency: Celiac disease, lymphoproliferative** disease, GI **malignancy** (gastric cancer, small bowel lymphoma), **autoimmune** disease.

CHAPTER 2

Ambulatory Medicine

Cindy Lai, MD

Screening for Hyperlipidemia

Hyperlipidemia is a risk factor for CAD, stroke, and peripheral vascular disease. Other major risk factors for CAD are as follows:

- Age (men ≥ 45, women ≥ 55), cigarette smoking, hypertension, a family history of premature CAD, HDL < 40 (> 60 protective), elevated LDL.
- Risk factor equivalents to CAD include DM, symptomatic carotid artery disease, peripheral arterial disease, abdominal aortic aneurysm, and renal insufficiency (Cr ≥ 1.5).

DIAGNOSIS

- Obtain a fasting total cholesterol, LDL, HDL, and TG.
- If there are no risk factors for CAD, recommendations for screening are as follows:
  - Men ≥ 35 years; women ≥ 45 years (according to the United States Preventive Services Task Force [USPSTF] and the American College of Physicians).
  - Adults ≥ 20 years at least once every five years (per the National Cholesterol Education Program Adult Treatment Panel III).
  - There is insufficient evidence supporting the benefit of screening patients > 65 years of age unless multiple cardiovascular risk factors are present.

TREATMENT

- Tables 2-1 and 2-2 list guidelines for the treatment of hyperlipidemia.
- There are three categories of risk that modify LDL cholesterol goals (see Table 2-3).

Combining statins and fibrates may lead to increased rates of myositis.

TABLE 2-1. Classes of Drugs for the Treatment of Hyperlipidemia

DRUG	LDL	HDL	TG	SIDE EFFECTS	BEST FOR	MONITOR
Nicotinic acid (niacin)	↓	↑	↓	Flushing, gout, GI distress, elevated LFTs, pruritus, increased blood glucose.	Elevated LDL and TG; low HDL ("jack of all trades").	LFTs
Statins (atorvastatin, simvastatin, pravastatin)	↓	↑	↓	GI distress, elevated LFTs, myositis.	Elevated LDL only; elevated LDL and TG.	LFTs, CK
Bile acid–binding resins (cholestyramine)	↓	↑	↑	GI distress, decreased absorption of fat-soluble vitamins and other drugs, **increased TG.**	Elevated LDL only.	
Fibrates (gemfibrozil)	↓	↑	↓	GI distress, **myositis (especially in combination with statins).**	Elevated LDL and TG.	LFTs

TABLE 2-2. Initial Drugs for Specific Cholesterol Panels

Findings	Treatment
Elevated LDL	Statins
Elevated TG	Fibrates
Elevated LDL and TG	Statin or fibrate; add niacin if necessary
Low HDL	Exercise + any agent
Elevated TG and low HDL	Fibrates

Screening for Diabetes Mellitus (DM)

Diagnosis

- Begin screening for DM at age 45 and repeat every three years (per the American Diabetes Association, or ADA). Consider screening earlier in high-risk patients, including African-Americans, Hispanics, Asians, Native Americans, and those with cardiac risk factors, a family history of DM, or obesity.
- The ADA's diagnostic criteria include any of the following (on more than one occasion):
  - **A fasting blood glucose ≥ 126 mg/dL.**
  - Symptoms of DM (polyuria, polydipsia, weight loss) and random blood glucose ≥ 200 mg/dL.
  - A two-hour blood glucose **≥ 200 mg/dL during an oral glucose tolerance test.** (Note: "Impaired fasting glucose" is defined as a fasting blood glucose of 110–126 mg/dL.)

TABLE 2-3. Three Categories of Risk that Modify LDL Cholesterol Goals

Risk Category	LDL Goal	Level at Which to Initiate Therapeutic Lifestyle Changes	Level at Which to Consider Drug Therapy
CAD or CAD risk equivalents (10-year risk > 20%)	< 100 mg/dL	≥ 100 mg/dL	≥ 130 mg/dL (100–129 mg/dL: drug optional)[a]
2+ risk factors (10-year risk ≤ 20%)	< 130 mg/dL	≥ 130 mg/dL	10-year risk 10–20%: ≥ 130 mg/dL 10-year risk < 10%: ≥ 160 mg/dL
0–1 risk factor	< 160 mg/dL	≥ 160 mg/dL	≥ 190 mg/dL (160–189 mg/dL: LDL-lowering drug optional).

[a]Some authorities recommend use of LDL-lowering drugs in this category if an LDL cholesterol < 100 mg/dL cannot be achieved by therapeutic lifestyle changes.

Adapted, with permission, from the Third Report of the National Cholesterol Education Program, Panel on Detection, Evaluation, and Treatment of High Blood Cholesterol in Adults (Adult Treatment Panel III) Executive Summary. Washington, DC: National Institutes of Health, NIH Publication No. 01-3670, May 2001, www.nhlbi.nih.gov/guidelines/cholesterol/index.htm.

- Hemoglobin A_{1c} (HbA_{1c}) is not included in the diagnostic criteria because of standardization difficulties.

Cancer Screening

The guidelines that follow are based on recommendations by the USPSTF. For breast cancer and cervical cancer screening, see Chapter 18.

- Colorectal cancer:
  - Screening should begin at age 50 but should be initiated at an earlier age if there are colorectal cancer risks—e.g., a personal or strong family history of colorectal cancer or adenomatous polyps, or a family history of hereditary syndromes (familial adenomatous polyposis and hereditary nonpolyposis colon cancer).
  - Screening should consist of annual fecal occult blood testing (FOBT) in combination with flexible sigmoidoscopy every 3–5 years **or** colonoscopy every 10 years.
- Prostate cancer:
  - Consider screening in men ≥ 50 years of age if the patient is expected to live at least 10 years. Begin at a younger age if patients are at increased risk (e.g., African-American men or those with a first-degree relative with prostate cancer).
  - Serum PSA testing and DRE are controversial because of their lack of proven effectiveness.
  - Most groups recommend that physicians discuss both the potential advantages of PSA screening (early detection) and its disadvantages (false-positive results, more biopsies, anxiety).

IMMUNIZATIONS

Table 2-4 describes the indications for and uses of some common vaccines.

EXERCISE AND OBESITY

Athletic Screening for Adolescents

*Live attenuated vaccines are contraindicated in pregnancy. Do **not** give MMR, varicella, or oral polio vaccines to pregnant women!*

Although rare, sudden death may occur in competitive athletes as a result of **hypertrophic cardiomyopathy** (36%), **coronary anomalies** (19%), and LVH. It is therefore recommended that students be evaluated prior to participation in high school and college athletics as well as every two years during competition. Evaluation should include the following:

- A careful history and physical exam focusing on cardiovascular risk factors and findings.
- An ECG and an echocardiogram in the presence of the following:
  - A family history of premature sudden death or cardiovascular disease.
  - Symptoms of chest pain, syncope, or near-syncope.
  - A Marfan's-like appearance—e.g., tall stature with long arms/legs/fingers (associated with an increased risk of aortic rupture).

TABLE 2-4. Indications for Immunization

MEASLES, MUMPS, RUBELLA (MMR)	TETANUS AND DIPHTHERIA (TD)	PNEUMOVAX (PVX)	VARICELLA	INFLUENZA
If born before 1957, patients are considered immune and do not need vaccine. If born in or after 1957, patients are not considered immune and should receive two doses of MMR at least one month apart.	Every 10 years. In the presence of a "dirty wound," every five years.	All patients > 65 years of age. Patients < 50 years of age should receive PVX if they are immunocompromised or have a chronic illness (cardiopulmonary disease, alcoholism, cirrhosis, asplenia). Revaccinate patients ≥ 65 years of age if they received their primary vaccine > 5 years ago or are at high risk.	All susceptible adults should receive two doses given 1–2 months apart. A history of **chickenpox** is an acceptable criterion for assuming immunity.	Yearly for all patients with cardiopulmonary disease, residents in chronic care facilities, adults ≥ 50 years of age, patients with chronic diseases (e.g., diabetes, chronic renal disease, HIV or other immunosuppression), or women who will be in their second or third trimester of pregnancy during influenza season.

Obesity

Affects approximately one-quarter of Americans. Associated with an increased risk of hypertension, type 2 DM, hyperlipidemia, CAD, degenerative joint disease, sleep apnea, steatohepatitis, and psychosocial disorders.

DIFFERENTIAL

Hypothyroidism, Cushing's syndrome, medications (steroids, insulin, sulfonylurea, SSRIs, atypical antipsychotics).

DIAGNOSIS

The **body mass index (BMI)** reflects excess adipose tissue and is calculated by dividing measured body weight (kg) by height (meters squared):

$$\text{BMI} = \text{weight (kg)} / \text{height (m}^2)$$

BMI is interpreted as follows: 25.0–29.9 = overweight; > 30 = obesity; > 40 = extreme obesity.

TREATMENT

- Weight loss improves type 2 DM, hypertension, cardiovascular risk, and hyperlipidemia (HDL, TG).
- A multidisciplinary approach combining a reduction in caloric intake, increased aerobic exercise, and social support optimizes the maintenance of weight loss.
- Diets include very low calorie diets (< 800 kcal/day) and low-carbohydrate diets (e.g., Atkins). Dietary interventions should be coordinated with a nutritionist to circumvent the pitfalls of problematic "fad" diets.

TABLE 2-5. Commonly Used (FDA-Approved) Obesity Medications

Drug	Mechanism of Action	Side Effects
Sibutramine	Inhibits the uptake of serotonin and norepinephrine in the CNS **(catecholaminergic).**	**Hypertension,** dry mouth, anorexia, constipation, insomnia, dizziness.
Orlistat	Inhibits intestinal lipase; **decreases fat absorption.**	Fatty stools, gas, cramping.

Consider surgery for patients with a BMI > 40 or a BMI > 35 plus obesity-related medical complications.

- Although pharmacotherapy leads to short-term weight loss, surgery is the only proven method for achieving long-term weight loss.
- In recent years, several obesity medications **(fenfluramine, dexfenfluramine)** have been removed from the market following reports of **valvular heart disease** and **pulmonary hypertension.**
- Indications for pharmacotherapy (see Table 2-5) are as follows:
  - Consider in patients with a BMI > 30 or in those with a BMI > 27 and obesity-related medical complications.
  - A course of medication for 6–12 months leads to increased weight loss compared to a placebo, but the **long-term efficacy of such treatment has not been proven.**
- The long-term efficacy of gastric surgery for weight reduction has been established. Indications are as follows:
  - Consider in patients with a BMI > 40 (severely obese) or in those with a BMI > 35 and obesity-related medical complications.
  - Complications of surgery include dumping syndrome, anastomotic stenosis, vitamin B_{12}/iron/vitamin D deficiencies, and perioperative mortality (0.3%).

NUTRITIONAL AND HERBAL SUPPLEMENTS

Vitamin and other nutritional deficiencies are discussed at length in Chapter 9. Table 2-6 lists the potential benefits of some common nutritional supplements. Table 2-7 outlines some common herbal supplements along with their indications and side effects.

OPHTHALMOLOGY

Red Eye

Table 2-8 outlines the most frequent causes of red eye. The following are some additional etiologies:

All patients with red eye and any of the following should be referred to an ophthalmologist emergently: moderate to severe eye pain, decreased visual acuity, photophobia, pupillary abnormalities, or ciliary flush.

- **Foreign body:** Characterized by a sharp superficial pain. Perform a fluorescein test.
- **Gonorrheal conjunctivitis:** Presents as a purulent discharge in sexually active adults.
- **Chlamydial conjunctivitis:** Associated with chronic red eye in sexually active adults.
- **HSV keratitis:** Usually unilateral; suggested by decreased vision. Branching (dendritic) ulcers on fluorescein stain test are diagnostic.

TABLE 2-6. Effects of Selected Nutritional Supplements

VITAMIN C	VITAMIN E	FIBER	FOLIC ACID
Antioxidant.	Antioxidant; may delay the progression of Alzheimer's dementia.	Decreases cholesterol; may decrease the risk of colon cancer and diverticular disease.	A dose of 0.4 mg/day decreases neural tube defects in fetuses whose mothers take folic acid near conception. Women on anticonvulsants may benefit from taking 1 mg/day during pregnancy.

Causes of red eye—
GO SUCK

Glaucoma
Orbital disease
Scleritis
Uveitis
Conjunctivitis (viral, bacterial, allergic)
Keratitis (HSV)

- **Subconjunctival hemorrhage:** Spares the limbus; common with trauma and anticoagulants.

See Figures 2-1 through 2-5 for images of conjunctivitis, uveitis/keratitis, subconjunctival hemorrhage, and acute angle-closure glaucoma.

Loss of Vision

Painless loss of vision is categorized as either acute or chronic. The etiologies of **acute loss of vision** include the following:

- **Retinal artery occlusion:** Commonly due to an embolus. Characterized by sudden, **painless,** unilateral blindness and by a **"cherry-red spot"** in the macula. Constitutes an emergency.
- **Retinal vein occlusion:** Commonly due to hypertension, hyperviscosity syndromes, hypercoagulable diseases, or Behçet's disease. Onset is sudden and **painless** with varying degrees of visual loss. There is no effective acute treatment, so referral is urgent (but not emergent).
- **Vitreous hemorrhage:** Due to vitreous detachment, proliferative diabetic retinopathy, or retinal tears. Visual acuity may be normal or reduced. Warrants urgent referral.
- **Retinal detachment:** May be spontaneous or due to trauma. Presents with

TABLE 2-7. Common Herbal Supplements

HERB	CONDITION	EFFICACY	SIDE EFFECTS
Gingko biloba	Dementia, claudication.	Suggested benefit in memory compared to a placebo. Benefit for other conditions is unclear.	May have an anticoagulant effect.
Echinacea	Prevention and treatment of the common cold.	Benefit is unclear.	Rash, pruritus, nausea.
Saw palmetto	BPH.	Improved urinary symptoms and flow.	Mild GI upset, headaches (rare).
St. John's wort	Depression.	Improved symptoms in mild to moderate depression.	Induces cytochrome P-450, thus decreasing some drug levels (e.g., warfarin, digoxin, OCPs).

TABLE 2-8. Common Causes of Red Eye

	Viral Conjunctivitis	Allergic Conjunctivitis	Bacterial Conjunctivitis	Acute Keratitis or Uveitis	Acute Angle-Closure Glaucoma
Incidence	Extremely common, especially after **URI** (adenovirus).	Common.	Common.	Common.	Uncommon.
Conjunctival injection and discharge	Unilateral or bilateral redness; watery discharge.	Bilateral redness, itching, and tearing; ropy discharge.	Unilateral redness; morning crustiness.	Circumcorneal redness (ciliary flush); no discharge.	Circumcorneal redness (ciliary flush); no discharge.
Pain, photophobia, vision changes	None.	None.	None.	**Moderate pain, photophobia, decreased visual acuity.**	**Severe pain, nausea, vomiting, decreased visual acuity.**
Cornea	Clear.	Clear.	Clear.	Usually clear.	**Steamy.**
Pupil	Normal.	Normal.	Normal.	**Constricted; poor light response.**	**Moderately dilated and fixed; no light response.**
Intraocular pressure	Normal.	Normal.	Normal.	Normal.	**High.**
Therapy	Symptomatic; cold compresses.	Cold compresses, antihistamine drops, topical ketorolac (NSAID), topical mast cell stabilizer.	Erythromycin ointment, polymyxin-trimethoprim drops.	**Emergency: refer to an ophthalmologist.**	**Emergency: refer to an ophthalmologist for laser iridectomy;** pupil constriction (topical pilocarpine), pressure reduction (topical β-blockers, acetazolamide).

unilateral blurred vision that progressively worsens (**floaters or lights in peripheral vision**). Considered an emergency.

- **Amaurosis fugax ("fleeting blindness")**: Due to retinal emboli from ipsilateral carotid disease or temporal arteritis (patients complain that "a curtain came down over my eye" for **only a few minutes**). Evaluate with carotid duplex ultrasonography or MRA and ESR +/– echocardiography. High-grade carotid stenoses may benefit from carotid endarterectomy. Lower-grade stenoses benefit from antiplatelet drugs.
- **Optic neuritis:** Unilateral, occasional pain that improves within 2–3 weeks. Associated with demyelinating diseases, especially MS.

The etiologies for **chronic loss of vision** include the following:

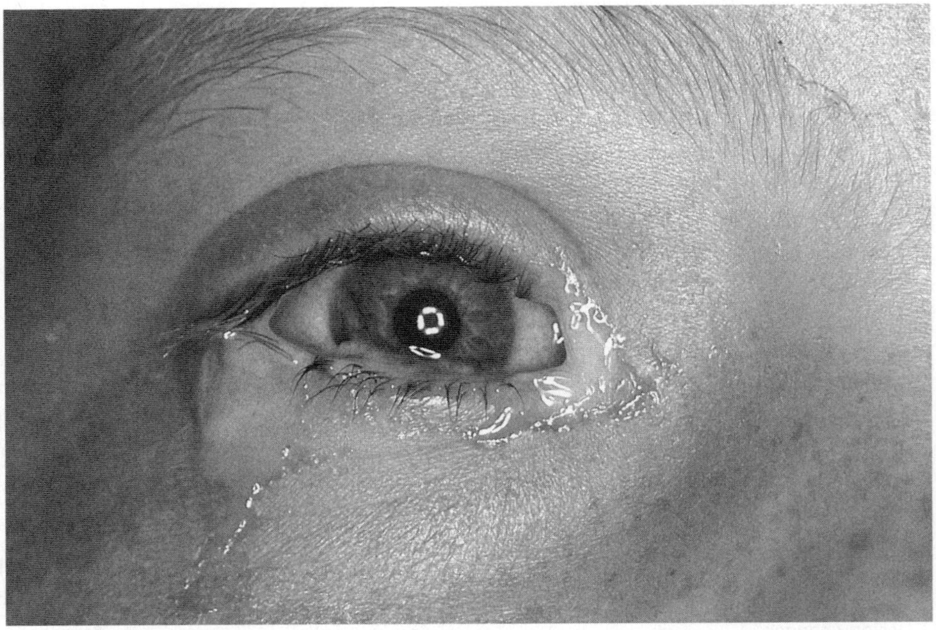

FIGURE 2-1. Bacterial conjunctivitis.

(Reproduced, with permission, from Knoop KJ, Stack LB, Storrow AB. *Atlas of Emergency Medicine*, 2nd ed. New York: McGraw-Hill, 2002:30.) (Also see Color Insert.)

- **Age-related macular degeneration:** The most common cause of permanent visual loss in the elderly. Characterized by loss of **central** vision only. Due to the development of retinal drusen (yellow spots on the macula).
- **Open-angle glaucoma:** Loss of **peripheral** vision ("tunnel vision") over a period of years. Characterized by increased intraocular pressure and an in-

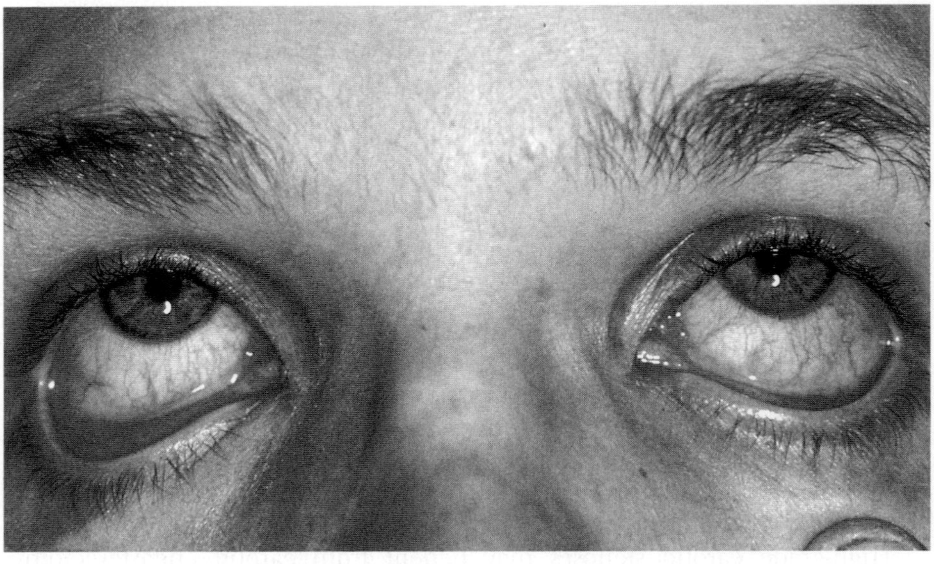

FIGURE 2-2. Viral conjunctivitis.

(Reproduced, with permission, from Knoop KJ, Stack LB, Storrow AB. *Atlas of Emergency Medicine*, 2nd ed. New York: McGraw-Hill, 2002:31.) (Also see Color Insert.)

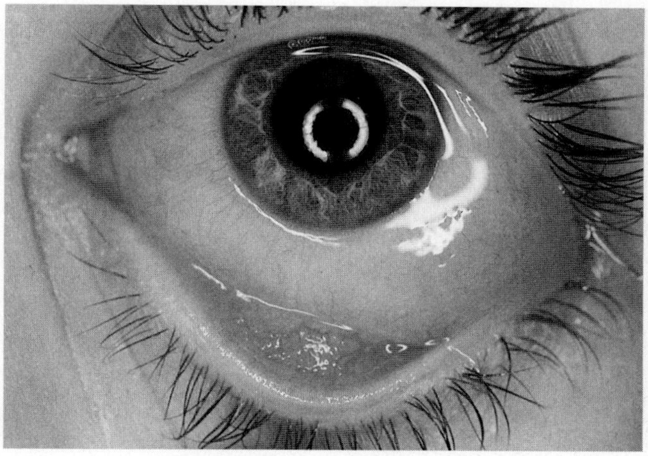

FIGURE 2-3. Allergic conjunctivitis.

(Courtesy of Timothy D. McGuirk, DO. Reproduced, with permission, from Knoop KJ, Stack LB, Storrow AB. *Atlas of Emergency Medicine*, 2nd ed. New York: McGraw-Hill, 2002: 36.) (Also see Color Insert.)

creased cup-to-disk ratio (**"cupping"**). **Treatment includes a combination of topical β-blockers,** α_2-agonists, and prostaglandin analogs.

- **Cataracts:** Visible lens opacities. Blurred vision occurs over months or years. Treatment consists of lens replacement.
- **Nonproliferative diabetic retinopathy:** The most common cause of legal blindness in adult-onset diabetes. Characterized by dilation of veins, microaneurysms, hard exudates, and retinal hemorrhages. Treat with intensive blood glucose control and laser photocoagulation.
- **Proliferative retinopathy:** Presents with neovascularization; vitreous hemorrhage is a common complication. Treat with laser photocoagulation.

Cataract causes—

ABCD

Aging
Bang (trauma)
Congenital
Diabetes and other metabolic diseases (steroids)

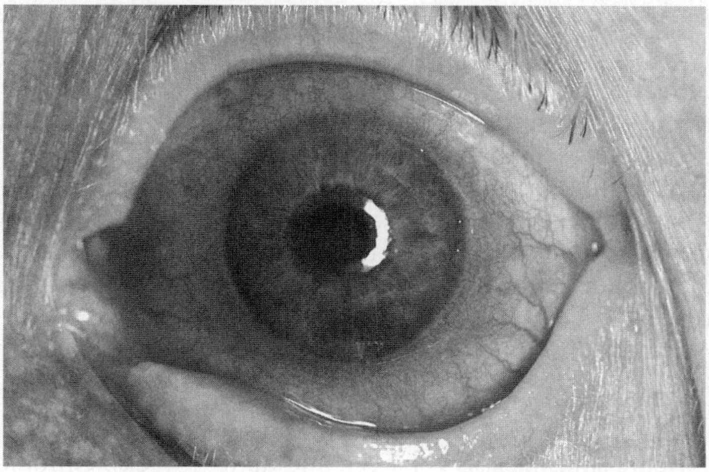

FIGURE 2-4. Anterior uveitis.

(Reproduced, with permission, from Knoop KJ, Stack LB, Storrow AB. *Atlas of Emergency Medicine*, 2nd ed. New York: McGraw-Hill, 2002:52.) (Also see Color Insert.)

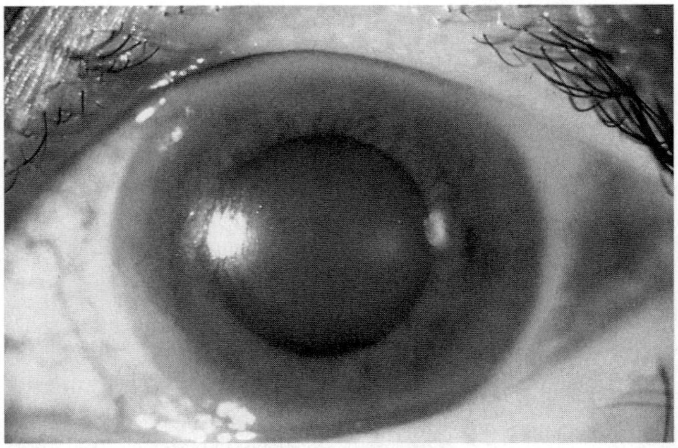

FIGURE 2-5. Acute angle-closure glaucoma.

(Courtesy of Gary Tanner, MD. Reproduced, with permission, from Knoop KJ, Stack LB, Storrow AB. *Atlas of Emergency Medicine*, 2nd ed. New York: McGraw-Hill, 2002:49.) (Also see Color Insert.)

Eye Findings in Systemic Diseases

Uveitis may be seen in the following conditions:

- Reiter's syndrome
- Behçet's disease
- IBD
- Wegener's granulomatosis
- Sarcoidosis
- HSV and herpes zoster
- TB
- Syphilis ("salt and pepper" fundus)
- HIV-associated diseases (toxoplasmosis, CMV, HSV, herpes zoster, *Mycobacterium, Cryptococcus, Candida*)

EAR, NOSE, AND THROAT

Bacterial Sinusitis

Eighty percent of sinusitis cases are due to viruses. Bacterial sinusitis results from impaired mucociliary clearance and obstruction of the osteomeatal complex. Viral and allergic rhinitis predisposes to acute sinusitis. Causative organisms of acute sinusitis include *Streptococcus pneumoniae,* other streptococci, *Haemophilus influenzae,* and, less commonly, *S. aureus* and *Moraxella catarrhalis.* Chronic sinusitis may also be caused by *Pseudomonas aeruginosa* and anaerobes.

Symptoms

Presents as unilateral or bilateral pain over the maxillary sinus or as a toothache. Acute sinusitis lasts > 1 week and up to 4 weeks. Chronic sinusitis lasts > 4 weeks.

EXAM

Purulent nasal discharge and tenderness over the maxillary sinus.

DIFFERENTIAL

- **Mucormycosis:** A rare but dangerous fungal disease that spreads through the blood vessels and primarily affects **immunocompromised** patients, including those with DM, end-stage renal disease, bone marrow transplant, lymphoma, and AIDS. It presents as sinusitis with more extreme facial pain, accompanied by **necrotic eschar** of the nasal mucosa and cranial neuropathies in the late stages. Early diagnosis is key. Treat emergently with amphotericin B and ENT surgical debridement.
- **Other:** If sinusitis is chronic and resistant to treatment, consider anatomical sinus obstruction, common variable immunodeficiency, a CF variant, or Wegener's granulomatosis.

DIAGNOSIS

- Generally made through a history and clinical exam.
- Routine imaging is not indicated for uncomplicated acute sinusitis. In cases of chronic sinusitis, refractory sinusitis, or suspected intracranial or orbital complications, a CT scan is more sensitive and cost-effective than x-ray imaging and may identify air-fluid levels or bony abnormalities.

TREATMENT

- Oral and/or nasal decongestants—e.g., oral pseudoephedrine, nasal oxymetazoline.
- **Acute sinusitis:** Amoxicillin or TMP-SMX × 10 days; amoxicillin-clavulanate in the presence of risk factors for anaerobes or resistant β-lactamase organisms (some strains of *H. influenzae* and *M. catarrhalis*). Risk factors include DM, immunocompromised states, and recent antibiotic use.
- **Chronic sinusitis: Amoxicillin-clavulanate for at least 3–4 weeks along with intranasal glucocorticoids.**

Otitis Media

Common causative organisms include *S. pneumoniae*, *H. influenzae*, *M. catarrhalis*, *S. pyogenes*, and viruses.

SYMPTOMS/EXAM

Ear pain, ear fullness, decreased hearing, and an erythematous, bulging tympanic membrane (see Figure 2-6).

TREATMENT

- Amoxicillin × 10–14 days.
- For penicillin-allergic patients, give TMP-SMX or a macrolide (erythromycin, azithromycin, clarithromycin).

Otitis Externa

Water exposure or mechanical trauma (e.g., Q-tips) are predisposing factors. Often caused by gram-negative rods (e.g., *Pseudomonas*, *Proteus*) or by a fungus (e.g., *Aspergillus*).

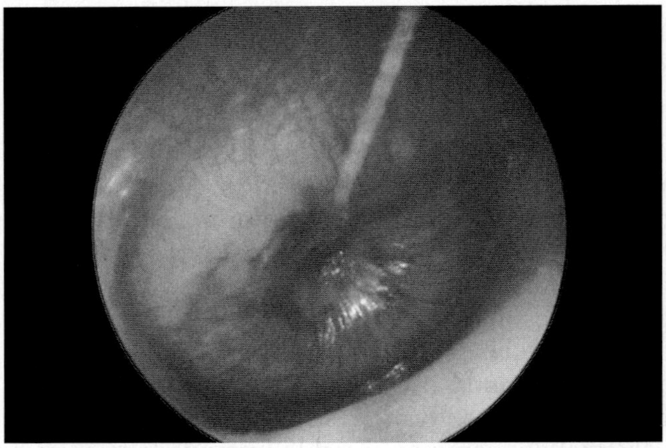

FIGURE 2-6. Acute otitis media.

(Courtesy of Richard A. Chole, MD, PhD. Reproduced, with permission, from Knoop KJ, Stack LB, Storrow AB. *Atlas of Emergency Medicine*, 2nd ed. New York: McGraw-Hill, 2002:118.) (Also see Color Insert.)

SYMPTOMS/EXAM

Presents with ear pain, often accompanied by pruritus and a purulent discharge. Erythema and edema of the ear canal with exudate may also be seen. Pain is elicited on manipulation of the ear.

DIFFERENTIAL

Malignant external otitis is seen in **diabetics** and other immunocompromised patients. Caused by ***P. aeruginosa*** and characterized by a foul discharge from the ear along with severe ear pain, evolving into osteomyelitis with cranial nerve palsies (CN VI, VII, IX, X, XI, and XII). Diagnose by CT scan; treat with prolonged antipseudomonal antibiotics, initially **IV but with a transition to oral administration.**

TREATMENT

- Avoid moisture and mechanical trauma.
- Give otic drops combining an aminoglycoside (neomycin sulfate, polymyxin B sulfate) and a corticosteroid.
- Use an ear wick to maintain an open canal.
- Add oral antibiotics to topical solutions if there is evidence of systemic spread (fever, regional lymphadenopathy).

Hearing Loss (HL)

Characterized as conductive (middle or external ear damage) or sensorineural (inner ear—cochlea or auditory nerve).

EXAM

- Differentiate between conductive and sensorineural HL in the following manner:
  - **Weber test:** With the tuning fork on the forehead, sound normally stays in the middle of the forehead. In conductive HL, the sound localizes to the affected side; in sensorineural HL, it localizes to the contralateral side.

- **Rinne test:** The tuning fork is first held on the mastoid. This sound on bone is then compared to that elicited with the tuning fork held near the ipsilateral ear. Normally, air-conducted sound is louder than bone-conducted sound, but with conductive HL, bone conduction is louder.
- Conduct an audiology test.

DIFFERENTIAL

Table 2-9 outlines the differential diagnosis of HL.

TREATMENT

- Prevention is the best treatment. Avoid excessive noise.
- Treat the underlying cause with antibiotics, removal of middle or outer ear blockages, repair of the tympanic membrane, or replacement of ossicles (in otosclerosis).
- For persistent sensorineural or conductive HL, consider hearing aids or, in cases of profound HL, cochlear implants.

Tinnitus

Perception of abnormal ear noises, usually due to sensory HL. Although bothersome, it is benign in the absence of other symptoms.

DIFFERENTIAL

Ménière's disease (episodic vertigo, sensorineural HL, tinnitus, and ear pressure).

TREATMENT

- Avoid exposure to excessive noise (e.g., rock concerts) and ototoxic drugs (aminoglycosides, salicylates, loop diuretics, cisplatin).
- Background noise (music) can be used to mask the tinnitus.
- Oral TCAs (e.g., nortriptyline) may be effective.

TABLE 2-9. Differential Diagnosis of Hearing Loss

	SENSORINEURAL HL	CONDUCTIVE HL
Areas of damage	Inner ear: cochlea or nerve (CN VIII).	Middle or external ear.
Rinne	Normal (air louder).	Abnormal **(bone louder).**
Weber	Sound lateralizes to (is louder in) the good ear.	Sound lateralizes to the bad ear.
Causes	Age (presbycusis), excessive noise exposure, ototoxic drugs, Ménière's disease, acoustic neuroma.	Otitis media, otosclerosis, eustachian tube blockage, perforated tympanic membrane, cerumen.

AMBULATORY MEDICINE

Pharyngitis

The main concern lies in identifying group A β-hemolytic streptococcal infection (GABHS). Adequate antibiotic treatment of GABHS usually prevents the complications of scarlet fever, glomerulonephritis, myocarditis, and local abscess formation. Rheumatic heart disease can still occur despite treatment.

SYMPTOMS/EXAM

The four classic features of GABHS (Centor criteria) are fever > 38°C, tender anterior cervical lymphadenopathy, the absence of cough, and pharyngotonsillar exudate. The presence of cough, hoarseness, and rhinorrhea makes GABHS less likely.

DIFFERENTIAL

- **Mononucleosis:** Occurs primarily in young adults, accounting for 5–10% of sore throats; characterized by the triad of lymphadenopathy, fever, and tonsillar pharyngitis. Symptoms also include severe fatigue, headache, and malaise.
  - Diagnose with a positive heterophil antibody (Monospot) test or a high anti-EBV titer.
  - EBV, the etiologic virus, can be transmitted through saliva (kissing) up to 18 months after primary infection but is not very contagious.
  - Complications include hepatitis, a morbilliform rash after **ampicillin** administration, and splenomegaly occurring within the first three weeks.
  - To decrease the risk of splenic rupture, noncontact sports must be avoided for 3–4 weeks and contact sports for 4–6 weeks after symptom onset.
- **Diphtheria:** Common in alcoholics; presents as malaise with gray pseudomembranes on the tonsils.
- **Viruses:** Viral infection is suggested by rhinorrhea and cough, other upper respiratory tract symptoms, and the absence of tonsillar exudate.

DIAGNOSIS

- **Test of choice:** The GABHS rapid antigen test has > 90% sensitivity. Routine cultures are not needed.
- **Algorithm:** In the presence of the Centor criteria:
  - **4 of 4:** Treat empirically without a rapid antigen test.
  - **2–3 of 4:** Test and treat positive results.
  - **0–1 of 4:** No test and no antibiotic treatment.

TREATMENT

- Penicillin V potassium or cefuroxime × 10 days.
- Erythromycin for penicillin-allergic patients.
- **All cases (bacterial, viral):** Acetaminophen or NSAIDs and salt-water gargling.
- **Viral pharyngitis:** Patients may return to work when fever resolves and they are well enough to participate in normal activities.
- **Strep throat:** Patients may return to work after 24 hours of antibiotics.

Acute Bronchitis

A nonspecific term used to describe patients with normal underlying lungs who develop an acute cough with no clinical evidence of pneumonia. The most common causative organisms are respiratory **viruses** (rhino, corona, adeno) and, to a lesser extent, atypical bacteria (*Mycoplasma pneumoniae, Chlamydia pneumoniae, Bordetella pertussis*).

SYMPTOMS/EXAM

Cough (productive or not) may persist for 1–3 weeks, often with initial URI symptoms (rhinorrhea, sore throat). Exam ranges from clear to wheezes or rhonchi (from bronchospasm).

DIFFERENTIAL

- It is important to rule out community-acquired pneumonia.
- Consider other URIs.

DIAGNOSIS

Diagnosis is made clinically. CXR is not routinely indicated.

TREATMENT

- **Antibiotics are not indicated** given the common viral etiology.
- Expectorants for symptomatic treatment.
- Bronchodilators (albuterol inhaler).

Oral Lesions

Tables 2-10 and 2-11 outline the differential diagnosis of common oral lesions.

UROLOGY

Benign Prostatic Hypertrophy (BPH)

Prevalence increases with age; > 90% of men > 80 years of age have an enlarged prostate. BPH symptoms do not occur in all cases, but there is an increased likelihood with advancing age.

SYMPTOMS

Obstructive symptoms include difficulty initiating a stream, terminal dribbling, and a weak stream. Irritative symptoms include urgency, frequency, and nocturia. DRE may reveal an enlarged, symmetrically firm prostate, but the **size of the prostate does not correlate with symptom severity.**

DIFFERENTIAL

Prostate cancer, bladder cancer, bladder stones, UTI, interstitial cystitis, prostatitis, prostatodynia, neurogenic bladder.

DIAGNOSIS

- Diagnose mainly by history and exam.
- Obtain UA and serum creatinine.
- PSA may be elevated in BPH but is not needed for diagnosis and is optional for prostate cancer screening (see the cancer screening discussion above).

TABLE 2-10. Differential of White Oral Lesions

	THRUSH	LEUKOPLAKIA	LICHEN PLANUS
Definition/ epidemiology	Oral candidiasis, often in **immunocompromised patients** (diabetes, chemotherapy, local radiation, steroids, antibiotics).	Hyperkeratoses due to chronic irritation (dentures, tobacco), but ~2–6% represent **dysplasia or early invasive squamous cell carcinoma (SCC).**	Common, chronic inflammatory autoimmune disease.
Symptoms	Pain.	None.	Discomfort; often confused with candidiasis, leukoplakia, or SCC.
Exam	Creamy white patches over red mucosa (see Figure 2.7).	White lesions **cannot be rubbed off.**	Reticular or erosive.
Diagnosis	Clinical; can do KOH wet prep (spores).	**Biopsy.**	Biopsy.
Treatment	Fluconazole × 7–14 days; clotrimazole troches 5×/day.	Treat if cancer.	Steroids (oral or topical).

α-blockers are more effective than finasteride in improving BPH symptoms. Surgery is most effective in patients with severe symptoms.

TREATMENT

- **Treatment options** include watchful waiting, pharmacologic therapy, and surgery (see Tables 2-12 and 2-13).
- Based on the severity of symptoms:
  - **Mild:** Watchful waiting only, as some men may have resolution of their symptoms.

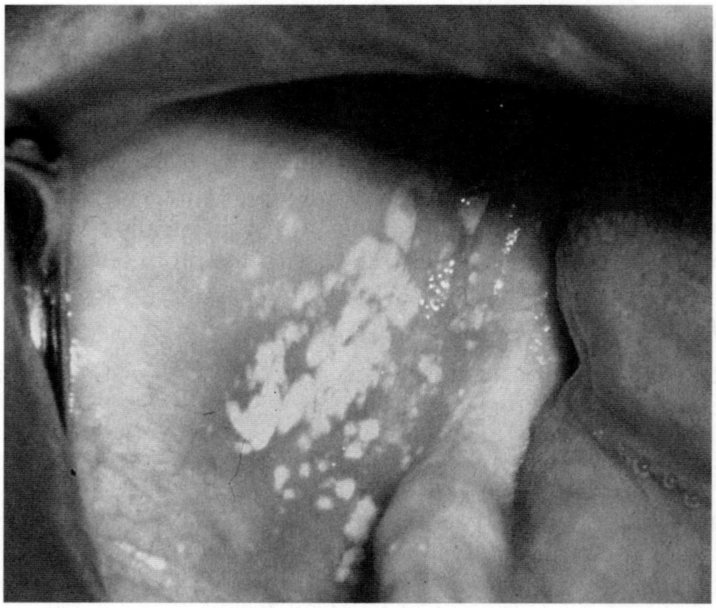

FIGURE 2-7. Thrush on buccal mucosa.

(Courtesy of James F. Steiner, DDS. Reproduced, with permission, from Knoop KJ, Stack LB, Storrow AB. *Atlas of Emergency Medicine*, 2nd ed. New York: McGraw-Hill, 2002:177.)

TABLE 2-11. Differential of Common Mouth Ulcers

	APHTHOUS ULCER (CANKER SORE)	HERPES STOMATITIS
Cause	Common; unknown cause (possible association with HHV-6).	Common; HSV.
Symptoms	Pain up to 1 week; heals within a few weeks.	Initial burning followed by small vesicles and then scabs.
Exam	Small ulcerations with yellow centers surrounded by red halos on **nonkeratinized** mucosa (buccal and lip mucosa; see Figure 2-8).	Vesicles, scabs.
Treatment	Anti-inflammatory: topical steroids.	No need, but oral **acyclovir** × 7–14 days may shorten the course and postherpetic pain.
Prognosis	Recurrent.	Resolves quickly; frequent reactivation in immunocompromised patients.
Differential diagnosis	If large or persistent, consider erythema multiforme, HSV, pemphigus, Behçet's disease, IBD, or SCC.	Aphthous ulcer, erythema multiforme, syphilis, cancer.

- **Moderate to severe:** Medications or surgery. Patients with severe symptoms benefit most from surgery, particularly after medication failure.
- Saw palmetto is a popular plant extract that appears to reduce symptoms. However, its efficacy and safety have not yet been rigorously tested.

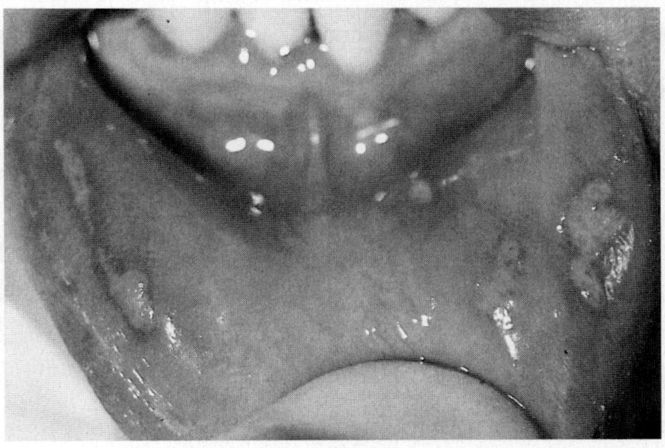

FIGURE 2-8. Aphthous ulcers on lip and gingival mucosa.

(Courtesy of James F. Steiner, DDS. Reproduced, with permission, from Knoop KJ, Stack LB, Storrow AB. *Atlas of Emergency Medicine*, 2nd ed. New York: McGraw-Hill, 2002:180.)

TABLE 2-12. Medications for BPH

	α_1-Blockers	5α-Reductase Inhibitors
Drugs	Prazosin, doxazosin, terazosin, tamsulosin.	Finasteride.
Mechanism	Reduce contractility of the prostate and bladder neck.	Block testosterone conversion to more potent dihydrotestosterone.
Results	Improve symptoms and urinary flow rates; **more effective than 5α-reductase inhibitors.**	Improve symptoms; reduce prostate size and PSA, especially in men with larger prostates.
Side effects	Orthostatic hypotension, nasal congestion, dizziness, fatigue.	Decreased libido, ejaculatory dysfunction, impotence.

Erectile Dysfunction (ED)

Defined as an inability to acquire or maintain an erection sufficient for sexual intercourse in > 75% of attempts. Evaluation is directed at distinguishing organic from psychogenic causes. In determining the etiology focus on identifying hyperlipidemia, hypertension, DM, neurologic disorders, pelvic surgical or trauma history, and drug use (see Table 2-14).

Diagnosis

- **Screening labs to rule out an organic etiology:** Glucose, cholesterol, TSH, testosterone, prolactin.
- If testosterone or prolactin is abnormal, check FSH and LH (pituitary abnormality).
- Urology referral if there is a plan for duplex ultrasonography or direct injection of vasoactive peptides.

TABLE 2-13. Urology Referral and Surgical Options for BPH

Indications for Urology Referral and Surgery	Surgical Options
Acute retention	Transurethral resection of the prostate (TURP)[a]
Hydronephrosis	Transurethral incision of the prostate (TUIP)
Recurrent UTIs	Open prostatectomy (gold standard)
Recurrent or refractory gross hematuria	Minimally invasive therapies
Renal insufficiency due to BPH	
Bladder stones	
Persistent severe symptoms despite maximal medical therapy	

[a] Side effects of TURP include retrograde ejaculation, impotence (10–40%, operator dependent), urinary incontinence, and hypervolemic hyponatremia.

TREATMENT

- Correct the underlying disorder (testosterone replacement for hypogonadism); eliminate medication- and drug-related causes.
- **Empiric therapy** is often indicated in the **absence of a suspected organic etiology. Oral sildenafil** is first-line therapy but is **contraindicated with nitrates or active cardiac disease** (hypotension, death).
- Psychosexual counseling is first-line therapy for psychogenic ED.
- Second-line therapies include intraurethral alprostadil suppositories, vacuum constrictive pump, and penile prostheses.

Up to one-quarter of all cases of ED may be related to drug or medication use.

Prostatitis

Includes acute bacterial prostatitis, chronic bacterial prostatitis, nonbacterial prostatitis, and prostatodynia.

SYMPTOMS/EXAM

Irritative voiding symptoms and perineal or suprapubic pain. Acute bacterial prostatitis is notable for the presence of fever and an exquisitely tender prostate.

TREATMENT

Table 2-15 outlines the treatment of prostatitis and prostatodynia.

TABLE 2-14. Etiologies of ED

■ Psychogenic disorders: performance anxiety, depression, mental stress
■ Diabetes mellitus: ED is seen in up to 50% of DM cases
■ Peripheral vascular disease
■ Endocrine disorders: hypogonadism, hyperprolactinemia, thyroid abnormalities
■ Pelvic surgery
■ Spinal cord injury
■ Drugs of abuse: amphetamines, cocaine, marijuana, chronic alcoholism
■ Medications:
■ Antihypertensives: **thiazides,** β-blockers, clonidine, methyldopa
■ Antiandrogens: spironolactone, H_2 blockers, finasteride
■ Antidepressants (TCAs, SSRIs)
■ Antipsychotics
■ Benzodiazepines
■ Opiates

All patients with genital lesions should be screened for syphilis (serology).

Genital Lesions

Table 2-16 outlines the differential diagnosis of genital lesions.

ORTHOPEDICS

Shoulder Pain: Rotator Cuff Tendinitis or Tear

Ranges from subacromial bursitis and rotator cuff tendinitis to partial or full rotator cuff tear. Due to excessive overhead motion (e.g., baseball players).

Symptoms

Nonspecific pain in the shoulder with occasional radiation down the lateral arm; worsens at night or with overhead movement. Motor weakness with abduction is seen in the presence of a tear.

Exam

- Decreased range of motion between 60 and 120 degrees. Tears lead to weakness on abduction.

TABLE 2-15. Treatment of Prostatitis and Prostatodynia

	Acute Bacterial Prostatitis	Chronic Bacterial Prostatitis	Nonbacterial Prostatitis	Prostatodynia
Fever	+	–	–	–
Urinalysis	+	–	–	–
Expressed prostatic secretions	Contraindicated.	+	+	–
Bacterial culture	+	+	–	–
Prostate exam	Very tender.	Normal, boggy, or indurated.	Normal, boggy, or indurated.	Usually normal.
Etiology	Gram-negative rods (*E. coli*); less commonly gram-positive (enterococcus).	Gram-negative rods; less commonly enterococcus.	Unknown; perhaps *Ureaplasma*, *Mycoplasma*, *Chlamydia*.	Varies; includes voiding dysfunction and pelvic floor musculature dysfunction.
Treatment	IV ampicillin and aminoglycoside until organism sensitivities are obtained; then switch to fluoroquinolones × 4–6 weeks.	TMP-SMX; fluoroquinolones × 6–12 weeks.	Erythromycin × 3–6 weeks if response at two weeks.	α-blocking drugs (e.g., terazosin) for bladder neck and urethral spasms; benzodiazepine and biofeedback for pelvic floor dysfunction.

Adapted, with permission, from Tierney LM et al (eds). *Current Medical Diagnosis & Treatment 2004,* 43rd ed. New York: McGraw-Hill, 2003:914.

TABLE 2-16. Differential Diagnosis of Genital Lesions

	HSV	Genital Warts (Condylomata Acuminata)	Primary Syphilis	Chancroid
Cause	HSV-2 > HSV-1.	HPV.	*Treponema pallidum.*	*Haemophilus ducreyi.*
Incubation period/ triggers	Primary: +/– asymptomatic; prodrome consists of malaise, genital paresthesias, and fever. Reactivation most commonly occurs with symptoms; triggers include stress, fever, and infection.	1–6 months; triggers include pregnancy and immunosuppression.	2–6 weeks.	3–5 days.
Symptoms	**Painful, grouped vesicles;** tingling, dysesthesias.	Warty "cauliflower" growths or none.	**Painless, clean-based** ulcer **("chancre").**	Pustule or pustules erode to form a **painful** ulcer with a necrotic base.
Exam	Groups of multiple, small vesicles.	Warty growths or none.	Ulcer on genitalia; nontender regional lymph nodes.	Usually unilateral, tender, fluctuant, matted nodes with overlying erythema.
Diagnosis	Mostly clinical; positive viral culture or direct fluorescent antibody or Tzanck smear with positive intranuclear inclusions and multinucleated giant cells.	Clinical if wartlike; 4% acetic acid applied to the lesion turns tissue white with papillae.	Serology: RPR positive 1–2 weeks after the primary lesion is first seen. Immunofluorescence or darkfield microscopy of fluid with treponemes.	Culture of lesion on special media.
Treatment	Acyclovir 200 mg 5×/day; famciclovir 250 mg TID; valacyclovir 1000 mg BID × 7 days **(asymptomatic shedding is common).**	Trichloroacetic acid; podophyllum (contraindicated in pregnancy); imiquimod.	**Benzathine penicillin G IM ×1;** in penicillin-allergic patients, doxycycline or tetracycline PO × 2 weeks.	Azithromycin 1 g PO ×1 or ceftriaxone 250 mg IM ×1.

- **Impingement sign:** Pain elicited by 60–120 degrees of passive abduction suggests impingement or trapping of an **inflamed rotator cuff** on the overlying acromion.

DIFFERENTIAL

- **Bicipital tendinitis:** Due to repetitive overhead motion (e.g., throwing, swimming). Exam reveals tenderness along the biceps tendon or muscle.
- Degenerative joint disease.
- **Systemic arthritis:** RA, pseudogout.
- Referred pain from a pulmonary process (e.g., pulmonary embolism, pleural effusion), a subdiaphragmatic process, cervical spine disease, or brachial plexopathy.

DIAGNOSIS

- Diagnosis is made by history and exam.
- MRI can be done if a complete tear is suspected or if no improvement is seen despite conservative therapy and the patient is a surgical candidate.

TREATMENT

- Rest; decrease exacerbating activities; NSAIDs.
- Steroid injection if no improvement.
- Range-of-motion exercises to strengthen rotator cuff muscles once acute pain has resolved.
- Refer to orthopedics for possible surgery if there is a complete tear or if no improvement is seen with conservative therapy after several months.

Knee Pain

Table 2-17 outlines the etiologies of common knee injuries.

DIAGNOSIS

- **X-ray imaging** is necessary to rule out a knee fracture in the following situations:
  - Effusion that occurs within 24 hours of traumatic injury.
  - Patellar tenderness.
  - Inability to bear weight either immediately after trauma or on examination.
  - Inability to completely flex the knee.
- **MRI** is most sensitive for soft tissue injuries (e.g., meniscal and ligament tears).

Stress Fractures

Often seen in runners, especially thin females who run long distances; also seen in military recruits and ballet dancers. Most occur in the **distal tibia, femoral neck,** and **second metatarsal of the foot.** Risk factors include low body weight, lower limb misalignment, muscle fatigue, menstrual irregularities, smoking, and excess volume or intensity of training.

SYMPTOMS/EXAM

Patients present with pain at the injury site that is reproducible upon running as well as with difficulty weight bearing. Tenderness is seen over the fracture site.

DIFFERENTIAL

- **Shin splints (medial tibial stress syndrome):** Commonly seen in runners. Can progress to stress fracture. Aches and tenderness are seen over the anteromedial distal tibia.
- **Plantar fasciitis:** Due to excessive standing, running without arch support, and poor footwear. Presents with severe pain on the bottoms of the feet upon standing in the morning; pain improves with activity. Exam shows tenderness over insertion of the fascia on the medial heel. No x-ray is necessary for diagnosis. Treat with arch supports, reduction of running, and stretching of the Achilles tendon and plantar fascia.

TABLE 2-17. Common Knee Injuries

	Iliotibial Band Syndrome	Anserine Bursitis	Patellofemoral Pain Syndrome	Medial Meniscus Tear	Anterior Cruciate Ligament (ACL) Tear
Those affected/ mechanism	Runners, deconditioned patients.	Runners, obese or deconditioned patients, washwomen, carpet layers.	Runners, deconditioned patients, often with chondromalacia of the patella.	Twisting of the knee while the foot is firmly planted on the ground (soccer, football).	Twisting trauma, often in noncontact sports (e.g., skiing).
Symptoms	**Lateral** knee pain that is gradual; tightness after running.	Pain **medial** and inferior to the knee joint.	**Anterior** knee pain behind the patella; occurs gradually during running.	Severe pain with **"locking," "catching,"** and swelling that peaks the next day.	**Audible "pop" and giving way; immediate swelling.**
Exam	Tenderness over the lateral femoral epicondyle.	Localized tenderness.	Pain on patellar compression; diffuse tenderness.	Medial joint line tenderness; pain on hyperflexion and hyperextension; swelling; **positive McMurray's** test; difficulty walking in a squatting position.	Positive anterior drawer sign, **positive Lachman's** test, swelling.
Treatment	Rest and abstain from running for a few weeks; then resume gentle stretching, especially before running.			Treat conservatively: RICE (rest, ice, coimpression, elevation); quadriceps strengthening with physical therapy; surgery only if symptoms persist.	Conservative; ACL reconstruction if the patient has a high activity level.

- **Metatarsalgia:** A nonspecific term for pain around the metatarsal heads, usually caused by callus or chronic pressure (e.g., overuse from running, high heels).

DIAGNOSIS

Usually diagnosed by history and exam. X-ray imaging **may miss early fracture;** MRI and nuclear scintigraphy are more sensitive and can confirm fracture.

TREATMENT

Activity modification with no running for at least 2–3 months; physical therapy.

The thin female teenager who is an "exercise nut" is particularly prone to stress fractures.

Back pain causes–

DISC MASS

Degeneration (DJD, osteoporosis, spondylosis)
Infection/**I**njury
Spondylitis
Compression fracture
Multiple myeloma/**M**ets (cancer of breast, kidney, lung, prostate, thyroid)
Abdominal pain/**A**neurysm
Skin (herpes zoster), **S**train, **S**coliosis, and lordosis
Slipped disk/ **S**pondylolisthesis

New-onset back pain in a patient with a previous diagnosis of cancer represents metastasis until proven otherwise. Cord compression is a neurosurgical emergency.

"Red flags" in the history of a patient with new-onset back pain:

- *Age > 50*
- *History of cancer*
- *Fever*
- *Weight loss*
- *IV drug use*
- *Osteoporosis*
- *Lower extremity weakness*
- *Bowel or bladder dysfunction*

Lower Back Pain (LBP)

Extremely common, with up to 80% of the population affected at some time. Three-quarters of LBP patients improve within one month. Most have self-limited, nonspecific mechanical causes of LBP.

Exam

- The goal of evaluation is to rule out serious conditions (fracture, cancer, infection, cauda equina syndrome). Fever and spinal process tenderness suggest infection; bilateral leg weakness, bladder fullness, saddle anesthesia, and decreased anal tone suggest cauda equina syndrome. "Red flag" symptoms for all patients include duration of pain > 1 month and no relief despite bed rest.
- Straight leg raise is a positive test for nerve root irritation if a passive leg raise in the supine position causes radicular pain at less than a 60-degree angle. Poor specificity (40%) but excellent sensitivity (95%).
- Exam may also localize the origin of nerve root syndrome (see Table 2-18).

Differential

- **Serious causes** of back pain can be distinguished as follows:
  - **Cancer:** Age ≥ 50 years, previous cancer history, unexplained weight loss.
  - **Compression fracture:** Age ≥ 50 years, significant trauma, history of osteoporosis, corticosteroid use.
  - **Infection (epidural abscess, diskitis, osteomyelitis, or endocarditis):** Fever, recent skin or urinary infection, immunosuppression, **IV drug use.**
  - **Cauda equina syndrome:** Bilateral leg weakness, decreased urinary retention.
- **Less urgent** causes of back pain include herniated disk; spinal stenosis; sciatica; musculoskeletal strain; and referred pain from a kidney stone, an intra-abdominal process, or herpes zoster. Table 2-19 outlines the differential diagnosis of herniated disk and spinal stenosis.

Diagnosis

- History and clinical exam are helpful in identifying the cause.
- A plain x-ray is indicated only if serious causes of back pain are considered (e.g., fracture, cancer, infection, cauda equina) or if pain persists despite conservative therapy for four weeks.
- MRI can initially be deferred unless features of high-risk conditions are present.

Treatment

- For mechanical causes of LBP, conservative therapy with NSAIDs, education, and early return to ordinary activity are indicated in the absence of major neurologic deficits or other alarm symptoms, as most cases of LBP resolve within four weeks. Bed rest should be limited to < 2 days.
- Back manipulation by a chiropractor or physical therapist is safe and effective for benign, mechanical causes of LBP.
- Spinal stenosis can be treated with exercises to decrease lumbar lordosis. Decompressive laminectomy may provide at least short-term relief.

TABLE 2-18. Nerve Root Syndromes (Sciatica)

NERVE ROOT	STRENGTH	SENSORY	REFLEXES
S1	Ankle plantar flexion (toe walking)	Lateral foot	Achilles
L5	Great toe dorsiflexion	Medial forefoot	None
L4 (less common)	Ankle dorsiflexion (heel walking)	Medial calf	Knee jerk

CARDIOPULMONARY

Hypertension

High blood pressure is defined as a systolic BP ≥ 140 or a diastolic BP ≥ 90 (see Table 2-20). Hypertension is associated with MI, heart failure (HF), stroke, and kidney disease. The control of hypertension is associated with a decreased risk of stroke, MI, and heart failure.

TABLE 2-19. Herniated Disk vs. Spinal Stenosis

	HERNIATED DISK	SPINAL STENOSIS
Etiology	Degeneration of ligaments leads to disk prolapse, leading in turn to compression or inflammation of the nerve root. Nearly all involve the L4–L5 or L5–S1 interspace.	Narrowing of the spinal canal from osteophytes at facet joints, bulging disks, or a hypertrophied ligamentum flavum.
Symptoms	**"Sciatica":** Pain and paresthesias in the dermatome from the buttock radiating down to below the knee. **Worsens with sitting** (lumbar flexion).	**"Neurogenic claudication"/ "pseudoclaudication":** Pain radiating to the buttocks, thighs, or lower legs. **Worsens with prolonged standing or walking** (extension of spine); improves with sitting or walking uphill (flexion of the spine).
Exam/ diagnosis	See Table 2-18. Positive straight leg raise (pain at 60 degrees or less) is seen.	Unremarkable. MRI confirms the diagnosis.
Therapy	Limited bed rest < 2 days; ordinary activity; NSAIDs; chiropractic for benign, mechanical LBP is as effective as therapy prescribed by physicians.	Exercise to reduce lumbar lordosis; decompressive laminectomy.

DIAGNOSIS

- BP should be checked at least every two years starting at age 18.
- Three goals of evaluation: (1) assess lifestyle and other cardiovascular risk factors or other disease that will affect management (e.g., diabetes); (2) identify secondary causes of hypertension; and (3) assess for the presence of target-organ damage and cardiovascular disease (heart, brain, kidney, peripheral vascular disease, retinopathy).

TREATMENT

- The goal of BP management is **< 140/90**, or **< 130/80** in patients with **diabetes, renal disease,** or cardiovascular disease.
- All patients with prehypertension and stages 1 and 2 hypertension should be counseled about lifestyle modification (see Table 2-21). If necessary, pharmacotherapy can be added (see Table 2-22).

Smoking and Smoking Cessation

A combination of pharmacotherapy and behavioral counseling is most effective in promoting smoking cessation.

Smoking is the leading cause of preventable death in the United States. Treat as follows:

- Apply the **"four A" approach** advocated by the National Cancer Institute: Ask, Advise, Assist, Arrange.
- Physician counseling at each visit is effective.
- Offer all patients pharmacotherapy, which is **twice as effective** in promoting cessation as behavioral counseling alone (see Table 2-23).
- Treat nicotine withdrawal symptoms—e.g., cravings, irritability, decreased concentration, and increased appetite leading to weight gain (decreased with gum).

TABLE 2-20. Classification of Blood Pressure

BP CLASS	SYSTOLIC BP (mmHg)	DIASTOLIC BP (mmHg)	INITIAL DRUG THERAPY
Normal	< 120	and < 80	
Prehypertension	120–139	or 80–89	No drug therapy, but increased risk of hypertension.
Stage 1 hypertension	140–159	or 90–99	Thiazides for most; may consider ACEIs, angiotensin II (AT II) receptor blockers, β-blockers, calcium channel blockers, or a combination.
Stage 2 hypertension	≥ 160	or ≥ 100	Two-drug combination for most (usually thiazide first; then ACEIs, AT II receptor blockers, β-blockers, or calcium channel blockers).

Adapted from The Seventh Report of the Joint National Committee on Prevention, Detection, Evaluation, and Treatent of High Blood Pressure. *JAMA* 290:1314, 2003.

TABLE 2-21. Lifestyle Modifications for Hypertension

- **Sodium restriction:** No added salt or low-sodium diet.
- **DASH diet (Dietary Approaches to Stop Hypertension):** Diet rich in fruits, vegetables, and low-fat dairy products with decreased saturated and unsaturated fat.
- **Weight reduction:** If over ideal BMI.
- **Aerobic physical activity.**
- **Limit alcohol consumption:** < 2 drinks/day (men), < 1 drink/day (women).

TABLE 2-22. Antihypertensive Medications

	THIAZIDES	β-BLOCKERS	ACEIs	AT II RECEPTOR BLOCKERS	CALCIUM CHANNEL BLOCKERS
Drug examples	Hydrochlorothiazide, chlorthalidone.	Atenolol, metoprolol.	Captopril, enalapril, ramipril.	Irbesartan, losartan, valsartan.	Nondihydropyridines: diltiazem, verapamil; dihydropyridines: amlodipine, felodipine, nifedipine.
Side effects	Hypokalemia, ED, increased insulin resistance, hyperuricemia, increased TG.	Bronchospasm, depression, fatigue, impotence, increased insulin resistance.	Cough (10%), hyperkalemia, renal failure.	Less cough, hyperkalemia, renal failure.	Conduction defects (nonhydropyridines); lower extremity edema (dihydropyridines).
Indications for use as first-line drug	**Most patients** as mono- or combination therapy (stage 1 or 2 hypertension), including **isolated systolic hypertension in elderly, osteoporosis.**	**MI,** high CAD risk.	**DM with microalbuminuria; MI** with systolic dysfunction or anterior infarct); mild with non-DM-related **proteinuria.**		
Other indications	Recurrent stroke prevention.	CHF.	CHF.	CHF, DM, chronic renal failure, ACEI-related cough.	Atrial arrhythmias (nonhydropyridines), isolated systolic hypertension in elderly (dihydropyridines).
Contra-indications		Bronchospasm; high-degree (type II second- or third-degree) heart block.	**Pregnancy.**	**Pregnancy.**	High-degree heart block.

TABLE 2-23. **Smoking Cessation Methods**

METHOD	TYPES	MECHANISMS/TREATMENT	SIDE EFFECTS	CONTRAINDICATIONS
Pharmaco-therapy	Nicotine replacement (patch, gum, inhaler, nasal spray).		Skin irritation (patch), mucosal irritation (nasal spray), cough (inhaler).	Recent MI, unstable angina, life-threatening arrhythmia, pregnancy (although nicotine replacement may be preferable to continued smoking).
	Sustained-release bupropion.	Atypical antidepressant. Begin one week before quit date to build up nicotine levels and continue for 2–3 months.		**Seizures,** head trauma, heavy alcohol use, history of eating disorders.
Behavioral counseling	Individual, group, telephone hotlines.			

COMMON SYMPTOMS

Vertigo

An illusion of motion ("head is spinning," "room is whirling") can be categorized as peripheral or central. Other forms of dizziness include the following:

- **Presyncope:** Impending loss of consciousness ("I'm going to faint"). See Chapter 13.
- **Disequilibrium:** Unsteadiness ("My balance is off").
- **Lightheadedness:** Anxiety ("I'm just dizzy").

SYMPTOMS

A sensation of exaggerated motion when there is no or little motion. Peripheral vertigo is often accompanied by nausea and vomiting. Central vertigo often presents with gait imbalance. Ipsilateral facial numbness or weakness or limb ataxia suggests a lesion of the cerebellopontine angle.

EXAM

- Orthostatics.
- **Dix-Hallpike maneuver (positional testing):** Used to diagnose benign positional vertigo (BPV). Quickly bring the patient from a sitting to a supine position with the head tilted 45 degrees. A positive test indicates the presence of fatigable, rotatory nystagmus with a vertical component toward the forehead, which occurs after a latent period.

Diagnosis/Treatment

Differentiate between central and peripheral vertigo as indicated below and in Tables 2-24 and 2-25:

- **Central** (indicates brain stem or cerebellar etiology):
  - Suggested by other symptoms consistent with vertebrobasilar insufficiency or cerebellar dysfunction (e.g., diplopia, dysarthria, sensory or motor dysfunction).
  - **Vertical nystagmus** is always abnormal and always central.
- **Peripheral:** Suggested by horizontal or rotatory nystagmus.

> ***Causes of vertigo—***
>
> **VOMItS**
>
> **V**estibulitis
> **O**totoxic drugs (aminoglycoside, furosemide)
> **M**énière's
> **I**njury
> **S**pin (benign positional vertigo)

Unintentional Weight Loss

Defined as an unintended weight loss > 5% or more of usual body weight over 6–12 months. Unintentional weight loss is associated with excess morbidity and mortality. Etiologies are as follows:

- **Cancer** and **GI disorders** (malabsorption, pancreatic insufficiency) and **psychiatric disorders** (depression, anxiety, dementia, anorexia nervosa) account for up to two-thirds of cases.
- Other causes include hyperthyroidism, DM, chronic diseases, and infections.
- Idiopathic in up to one-third of cases.

Diagnosis

- History and exam often provide clues.
- Initial evaluation should include CBC, TSH, electrolytes, UA, FOBT, CXR, and age-appropriate cancer screening tests.
- The second evaluation (if the initial is negative) should consist of observation or, if the symptoms/exam are suggestive, further cancer screening or GI evaluation.

Treatment

- Treat the underlying disorder.
- Caloric intake goals; give caloric supplementation.

TABLE 2-24. Causes of Central Vertigo

	Acoustic Neuroma (CN VIII Schwannoma)	Brain Stem Ischemia	Basilar Migraine	Multiple Sclerosis
Symptoms	Unilateral hearing loss.	Symptoms of vertebrobasilar insufficiency: diplopia, dysarthria, numbness.	Occipital headache, visual disturbances, sensory symptoms.	Chronic imbalance.
Duration	Continuous.	Varies.	Varies.	Fluctuating.
Signs/diagnosis	MRI.	MRI/CT, angiogram.	Diagnosis of exclusion.	MRI/CT.
Treatment	Surgery.	Stroke treatment.	β-blockers, ergots.	See Chapter 13.

TABLE 2-25. Causes of Peripheral Vertigo

	Benign Positional Vertigo (BPV)	Ménière's Syndrome	Vestibular Neuronitis/Acute Labyrinthitis	Post-traumatic
Symptoms	A few seconds following head motion; nausea/vomiting.	**Four classic symptoms: episodic vertigo, sensorineural hearing loss, tinnitus, and ear fullness.**	May be preceded by URI; sudden, continuous.	
Duration	Up to one minute.	One to several hours.	A few days to one week.	A few days to one month.
Signs/diagnosis	**Positive Dix-Hallpike.**	Clinical; MRI to rule out acoustic neuroma.	Clinical.	Clinical.
Etiology	Dislodging of otolith into the semicircular canal.	Distention of the endolymphatic compartment of the inner ear.	Unknown; often occurs after URI.	Post–head trauma.
Treatment	Epley's maneuver (head-positioning maneuvers); physical therapy to reposition otoliths; ? trial of an anticholinergic such as meclizine.	Bed rest, low-salt diet +/– diuretics; symptomatic treatment with antihistamines, anticholinergics, and benzodiazepines.	Symptomatic.	Symptomatic; occasionally surgery.

Causes of fatigue/malaise–

FATIGUED

Fat/**F**ood (poor diet)
Anemia
Tumor
Infection (HIV, endocarditis)
General joint or liver disease
Uremia
Endocrine (hypothyroidism, cortisol deficiency)
Diabetes mellitus, **D**epression, **D**rugs

- Appetite stimulants (megestrol acetate, dronabinol) in the presence of low appetite.

Fatigue

A common symptom that is most often due to stress, sleep disturbance, viral infection, or other illnesses. Causes include the following:

- Thyroid abnormalities (hypo- and hyperthyroidism), infections (hepatitis, endocarditis), COPD, CHF, anemia, sleep apnea, psychiatric disorders (depression, alcoholism), drugs (β-blockers, sedatives), and autoimmune disorders.
- **Chronic fatigue syndrome:** Fatigue lasting at least six months that interferes with daily activities, in combination with four or more of the following: impaired memory or concentration, sore throat, tender cervical or axillary lymph nodes, muscle pain, multijoint pain, new headaches, unrefreshing sleep, and postexertion malaise.

TREATMENT

The treatment of chronic fatigue syndrome should center on a multidisciplinary approach involving the following:

- Continuing psychiatric treatment.
- Cognitive behavior therapy (promotes self-help).
- Graded exercise (improves physical function).
- A supportive patient-physician relationship.

Chronic Cough

Defined as a cough lasting > 3 weeks. The three most common causes (excluding postinfectious and ACEI use) are as follows:

- **Postnasal drip.**
- **Cough-variant asthma:** Exacerbated by seasonal allergies, exercise, and cold.
- **GERD:** Asymptomatic in 75% of cases.
- Other causes include post-URI cough (may persist for 2 months), *Bordetella pertussis*, chronic bronchitis, and ACEI use (may last for a few weeks after cessation).

> ***Causes of chronic cough–***
>
> **GASPS AND COUgh**
>
> **G**ERD
> **A**sthma
> **S**moking, chronic bronchitis
> **P**ostinfection
> **S**inusitis, postnasal drip
> **A**CEIs
> **N**eoplasm
> **D**iverticulum
> **C**HF
> **O**uter ear disease
> **U**pper airway obstruction

DIAGNOSIS

- Findings suggestive of chronic cough include nasal bogginess, a "cobblestoning" oropharynx, wheezes, a prolonged expiratory phase, and rales.
- Trial of empiric therapy.
- Consider CBC, CXR, and PFTs (+/– methacholine challenge and spirometry) if no improvement is seen following a therapeutic trial.

TREATMENT

Empirically treat the most likely causes—e.g., inhaled nasal corticosteroids, bronchodilators +/– inhaled steroids, acid suppressants.

Insomnia

The most common of all sleep disorders, affecting roughly 15% of patients at some point. Chronic insomnia is defined as > 3 weeks of difficulty falling or staying asleep, frequent awakenings during the night, and a feeling of insufficient sleep (daytime fatigue, forgetfulness, irritability). Exacerbating factors include stress, pain, daytime napping, early bedtimes, drug withdrawal (alcohol, benzodiazepines, opiates), and alcoholism.

DIFFERENTIAL

Restless leg syndrome (RLS), periodic limb-movement disorder (PLMD; see Table 2-26).

DIAGNOSIS

- Diagnosis is mainly clinical.
- Rule out psychiatric and medical conditions—e.g., depression, posttraumatic stress disorder, delirium, chronic pain, and Cheyne-Stokes respiration in CHF.
- Labs for RLS include CBC, ferritin, and BUN/creatinine.

TABLE 2-26. **Differential Diagnosis of Insomnia**

	Restless Leg Syndrome	Periodic Limb-Movement Disorder	Insomnia
Symptoms	A painless, "creepy-crawling" sensation that is relieved by leg movement but worsens at night and at rest.	Intermittent limb movements during non-REM sleep; seen in > 75% of patients with RLS.	Difficulty going to sleep without "physical" symptoms.
Disease associations	**Iron deficiency** (even in the absence of anemia), uremia, DM; idiopathic in most.	Uremia, TCAs, MAOIs.	Depression, anxiety, stimulants, chronic pain, alcohol.
Pathophysiology	Unknown; perhaps abnormal dopamine transmission.		Unknown vs. disease specific.
Treatment	Correct the underlying disorder (e.g., iron supplementation in RLS); give **dopaminergic agonists** (carbidopa-levodopa, pramipexole) or benzodiazepine if dopaminergic agonists fail.		Correct the underlying disorder; sleep hygiene; medications.

- Polysomnography may help diagnose PLMD and RLS and may rule out other causes of sleep disorders.

Treatment

- Treat the underlying disorder.
- Sleep hygiene and relaxation techniques.
- Short-acting benzodiazepines (< 4 weeks) are acceptable as first-line therapy in short-term insomnia due to stress, grief, etc.
- For chronic insomnia, avoid benzodiazepines and consider trazodone.

Chronic Lower Extremity Edema

Symptoms

- Pain, difficulty walking, lower extremity swelling.
- Distribution may be isolated or systemic (periorbital, ascites, anasarca, pulmonary edema).

Differential

- The differential for **unilateral lower extremity edema** includes the following:
  - **Venous insufficiency:** Post–vein graft for CABG.
  - **Reflex sympathetic dystrophy:** Hyperesthesia and hyperhidrosis that occurs a few weeks after trauma; trophic skin changes and pain out of proportion to exam.
  - **Deep venous thrombosis:** Usually acute edema.
  - **Infection:** Cellulitis.
  - **Inflammation:** Gout; ruptured Baker's cyst (posterior knee).
- The differential for **bilateral lower extremity edema** is given in Table 2-27.

TABLE 2-27. Chronic Bilateral Lower Extremity Edema

MECHANISM	CAUSES
Elevated capillary hydrostatic pressure	Venous insufficiency: a heavy, achy feeling that worsens as the day progresses; "brawny" edema. CHF, constrictive pericarditis. IVC compression (tumor, clot, lymph nodes). Pregnancy. Filariasis (lymph node obstruction by *Wuchereria bancrofti* and *Brugia malayi*). Drugs (affect salt): NSAIDs, glucocorticoids, estrogen.
Increased capillary permeability	Hypothyroid myxedema, drugs (calcium channel blockers, hydralazine), vasculitis.
Decreased oncotic pressure	Nephrotic syndrome, protein-losing enteropathy, cirrhosis, malnutrition.

DIAGNOSIS

- The etiology can often be determined without diagnostic testing.
- Depending on the history and physical exam, obtain an echocardiogram, UA for protein, liver enzymes, and abdominal/pelvic imaging.
- Lower extremity Dopplers.

TREATMENT

- Treat the underlying causes, including discontinuation of contributing medications.
- Support stockings.
- Lifestyle modification (decrease salt) and leg elevation.
- Surgery for varicosities.

MEDICAL ETHICS

Based on a group of fundamental principles that should guide the best practice:

- **Beneficence:** Be of benefit to your patient.
- **Nonmaleficence:** Do no harm to your patient.
- **Justice:** The equitable distribution of resources within a population.
- **Autonomy:** A patient's right for self-determination of health care.
- **Fidelity:** A proposed fifth principle—truthful disclosure to patients.

GAY AND LESBIAN HEALTH

Sexual practices, not orientation, determine the risk of infections and cancers. Remember that patients in homosexual relationships may have had heterosexual relationships in the past (and vice versa) and thus remain at risk for certain diseases.

Risks

- There is an increased risk of anal cancer in gay men, particularly in those who are HIV positive.
- There is a **decreased** risk of cervical cancer and HPV among gay women; however, a history of sex with men puts gay women at higher risk of cervical cancer than women with no heterosexual contact.
- There is a decreased risk of gonorrhea, syphilis, and chlamydia among women not having sex with men.
- HIV and hepatitis B are increased among men who have sex with men.

Screening

- **In men:**
  - Screen for HIV and HBV.
  - **Urethritis:** Screen for *Neisseria gonorrhoeae* and *Chlamydia trachomatis* urethritis.
  - **Proctitis:** Screen for *N. gonorrhoeae*, *C. trachomatis*, HSV, and syphilis.
  - Offer HBV and HAV vaccines.
  - **Anal Pap smear:** In HIV-positive gay men, this test has characteristics similar to those of the cervical Pap.
- **In women,** obtain a Pap smear if the patient is sexually active with men.

STATISTICS

Major Study Types

Table 2-28 outlines the major types of studies used in statistical analysis.

Test Parameters

Test \ Disease	+	–
+	a	b
–	c	d

$$Sn = \frac{a}{a+c}$$

$$Sp = \frac{d}{b+d}$$

Test parameters measure the clinical usefulness of a test. These include:

- **The sensitivity of a test (Sn)—"PID" (Positive in Disease):** The probability that a test will be positive in someone with the disease (i.e., the test's ability to correctly identify persons who truly have the disease) when compared to a gold standard test.
- **The specificity of a test (Sp)—"NIH" (Negative in Health):** The probability that a test will be negative in someone who truly does not have the disease (i.e., the test's ability to correctly identify persons who do not have the disease) when compared to a gold standard test.
- **Positive predictive value (PPV):** The proportion of persons testing positive who have the condition (i.e., of all people who test positive, the probability that they truly have the disease).
- **Negative predictive value (NPV):** The proportion of persons testing negative who do not have the condition (i.e., of all people who test negative, the probability that they truly do not have the disease).
- **Likelihood ratio (LR): LR = sensitivity / (1 – specificity)**—i.e., the proportion of patients **with** a disease who have a certain test result over the proportion of patients **without** the disease in question who have the given test result ("WOWO"—With over Without). **Example:** A high-probability V/Q scan has an LR of 14. This implies that a positive V/Q scan is 14 times more likely to be seen in patients **with** pulmonary embolism than in patients **without** pulmonary embolism.

$$PPV = \frac{a}{a+b}$$

$$NPV = \frac{d}{d+c}$$

TABLE 2-28. Statistical Study Types

Study Type	Explanation	Example	Advantages	Disadvantages
Randomized controlled trial	Intervene by **assigning** exposure to subjects and observing disease outcome.	Assigning patients with hypertension to receive one of two treatments: diuretics vs. ACEIs.	True experiment erases unforeseen confounders.	Expensive.
Cohort study	Identify exposure subjects and then **follow** for disease outcomes.	Identifying obese adults and following them for the development of hypertension.	The most robust observational study type; evaluates multiple exposures.	May take a long time to develop disease.
Case-control study	Identify cases and noncases of the disease outcome **before** determining exposure.	Identifying children born with a rare birth defect and looking at possible in utero exposures.	Cheap; fast; good for rare diseases.	Prone to biases.
Cross-sectional study	Identify exposure and outcome **at the same time** for each subject **within a specified population.**	Checking for hypertension and concurrently obtaining data on obesity in all persons seen in San Francisco county clinics.	Often survey data.	No ability to detect temporal relationship of outcome.

- **Lead-time bias:** The time by which a screening test advances the date of diagnosis from the usual symptomatic phase to an earlier presymptomatic phase. It occurs because the time between diagnosis and death will always increase by the amount of lead time (see Figure 2-9). **Example:** A new screening test for pancreatic cancer is able to detect disease in a presymptomatic stage. Unfortunately, the poor overall prognosis for the disease re-

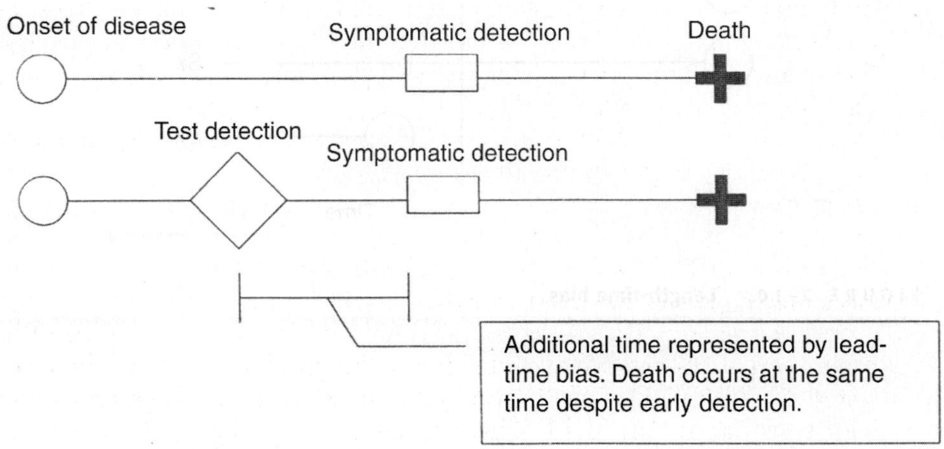

FIGURE 2-9. Lead-time bias.

mains the same. Thus, screened patients know about their disease sooner and live with disease longer because of this knowledge but still die of pancreatic cancer.

- **Length-time bias:** Because cases vary in the lengths of their asymptomatic phase, screening will overdetect cases of slowly progressing disease (longer duration in the asymptomatic phase) and miss rapidly progressing cases. **Example:** Diseases have variable latency periods in different individuals with the same disease. Length-time bias reflects the propensity of screening tests to detect slower, less serious tumors. In Figure 2-10, mammography is able to detect two cases of slowly growing breast cancer due to the long period between disease onset and symptoms, but two cases with rapid change from onset to symptoms are missed (see Figure 2-10).

Sensitivity and specificity are ***independent*** *of disease prevalence in the tested population. PPV and NPV depend on disease prevalence.*

Threats to Validity

Table 2-29 lists factors that can adversely affect the outcome of a statistical study.

Hypothesis Testing

- **P-value:** A quantitative estimate of the probability that a study's outcome could occur by chance alone. A study with a $p < 0.05$ signifies that the probability of the results occurring by chance is < 1 in 20 and is thus "statistically significant."
- **Type 1 error** (α): The probability of detecting a difference when none exists (rejecting the null hypothesis).
- **Type 2 error** (β): The probability of failing to detect a difference when it exists (failing to reject the null hypothesis).

Screen-detected patients will always live longer than clinically detected patients even if early detection and treatment confer no benefit because of lead-time and length biases.

Type ***I*** *(****A****lpha)* ***E****rror: "There* ***I****s* ***A****n* ***E****ffect" where in reality there is none.*

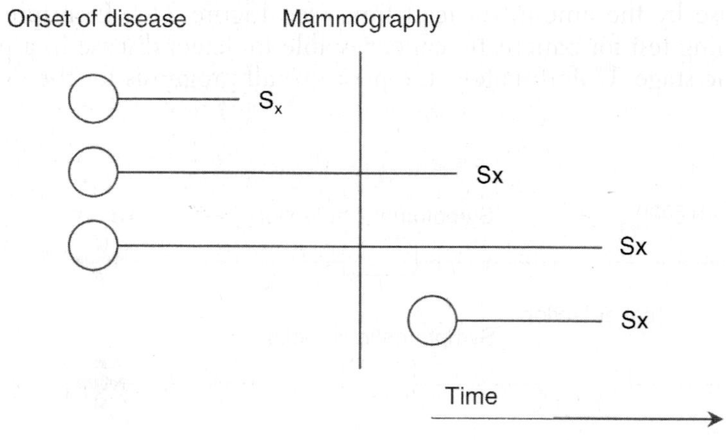

FIGURE 2-10. Length-time bias.

Disease

Test	+	−
+	Correct	Type I (α)
−	Type II (β)	Correct

TABLE 2-29. Threats to the Validity of Statistical Studies

	EXPLANATION	EXAMPLE
Confounding	Another variable (confounding factor) is associated with the predictor variable and the outcome variable without being in the causal pathway.	Coffee as a confounding variable in MI: Smoking is associated with coffee drinking, and smoking is a cause of MI. This does not mean that coffee causes MI; rather, coffee is a confounder in this case, as it is associated with both the predictor (smoking) and the outcome (MI) without being causal.
Measurement biases	When the method of measuring misleadingly changes the degree of an association.	
	Recall bias: Self-reporting by study subjects is influenced by knowledge of the study hypothesis.	In a case-control study, cancer patients may think harder than controls about certain toxic exposures.
	Misclassification bias: When a person without disease is "misclassified" into the diseased group or vice versa.	
	Random misclassification: When participants are placed in the wrong group (either with or without disease) in a random fashion. This biases the results to the null.	
	Nonrandom misclassification: When participants are placed selectively in the wrong group (e.g., many disease patients are mistakenly placed in the control group). This can bias findings either toward or away from the null.	
Selection bias	Study subjects are selected into (or drop out of) a study in a way that misleadingly changes the degree of association.	Control patients chosen from a hospital may be more likely to have unhealthy behaviors than ambulatory controls.

NOTES

CHAPTER 3

Cardiovascular Medicine

Sanjiv Shah, MD
Josh Cohen, MD

Physical Exam

ARTERIAL PULSATIONS

- **Diminished pulses:** Atherosclerotic peripheral vascular disease (listen for bruits) and conditions associated with low cardiac output (e.g., heart failure, cardiac tamponade, critical aortic stenosis).
- **Exaggerated pulses:** Aortic regurgitation, coarctation (upper extremities only), patent ductus arteriosus (PDA), hyperthyroidism, and arteriovenous fistulas.
- **Asymmetric pulses:** Severe atherosclerotic vascular disease, aortic dissection, Takayasu's arteritis, coarctation of the aorta (palpate for femoral pulses that are delayed when compared with radial pulses).
- **Carotid pulsations:**
  - **Delayed upstroke:** Aortic stenosis.
  - **Bisferiens pulse:** Two palpable peaks during systole; occurs in mixed aortic stenosis and aortic regurgitation as well as in hypertrophic cardiomyopathy.
  - **Dicrotic pulse:** Two palpable peaks (one in systole, one in diastole); most commonly occurs in young patients with severe heart failure and very low ejection fraction (e.g., dilated cardiomyopathy secondary to alcoholism).
- **Peripheral pulses:**
  - **Corrigan (water-hammer) pulse:** Occurs in chronic, hemodynamically significant aortic regurgitation. Characterized by a rapid rise and fall of the radial pulse accentuated by wrist elevation.
  - **Pulsus paradoxus:** Defined as a **BP decrease of > 10 mmHg** during normal inspiration. Occurs in cardiac tamponade, constrictive pericarditis, severe asthma, and COPD.
  - **Pulsus alternans:** Amplitude alternates with every other heartbeat. Occurs in severe systolic heart failure.
- See Figure 3-1 for illustrations of arterial pulse waveforms.

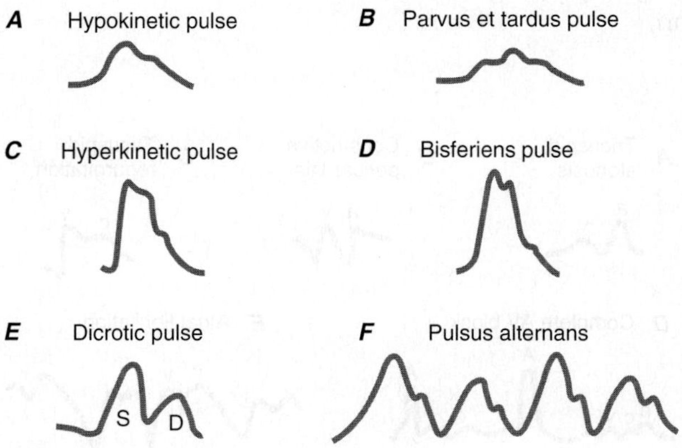

FIGURE 3-1. Arterial pulse waveforms.

(Adapted, with permission, from Fuster V et al [eds]. *Hurst's the Heart,* 10th ed. New York: McGraw-Hill, 2001.)

VENOUS PULSATIONS

- **Normal jugular venous pulsations:**
  - **a wave:** Atrial systole.
  - **c wave:** Closure of the tricuspid valve.
  - **x descent:** Atrial relaxation.
  - **v wave:** Ventricular systole (with passive venous filling of the atrium).
  - **y descent:** Opening of the tricuspid valve with rapid emptying of the right atrium.
- **Abnormal patterns of jugular venous pulsations** (see Figure 3-2):
  - **Cannon a waves:** Atrioventricular (AV) dissociation (the atrium contracts against a closed tricuspid valve).
  - **Large a wave:** Tricuspid stenosis, pulmonary hypertension, pulmonary stenosis.
  - **Absent a waves:** Atrial fibrillation (AF).
  - **Large cv wave:** Tricuspid regurgitation.
  - **Rapid y descent:** Constrictive pericarditis, restrictive cardiomyopathy.
  - **Blunted y descent:** Cardiac tamponade.

HEART MURMURS

Table 3-1 illustrates the differential diagnosis of valvular heart disease. Table 3-2 shows the effect of various interventions on systolic murmurs.

HEART SOUNDS

- S1:
  - Denotes closure of the mitral and tricuspid valves.
  - Diminished with severe left ventricular systolic dysfunction, mitral regurgitation, and long PR interval.
  - Accentuated with mitral stenosis, short PR interval, and atrial myxoma.
- S2:
  - Denotes closure of the aortic and pulmonic valves.
  - In normal hearts, the aortic component (A2) comes before the pulmonic component (P2).
  - A2 is diminished in severe aortic stenosis.
  - **Physiologic splitting:** The time between A2 and P2 widens during inspiration.

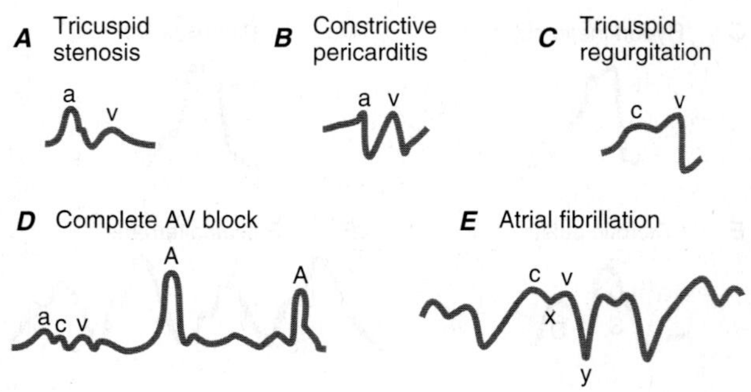

FIGURE 3-2. Abnormal jugular venous pulse waveforms.

(Adapted, with permission, from Fuster V et al [eds]. *Hurst's the Heart,* 10th ed. New York: McGraw-Hill, 2001.)

TABLE 3-1. Differential Diagnosis of Valvular Heart Disease

	Mitral Stenosis	Mitral Regurgitation	Aortic Stenosis	Aortic Regurgitation	Tricuspid Stenosis	Tricuspid Regurgitation
Inspection	Malar flush, precordial bulge, and diffuse pulsation in young patients.	Usually prominent and hyperdynamic apical impulse to the left of the midclavicular line (MCL).	Sustained point of maximal impulse (PMI); prominent atrial filling wave.	Hyperdynamic PMI to the left of the MCL and down. Visible carotid pulsations.	Giant a wave in jugular pulse with sinus rhythm. Often olive-colored skin (mixed jaundice and local cyanosis).	Large v wave in jugular pulse.
Palpation	"Tapping" sensation over the area of expected PMI. Mid-diastolic or presystolic thrill at the apex. Small pulse. Right ventricular pulsation in the left third to fifth intercostal space (ICS) parasternally when pulmonary hypertension is present.	Forceful, brisk PMI; systolic thrill over PMI. Pulse normal, small, or slightly collapsing.	Powerful, heaving PMI to the left and slightly below the MCL. Systolic thrill over the aortic area, sternal notch, or carotids. Small and slowly rising carotid pulse.	Apical impulse forceful and displaced significantly to the left and down. Prominent carotid pulses. Rapidly rising and collapsing pulses.	Mid-diastolic thrill between the lower left sternal border and PMI. Presystolic pulsation of the liver (sinus rhythm only).	Right ventricular pulsation. Occasionally systolic thrill at the lower left sternal edge. Systolic pulsation of the liver.
Heart sounds, rhythm, and blood pressure	Loud snapping M1. Opening snap following S2 along the left sternal border or at the apex. AF is common. Blood pressure is normal.	M1 is normal or buried in murmur. Prominent third heart sound. AF is common. Blood pressure is normal. Midsystolic clicks may be present.	A2 is normal, soft, or absent. Paradoxic splitting of S2 if A2 is audible. Prominent S4. Blood pressure is normal, or systolic pressure is normal with high diastolic.	S1 is normal or reduced; A2 is loud. Wide pulse pressure with diastolic pressure < 60 mmHg.	S1 is often loud.	AF is usually present.
Murmurs						
Location and transmission	Localized at or near the apex. Rarely, short diastolic (Graham Steell) murmur along the lower left sternal border in severe pulmonary hypertension.	Loudest over PMI; transmitted to the left axilla and left infrascapular area. With posterior papillary muscle dysfunction, may transmit to the base.	Right second ICS parasternally or at the apex, heard in the carotids and occasionally in the upper interscapular area.	Diastolic: louder along the left sternal border in the third to fourth ICS. Heard over the aortic area and apex. May be associated with a low-pitched mid-diastolic murmur at the apex (Austin Flint) in nonrheumatic disease.	Third to fifth ICS along the left sternal border out to the apex.	As for tricuspid stenosis.

TABLE 3-1. **Differential Diagnosis of Valvular Heart Disease (continued)**

	Mitral Stenosis	Mitral Regurgitation	Aortic Stenosis	Aortic Regurgitation	Tricuspid Stenosis	Tricuspid Regurgitation
Timing	Onset at the opening snap ("mid-diastolic") with presystolic accentuation if in sinus rhythm. Graham Steell begins with P2 (early diastole).	Pansystolic: begins with M1 and ends at or after A2. May be late systolic in papillary muscle dysfunction.	Midsystolic: begins after M1, ends before A2, and reaches maximum intensity in midsystole.	Begins immediately after the aortic second sound and ends before the first sound.	As for mitral stenosis.	As for mitral regurgitation.
Character	Low pitched, rumbling; presystolic murmur merges with loud M1 and ends at or after A2. May be late systolic in papillary muscle dysfunction.	Blowing, high pitched; occasionally harsh or musical.	Harsh, rough.	Blowing, often faint.	As for mitral regurgitation.	Blowing, coarse, or musical.
Optimum auscultatory conditions	After exercise, left lateral recumbency. Bell chest piece is lightly applied.	After exercise; diaphragm chest piece. In prolapse, findings are most prominent while standing.	Patient resting, leaning forward; breath held in full expiration.	Patient leaning forward; breath held in expiration.	Murmur is usually louder and at a peak during inspiration. Patient is recumbent.	Murmur usually becomes louder during inspiration.
X-ray	Straight left heart border. Large left atrium sharply indenting the esophagus. Elevation of the left main stem bronchus. Large right ventricle and pulmonary artery if pulmonary hypertension is present. Calcification is occasionally seen in the mitral valve.	Enlarged left ventricle and left atrium.	Concentric left ventricular hypertrophy (LVH). Prominent ascending aorta; small knob. Calcified valve is common.	Moderate to severe left ventricular enlargement. Prominent aortic knob.	Enlarged right atrium only.	Enlarged right atrium and ventricle.
Electrocardiography	Broad P waves in standard leads; broad negative phase of diphasic P in V_1. If pulmonary hypertension is present, tall peaked P waves, right axis deviation, or right ventricular hypertrophy (RVH) appears.	Left axis deviation or frank LVH. P waves are broad, tall, or notched in standard leads. Broad negative phase of diphasic P in V_1.	LVH.	LVH.	Tall, peaked P waves. Normal axis.	Right axis usual.

TABLE 3-1. Differential Diagnosis of Valvular Heart Disease (continued)

	Mitral Stenosis	Mitral Regurgitation	Aortic Stenosis	Aortic Regurgitation	Tricuspid Stenosis	Tricuspid Regurgitation
Echocardiography						
M mode	Thickened, immobile mitral valve with anterior and posterior leaflets moving together. Slow early diastolic filling slope, left atrial enlargement, and normal to small left ventricle.	Thickened mitral valve in rheumatic disease; mitral valve prolapse; flail leaflet or vegetations may be seen. Enlarged left ventricle with above-normal, normal, or decreased function.	Dense persistent echoes from the aortic valve with poor leaflet excursion; LVH with preserved contractile function.	Diastolic vibrations of the anterior leaflet of the mitral valve and septum; early closure of the mitral valve when severe; dilated left ventricle with normal or decreased contractility.	Tricuspid valve thickening; decreased early diastolic filling slope of the tricuspid valve. The mitral valve is usually abnormal as well.	Enlarged right ventricle; prolapsing valve; mitral valve is often abnormal.
Two-dimensional	Maximum diastolic orifice size reduced; subvalvular apparatus foreshortened; variable thickening of other valves.	Same as M mode but more reliable.	Above plus poststenotic dilation of the aorta, restricted opening of the aortic leaflets, and bicuspid aortic valve in about 30%.	Above plus may show vegetations in endocarditis, bicuspid valve, and root dilation.	Above plus enlargement of the right atrium.	Same as above.
Doppler	Prolonged pressure half-time across the mitral valve; indirect evidence of pulmonary hypertension.	Regurgitant flow mapped into the left atrium; indirect evidence of pulmonary hypertension.	Increased transvalvular flow velocity, yielding calculated gradient. Valve area estimate using continuity equation.	Demonstrates regurgitation and qualitatively estimates severity.	Prolonged pressure half-time across the tricuspid valve.	Regurgitant flow mapped into the right atrium and venae cavae; right ventricular systolic pressure estimated.

- **Normal splitting with loud P2:** Pulmonary hypertension.
- **Fixed splitting:** Atrial septal defect (ASD).
- **Wide splitting:** Right bundle branch block (RBBB).
- **Paradoxical splitting:** Increased splitting **with expiration.** Etiologies include aortic stenosis, left bundle branch block (LBBB), paced rhythm, and left ventricular systolic dysfunction.

- S3:
  - A low-pitched sound heard in diastole just after S2.
  - Occurs as a result of sudden limitation of blood flow during ventricular filling.
  - Can be a normal finding in healthy young adults.
  - Abnormal in older adults; suggests enlargement of the ventricle and is usually due to systolic dysfunction of the left ventricle and/or hemodynamically significant mitral regurgitation.

TABLE 3-2. The Effect of Various Interventions on Systolic Murmurs

Intervention	Hypertrophic Obstructive Cardiomyopathy	Aortic Stenosis	Mitral Regurgitation	Mitral Prolapse
Valsalva	↑	↓	↓ or ↔	↑ or ↓
Standing	↑	↑ or ↔	↓ or ↔	↑
Hand grip or squatting	↓	↓ or ↔	↑	↓
Supine position with legs elevated	↓	↑ or ↔	↔	↓
Exercise	↑	↓ or ↔	↓	↑
Amyl nitrite	↑↑	↑	↓	↑
Isoproterenol	↑↑	↑	↓	↑

↑, increased; ↑↑, markedly increased; ↓, decreased; ↔, unchanged.

Reproduced, with permission, from Tierney LM et al (eds). *Current Medical Diagnosis & Treatment 2005,* 44th ed. New York: McGraw-Hill, 2005:321. As modified from Paraskos JA, Combined valvular disease. In Dalen JE, Alpert JS (eds). *Valvular Heart Disease,* 2nd ed. Boston: Little, Brown, 1987.

CARDIOVASCULAR MEDICINE

- S4:
  - A low-pitched sound heard in diastole just before S1.
  - Coincides with atrial systole ("atrial kick").
  - Occurs as a result of a stiff left ventricle with increased ventricular filling during atrial systole.
  - A normal finding with advancing age due to loss of ventricular compliance.
  - Pathologic causes include long-standing hypertension, aortic stenosis, hypertrophic cardiomyopathy, and other causes of a stiff left ventricle.
  - **Absent in AF.**
- **Systolic clicks:**
  - **Aortic ejection click:** A high-frequency sound in early systole. Occurs in the setting of aortic stenosis, aortic regurgitation, and aortic root dilatation (e.g., aneurysm of the ascending aorta, long-standing systemic hypertension).
  - **Pulmonic ejection click:** A high-frequency sound in early systole. Decreases in intensity during inspiration; occurs in the setting of pulmonary stenosis and pulmonary hypertension.
  - **Midsystolic click:** A high-frequency sound that occurs in the middle of systole. Most often due to mitral valve prolapse; may not be associated with a systolic murmur.
- **Additional diastolic sounds:**
  - **Opening snap:** A high-frequency, early diastolic sound most frequently caused by mitral stenosis.
  - **Pericardial knock:** A low-frequency sound due to abrupt termination of ventricular filling in early diastole in the setting of constrictive pericarditis.
  - **Tumor plop:** Occasionally heard in patients with atrial myxoma.

Noninvasive Cardiac Testing

EXERCISE TREADMILL TEST (ETT)

- A screening test for patients with symptoms suggestive of CAD **who have a normal resting ECG** and the ability to undergo vigorous exercise testing.
- Exercise increases myocardial O_2 demand and unmasks reduced coronary flow reserve in patients with hemodynamically significant coronary stenoses.
- ST-segment depression (especially if horizontal or down-sloping) has very high sensitivity and specificity for CAD if peak heart rate is at least **85%** of the maximum predicted rate (220 – age).
- **False positives:** More common in women and in those with atypical chest pain, no chest pain, and anemia.
- **False negatives:** More common in patients with preexisting CAD.
- An abnormal resting ECG (e.g., digoxin or LVH) may also reduce the sensitivity and specificity of results.

ECHOCARDIOGRAPHY

- A noninvasive ultrasound imaging modality used to identify anatomic abnormalities of the heart and great vessels, to assess the size and function of cardiac chambers, and to evaluate valvular function.
- **Resting** regional left ventricular wall motion abnormalities (hypokinesis, akinesis) are highly suggestive of ischemic heart disease. The **distribution** of wall motion abnormalities suggests the culprit coronary artery.
- **Stress echocardiography:** Used to determine regional wall motion abnormalities in patients with a normal resting echocardiogram and signs or symptoms of ischemic heart disease. Stress with exercise or dobutamine.
- **Doppler:** Used to investigate blood flow in the heart and great vessels. Very useful for detecting stenotic or regurgitant blood flow across the valves as well as any abnormal communications within the heart. Doppler velocities across a valve can be converted to pressure gradients. Cardiac output and pressure gradient data can be used to calculate stenotic valve areas.
- **Bubble study:** Injection of agitated normal saline to diagnose right-to-left shunts. Consider patent foramen ovale if bubbles flow directly from the right to the left atrium; consider intrapulmonary shunt with delayed appearance of bubbles in the left atrium.
- **Transesophageal echocardiography (TEE):** A small ultrasound probe placed into the esophagus allows for higher-resolution images of **posterior** cardiac structures. Common indications include the detection of left atrial thrombi, valvular vegetations, and thoracic aortic dissection.

MYOCARDIAL PERFUSION IMAGING

- A nuclear medicine study that looks for the presence and distribution of areas of myocardial ischemia based on differences in myocardial perfusion.
- Exercise or pharmacologic stress (dipyridamole or adenosine) is used to induce coronary vasodilation, which increases flow to the myocardium perfused by healthy coronary arteries but fails to increase flow in the distribution of a hemodynamically significant stenosis.
- Perfusion images show defects in areas where blood flow is relatively reduced. If a perfusion defect on the initial (stress) imaging improves on repeat (rest) imaging after 3–24 hours, the area is presumably still viable (i.e., it is a reversible defect).

- A fixed defect suggests myocardial scar tissue. Redistribution images can be performed after 24 hours to look for additional areas of viable myocardium.

Electrocardiography (ECG)

- **Dimensions (one small box):** Height: 0.1 mV = 1 mm; duration: 40 msec = 1 mm.
- **Rate:** Normal rate is 60–100 bpm.
- **QRS axis:** Normal axis is –30° to +90°. An axis < –30° is left axis deviation; an axis > +90° is right axis deviation. Use QRS in leads I and II to determine axis. Upright in I and II = normal axis; upright in I and downward in II = left axis deviation; downward in I and upright in II = right axis deviation; downward in I and II = extreme axis deviation.
- **The differential diagnosis of axis deviations (in order of likelihood)** is outlined in Table 3-3.
- Intervals:
  - **PR:** Normal 120–200 msec (3–5 small boxes).
  - **QRS:** Abnormal > 120 msec (> 3 small boxes).
  - **QT:** Normal < ½ RR interval (rule of thumb).
  - **QTc:** Abnormal > 440 msec.
- **Right atrial abnormality (only one criterion needed):**
  - **Lead II:** P > 2.5 mm (P-wave height > 2.5 small boxes).
  - **Lead V_1:** P > 1.5 mm (P-wave height > 1.5 small boxes).
- **Left atrial abnormality (only one criterion needed):**
  - **Lead II:** P > 120 msec with notches separated by at least one small box.
  - **Lead V_1:** P wave has a negative terminal deflection that is ≥ 40 msec by 1 mm (one small box by one small box).
- **LVH:** There are numerous criteria, three of which are listed below. All are specific but insensitive, so fulfillment of one criterion is sufficient for LVH in patients > 35 years of age. Specificity decreases significantly in younger patients (those < 35 years of age).
  - RaVL > 9 mm (women), > 11 mm (men).
  - RaVL + SV_3 > 20 mm (women), > 25 mm (men).
  - SV_1 + (RV_5 or RV_6) > 35 mm.
- **RVH:** The following findings suggest RVH (there are several others):
  - Right axis deviation.
  - $RV_1 + SV_6$ > 11 mm (or simply look for deep S wave in V_6).
  - R:S ratio > 1 in V_1 (in the absence of RBBB or posterior MI).
- **RBBB** (see Figure 3-3):
  - QRS > 120 msec.
  - Wide S wave in I, V_5, and V_6.

TABLE 3-3. Differential Diagnosis of Axis Deviations

Right Axis	Left Axis
RVH	Left anterior fascicular block
Lateral or anterolateral MI	Inferior MI
Wolfe-Parkinson-White (WPW) syndrome with left-lateral free wall pathway	WPW with posteroseptal pathway
	COPD
Left posterior fascicular block	

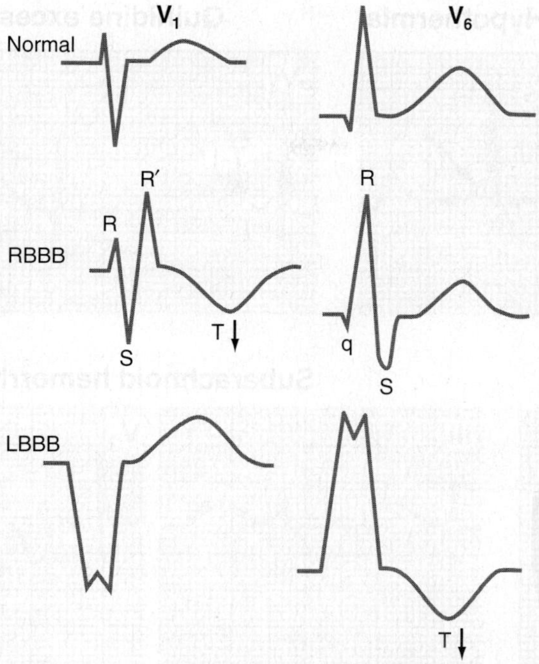

FIGURE 3-3. Bundle branch blocks.

(Reproduced, with permission, from Kasper DL et al [eds]. *Harrison's Principles of Internal Medicine,* 16th ed. New York: McGraw-Hill, 2005:1315.)

- Secondary R wave (R′) in right precordial leads, with R′ greater than initial R (look for "rabbit ears" in V_1 and V_2).
- **LBBB** (see Figure 3-3):
  - QRS > 120 msec, broad R wave in I and V_6, broad S wave in V_1, and normal axis **or**
  - QRS > 120 msec, broad R wave in I, broad S wave in V_1, RS in V_6, and left axis deviation.
- **Left anterior fascicular block:** There are several sets of criteria for left anterior fascicular block:
  - The axis is more negative than –45°.
  - Q in aVL, and time from onset of QRS to peak of R wave is > 0.05 sec.
  - Also look for Q in lead I and S in lead III.
- **Left posterior fascicular block: Must exclude anterolateral MI, RVH, and RBBB:** Axis > 100° and Q in lead III; S in lead I pattern.
- Figure 3-4 illustrates the appearance on ECG of a range of medical conditions and drug effects. Table 3-4 outlines wide-complex tachycardia.

Cardiac Catheterization and Coronary Angiography

Cardiac Catheterization Indications

Indications include heart failure, pulmonary hypertension, suspected valvular disease, and congenital heart disease; also performed to assess the severity of disease and guide further therapy. Table 3-5 lists contraindications to cardiac catheterization; Table 3-6 outlines patient characteristics associated with increased mortality from the procedure.

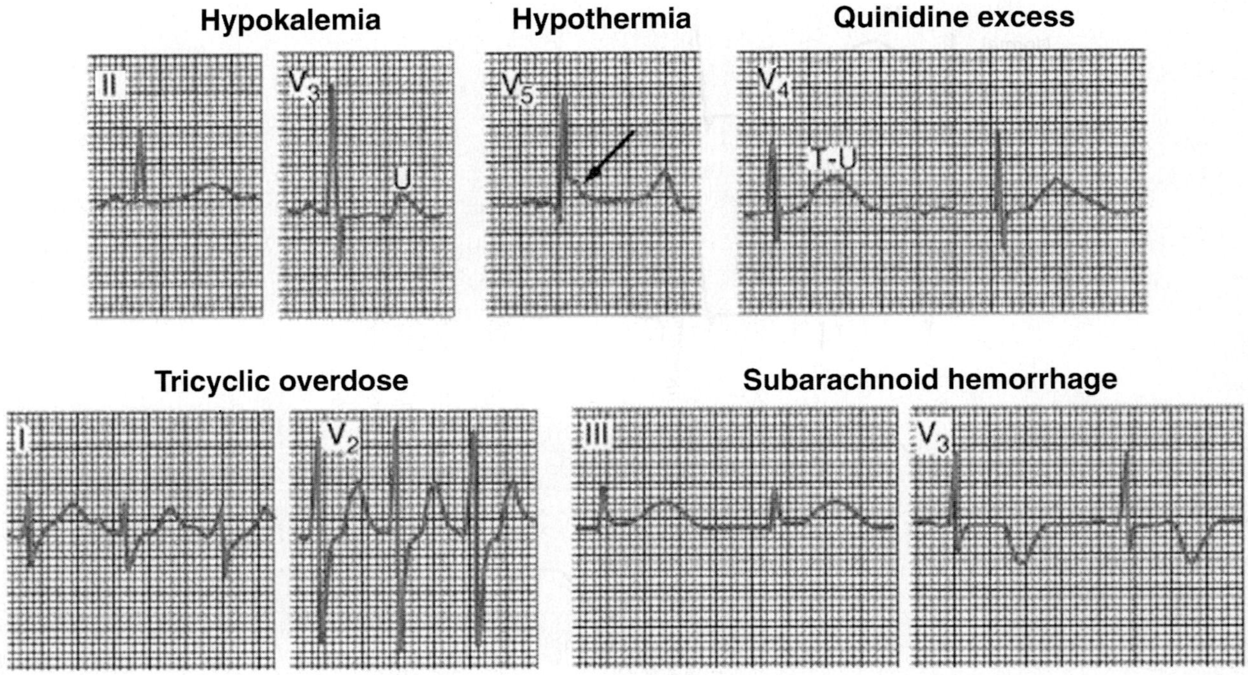

FIGURE 3-4. Electrocardiographic manifestations of various of medical conditions and drug effects.

(Reproduced, with permission, from Braunwald E [ed]. *Harrison's Principles of Internal Medicine,* 15th ed. New York: McGraw-Hill, 2001.)

CORONARY ANGIOGRAPHY INDICATIONS

- **Elective (diagnostic):** For patients with known or suspected CAD who are candidates for coronary revascularization.
- **Primary:** Initial reperfusion therapy for acute ST-segment-elevation MI (STEMI).
- **Rescue:** After failed thrombolysis (if there is ongoing chest pain and/or a < 50% decrease in ST-segment elevation 60–90 minutes after thrombolysis).

CORONARY STENTS

- Currently the standard of care for the treatment of CAD.
- Patients treated with coronary stents must be treated with aspirin and **clopidogrel** for at least four weeks for bare-metal stents and for at least 3–6 months for drug-eluting stents. If there are no contraindications, continuing clopidogrel for one year following stenting reduces the risk of death and MI.
- Preprocedural loading with clopidogrel should be avoided if there is a chance that the patient will undergo coronary artery bypass grafting (CABG) in the next 5–7 days (associated with increased bleeding complications).
- Drug-eluting stents decrease the incidence of restenosis with the use of antiproliferative agents (e.g., sirolimus and paclitaxel) but require more prolonged treatment with clopidogrel.

TABLE 3-4. Wide-Complex Tachycardia

ECG criteria that favor ventricular tachycardia:

1. AV dissociation
2. QRS width: > 0.14 sec with RBBB configuration
   > 0.16 sec with LBBB configuration
3. QRS axis: Left axis deviation with RBBB morphology
   Extreme left axis deviation (northwest axis) with LBBB morphology
4. Concordance of QRS in precordial leads
5. Morphologic patterns of the QRS complex
   RBBB: Mono- or biphasic complex in V_1
   RS (*only with left axis deviation*) or QS in V_6

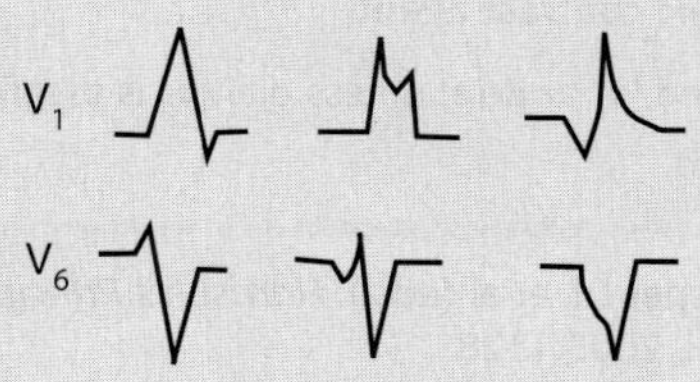

LBBB: Broad R wave in V_1 or $V_2 \geq 0.04$ sec
Onset of QRS to nadir of S wave in V_1 or V_2 of ≥ 0.07 sec
Notched downslope of S wave in V_1 and V_2
Q wave in V_6

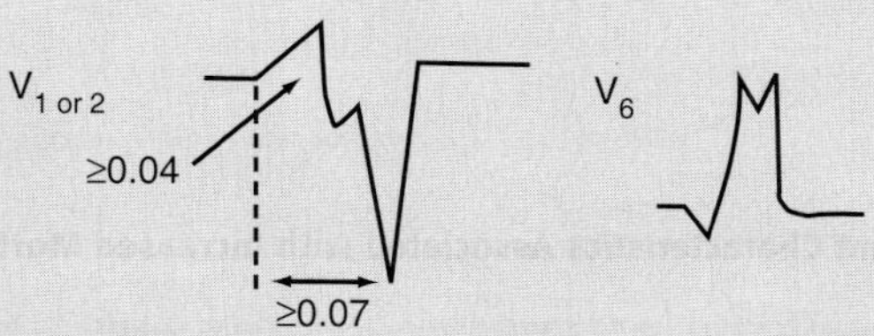

Reproduced, with permission, from Kasper DL et al (eds). *Harrison's Principles of Internal Medicine,* 16th ed. New York: McGraw-Hill, 2005:1352.

Coronary Arterial Complications During Percutaneous Coronary Intervention (PCI)

- Distal microembolization of the coronary artery (5%).
- Vessel perforation or dissection (1%).
- **Abrupt closure (< 1% with stenting):** Of all cases, 75% occur within minutes of angioplasty and 25% within 24 hours. Usually due to dissection or thrombosis. One-third have major ischemic complications requiring emergent revascularization.
- **Subacute thrombotic occlusion of coronary stent (1–4%) within 2–14 days:** Often results in MI or death.
- **Gradual restenosis:** Defined as ≥ 50% narrowing of the luminal diameter within 1–6 months. There is a decreased risk of in-stent restenosis with drug-eluting stents.

Other Complications

- Retroperitoneal bleeding.
- Femoral artery hematoma, pseudoaneurysm, or fistula formation.

TABLE 3-5. Relative Contraindications to Cardiac Catheterization and Angiography

- **Uncontrolled ventricular irritability:** Increased risk of ventricular tachycardia and fibrillation during catheterization if ventricular irritability is uncontrolled.
- **Uncorrected hypokalemia or digitalis toxicity.**
- **Uncorrected hypertension:** Predisposes to myocardial ischemia and/or heart failure during angiography.
- **Intercurrent febrile illness.**
- **Decompensated heart failure:** Especially acute pulmonary edema, unless catheterization can be done with patient sitting up.
- **Anticoagulated state:** Prothrombin time > 18 sec.
- **Severe allergy to radiographic contrast agent.**
- **Severe renal insufficiency and/or anuria:** unless dialysis is planned to remove fluid and radiographic contrast load.

Reprinted, with permission, from Kasper DL et al (eds.). *Harrison's Principles of Internal Medicine,* 16th ed. New York: McGraw-Hill, 2005:1328.

TABLE 3-6. Patient Characteristics Associated with Increased Mortality from Cardiac Catheterization

Age: Infants (< 1 month old) and the elderly (> 85 years old) are at increased risk of death during cardiac catheterization. Elderly women appear to be at higher risk than elderly men.
Functional class: Mortality in class IV patients is > 10 times greater than that of class I–II patients.
Severity of coronary obstruction: Mortality for patients with left main coronary artery disease is > 10 times greater than that of patients with one- or two-vessel disease.
Valvular heart disease: Especially when severe and combined with coronary disease, associated with a higher risk of death at cardiac catheterization than CAD alone.
Left ventricular dysfunction: Mortality in patients with a left ventricular ejection fraction < 30% > than 10 times greater than that of patients with an ejection fraction of 50%.
Severe noncardiac disease: Patients with renal insufficiency, insulin-requiring diabetes, advanced cerebrovascular and/or peripheral vascular disease, or severe pulmonary insufficiency have an increased incidence of death and other major complications from cardiac catheterization.

Reproduced, with permission, from Kasper DL et al (eds). *Harrison's Principles of Internal Medicine,* 16th ed. New York: McGraw-Hill, 2005:1328.

- **Contrast nephropathy:** Usually occurs 24–48 hours after contrast load. Diabetes and preexisting renal insufficiency are the most important risk factors. Prevent with pre- and postprocedural hydration. Acetylcysteine, decreased volume of contrast, and low osmolar contrast are other preventive measures.
- **Atheroembolic kidney disease:** Look for eosinophilia, eosinophiluria, hypocomplementemia, and distal embolic complications ("blue toes").
- **Anaphylaxis or allergic reaction to contrast media:** In the presence of known contrast allergy, premedicate with diphenhydramine and steroids.
- **Hyperthyroidism in patients with known (or unknown) Graves' disease or toxic thyroid nodule:** Can present weeks to months after iodinated contrast load.

CARDIAC HEMODYNAMICS

Table 3-7 lists the normal values for cardiac hemodynamic parameters.

CORONARY ARTERY DISEASE (CAD)

Acute Coronary Syndromes

Acute coronary syndromes encompass STEMI, non-ST-segment-elevation MI (NSTEMI), and unstable angina. Etiologies include unstable plaques with nonocclusive thrombosis (unstable angina and NSTEMI) and thrombotic occlusion of an epicardial coronary artery (STEMI).

SYMPTOMS

Ischemic chest pain is often described as dull or squeezing substernal or left-sided discomfort associated with dyspnea and diaphoresis, with radiation down the left arm or into the neck.

EXAM

Acute ischemia may be associated with an S4. Ischemic systolic dysfunction can cause pulmonary edema and an S3. Elevation of jugular venous pulsation is uncommon in the absence of right ventricular involvement.

DIFFERENTIAL

Aortic dissection, pulmonary embolism, acute pericarditis, tension pneumothorax.

DIAGNOSIS

- Based primarily on **risk factors** and **initial ECG during chest pain.**
- In patients with chest pain, the initial goal is to rule out STEMI that requires immediate reperfusion therapy.
- In patients without ST-segment elevation, cardiac enzymes will determine if patients have NSTEMI or unstable angina.

TREATMENT

- **Immediate reperfusion** is the goal for STEMI.
  - Primary PCI is generally preferred if available.
  - Pharmacologic thrombolysis is also considered first-line therapy if ad-

TABLE 3-7. Normal Values for Cardiac Hemodynamic Parameters

Parameter	Values
Pressures (mmHg)	
Systemic arterial	
Peak systolic/end-diastolic	100–140/60–90
Mean	70–105
Left ventricle	
Peak systolic/end-diastolic	100–140/3–12
Left atrium (or pulmonary capillary wedge)	
Mean	2–10
a wave	3–15
v wave	3–15
Pulmonary artery	
Peak systolic/end-diastolic	15–30/4–12
Mean	9–18
Right ventricle	
Peak systolic/end-diastolic	15–30/2–8
Right atrium	
Mean	2–8
a wave	2–10
v wave	2–10
Resistances [(dyn·s)/cm^5]	
Systemic vascular resistance	700–1600
Pulmonary vascular resistance	20–130
Cardiac index [(L/min)/m^2]	2.6–4.2
O_2 consumption index [(L/min)/m^2]	110–150
Arteriovenous oxygen difference (mL/L)	30–50

Reprinted, with permission, from Kasper DL et al (eds). *Harrison's Principles of Internal Medicine*, 16th ed. New York: McGraw-Hill, 2005:1329.

ministered **within 12 hours** of chest pain onset (especially at medical centers that do not have access to 24-hour PCI).

- **Medical therapy for NSTEMI and unstable angina:** Aspirin, β-blockers, ACEIs, and low-molecular-weight or unfractionated heparin. The addition of clopidogrel and glycoprotein IIB/IIIA inhibitors should be considered for high-risk patients.
- Increasing evidence supports an early aggressive strategy (cardiac catheterization within 48 hours) for moderate- to high-risk patients who present with acute coronary syndromes. Patients with recurrent angina, elevated cardiac biomarkers, or ST-segment depression should be considered for early coronary angiography.

COMPLICATIONS

- **Delayed therapy:** Ischemic arrhythmias (VT/VF); extension of infarction resulting in chronic heart failure.
- **Complications of thrombolysis and aggressive anticoagulation/antiplatelet regimens:** Hemorrhagic stroke, GI bleeding, spontaneous retroperitoneal bleeding.
- **Hemodynamic complications of acute MI:** See Table 3-8.

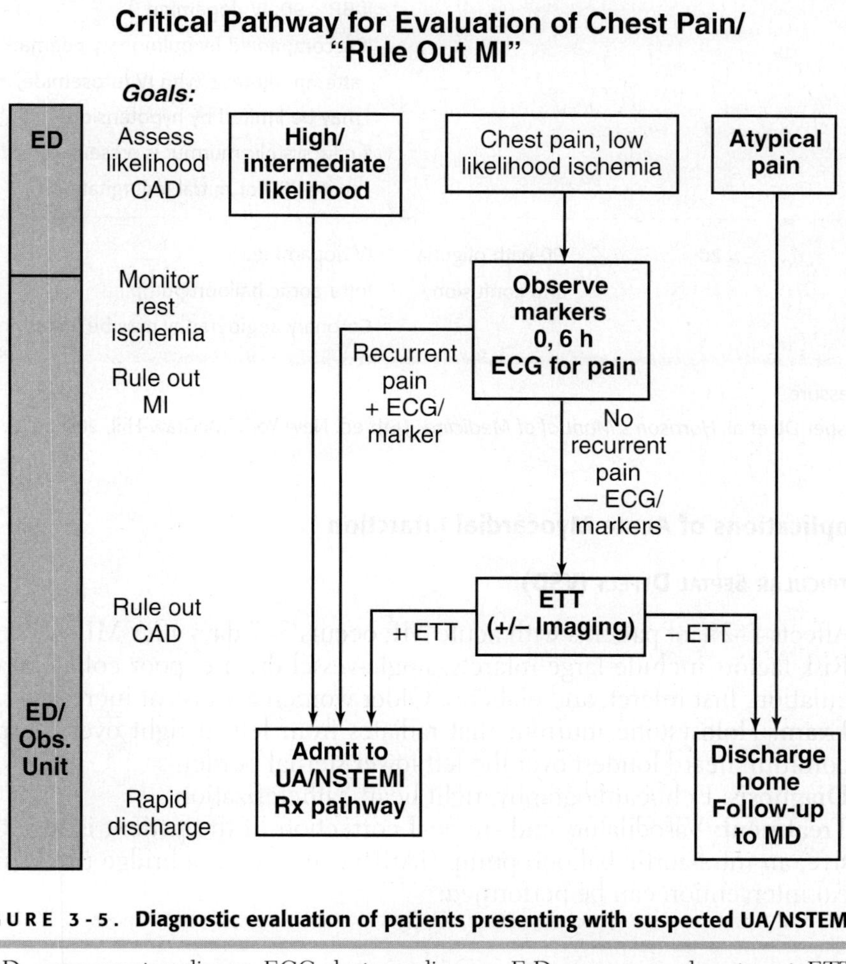

FIGURE 3-5. Diagnostic evaluation of patients presenting with suspected UA/NSTEMI.

(CAD, coronary artery disease; ECG,electrocardiogram; E.D., emergency department; ETT, exercise tolerance test; MI, myocardial infarction; OBS, observation unit.) (Reproduced, with permission from Kasper DL [ed]. *Harrison's Principles of Internal Medicine,* 16th ed. New York: McGraw-Hill, 2005).

TABLE 3-8. Hemodynamic Complications of Acute MI

Condition	Cardiac Index, ([L/min]/m²)	PCW[a] (mmHg)	Symbolic BP (mmHg)	Treatment
Uncomplicated	> 2.5	≤ 18	> 100	—
Hypovolemia	< 2.5	< 15	< 100	Successive boluses of normal saline. In setting of inferior wall MI, consider right ventricular infarction (especially if right atrial pressure > 10)
Volume overload	> 2.5	> 20	> 100	Diuretic (e.g., furosemide 10–20 mg IV). Nitroglycerin, topical paste or IV.
Left ventricular failure	< 2.5	> 20	> 100	Diuretic (e.g., furosemide 10–20 mg IV). IV nitroglycerin (or if hypertensive, use IV nitroprusside).
Severe left venticular failure	< 2.5	> 20	< 100	If BP ≥ 90: IV dobutamine +/– IV nitroglycerin or sodium nitroprusside. If BP < 90: IV dopamine. If accompanied by pulmonary edema: attempt diuresis with IV furosemide; may be limited by hypotension. If new systolic murmur is present, consider acute VSD or mitral regurgitation.
Cardiogenic shock	< 1.8	> 20	< 90 with oliguria and confusion	IV dopamine. Intra-aortic balloon pump. Coronary angiography may be life-saving.

[a]PCW = pulmonary capillary wedge pressure.

Reproduced, with permission, from Kasper DL et al. *Harrison's Manual of Medicine,* 16th ed. New York: McGraw-Hill, 2005:628.

Complications of Acute Myocardial Infarction

Ventricular Septal Defect (VSD)

- Affects 1–2% of patients with acute MI; occurs 3–7 days after MI.
- Risk factors include large infarcts, single-vessel disease, poor collateral circulation, first infarct, and diabetes. Older women are also at increased risk.
- **Exam:** Holosystolic murmur that radiates from left to right over the precordium, heard loudest over the left lower sternal border.
- **Diagnosis:** Echocardiography, right heart catheterization.
- **Treatment:** Vasodilators and surgical correction. If the patient is hypotensive, an intra-aortic balloon pump (IABP) can serve as a bridge until surgical intervention can be performed.

Papillary Muscle Rupture

- Affects 1% of patients with acute MI; occurs 2–7 days after MI.
- Risk factors include inferior MI and VSD.

- **Exam:** New systolic murmur, loudest at the apex, that radiates to the axilla. The intensity of the murmur does not correlate with the severity of mitral regurgitation.
- **Diagnosis:** Echocardiography; right heart catheterization.
- **Treatment:** Vasodilators and surgical correction. If the patient is hypotensive, an IABP can serve as a bridge until surgical intervention can be performed.

LEFT VENTRICULAR FREE WALL RUPTURE

- Affects < 1% of patients with acute MI; accounts for up to 15% of early MI deaths. Occurs 5–14 days after MI or earlier in patients who receive thrombolysis.
- Risk factors include transmural MI, first MI, single-vessel disease, lack of collaterals, and female gender.
- **Exam:** Acute decompensation related to cardiac tamponade (elevated JVP, pulsus paradoxus, diminished heart sounds).
- **Diagnosis:** Echocardiography, right heart catheterization.
- **Treatment:** Urgent pericardiocentesis and thoracotomy. **Cardiac rupture is a true cardiothoracic surgical emergency.**

CARDIOGENIC SHOCK

- Risk factors include anterior MI, diabetes, and older age.
- **Exam:** Look for signs of heart failure with associated hypotension. Decreased urine output is common.
- **Diagnosis:** CXR, echocardiography, right heart catheterization.
- **Treatment:** Revascularization, IABP, ventilatory support, dopamine/dobutamine.

LEFT VENTRICULAR ANEURYSM

- Affects 10–30% of patients after acute MI; incidence is decreasing in the era of PCI. Can occur acutely, but most are chronic and persist for > 6 weeks after MI.
- Anterior MI is a risk factor.
- **Exam:** Large, diffuse PMI; S3 may be present.
- **Diagnosis:** ECG (Q waves in V_{1-3} with persistent ST-segment elevation), echocardiography, cardiac MRI.
- **Treatment:**
  - **Acute:** Treat associated cardiogenic shock.
  - **Chronic:** Anticoagulate with heparin/warfarin if mural thrombus is present; consider a defibrillator if the left ventricular ejection fraction < 35% or there are documented ventricular arrhythmias.
- **Prevention:** Early revascularization.

EARLY PERICARDITIS

- Affects 10% of patients with acute MI; occurs 1–4 days after MI.
- Transmural MI is a risk factor.
- **Symptoms:** Pain worsens when patients are supine and radiates to the trapezius ridge.
- **Exam:** Pericardial friction rub.
- **Diagnosis:** ECG may show evidence of pericarditis; echocardiography may reveal pericardial effusion.

- **Treatment:** Aspirin. Avoid NSAIDs and corticosteroids (may interfere with healing of infarcted myocardium). Avoid heparin to reduce the risk of pericardial hemorrhagic transformation.

LATE PERICARDITIS (DRESSLER'S SYNDROME)

- Affects 1–3% of patients with acute MI; thought to be secondary to immune-mediated injury. Occurs 1–8 weeks after MI.
- **Exam:** Pericardial rub, fever.
- **Diagnosis:** ECG may show evidence of pericarditis; echocardiography may show pericardial effusion.
- **Treatment:** Aspirin. If > 4 weeks after MI, NSAIDs and/or corticosteroids can be used.

ARRHYTHMIAS

- Can occur at any time post-MI. Reperfusion arrhythmias within 24–48 hours of MI generally do not mandate aggressive therapy.
- **Diagnosis**: ECG, telemetry. **Routine electrophysiologic or signal-average ECG testing is not recommended.**
- **Treatment:** If ventricular arrhythmias persist > 48 hours post-MI and are symptomatic or hemodynamically significant, implantation of a defibrillator is more effective than antiarrhythmics.

ISCHEMIC COMPLICATIONS

- Infarct extension, postinfarction angina, or reinfarction.
- **Diagnosis and treatment:** Cardiac catheterization with PCI when indicated.

EMBOLIC COMPLICATIONS

- Nonhemorrhagic stroke occurs in approximately 1% of patients post-MI. Occurs within 10 days after MI.
- Risk factors include anterior MI, large MI, and left ventricular aneurysm.
- **Exam:** Depends on the site of embolization. Look for signs of stroke or signs of limb or intestinal ischemia.
- **Treatment:** Anticoagulation with heparin/warfarin.

Cardiogenic Shock

Occurs in approximately 5–7% of patients with acute MI and is the **leading cause of death related to acute MI.** See Figure 3-6 for the approach to hypotensive patients with acute MI. Etiologies are as follows:

- **Left ventricular systolic dysfunction:**
  - The most common cause of cardiogenic shock (75% of patients).
  - STEMI causes cardiogenic shock more frequently than does NSTEMI.
- Acute, severe valvular insufficiency (most often due to acute mitral regurgitation).
- Isolated right ventricular MI.
- Cardiac tamponade.

- Left ventricular free wall rupture.
- Ventricular septal rupture.
- Left ventricular outflow tract obstruction (aortic stenosis, hypertrophic cardiomyopathy).
- Obstruction to left ventricular filling (mitral stenosis, left atrial myxoma).

SYMPTOMS/EXAM

- Hypotension (systolic BP < 90 mmHg) or relative hypotension (decrease in systolic BP > 30 mmHg in a chronically hypertensive patient). Note that some patients with severe end-stage heart failure will have chronically low BP (look for evidence of hypoperfusion in these patients).
- Tachycardia.
- Hypoperfusion (cyanosis, poor peripheral pulses) despite adequate filling pressures.
- Dyspnea.
- Altered mental status (acute delirium).
- Decreased urine output.

TREATMENT

- If the underlying etiology is ischemic, proceed immediately to revascularization (PCI or CABG).

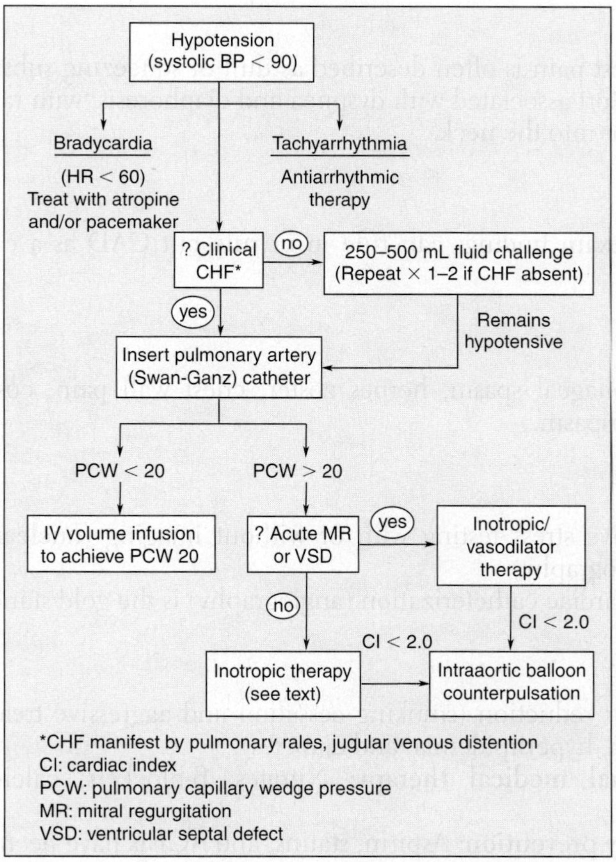

FIGURE 3-6. Approach to hypotensive patients with acute MI.

(Reproduced, with permission, from Braunwald E [ed]. *Harrison's Principles of Internal Medicine*, 15th ed. New York: McGraw-Hill, 2001.)

- Urgent revascularization is superior to medical management (thrombolysis) alone.
- **Supportive care:** Vasopressors, mechanical ventilation, IABP counterpulsation.
  - Vasopressor therapy usually consists of dopamine and dobutamine. Norepinephrine can also be used in cases of refractory hypotension.
  - Placement of an IABP decreases afterload and improves coronary perfusion in diastole. It is contraindicated in patients with severe peripheral vascular disease and hemodynamically significant aortic insufficiency.
  - For ischemia-induced cardiogenic shock, nitrates and nitroprusside can be used, but only with extreme caution. IABP is a more effective therapy for coronary ischemia in these patients.
- Ventricular assist devices can serve as a bridge to cardiac transplantation.

Chronic Stable Angina

The hallmark is chronic, reproducible, exercise-induced chest discomfort that is relieved by rest and nitroglycerin. Unlike unstable angina and MI, stable angina is thought to involve a **fixed** coronary stenosis that limits myocardial O_2 delivery. Angina results when demand outstrips supply. The most important CAD risk factors are diabetes, smoking, hyperlipidemia, hypertension, age, and a family history of premature CAD.

Symptoms

Ischemic chest pain is often described as dull or squeezing substernal or left-sided discomfort associated with dyspnea and diaphoresis, with radiation down the left arm or into the neck.

Exam

No specific exam findings can rule in or rule out CAD as a cause of chest pain.

Differential

GERD, esophageal spasm, herpes zoster, chest wall pain, costochondritis, coronary vasospasm.

Diagnosis

Flow-limiting stenoses that are responsible for stable angina are less likely to rupture and cause acute coronary syndromes than nonocclusive unstable plaques.

- Noninvasive stress testing with or without imaging (nuclear imaging or echocardiography).
- Invasive cardiac catheterization (angiography) is the gold standard.

Treatment

- Risk factor reduction (smoking cessation and aggressive treatment of hypertension, hyperlipidemia, and diabetes).
- **Antianginal medical therapy:** Nitrates, β-blockers, calcium channel blockers.
- **Secondary prevention:** Aspirin, statins, and ACEIs have been shown to reduce cardiovascular events in patient with chronic CAD.
- **Revascularization:** PCI or CABG.

- **Enhanced external counterpulsation (EECP):** Used in patients with angina that is refractory to medical therapy in whom revascularization is not possible.

COMPLICATIONS

Reduction in quality of life; limitation of activities of daily living.

Diagnostic Strategies and Risk Stratification for Chest Pain

EVALUATION OF PATIENTS WITH CHEST PAIN

- The most important single test in the initial evaluation of patients with chest pain is the **ECG** (should be obtained and interpreted within the first five minutes of presentation).
- The history, physical exam, and initial laboratory and radiographic assessment should focus on **excluding life-threatening causes of chest pain** (acute ischemic heart disease, aortic dissection, acute pericarditis, pulmonary embolism, tension pneumothorax, esophageal rupture).
- Troponins and CK-MB biomarkers typically become elevated **6–8 hours** after the onset of chest pain. Troponins remain elevated for several days; therefore, in patients with a recent MI, checking CK-MB can be useful to look for recurrent MI.

ACUTE TREATMENT

- All patients with chest pain should receive O_2, and an IV should be placed.
- Unless contraindicated, all patients with chest pain presumed to be ischemic in etiology should receive aspirin, β-blockers, nitrates, and heparin during the initial evaluation.

RISK STRATIFICATION

- All patients who present with chest pain should be risk stratified by the presence or absence of coronary risk factors (e.g., older age, hypertension, DM, hyperlipidemia, smoking, family history of premature CAD, chronic renal insufficiency).
- As the number of risk factors increases, the likelihood that the patient's chest pain is ischemic in origin also increases (even if the chest pain is atypical).
- Guidelines for stress testing are as follows:
  - High-risk patients with chest pain (e.g., ST-segment elevation on ECG or the presence of heart failure in the setting of ischemia or positive biomarkers) should proceed directly to cardiac catheterization.
  - Lower-risk patients with a high likelihood of ischemia (as determined primarily by the presence of coronary risk factors, a history of CAD, ECG findings, or a positive troponin result) should undergo future cardiac stress testing (ideally prior to discharge from the hospital).
- Patients with an elevated troponin and ≥ 2 high-risk prognostic variables (age ≥ 65 years, ≥ 3 traditional CAD risk factors, documented CAD with ≥ 50% stenosis, ST-segment deviation, ≥ 2 anginal episodes within the last 24 hours, positive biomarkers, or aspirin use within the last week) should undergo cardiac catheterization within 24 hours.

Management of Coronary Artery Disease

Risk Factor Reduction

- **Modifiable risk factors** such as DM, hypertension, hyperlipidemia, and smoking should be aggressively treated.
- Other risk factors (e.g., chronic renal insufficiency, cocaine use) should also be addressed.

Pharmacologic Therapy

- **Aspirin:** Decreases mortality. Give 81 mg daily. If aspirin is absolutely contraindicated, clopidogrel can be used effectively.
- **Clopidogrel:** Decreases mortality in patients who have had recent acute coronary syndromes or who have had a coronary stent placed.
- **Statins:** Decrease mortality and the risk of acute cardiac events. Recent guidelines state that LDL should be < 100 mg/dL in patients with a history of CAD. However, recent trials indicate that patients may have better outcomes with even lower LDL levels (the newest guidelines indicate that LDL should be < 70 mg/dL in patients with a history of CAD).
- **β-blockers:** Decrease mortality. **All patients with CAD** should be on β-blockers unless absolutely contraindicated. In patients with reactive airway disease, cardioselective β-blockers should be tried and discontinued only if bronchospasm occurs. **DM is not a contraindication to β-blocker use.**
- **ACEIs:** Decrease mortality and the risk of MI and stroke. If not tolerated, an angiotensin receptor blocker should be prescribed.

Indications for Elective Revascularization

- Chronic stable angina with three-vessel disease.
- Two-vessel disease with proximal left anterior descending artery involvement.
- One- or two-vessel disease with high-risk features on noninvasive testing.
- Significant left main CAD (> 50% stenosis).
- Refractory symptoms of chronic angina.

CONGESTIVE HEART FAILURE (CHF)

Table 3-9 outlines the stages of CHF.

Systolic vs. Diastolic Dysfunction

Most patients with heart failure have a combination of systolic and diastolic dysfunction of the left ventricle.

Heart Failure with Reduced Systolic Function

- **Clinical definition:** Evidence of decreased ejection fraction (by physical exam or echocardiogram) in the setting of symptoms and signs of heart failure.
- **Epidemiology:** Affects all ages; more common in males. CAD is present in approximately 70% of patients with reduced systolic dysfunction.
- **Exam:** S3 present.

Table 3-9. Stages of Heart Failure[a]

Stage A: Patients at risk of developing heart failure because of comorbid conditions that are strongly associated with the development of heart failure. Such patients have no signs or symptoms of heart failure and have never manifested signs or symptoms of heart failure. There are no structural or functional abnormalities of the valves or ventricles. Examples include systemic hypertension, CAD, and DM.
Stage B: Patients who have developed structural heart disease that is strongly associated with the development of heart failure but have no symptoms of heart failure and have never manifested signs or symptoms of heart failure. Examples include LVH; enlarged, dilated ventricles; asymptomatic valvular heart disease; and previous MI.
Stage C: Patients who have current or prior symptoms of heart failure associated with underlying structural heart disease. This represents the largest group of patients with clinical evidence of heart failure.
Stage D: Patients with marked symptoms of heart failure at rest despite maximal medical therapy and who require specialized interventions. Examples include patients who cannot be safely discharged from the hospital, are repeatedly hospitalized, are in the hospital awaiting heart transplantation, are residing in a hospice setting, are living at home and receiving continuous IV support for symptom relief, or are being supported with a mechanical circulatory assist device.

[a]Derived from the 2001 American College of Cardiology/American Heart Association guidelines. Adapted, with permission, from Fuster V (ed). *Hurst's the Heart,* 11th ed. New York: McGraw-Hill, 2004.

- **Diagnosis:** Echocardiogram shows decreased ejection fraction (≤ 40%) with an enlarged, dilated left ventricle.

HEART FAILURE WITH PRESERVED SYSTOLIC FUNCTION

- Clinically defined as normal ejection fraction (by echocardiogram) in the setting of symptoms and signs of heart failure.
- Affects elderly patients; occurs more often in females. Comorbidities include hypertension, DM, obesity, obstructive sleep apnea, and chronic kidney disease.
- **Exam:** S4 is present.
- **Diagnosis:** Echocardiogram shows normal or near-normal ejection fraction (> 40%); LVH is common.

Diastolic Dysfunction

Very common. Often coexists with systolic dysfunction; frequently associated with hypertension and ischemic heart disease. Etiologies are as follows:

- **Myocardial:** Impaired relaxation (ischemia, hypertrophy, cardiomyopathies, hypothyroidism, aging); increased passive stiffness (diffuse fibrosis, scarring, hypertrophy, infiltrative).
- **Endocardial:** Fibrosis, mitral stenosis.
- **Pericardial:** Constrictive pericarditis, cardiac tamponade.
- **Other:** Volume overload of the right ventricle, extrinsic compression (e.g., tumor).

SYMPTOMS

Indistinguishable from systolic dysfunction based on symptoms. May be asymptomatic, although patients have a higher mortality when compared to controls.

EXAM

Look for evidence of heart failure (elevated jugular venous pulsations, crackles on lung exam, lower extremity edema). On cardiac exam, listen for an S4. **An S3 should not be present in isolated diastolic dysfunction** (however, many patients have mixed systolic and diastolic dysfunction).

DIAGNOSIS

- No gold standard.
- **Echocardiography:** Normal **ejection fraction** in the setting of signs and symptoms of heart failure. Also look for other causes of diastolic dysfunction (hypertrophy, right ventricular enlargement, pericarditis, infiltrative diseases).
- **Cardiac catheterization:** Elevated A wave in left ventricular pressure tracing (represents left atrial contraction) and elevated left ventricular end-diastolic pressure (≥ 15 mmHg).

In patients with isolated diastolic dysfunction, always consider underlying myocardial or pericardial causes of a stiff left ventricle (e.g., infiltrative diseases, constrictive pericarditis, restrictive cardiomyopathies).

TREATMENT

- **Avoid exacerbating factors:** AF, tachycardia, ischemia, hypertension, fluid overload, anemia.
- **Slow the heart rate: β-blockers, nondihydropyridine calcium channel blockers (e.g., diltiazem, verapamil).**
- ACEIs and angiotensin receptor blockers may help with cardiac remodeling.

Treatment of Congestive Heart Failure

SYSTOLIC DYSFUNCTION

- **Diuretics:** Acutely used to reduce symptoms of pulmonary edema; **no mortality benefit.** Maintenance doses of diuretics may need to be weight adjusted.
- **ACEIs:** Proven mortality benefit. If ACEIs are not tolerated because of cough, substitute with an angiotensin receptor blocker.
- **Hydralazine with nitrates:** Useful in an acute setting to reduce pulmonary edema by decreasing preload. Associated with a mortality benefit when used, but less benefit than ACEIs.
- **Spironolactone:** Mortality benefit in class III–IV heart failure.
- **β-blockers:** Mortality benefit in all classes of heart failure. However, do not start in the setting of acutely decompensated heart failure. Proven benefit is limited to carvedilol, metoprolol, and long-acting metoprolol.
- **B-type natriuretic peptide:** Acts primarily as a vasodilator. Can be considered in severe heart failure requiring ICU stay. May provide additional improvement in clinical status and symptoms.
- **Mechanical therapy:** For severe heart failure due to ischemia, consider an IABP. For very poor cardiac output, consider a ventricular assist device as a bridge to cardiac transplantation.
- **Cardiac resynchronization:** Pacemaker-based therapy is used in patients with severe systolic heart failure and wide QRS on ECG. Improves ventricular synchrony and cardiac output.
- Cardiac transplantation (see Table 3-10).

TABLE 3-10. Indications and Contraindications for Cardiac Transplantation

Indications
1. End-stage heart disease that limits the prognosis for survival > 2 years or severely limits daily quality of life despite optimal medical and other surgical therapy.
2. No secondary exclusion criteria.
3. Suitable psychosocial profile and social support system.
4. Suitable physiologic/chronologic age.
Exclusion Criteria
1. Active infectious process.
2. Recent pulmonary infarction.
3. Insulin-requiring diabetes with evidence of end-organ damage.
4. Irreversible pulmonary hypertension (pulmonary vascular resistance [PVR] poorly responsive to nitroprusside with PVR > 2 or pulmonary systolic pressure > 50 mmHg at peak dose or at mean arterial pressure of 65–70 mmHg).
5. Presence of circulating cytotoxic antibodies.
6. Presence of active PUD.
7. Active or recent malignancy.
8. Presence of severe COPD or chronic bronchitis.
9. Substance or alcohol abuse.
10. Presence of peripheral or cerebrovascular disease.
11. Other systemic diseases that would jeopardize rehabilitation post-transplant.

Reproduced, with permission, from Braunwald E (ed). *Harrison's Principles of Internal Medicine*, 15th ed. New York: McGraw-Hill, 2001.

DIASTOLIC DYSFUNCTION

- **Goals:** Improve ventricular relaxation, decrease heart rate, maintain sinus rhythm, treat hypertension aggressively.
- β-blockers and nondihydropyridine calcium channel blockers (diltiazem, verapamil) are the mainstays of treatment.
- ACEIs and diuretics are also effective.

CARDIOMYOPATHIES AND MYOCARDITIS

Tables 3-11 through 3-13 outline the etiologies, classification, and evaluation of cardiomyopathies.

Restrictive Cardiomyopathy

Infiltration or fibrosis of the myocardium, causing impaired ventricular filling with preserved systolic function. In end-stage disease, systolic dysfunction may develop. Causes include amyloidosis, sarcoidosis, radiation, and fibrosis following cardiac surgery.

TABLE 3-11. Etiologic Classification of Cardiomyopathies[a]

Primary Myocardial Involvement
Idiopathic (D, R, H)
Familial (D, R, H)
Eosinophilic endomyocardial disease (R)
Endomyocardial fibrosis (R)
Secondary Myocardial Involvement
Infective (D) Viral myocarditis Bacterial myocarditis Fungal myocarditis Protozoal myocarditis Metazoal myocarditis Spirochetal Rickettsial
Metabolic (D)
Familial storage disease (D, R) Glycogen storage disease Mucopolysaccharidoses Hemochromatosis Fabry's disease
Deficiency (D) Electrolytes Nutritional
Connective tissue disorders (D) SLE Polyarteritis nodosa RA Progressive systemic sclerosis Dermatomyositis
Infiltrations and granulomas (R, D) Amyloidosis Sarcoidosis Malignancy
Neuromuscular (D) Muscular dystrophy Myotonic dystrophy Friedreich's ataxia (H, D)
Sensitivity and toxic reactions (D) Alcohol Radiation Drugs
Peripartum heart disease (D)

[a]The principal clinical manifestations of each etiologic grouping are denoted by D (dilated), R (restrictive), or H (hypertrophic) cardiomyopathy.

Reproduced, with permission, from Kasper DL et al (eds). *Harrison's Principles of Internal Medicine,* 16th ed. New York: McGraw-Hill, 2005:1408, as adapted from the WHO/ISFC task force report on the definition and classification of cardiomyopathies, 1980.

TABLE 3-12. Clinical Classification of Cardiomyopathies

Dilated: Left and/or right ventricular enlargement, impaired systolic function, CHF, arrhythmias, emboli.
Restrictive: Endomyocardial scarring or myocardial infiltration resulting in restriction to left and/or right ventricular filling.
Hypertrophic: Disproportionate LVH, typically involving the septum more than the free wall, with or without an intraventricular systolic pressure gradient; usually of a nondilated left ventricular cavity.

Reproduced, with permission, from Kasper DL et al (eds). *Harrison's Principles of Internal Medicine,* 16th ed. New York: McGraw-Hill, 2005:1408.)

SYMPTOMS

Dyspnea, fatigue, peripheral edema.

EXAM

Elevated JVP that increases with inspiration (**Kussmaul's sign**); normal left ventricular impulse; hepatosplenomegaly and ascites in advanced disease.

TABLE 3-13. Laboratory Evaluation of Cardiomyopathies

	DILATED	RESTRICTIVE	HYPERTROPHIC
CXR	Moderate to marked cardiac silhouette enlargement. Pulmonary venous hypertension.	Mild cardiac silhouette enlargement.	Mild to moderate cardiac silhouette enlargement.
ECG	ST-segment and T-wave abnormalities.	Low voltage, conduction defects.	ST-segment and T-wave abnormalities. LVH. Abnormal Q waves.
Echocardiogram	Left ventricular dilatation and dysfunction.	Increased left ventricular wall thickness. Normal or mildly reduced systolic function.	Asymmetric septal hypertrophy. Systolic anterior motion of the mitral valve.
Radionuclide studies	Left ventricular dilatation and dysfunction (RVG).[a]	Normal or mildly reduced systolic function (RVG).	Vigorous systolic function (RVG). Perfusion defect (^{201}Tl).[a]
Cardiac catheterization	Left ventricular dilatation and dysfunction. Elevated left- and often right-sided filling pressures. Diminished cardiac output.	Normal or mildly reduced systolic function. Elevated left- and right-sided filling pressures.	Vigorous systolic function. Dynamic left ventricular outflow obstruction. Elevated left- and right-sided filling pressures.

[a]RVG = radionuclide ventriculogram; ^{201}Tl = thallium 201.

Reproduced, with permission, from Kasper DL et al (eds). *Harrison's Principles of Internal Medicine,* 16th ed. New York: McGraw-Hill, 2005:1409.

DIFFERENTIAL

- **Hypertrophic cardiomyopathy.**
- **Dilated cardiomyopathy.**
- **Constrictive pericarditis:** Clinical presentation and physical exam may be identical to those of restrictive cardiomyopathy. MRI shows pericardial thickening (> 5 mm), and right heart catheterization demonstrates equalization of diastolic pressures in constrictive pericarditis.

DIAGNOSIS

Restrictive cardiomyopathy causes severe diastolic dysfunction with preserved systolic function.

- **ECG:** Conduction system disease, low QRS voltage, nonspecific ST-T-wave changes.
- **Echocardiogram:** Restrictive filling pattern with preserved systolic function and biatrial enlargement. Infiltrative causes can present with the characteristic granular appearance of myocardium.
- **Right heart catheterization:** Dip-and-plateau ventricular filling pressure ("**square root sign**"), pulmonary hypertension, respiratory concordance of the right and left ventricles.
- **Myocardial biopsy:** Detects infiltrative diseases such as amyloidosis and sarcoidosis.

TREATMENT

- **Treat the underlying disease process** (e.g., amyloidosis, sarcoidosis).
- **Diuretics:** Reduce symptoms from venous congestion, but **overdiuresis leads to decreased cardiac output due to preload dependence.**
- **β-blockers/calcium channel blockers:** Improve diastolic function by slowing heart rate and increasing ventricular filling time. Caution should be used in administration, as this may result in a fall in cardiac output. **Avoid use of calcium channel blockers in amyloid heart disease.**
- **Cardiac transplantation:** Remains an option for patients with intractable heart failure without severe systemic disease.

Hypertrophic Cardiomyopathy

An autosomal-dominant disorder of myocardial structural proteins that causes premature, severe LVH. A subset of hypertrophic cardiomyopathy cases may have asymmetric septal hypertrophy and dynamic outflow tract obstruction.

SYMPTOMS

Dyspnea, chest pain, syncope.

EXAM

The obstructive form presents with a systolic crescendo-decrescendo murmur that **intensifies with reduction in left ventricular volume (e.g., standing upright, Valsalva maneuver)** and **decreases with increase in left ventricular volume (e.g., hand grip, raising legs when the patient is in a supine position).** An S4 and a sustained apical impulse are characteristic. Carotid upstrokes are **bifid** owing to midsystolic obstruction.

DIFFERENTIAL

- **Valvular aortic stenosis:** The murmur of aortic stenosis radiates to the neck. Aortic stenosis also has weak and delayed carotid upstrokes (parvus et tardus).

- **Hypertensive heart disease:** Not associated with asymmetric septal hypertrophy or outflow tract obstruction.

DIAGNOSIS

- **ECG:** LVH and left atrial enlargement. The apical form of the disease can have giant anterior T-wave inversions.
- **Echocardiogram:** LVH with systolic anterior motion of the mitral valve and left ventricular outflow tract obstruction. The pattern of hypertrophy varies. In the classic obstructive phenotype, the septum is asymmetrically hypertrophied. The left ventricular cavity is small and hypercontractile, often with diastolic dysfunction.
- **Holter monitor:** Detects ventricular arrhythmias as the cause of syncope.
- **Genetic testing:** Not routinely done, but has the potential to identify the genotype (which has prognostic value) and screen family members.

TREATMENT

- **Avoid high-intensity sports.**
- **β-blockers or verapamil:** Improve symptoms by negative inotropy, which decreases the outflow tract gradient and slows heart rate to increase filling time.
- **Electrophysiologic study and implantable cardioverter defibrillator (ICD) placement:** Indicated for patients with syncope or a family history of sudden cardiac death.
- **Surgical myectomy:** Removes tissue from hypertrophic septum and relieves outflow tract obstruction. Improves symptoms but does not reduce the rate of sudden cardiac death.
- **Percutaneous alcohol septal ablation:** Has the same objective as surgical myectomy by injection of alcohol into hypertrophic septum, causing local infarction.

Agents that decrease left ventricular volume, such as nitrates and diuretics, increase the outflow tract gradient, increase murmur intensity, and are contraindicated in patients with hypertrophic cardiomyopathy.

Dilated Cardiomyopathy

Most commonly occurs in the setting of ischemic heart disease. *Idiopathic dilated cardiomyopathy* is a term used to describe a dilated left ventricle with decreased ejection fraction in the absence of systemic hypertension, CAD, chronic alcoholism, congenital heart disease, or other systemic diseases known to cause dilated cardiomyopathy. Etiologies are as follows:

- **Idiopathic:** A genetic predisposition may exist.
- **Secondary to a known etiologic agent:**
  - **Acute myocarditis:** Infectious, toxic, or immune mediated.
  - **Drugs/toxins:** Anthracyclines, cocaine, amphetamines, alcohol.
  - **Nutritional:** Thiamine, carnitine deficiency.
  - **Collagen vascular disease** (e.g., Churg-Strauss syndrome).
  - **Chronic viral infections:** HIV, HCV.
  - **Endocrine:** Thyroid disorders, hypocalcemia, hypophosphatemia.
  - **Hemochromatosis.**
  - **X-linked muscular dystrophies.**

SYMPTOMS

Exertional dyspnea, fatigue, syncope, decreased exercise tolerance, edema.

EXAM

Elevated JVP, diffuse PMI, S3, S4, holosystolic murmur of mitral regurgitation, evidence of fluid overload (e.g., crackles on lung exam, lower extremity edema, ascites), evidence of AF or other arrhythmias.

DIAGNOSIS

- **ECG:** Can be normal. If abnormal, look for evidence of left ventricular enlargement, conduction disorders (wide QRS, LBBB), or arrhythmias (AF, nonsustained VT).
- **Echocardiogram:** Decreased ejection fraction, dilated left ventricle.
- **Laboratory evaluation:** Can be helpful to diagnose specific etiologies (e.g., HIV).
- **Coronary angiography:** Excludes ischemic heart disease.
- **Endomyocardial biopsy:** Not routinely recommended and generally low yield.

TREATMENT

- Similar to that for systolic heart failure.
- Revascularization in patients with ischemic dilated cardiomyopathy.
- **Neurohormonal blockade: β-blockers, ACEIs** (or angiotensin receptor blockers), spironolactone (for patients with stage III or IV heart failure).
- **Symptom control:** Diuretics, nitrates.
- **Anticoagulation: Controversial;** generally used only in patients with a history of systemic thromboembolism, AF, or evidence of an intracardiac thrombus.
- **Other:** Hemofiltration (for patients with oliguria or renal dysfunction), cardiac resynchronization, ventricular assist devices, cardiac transplantation.

Acute Myocarditis

A common cause of "idiopathic" dilated cardiomyopathy. Patients are typically young and healthy, and many present after a viral upper respiratory illness. Can be a cause of sudden cardiac death. Etiologies are as follows:

- **Infectious: Most commonly viral** (coxsackievirus, HIV), but can be caused by numerous pathogens (including *Trypanosoma cruzi*, or Chagas' disease).
- **Immune mediated:** Allergic reaction to medications, sarcoidosis, scleroderma, SLE, and others.
- **Toxic:** Medications (anthracyclines), alcohol, heavy metals, and others.

SYMPTOMS

Can be nonspecific. Look for flulike symptoms, fever, arthralgias, and malaise. In more severe cases, patients can present with chest pain, dyspnea, and symptoms of heart failure (e.g., orthopnea, edema, decreased exercise tolerance).

EXAM

Can be normal. If abnormal, look for evidence of heart failure.

DIFFERENTIAL

CAD, aortic dissection, pericarditis, pulmonary embolism, and pulmonary and GI illnesses.

DIAGNOSIS

- The gold standard is **endomyocardial biopsy,** but because of patchy involvement of the myocardium, yield is not great and the test can be insensitive. By the time most patients seek medical care, fibrosis is the only finding on biopsy.
- **ECG:** Can be abnormal but is neither sensitive nor specific.
- **Cardiac biomarkers:** Elevated in the acute phase.
- **Echocardiography:** Can be helpful to look for focal wall motion abnormalities and decreased ejection fraction, but findings are nonspecific.
- **Cardiac catheterization:** To exclude CAD.

TREATMENT

- No specific therapy. Steroids have not been shown to be helpful.
- Treat heart failure.
- Cardiac transplantation for severe cases.

Consider the diagnosis of myocarditis in young patients who present after a viral illness. They commonly have no coronary risk factors and have positive cardiac enzymes but normal coronary arteries on cardiac catheterization.

PERICARDIAL DISEASE

Acute Pericarditis

Pericardial inflammation that results in chest pain, pericardial friction rub, and diffuse ST-segment elevation. Common etiologies are viral, connective tissue disease, post-MI, and idiopathic.

SYMPTOMS

Classically described as sharp, pleuritic chest discomfort that **worsens while supine and eases while leaning forward.** Dull pain similar in quality to angina pectoris is also possible. A prodrome of flulike symptoms with fever and myalgias is often present in patients with viral pericarditis.

EXAM

Pericardial **friction rub** is the hallmark. Classically described as having three components: atrial contraction, ventricular contraction, and ventricular filling.

DIFFERENTIAL

- **Acute myocardial ischemia/infarction:** Reciprocal ST-segment depressions are key in distinguishing the ECG changes of STEMI from those of pericarditis.
- **Aortic dissection.**
- **Pneumothorax.**
- **Early repolarization:** A normal variant pattern of ST-segment elevation, usually with a "fishhook" configuration of the J point.
- **Costochondritis:** A diagnosis of exclusion.

DIAGNOSIS

- A consistent history of chest pain typical of acute pericarditis.
- Presence of friction rub on exam. May not have the classic three components described above.
- Presence of typical ECG changes (diffuse ST-segment elevation, PR-segment depression) **not compatible with a single coronary distribution** (see Figure 3-7 and Table 3-14); PR-segment elevation in aVR.

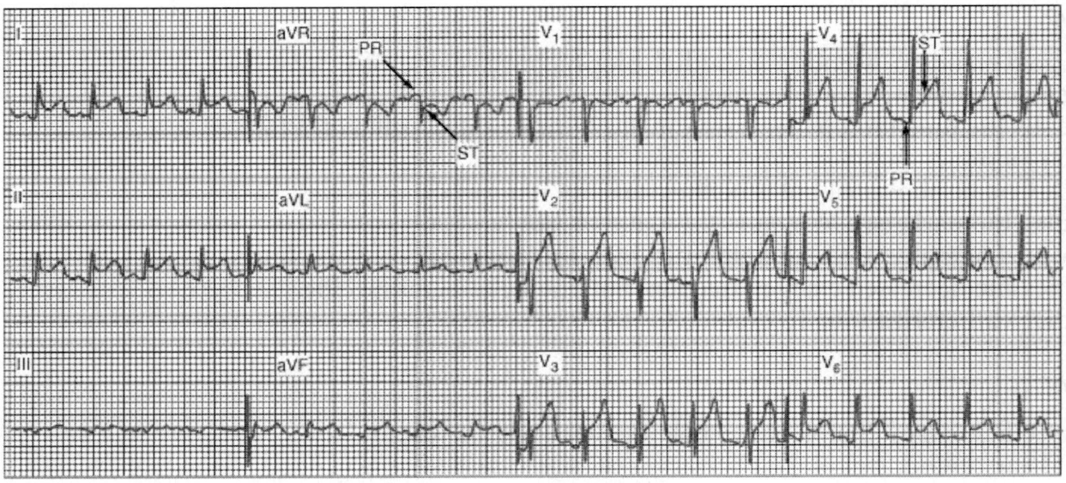

FIGURE 3-7. Acute pericarditis on ECG.

(Reproduced, with permission, from Kasper DL et al [eds]. *Harrison's Principles of Internal Medicine,* 16th ed. New York: McGraw-Hill, 2005:1318.)

In acute pericarditis, the atrial current of injury is reflected in aVR as PR-segment elevation, also known as the "knuckle sign" (the PR segment appears as if a knuckle is pushing it up).

- Echocardiography is useful to exclude a large pericardial effusion, but many patients will have only a small effusion or a normal echocardiogram.

TREATMENT

- NSAIDs.
- Colchicine can be useful for patients with multiple recurrent episodes.
- Steroids are often used as a last resort, when patients do not respond to other therapies.

TABLE 3-14. ECG in Acute Pericarditis vs. Acute (Q-Wave) MI

ST-Segment Elevation	ECG Lead Involvement	Evolution of ST and T Waves	PR-Segment Depression
Pericarditis			
Concave upward	All leads involved except aVR and V_1.	ST remains elevated for several days; after ST returns to baseline, T waves invert.	Yes, in majority.
Acute MI			
Convex upward	ST elevation over infarcted region only; reciprocal ST depression in opposite leads.	T waves invert within hours, while ST is still elevated; followed by Q-wave development.	No.

Reproduced, with permission, from Kasper DL et al (eds). *Harrison's Manual of Medicine,* 16th ed. New York: McGraw-Hill, 2005:613.

Complications

- Anticoagulation should be avoided, but conversion to hemorrhagic pericarditis is rare.
- Echocardiography to rule out tamponade in patients with hypotension and elevated JVP.

Pericardial Effusion

Symptoms

Slowly developing effusions can be asymptomatic. Rapidly developing effusions can lead to tamponade, causing severe chest pain and dyspnea. Etiologies include pericarditis, infections, uremia, malignancy, myxedema, nephrotic syndrome, cirrhosis, post–cardiac surgery, and medications.

Exam

Pericardial friction rub may be present. However, there may be a lack of findings in small effusions. Larger effusions can cause muffled heart sounds and elevated jugular venous pulsations. Rapidly evolving effusions can cause symptoms of cardiac tamponade.

Diagnosis

- **ECG:** Low voltage, electrical alternans (beat-to-beat variation in the height of the QRS complex).
- **CXR:** Cardiomegaly with characteristic "boot-shaped heart."
- **Echocardiography:** Useful for visually detecting the effusion as well as for ruling out tamponade physiology.
- **Pericardiocentesis:** Can help diagnose the underlying cause of the effusion (e.g., transudate vs. exudate).

Treatment

- If unstable, follow guidelines for the treatment of **cardiac tamponade.**
- Drainage of fluid via pericardiocentesis or pericardial window may be necessary in slowly evolving effusions that become symptomatic.

If fluid from a bloody pericardial effusion clots on drainage, the fluid is likely coming from an acute or subacute ruptured myocardium or blood vessel. In other forms of bloody pericardial fluid (e.g., renal failure or malignancy), the fluid does not clot.

Constrictive Pericarditis

Impaired ventricular filling due to thickening and scarring of pericardium. Commonly associated with recurrent episodes of acute pericarditis, prior radiation therapy, neoplasm, collagen vascular disease, and post–cardiac surgery.

Symptoms

Insidious onset of pulmonary and systemic venous congestion and reduced cardiac output (fatigue, dyspnea, peripheral edema).

Exam

Elevated JVP with prominent y descent and **Kussmaul's sign** (absence of normal fall in JVP during inspiration). Pulsus paradoxus may be present. A pericardial knock may be heard following S2, representing rapid cessation of early diastolic filling.

DIFFERENTIAL

- **Restrictive cardiomyopathy:** A similar presentation that may require MRI and/or myocardial biopsy to distinguish. On hemodynamic study, right and left ventricular pressures are concordant with respiration in restriction and discordant in constriction.
- **Cardiac tamponade:** Blunted y descent on right atrial pressure tracing, absence of Kussmaul's sign, and more frequent presence of **pulsus paradoxus.** Right heart catheterization shows diastolic equalization of pressures in both disorders, but a dip-and-plateau pattern is seen only in constriction (and restriction). Table 3-15 further outlines the distinctions between tamponade and pericardial restriction.
- **Cirrhosis:** Patients with hepatic congestion and ascites due to constriction can be incorrectly diagnosed as having cryptogenic cirrhosis.

DIAGNOSIS

- **ECG:** No specific findings, but low voltage may be present.
- **CXR:** Pericardial calcifications (on lateral view) in approximately 25% of patients; bilateral pleural effusions are often present.
- **Echocardiogram:** Pericardial thickening and adhesions, septal bounce, plethoric inferior vena cava without inspiratory collapse.
- **Right heart catheterization:** Equalization of diastolic pressures and dip-and-plateau pattern ("**square root sign**") that reflects early diastolic filling followed by constraint from fixed pericardial volume. Interventricular discordance is specific for pericardial constriction.
- **MRI:** The most sensitive imaging modality for measuring abnormal pericardial thickness.

TREATMENT

Surgical pericardectomy is the treatment of choice, but mortality ranges from 5% to 12%, and symptom relief may not occur for several months following the procedure.

Cardiac Tamponade

An accumulation of pericardial fluid under pressure that impedes ventricular filling. Most commonly associated with malignancy, trauma, and ventricular rupture following MI.

SYMPTOMS

Dyspnea, chest pain, lightheadedness.

EXAM

Tachycardia and hypotension with diminished heart sounds and clear lungs; elevated JVP with blunting or absence of the y descent. Pulsus paradoxus > 10 **mmHg.**

DIFFERENTIAL

- **Constrictive pericarditis:** Slow, insidious onset. Kussmaul's sign is usually present. Echocardiogram shows pericardial thickening without large effusion.

- **Echocardiogram:** Look for structural heart disease. Consider in patients with a history of heart disease, those with an abnormality on physical exam or ECG, or elderly patients.
- **Holter monitoring:** Use when the patient has symptoms that suggest arrhythmia (cluster of spells, sudden loss of consciousness, palpitations, use of medications associated with arrhythmia, patients with known heart disease, abnormal ECG).
- **Tilt-table testing:** Use in patients with normal hearts and relatively infrequent syncope, nondiagnostic Holter monitoring, or symptoms that suggest vasovagal spells (warmth, nausea) but lack an obvious precipitating event.

Bradycardia

Incidence increases with age. Etiologies are as follows:

- **Intrinsic causes:** Idiopathic senile degeneration; ischemia (usually involving the inferior wall); infectious (endocarditis, Chagas' disease, Lyme disease); infiltrative diseases (sarcoidosis, amyloidosis, hemochromatosis); autoimmune disease (SLE, RA, scleroderma); iatrogenic (heart transplant, surgery); inherited/congenital disease (myotonic muscular dystrophy); conditioned heart (trained athletes).
- **Extrinsic causes:** Autonomic (neurocardiac, carotid-sinus hypersensitivity, situational), medications (β-blockers, calcium channel blockers, clonidine, digoxin, antiarrhythmics), metabolic (electrolyte abnormalities, hypothyroidism, hypothermia), neurologic (increased ICP, obstructive sleep apnea).

Anatomically, type II second-degree heart block is most commonly due to a lesion in the bundle of His and is therefore higher grade than type I second-degree heart block, which is due to a problem within the AV node.

Symptoms

Patients may be asymptomatic or they may present with dizziness, weakness, fatigue, heart failure, or loss of consciousness (syncope). Symptoms can also be related to the underlying cause of the bradycardia.

Exam

Look for evidence of decreased pulse rate and evidence of the underlying cause of bradycardia. Look for **cannon A** waves in cases of complete AV dissociation (complete heart block).

Diagnosis

- **ECG:** Look for the origin of the rhythm and whether dropped beats or AV dissociation are present (evidence of AV block; see Table 3-17).
- **Telemetry,** event monitors, tilt-table testing, and electrophysiology studies can also be helpful.

Treatment

- If the patient is **unstable,** follow ACLS protocols.
- If possible, treat the underlying cause (e.g., endocarditis).
- **Medications:** Atropine, **glucagon** (for β-blocker overdose), calcium (for calcium channel blocker overdose). **Note:** Calcium is **contraindicated** in digoxin toxicity.
- Transcutaneous or transvenous pacing if medical therapy is ineffective.
- **Indication for permanent pacemakers:** Documented symptomatic bradycardia. If the patient is asymptomatic, pacemakers may be considered in patients with third-degree AV block with > 3 seconds of asystole or a heart rate < 40 bpm while the patient is awake. In second-degree type II AV

If left untreated, Lyme disease can cause varying degrees of AV conduction block at any time in the course of the disease.

TABLE 3-17. ECG Findings with AV Block

Type of AV Block	Findings on ECG
First degree	Prolonged PR interval (> 200 msec)
Second degree type I (Wenckebach)	Progressive prolongation of the PR interval until there is a dropped QRS. Progressive shortening of the RR interval and a constant PP interval are other signs.
Second degree type II	Regularly dropped QRS (e.g., every third QRS complex dropped). Constant PR interval (no prolongation). Usually associated with bundle branch blocks.
Third degree	Complete dissociation of P waves and QRS complexes (P-wave rate > QRS rate).

block, pacemakers have a class II indication (there is conflicting evidence and opinion regarding the need for permanent pacing).

Indications for Permanent Pacing

Indications for permanent cardiac pacing, based on expert guidelines, are classified as follows: I (definite indications), II (indications with conflicting evidence or opinion), or III (not indicated or harmful). **All indications assume that transient causes such as drugs, electrolytes, and ischemia have been corrected or excluded.**

Class I

- Third-degree AV block and advanced second-degree AV block associated with the following:
  - Symptomatic bradycardia.
  - Arrhythmias or other conditions requiring medications that result in symptomatic bradycardia.
  - Documented asystole of > 3 seconds or escape rates < 40 bpm in **awake,** asymptomatic patients.
  - After AV junction ablation.
  - Post–cardiac surgery when AV block is not expected to resolve.
  - Neuromuscular diseases with AV block due to the unpredictable progression of AV conduction disease in these patients.
- Second-degree AV block (regardless of type) associated with symptomatic bradycardia.

Class IIa

- Asymptomatic third-degree AV block with **awake** escape rates of > 40 bpm.
- Asymptomatic type II second-degree block with narrow QRS (with wide QRS, it becomes a class I indication).
- Asymptomatic type I second-degree block with intra- or infra-His levels found on an electrophysiologic study done for another indication.

- First- and second-degree AV block with symptoms suggestive of pacemaker syndrome.

Class IIb

- Marked first-degree AV block (PR > 300 msec) in patients with left ventricular dysfunction.
- Neuromuscular diseases with any level of AV block due to the unpredictable progression of block in these patients.

Class III

- Asymptomatic first-degree AV block.
- Asymptomatic type I second-degree AV block not known to be due to a problem within or below the bundle of His.
- AV block that is expected to resolve and/or is not likely to recur.

Sudden Cardiac Death

Approximately 450,000 sudden cardiac deaths occur annually in the United States. The etiologies include CAD, MI, pulmonary embolism, aortic dissection, cardiac tamponade, and other acute cardiopulmonary insults. Seventy-five percent of patients do not survive cardiac arrest.

Causes of Sudden Cardiac Death in Young Athletes

- In young athletes, the causes of sudden cardiac death are different from those in the overall population.
- Causes of sudden cardiac death in this population include (in order of decreasing incidence):
  - Hypertrophic cardiomyopathy.
  - **Commotio cordis:** A sudden blow to the precordium causing ventricular arrhythmia.
  - Coronary artery anomalies.
  - Myocarditis.
  - Ruptured aortic aneurysm (e.g., due to Marfan's syndrome or Ehlers-Danlos syndrome).
  - **Arrhythmogenic right ventricular dysplasia:** The right ventricle is replaced by fat and fibrosis, causing increased frequency of ventricular arrhythmias.
  - Aortic stenosis.
  - **Myocardial bridge:** Causes coronary ischemia during ventricular contraction.
  - Atherosclerotic CAD.
  - Coronary artery vasospasm.
  - **Brugada syndrome:** Caused by a sodium channel defect that predisposes to ventricular fibrillation. Baseline ECG shows incomplete RBBB and ST-segment elevation in the precordial leads.
  - Long QT syndrome.
- **Noncardiac precipitants of sudden cardiac death in young athletes:** Asthma, illicit drug use (e.g., cocaine, ephedra, amphetamines), and heat stroke.

SCREENING FOR SUDDEN CARDIAC DEATH IN YOUNG ATHLETES

- It is difficult to assess patients for risk factors of sudden cardiac death because these conditions are rare and because millions of young athletes need to be screened.
- Although screening usually involves history taking and physical examination, these measures alone lack the sensitivity to detect even the most common causes of sudden cardiac death in athletes (e.g., hypertrophic cardiomyopathy).
- In patients with a suggestive history or physical examination, further workup with ECG and echocardiography is warranted.

Implantable Cardiac Defibrillators (ICDs)

RISK FACTORS FOR VENTRICULAR ARRHYTHMIAS

Dilated cardiomyopathy (with reduced ejection fraction), hypertension, hyperlipidemia, tobacco, diabetes, a family history of sudden cardiac death, myocardial ischemia and reperfusion, toxins (e.g., cocaine).

SECONDARY PREVENTION

- **Goal:** To prevent recurrent sudden cardiac death in patients with a history of VT or VF.
- **Drugs:** Antiarrhythmic drugs have been disappointing in the secondary prevention of sudden cardiac death, especially in the large group of patients who are post-MI. Standard therapies for CAD alone (especially β-blockers) play a significant role in decreasing sudden cardiac death in these patients.
- **Devices: ICDs** are superior to amiodarone in patients with CAD who have survived cardiac arrest and have a **low** ejection fraction.
- There is no survival advantage of ICDs over amiodarone in patients who have an ejection fraction > 35%.

PRIMARY PREVENTION

- **Goal:** To prevent sudden cardiac death in patients who have no history of VT and/or VF.
- Studies have shown that in patients with a history of MI who have an ejection fraction < 30%, ICD therapy improves mortality and is superior to antiarrhythmic therapy.

INDICATIONS FOR ICD USE

- **Etiology of heart failure:** Recent studies indicate that ICD therapy appears effective for both ischemic and nonischemic cardiomyopathy.
- **Severity of heart failure:** Consider ICDs in patients with an ejection fraction < 30%.
- **Noninvasive testing:**
  - **T-wave alternans:** Microfluctuations in the morphology of T waves on ECG may indicate an increased risk for sudden cardiac death (requires specialized testing).
  - **Heart rate variability:** Decreased heart rate variability corresponds to worsening heart failure and may be associated with an increased risk of sudden cardiac death.

CARDIOVASCULAR MEDICINE

Aortic Stenosis

The most common causes are senile calcific aortic stenosis and congenital bicuspid aortic valve. Rheumatic aortic stenosis is usually not hemodynamically significant and **almost always occurs in the presence of mitral valve disease.**

Symptoms

A long asymptomatic period followed by the development of the classic triad of **angina, syncope, and heart failure.** The normal valve area is 3 cm^2, and symptoms usually do not develop until the area is < 1 cm^2.

Exam

A crescendo-decrescendo systolic murmur is heard at the base of the heart with radiation to the carotid arteries. Late-peaking murmurs signify more severe stenosis. Diminished carotid upstrokes (parvus et tardus) and a sustained PMI due to LVH may be present. A systolic ejection click can occur in patients with a bicuspid aortic valve. A2 diminishes in intensity, and S2 may be single.

Differential

- **Hypertrophic obstructive cardiomyopathy:** Murmur accentuated with Valsalva or standing and decreased by hand grip.
- **Sub- or supravalvular stenosis:** Due to left ventricular outflow tract membrane or fibromuscular ring (rare).

Diagnosis

- **Echocardiography:** A modified Bernoulli equation is used to derive the pressure gradient across the aortic valve. The aortic valve area is derived by the continuity equation.
- **Cardiac catheterization:** Required to exclude significant coronary stenoses in symptomatic patients who are scheduled for surgery and are at risk for CAD; also required to confirm the severity of aortic stenosis when there is a discrepancy between clinical and noninvasive data.
- **Dobutamine stress testing:** Used in cases of low-gradient aortic stenosis to distinguish true stenosis from pseudostenosis caused by decreased systolic function.

Treatment

- **Aortic valve replacement** is the only therapy for symptomatic aortic stenosis. Older patients do quite well after aortic valve replacement and should not be disqualified by age alone. Patients who are unlikely to outlive a bioprothesis can be spared the lifelong anticoagulation that is required for mechanical valves.
- **Antibiotic prophylaxis against subacute bacterial endocarditis is indicated for all patients.**
- **Aortic valvuloplasty may be effective in** young adults with congenital aortic stenosis. It is **less effective in patients with degenerative aortic stenosis and should be considered palliative therapy or a bridge to surgery.**

Aortic valve replacement should be performed as soon as symptoms develop in aortic stenosis to prevent cardiac death.

Aortic stenosis has been associated with an increased risk of GI bleeding, which is now thought to be due to acquired von Willebrand's disease from disruption of von Willebrand factor multimers as they pass through the stenotic aortic valve.

COMPLICATIONS

- Sudden death occurs but is uncommon (< 1% per year) in patients with severe asymptomatic aortic stenosis.
- In patients who have developed symptoms, survival is 2–5 years.

Aortic Regurgitation

Can be caused by destruction or malfunction of the valve leaflets (infective endocarditis, bicuspid aortic valve, rheumatic valve disease) or dilatation of the aortic root such that the leaflets no longer coapt (Marfan's syndrome, aortic dissection).

SYMPTOMS

- **Acute aortic regurgitation:** Rapid onset of cardiogenic shock.
- **Chronic aortic regurgitation:** A long asymptomatic period followed by progressive dyspnea on exertion and other signs of heart failure.

EXAM

- Soft S1 (usually due to a long PR interval) and soft or absent A2 with a decrescendo blowing diastolic murmur at the base.
- Wide pulse pressure with water-hammer peripheral pulses.
- **Other peripheral signs:** Bruit over the femoral artery (Duroziez's sign); nail-bed pulsations (Quincke's pulse); a popliteal-brachial BP difference of > 20 mmHg (Hill's sign).
- In acute aortic regurgitation, these signs are usually not present, and the only clues may be decreased intensity of S1 and a short, blowing diastolic murmur.
- In severe aortic regurgitation, the anterior mitral valve leaflet can vibrate in the aortic regurgitation jet, creating an apical diastolic rumble that mimics mitral stenosis (Flint murmur).

DIFFERENTIAL

Other causes of diastolic murmurs include mitral stenosis, tricuspid stenosis, pulmonic insufficiency, and atrial myxoma.

DIAGNOSIS

- **Echocardiography:** Essential for determining left ventricular size and function as well as the structure of the aortic valve. TEE is often necessary to rule out endocarditis in acute aortic regurgitation.
- **Cardiac catheterization:** Aortography can be used to estimate the degree of regurgitation if noninvasive studies are inconclusive. Coronary angiography is indicated to exclude CAD in patients at risk prior to surgery.

TREATMENT

- In asymptomatic patients with normal left ventricular function, afterload reduction is essential. ACEIs or other vasodilators can reduce left ventricular volume overload and progression to heart failure.
- **Aortic valve replacement:** Should be considered in symptomatic patients or in those without symptoms who develop worsening left ventricular dilatation and systolic failure.
- **Acute aortic regurgitation:** Surgery is the definitive therapy, since mortality is high in this setting. IV vasodilators may be used as a bridge to surgery.
- **Endocarditis prophylaxis:** Consider in all patients.

Complications

Irreversible left ventricular systolic dysfunction if valve replacement is delayed.

Mitral Stenosis

Almost exclusively due to **rheumatic heart disease,** with rare cases due to congenital lesions and calcification of the mitral annulus. The normal mitral valve area is 4–6 cm^2. Severe mitral stenosis occurs when the valve area is < 1 cm^2.

Symptoms

Characterized by a long asymptomatic period followed by gradual onset of dyspnea on exertion and findings of right heart failure and pulmonary hypertension. Hemoptysis and thromboembolic stroke are late findings.

Indications for valve replacement in aortic regurgitation include the development of symptoms or left ventricular systolic failure even in the absence of symptoms.

Exam

- Loud S1.
- Opening snap of stenotic leaflets after S2 followed by an apical diastolic rumble.
- Signs of pulmonary hypertension (loud P2) and right heart failure (elevated JVP and hepatic congestion) are present in advanced disease.

Differential

- **Left atrial myxoma:** Causes obstruction of mitral inflow.
- **Cor triatriatum:** Left atrial septations cause postcapillary pulmonary hypertension.
- **Aortic insufficiency:** Can mimic the murmur of mitral stenosis (Flint murmur) due to restriction of mitral valve leaflet motion by regurgitant blood from the aortic valve, but no opening snap is present.

Diagnosis

- **Echocardiography:** Used to estimate valve area and to measure the transmitral pressure gradient. Mitral valve morphology on echocardiography determines a patient's suitability for percutaneous valvuloplasty.
- **TEE:** Indicated to exclude left atrial thrombus in patients scheduled for balloon valvotomy.
- **Cardiac catheterization:** Can be used to directly measure the valve gradient through simultaneous recording of pulmonary capillary wedge pressure and left ventricular diastolic pressure. Rarely needed for diagnosis; performed prior to percutaneous balloon valvotomy.

Patients with rheumatic heart disease typically have involvement of the mitral valve. Isolated involvement of the aortic or tricuspid valve with sparing of the mitral valve is exceedingly rare in patients with rheumatic heart disease.

Treatment

- **Percutaneous mitral balloon valvotomy:** Unlike aortic valvuloplasty, balloon dilatation of the mitral valve has proven to be a successful strategy in patients without concomitant mitral regurgitation. Severe annular calcification, severe mitral regurgitation, and atrial thrombus are all contraindications to balloon valvuloplasty.
- **Mitral valve replacement:** For patients who are not candidates for valvotomy.
- Endocarditis prophylaxis is indicated for all patients.

Complications

- Left atrial enlargement and AF with resultant stasis is common and can result in left atrial thrombus formation and embolic stroke.
- Pulmonary hypertension and secondary tricuspid regurgitation.

Mitral Regurgitation

Common causes include mitral valve prolapse, myxomatous (degenerative) mitral valve disease, dilated cardiomyopathy (which causes functional mitral regurgitation due to dilatation of the mitral valve annulus), rheumatic heart disease (acute mitral valvulitis produces the Carey Coombs murmur of acute rheumatic fever), acute ischemia (due to rupture of a papillary muscle), mitral valve endocarditis, mitral valve prolapse, and trauma to the mitral valve.

Symptoms

- **Acute mitral regurgitation:** Abrupt onset of dyspnea due to pulmonary edema.
- **Chronic mitral regurgitation:** Can be asymptomatic. In severe cases, can present with dyspnea and symptoms of heart failure.

Exam

- Soft S1; holosystolic, blowing murmur heard best at the apex with radiation to the axilla. S3 can be due to mitral regurgitation alone (in the absence of systolic heart failure), and its presence suggests severe mitral regurgitation.
- Acute mitral regurgitation can be associated with hypotension and pulmonary edema; murmur may be early systolic.
- The intensity of the murmur does not generally correlate with mitral regurgitation severity as documented by echocardiogram.

Differential

- **Aortic stenosis:** Can mimic the murmur of mitral regurgitation (Gallavardin phenomenon).
- **Tricuspid regurgitation:** Holosystolic murmur best heard at the left sternal border; increases in intensity with inspiration

In patients with mitral regurgitation, the intensity of the murmur on physical examination does not correlate with disease severity. In patients with acute myocardial ischemia, even a low-intensity murmur of mitral regurgitation should alert the physician to the possibility of papillary rupture.

Diagnosis

- **Early detection of mitral regurgitation is essential because treatment should be initiated before symptoms occur.**
- **Exercise stress testing:** Document exercise limitation before symptoms occur at rest.
- **Echocardiography:** Transthoracic echocardiography is important for diagnosis as well as for grading the severity of mitral regurgitation. Transesophageal echocardiography is useful in patients who may need surgical repair or mitral valve replacement.
  - Echocardiography should be performed every 2–5 years in mild to moderate mitral regurgitation with a normal end-systolic diameter and an ejection fraction > 65%.
  - Echocardiography should be performed every 6–12 months in patients with severe mitral regurgitation, an end-systolic diameter > 4.0 cm, or an ejection fraction < 65%.
- **Catheterization:** To exclude CAD prior to surgery.

TREATMENT

- See Figure 3-9 for the treatment of advanced mitral regurgitation.
- **ACEIs:** Useful only in patients with left ventricular dysfunction or hypertension. Medical therapy is generally the only option in patients with an ejection fraction < 30%.
- **Surgical intervention:**
  - **Indications for surgery:** Symptoms related to mitral regurgitation, left ventricular dysfunction, AF, or pulmonary hypertension.
  - **Optimal timing of surgery is early in the course of the disease,** when patients progress from a chronic, compensated state to symptomatic mitral regurgitation.
  - Surgical outcomes are best in patients who have an ejection fraction > 60% and a left ventricular end-systolic diameter < 4.5 cm.
- **Mitral valve repair:** Associated with better outcomes than mitral valve replacement. Repair is most successful when mitral regurgitation is due to prolapse of the posterior mitral valve leaflet.
- **Mitral valve replacement:** For symptomatic patients with an ejection fraction > 30% when the mitral valve is not technically reparable (can be predicted by echocardiography).

Mitral Valve Prolapse

Defined by a displaced and abnormally thickened redundant mitral valve leaflet that projects into the left atrium during systole. Most recent studies

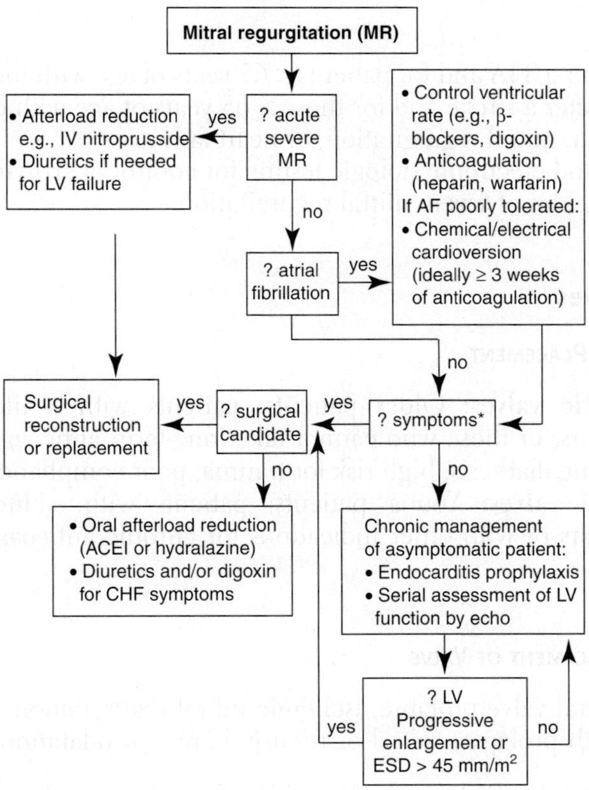

FIGURE 3-9. Management of advanced mitral regurgitation.

(Reproduced, with permission, from Braunwald E et al. *Harrison's Manual of Medicine,* 15th ed. New York: McGraw-Hill, 2001.)

demonstrate a prevalence of approximately 0.5–2.5% in the general population, with men and women affected equally. Mitral valve prolapse may be complicated by chordal rupture or endocarditis, both of which can lead to severe mitral regurgitation. Etiologies are as follows:

- **Primary:** Familial, sporadic, Marfan's syndrome, connective tissue disease.
- **Secondary:** CAD, rheumatic heart disease, "flail leaflet," reduced left ventricular dimension (hypertrophic cardiomyopathy, pulmonary hypertension, dehydration).

Endocarditis prophylaxis is not needed for patients with mitral valve prolapse unless they have evidence of mitral regurgitation, thickened mitral valves, or an audible systolic murmur associated with the midsystolic click.

Symptoms

Most patients have no symptoms, and the diagnosis is often found incidentally on physical exam or echocardiography. However, some patients may present with atypical chest pain, palpitations, or TIAs.

Exam

Midsystolic click and midsystolic murmur with characteristic response to maneuvers. In more severe cases, listen for the holosystolic murmur of mitral regurgitation.

Diagnosis

- There is no consensus from the most recent American Heart Association guidelines.
- **Echocardiography:** Use for initial assessment and then follow every 3–5 years unless symptomatic or associated with mitral regurgitation (check echocardiogram yearly).

Treatment

- **Aspirin:** After a TIA and for patients < 65 years of age with lone AF.
- **Warfarin:** After a stroke and for those > 65 years of age with coexistent AF, hypertension, mitral regurgitation, or heart failure.
- β-blockers and electrophysiologic testing for control of arrhythmias.
- Surgery for cases of severe mitral regurgitation.

Prosthetic Valves

Indications for Placement

- **Bioprosthetic valves:** Older patients; patients with a life expectancy < 10–15 years; or those who cannot take long-term anticoagulant therapy (e.g., bleeding diathesis, high risk for trauma, poor compliance).
- **Mechanical valves:** Young patients; patients with a life expectancy > 10–15 years or with other indications for chronic anticoagulation (e.g., AF).

Repair vs. Replacement of Valve

- **Repair:** Mitral valve prolapse, ischemic mitral regurgitation, bicuspid aortic valve with prolapse, mitral or tricuspid annular dilatation with normal leaflets.
- **Replacement:** Rheumatic heart disease, endocarditis, heavily calcified valve, restricted leaflet motion, extensive leaflet destruction.

ANTICOAGULATION

- None is needed for porcine valves after **three months** of warfarin therapy. Aspirin can be used in high-risk patients.
- For patients with mechanical valves, the level of anticoagulation depends on the location and type of valve (valves in the mitral and tricuspid position and older **caged-ball valves are most prone to thrombosis**).
- Risk factors for thromboembolic complications include AF, previous systemic emboli, left atrial thrombus, and severe left ventricular dysfunction.

COMPLICATIONS

- AF.
- Conduction disturbances.
- **Endocarditis:**
  - **Early prosthetic valve endocarditis:** Occurs during the first 60 days after valve replacement, most commonly due to *S. epidermidis*; often fulminant and associated with high mortality rates.
  - **Late prosthetic valve endocarditis:** Most often occurs in patients with multiple valves or bioprosthetic valves. Microbiology is similar to that of native valve endocarditis.
- **Hemolysis:** Look for schistocytes on peripheral smear. Usually occurs in the presence of perivalvular leak.
- **Thrombosis:**
  - At highest risk are those with mitral location of the valve and inadequate anticoagulation.
  - Presents clinically as heart failure, poor systemic perfusion, or systemic embolization.
  - Often presents acutely with hemodynamic instability.
  - Diagnose with echocardiogram.
  - For small thrombi (< 5 mm) that are nonobstructive, IV heparin should be tried initially. For large thrombi (> 5 mm), use more aggressive therapy (fibrinolysis or valve replacement).
- **Perivalvular leak:** Rare. In severe cases, look for hemolytic anemia and valvular insufficiency causing heart failure.
- **Emboli:** Typically present as stroke, but can present as intestinal or limb ischemia.
- **Primary valve failure:** Most common with bioprosthetic valves; usually occurs after 10 years.

ADULT CONGENITAL HEART DISEASE

Congenital heart disease comprises 2% of adult heart disease. Only the most common acyanotic heart defects will be presented. Table 3-18 outlines the extent to which patients with congenital cardiac malformations can tolerate pregnancy. Examples of adult congenital heart disease follow.

Atrial Septal Defect (ASD)

There are three major types: ostium secundum (most common), ostium primum, and sinus venosus.

TABLE 3-18. Tolerance of Pregnancy by Patients with Congenital Cardiac Malformations

WELL TOLERATED	INTERMEDIATE EFFECT	POORLY TOLERATED
NYHA class I.[a]	NYHA class II–III.	NHYA class IV.
Left-to-right shunts without pulmonary hypertension.	Repaired transposition of the great arteries.	Right-to-left shunt; unrepaired cyanotic heart disease.
Aortic or mitral valvular regurgitation (mild to moderate).	Fontan repairs.	Pulmonary hypertension and/or pulmonary vascular disease (e.g., Eisenmenger's, "primary pulmonary hypertension").
Pulmonic or tricuspid regurgitation (if low pressure, even severe).	Aortic or mitral stenosis (moderate).	Aortic or mitral stenosis (severe).
Pulmonic stenosis (mild-to-moderate).	Ebstein's anomaly.	Pulmonic stenosis (severe).
Well-repaired tetralogy of Fallot.		Marfan's or aortic coarctation.

[a]NYHA = New York Heart Association.

Reproduced, with permission, from Kasper DL et al (eds). *Harrison's Principles of Internal Medicine,* 16th ed. New York: McGraw-Hill, 2005:1383.)

SYMPTOMS

Most cases are asymptomatic and are either diagnosed incidentally on echocardiography or found during workup of paradoxical emboli. Large shunts can cause dyspnea on exertion and orthopnea.

EXAM

Fixed wide splitting of S2 with loud P2 as pulmonary hypertension develops. Systolic flow murmur; diastolic rumble across the tricuspid valve due to increased flow.

DIFFERENTIAL

Other shunts, including VSD and patent ductus arteriosus.

DIAGNOSIS

- ECG: Incomplete RBBB with right axis deviation in ostium secundum ASD. Left axis deviation suggests ostium primum ASD.
- Echocardiography with agitated saline bubble study can be used to visualize the intracardiac shunt and determine the ratio of pulmonary-to-systemic blood flow (Q_p/Q_s).
- TEE is extremely useful for documenting the location and size of the defect and for excluding associated lesions.
- Cardiac catheterization documenting a "step-up" in O_2 saturation between the superior vena cava and right atrium is the gold standard.

TREATMENT

- Percutaneous device closure is the treatment of choice for ostium secundum ASDs.
- Surgical correction is indicated for very large defects as well as for ostium primum and sinus venosus defects.
- Endocarditis prophylaxis is not indicated for isolated uncorrected ASDs but is indicated for six months after closure by device or surgery.

COMPLICATIONS

- Paradoxical embolization leading to transient ischemic attacks and strokes.
- AF and atrial flutter.
- Pulmonary hypertension and **Eisenmenger's syndrome.**
- Endocarditis is rare in patients with secundum ASD but can occur in other types.

Coarctation of the Aorta

Proximal narrowing of the descending aorta just beyond the left subclavian artery with development of collateral circulation involving the internal mammary, intercostal, and axillary arteries. A bicuspid aortic valve is present in > 50% of patients with coarctation of the aorta. More common in males than in females.

Surgical correction of ASD carries a long-term survival rate better than that of medical therapy alone and is recommended even for asymptomatic patients with significant shunts (Q_p/Q_s > 1.5:1).

SYMPTOMS

Headache, dyspnea, fatigue, leg claudication.

EXAM

Diminished femoral pulses with a radial-to-femoral-pulse delay. Continuous scapular murmur due to collateral flow.

DIFFERENTIAL

- Other causes of secondary hypertension, including renal artery stenosis.
- Peripheral arterial disease leads to diminished femoral pulses and claudication.

DIAGNOSIS

- **CXR:** Rib notching from enlarged collaterals.
- ECG: LVH.
- Cardiac catheterization with aortography to define stenosis and measure gradient.
- **MRI/MRA:** Offer excellent visualization of location and extent of coarctation.

TREATMENT

- Medical treatment of hypertension.
- Surgical correction for patients < 20 years of age and in older patients with upper extremity hypertension and a gradient of ≥ 20 mmHg.
- Balloon dilatation with or without stent placement is an alternative for native or recurrent coarctation.

COMPLICATIONS

- LVH and dilatation due to increased afterload.
- Severe hypertension.
- Aortic dissection or rupture.
- Subarachnoid hemorrhage due to rupture of aneurysms of the circle of Willis (rare).
- Premature CAD.

Coarctation of the aorta is commonly associated with congenital bicuspid aortic valve.

Patent Ductus Arteriosus (PDA)

Uncommon in adults. Risk factors include premature birth and exposure to rubella virus in the first trimester.

SYMPTOMS

Usually asymptomatic, but moderate to large shunts can cause dyspnea, fatigue, and eventually signs and symptoms of pulmonary hypertension and right heart failure.

Differential cyanosis of the fingers (pink) and toes (blue and clubbed) is pathognomonic for Eisenmenger's syndrome caused by an uncorrected PDA.

EXAM

Continuous "machinery-like" murmur at the left upper sternal border. Bounding peripheral pulses due to rapid aortic runoff to the pulmonary artery. In the presence of pulmonary hypertension (Eisenmenger's syndrome), the murmur is absent or soft, and there is differential cyanosis involving the lower extremities and sparing the upper extremities.

DIFFERENTIAL

Other shunts, including ASDs and VSDs.

DIAGNOSIS

- **ECG:** Nonspecific; LVH and left atrial enlargement in the absence of pulmonary hypertension can be seen.
- Echocardiography can be used to calculate the shunt fraction and to estimate pulmonary artery systolic pressure. Abnormal ductal flow can be visualized in the pulmonary artery.
- Cardiac catheterization can be used to document a "step-up" in O_2 saturation from the right ventricle to the pulmonary artery.

TREATMENT

Endocarditis prophylaxis, transcatheter coil closure, surgical correction.

COMPLICATIONS

- **Eisenmenger's syndrome** with pulmonary hypertension and shunt reversal.
- Infective endocarditis.

Ventricular Septal Defect (VSD)

Most VSDs occur in close proximity to the membranous portion of the intraventricular septum, but muscular, inlet, and outlet VSDs can also occur.

SYMPTOMS

Most patients diagnosed in adulthood are asymptomatic, but insidious dyspnea on exertion and orthopnea may develop.

EXAM

Holosystolic murmur at the left lower sternal border with a right ventricular heave and prolonged splitting of S2. As pulmonary arterial pressure increases, a loud P2 and tricuspid regurgitation can also be appreciated. Cyanosis, clubbing, and signs of right heart failure can appear with the development of Eisenmenger's syndrome.

DIFFERENTIAL

Other shunts, including ASD and PDA.

DIAGNOSIS

- Echocardiography with agitated saline bubble study can be used to visualize the intracardiac shunt and determine Q_p/Q_s.
- Cardiac catheterization documenting a "step-up" in oxygen saturation between the right atrium and right ventricle is the gold standard.
- **ECG:** Nonspecific; LVH and left atrial enlargement in the absence of pulmonary hypertension can be seen. Right atrial enlargement, RVH, and RBBB can develop with the development of pulmonary hypertension.
- **CXR:** Cardiomegaly and enlarged pulmonary arteries.

Surgical closure is contraindicated once Eisenmenger's syndrome develops because it can increase pulmonary hypertension and right heart failure.

TREATMENT

- Endocarditis prophylaxis.
- Diuretics and vasodilators to reduce left-to-right shunt and symptoms of right heart failure.
- Surgical correction for patients with significant shunt ($Q_p/Q_s > 1.7{:}1$).

COMPLICATIONS

- **Eisenmenger's syndrome:** Long-standing left-to-right shunting causes pulmonary vascular hyperplasia, resulting in pulmonary arterial hypertension and shunt reversal.
- Paradoxical embolism leading to TIAs or stroke.
- Infective endocarditis.

OTHER TOPICS

Aortic Dissection

Approximately 2000 cases are diagnosed each year in the United States. Aortic dissection is associated with uncontrolled hypertension, medial degeneration of the aorta (Marfan's syndrome, Ehlers-Danlos syndrome), cocaine use, coarctation, congenital bicuspid valve, trauma, cardiac surgery, pregnancy, and syphilitic aortitis. Type A = proximal dissection; type B = distal dissection (dissection flap originates distal to the left subclavian artery).

SYMPTOMS

- Classically presents as a sudden-onset "tearing" or "ripping" sensation originating in the chest and radiating to the back, but symptoms may not be classic.

- Unlike MI, pain is maximal at the onset and is not gradual in nature.
- Can present with organ hypoperfusion due to occlusion of arteries by the dissection flap (e.g., coronary ischemia, stroke, intestinal ischemia, renal failure, limb ischemia).
- Other presentations include cardiac tamponade and aortic insufficiency in cases of proximal aortic dissection.

EXAM

- Elevated BP (although hypotension can be seen with proximal dissections associated with tamponade).
- In proximal dissection, listen for the diastolic murmur of aortic insufficiency.
- Pulse deficits or unequal pulses between the right and left arms.
- Can present with focal neurologic deficits (from associated cerebrovascular infarct) or with paraplegia (from associated anterior spinal artery compromise).

DIFFERENTIAL

Acute MI, cardiac tamponade, thoracic or abdominal aortic aneurysm, pulmonary embolism, tension pneumothorax, esophageal rupture.

Proximal (type A) aortic dissection can present as acute inferior or right-sided MI due to involvement of the right coronary artery (prone to occlusion by the dissection flap).

DIAGNOSIS

- Three major clinical predictors are sudden, tearing chest pain; differential pulses or blood pressures between right and left arms; and abnormal aortic or mediastinal contour on CXR. If all three are present, the positive likelihood ratio is 0.66. The negative likelihood ratio if all three are absent is 0.07.
- **CXR:** Look for widened mediastinum (occurs in approximately 60% of all aortic dissections).
- **TEE:** The fastest and most portable method for unstable patients, but may not be available at all hospitals. Sensitivity is 98% and specificity 95%.
- **Chest CT:** Sensitivity is 94% and specificity 87%.
- **MRI:** Highly sensitive (98%) and specific (98%), but the test is slow and may not be available at many hospitals. Good for following patients with type B dissections.
- **Aortography:** Gold standard.

TREATMENT

- **Type A:** Surgical repair.
- **Type B:** Admit to the ICU for medical management of hypertension. Treat first with β-blockers (esmolol, labetalol) and then with IV nitroprusside. Avoid anticoagulation. Surgery is indicated for complications of dissection, end-organ damage, or failure to control hypertension.

Proximal (type B) aortic dissection can present as acute paraplegia due to occlusion of the anterior spinal artery.

COMPLICATIONS

- Acute MI from occlusion of the right coronary artery by dissection flap or dissection of the coronary artery.
- Acute aortic insufficiency, which can present as hemodynamic instability and heart failure.
- Cardiac tamponade due to dissection into the pericardium.
- Cardiac arrest.
- Cerebrovascular accident (due to concomitant carotid artery dissection).

- Occlusion of distal arteries can lead to end-organ damage (e.g., paraplegia, renal failure, intestinal ischemia, limb ischemia).

Peripheral Vascular Disease

Atherosclerosis of the peripheral arterial system is associated with the same clinical risk factors as coronary disease (smoking, diabetes, hypertension, and hyperlipidemia).

Symptoms

Intermittent claudication is reproducible pain in the lower extremity muscles that is brought on by exercise and relieved by rest; however, most peripheral vascular disease is asymptomatic.

Exam

Poor distal pulses, femoral bruits, loss of hair in the legs and feet, slow capillary refill, poor wound healing (chronic ulceration).

Differential

- Nearly all peripheral vascular disease is caused by atherosclerosis. Less common causes include coarctation, fibrodysplasia, retroperitoneal fibrosis, and radiation.
- Nonarterial causes of limb pain include spinal stenosis (pseudoclaudication), deep venous thrombosis, and peripheral neuropathy (often coexists with peripheral vascular disease in diabetics).

Diagnosis

- **Ankle-brachial index (ABI) < 0.90** (the highest ankle systolic pressure measured by Doppler divided by the highest brachial systolic pressure).
- **MRI** is a useful noninvasive diagnostic test.
- Lower extremity **angiography** is the gold standard.

Treatment

- Aggressive cardiac risk factor reduction, including control of smoking, hypertension, and hyperlipidemia.
- A structured exercise rehabilitation program.
- **Antiplatelet agents:** Aspirin is first-line therapy for overall cardiovascular event reduction, but data also support the use of ticlopidine, clopidogrel, and dipyridamole in peripheral vascular disease.
- ACEIs.
- **Pentoxifylline:** Increases RBC deformability to increase capillary flow.
- **Cilostazol:** Inhibits platelet aggregation and promotes lower arterial vasodilation.
- Percutaneous transluminal angioplasty and lower extremity revascularization bypass surgery (only for severe symptoms).
- Thrombolytic therapy for acute limb ischemia.

If defined as ABI < 0.90, most peripheral vascular disease is asymptomatic but still confers a high risk of adverse cardiovascular events and death.

Complications

- Critical leg ischemia leading to limb amputation.
- Even asymptomatic peripheral vascular disease is a major risk factor for adverse cardiovascular events.

NOTES

CARDIOVASCULAR MEDICINE

CHAPTER 4

Critical Care

Christian Merlo, MD, MPH

ACUTE RESPIRATORY DISTRESS SYNDROME (ARDS)

Acute-onset respiratory failure characterized by bilateral pulmonary infiltrates and hypoxemia in the setting of a pulmonary capillary occlusion pressure of ≤ 18 mmHg or in the absence of clinical evidence of left atrial hypertension. Thought to be due to both alveolar epithelial cell and vascular endothelial cell injury. Commonly associated with pneumonia, aspiration, sepsis, trauma, acute pancreatitis, cardiopulmonary bypass, transfusion of blood products, inhalational injury, and reperfusion injury after lung transplantation.

SYMPTOMS/EXAM

- Rapid onset of dyspnea, tachypnea, and diffuse crackles.
- Approximately 25% of survivors have no pulmonary impairment at one year; 50% have mild impairment, 25% moderate impairment, and a small fraction severe impairment. Reduced single-breath DL_{CO} is the most common pulmonary function abnormality.

DIFFERENTIAL

Cardiogenic pulmonary edema, pneumonia, diffuse alveolar hemorrhage.

DIAGNOSIS

Both acute lung injury and ARDS are clinically defined by means of rapidity of symptom onset, oxygenation, hemodynamic criteria, and CXR findings (see Table 4-1). Additional findings are as follows:

- **CT of the thorax:** May demonstrate alveolar filling and consolidation in dependent lung zones with sparing of other areas.
- **Bronchoalveolar lavage:** May help differentiate the etiology (e.g., *Pneumocystis* in the immunocompromised patient).

TREATMENT

- Search for and treat the underlying cause of acute respiratory failure (ARF).
- Most patients with ARDS require mechanical ventilation during the course of the disease.
  - Use of tidal volumes ≤ 6 cc/kg of predicted body weight has been shown to reduce mortality.
  - Positive end-expiratory pressure (PEEP) can help improve oxygenation and reduce high levels of inspired O_2, but no consensus exists on the optimum level.
- Corticosteroids have been given in the proliferative phase of ARDS, but

TABLE 4-1. Diagnosis of Acute Lung Injury and ARDS

	Onset of Symptoms	Oxygenation	Hemodynamics	CXR
Acute lung injury	Acute	$PaO_2/FiO_2 \le 300$	Low or normal left atrial pressure	Bilateral infiltrates
ARDS	Acute	$PaO_2/FiO_2 \le 200$	Low or normal left atrial pressure	Bilateral infiltrates

their use in this context is still considered experimental. Use of inhaled vasodilators, exogenous surfactant, high-frequency ventilation, liquid ventilation, and antioxidant therapy have been studied with no proven benefit.

ACUTE RESPIRATORY FAILURE (ARF)

Consists of failure in oxygenation characterized by hypoxemia or failure in ventilation characterized by hypercarbia. Oxygenation and ventilatory failure can occur simultaneously. However, failure in oxygenation may occur despite adequate ventilation (pulmonary hypertension and a newly patent foramen ovale), and failure in ventilation may occur despite adequate oxygenation (neuromuscular weakness).

SYMPTOMS/EXAM

Clinical presentation varies with the underlying disease process. Whereas dyspnea, tachypnea, respiratory alkalosis, and hypoxemia suggest hypoxic respiratory failure, decreased respiratory rate and unresponsiveness point to hypercarbic respiratory failure.

DIFFERENTIAL

The differential of ARF is outlined in Tables 4-2 and 4-3.

TABLE 4-2. Etiologies of Hypoxemic Respiratory Failure

CAUSE	MECHANISM	DISEASE STATES	COMMENTS
Decreased FiO_2 or low total O_2	O_2 is replaced by other gases (enclosed spaces, fire) or low O_2 from high altitudes and air travel results in reduced PaO_2.		
Diffusion abnormality	Reduction in diffusion capacity leads to low PaO_2.	Pulmonary alveolar proteinosis.	An uncommon cause of hypoxemic respiratory failure.
Hypoventilation	Decreased minute ventilation results in increased $PaCO_2$ and decreased PaO_2 according to the alveolar gas equation.	See Table 4-3.	Normal A-a gradient.
Ventilation-perfusion (V/Q) mismatch	Results when there is an altered ratio of perfusion to ventilation.	Pulmonary embolus, pulmonary hypertension, COPD, asthma.	Increased A-a gradient; PaO_2 corrects with supplemental O_2.
Shunt	Occurs when there is perfusion to the nonventilated lung or a communication between the arterial and venous systems.	ARDS, pneumonia, pulmonary AVM, congenital heart disease, patent foramen ovale with right-to-left flow.	Increased A-a gradient; PaO_2 does not correct with supplemental O_2.

TABLE 4-3. Etiologies of Hypercarbic Respiratory Failure

CAUSE	MECHANISM	DISEASE STATES
CNS disorders/decreased ventilatory drive	Decreased minute ventilation leads to increased $Paco_2$.	Drug overdose, CNS lesion/ infarction, central sleep apnea, hypothyroidism.
Peripheral nerve disorders	Same as above.	Guillain-Barré syndrome, ALS, poliomyelitis, West Nile virus, ICU-acquired paresis.
Neuromuscular junction disorders	Same as above.	Myasthenia gravis, botulism.
Muscle disorders	Same as above.	Muscular dystrophy, glycogen storage disease, ICU-acquired paresis.
Lung disorders	Decreased alveolar ventilation due to obstructive lung disease leads to increased $Paco_2$.	COPD, asthma, CF.
Chest wall disorders	Chest wall mechanics altered leading to decreased alveolar ventilation and increased $Paco_2$.	Kyphoscoliosis, massive obesity.

TREATMENT

- Treatment depends on the etiology. In all cases, focus on providing sufficient O_2 through use of supplemental oxygen and maintenance of adequate ventilation.
- In patients with COPD and ARF, evidence suggests that noninvasive positive-pressure mechanical ventilation decreases the need for intubation, shortens hospital stay, and reduces in-hospital mortality.
- For patients with pulmonary edema and ARF, evidence strongly suggests that the use of continuous positive airway pressure (CPAP) greatly reduces the need for intubation.
- Although noninvasive techniques have been studied in other causes of ARF, results have been controversial, and intubation with mechanical ventilation remains the standard of care.

VENTILATOR MANAGEMENT

A ventilator is a machine designed to reduce the mechanical work of breathing and to improve gas exchange. Invasive ventilatory support is provided through an airway such as an endotracheal or tracheostomy tube. The main indication for mechanical ventilation is **ARF** of any cause. Patients with ARF and COPD or pulmonary edema may respond to noninvasive techniques. Other indications include surgery with general anesthesia and airway protection with drug overdose.

Classification

Mechanical ventilation is categorized by the way the machine terminates an inspired breath:

- **Volume cycled (most common):** Terminates inspiration after a preset volume has been delivered.
- **Pressure cycled:** Ends inspiration when a preset pressure has been reached. The volume of the delivered breath will vary depending on lung/chest wall mechanics.
- **Flow cycled:** Stops inspiration when a flow rate has been reached. The ventilator delivers a breath with a preset pressure, and the cycle is terminated when the inspiratory flow rate falls to a predetermined level.
- **Time cycled:** Ceases inspiration after a preset inspiratory time has elapsed.

Mode

Full ventilatory support is provided using either conventional mechanical ventilation or alternative modes of ventilation.

- **Conventional modes** include the following:
  - **Assist control:** Senses an inspiratory effort and delivers a preset tidal volume. The physician sets a mandatory minimum machine-triggered rate and the tidal volume. If the patient attempts to spontaneously breathe above the set rate, the additional breaths will be delivered at the same tidal volume as the mandatory breaths. Tidal volume is determined by the physician, whereas respiratory rate is patient dependent.
  - **Synchronized intermittent mandatory ventilation:** Delivers a breath of set tidal volume at a set rate (like AC). Additionally, the patient may breathe spontaneously and will get the tidal volume they can pull spontaneously. The spontaneous breaths and mandatory breaths are synchronized to reduce breath stacking.
  - **Pressure support:** Delivers a breath with a set pressure; ends inspiration once flow rate has fallen to a percentage of its maximum value. Although many patients find this mode comfortable, it requires close monitoring, as tidal volume and respiratory rate are both patient determined. **Caution:** There is no set minute ventilation, so a non–spontaneously breathing patient will have apnea. Can be combined with syncronized intermittent mandatory ventilation.
- **Alternative modes** include the following:
  - **Pressure control:** Delivers a breath until a preset pressure is reached. Evidence suggests that there is no clear-cut advantage to this mode when compared to conventional mechanical ventilation.
  - **High-frequency oscillator ventilation:** Delivers rapid, low-tidal-volume breaths that oscillate around a mean airway pressure. The literature suggests that this is an acceptable alternative to conventional ventilator modes in patients with ARDS. However, the need for specialized equipment and training limits its use. Definitive demonstration of benefit over conventional ventilation is still lacking.
  - **Airway pressure release ventilation:** Provides continuous positive pressure to inflate the lungs. The pressure is cyclically **released** to allow for lung deflation and gas exchange. Remains an experimental mode of ventilation.

Settings and Measurements

After a patient has been intubated, a number of adjustments must be made and physiologic measurements obtained from the ventilator.

- **Mode:** The initial choice should be based on physician and staff familiarity with the ventilator mode as well as on the patient-specific disease process. Assist control is a good first choice in most clinical situations and is the most common ventilator mode used in the ICU.
- **Respiratory rate:** The minute ventilation needs prior to intubation should be approximated. Respiratory rate multiplied by tidal volume will determine minute ventilation. If the patient is paralyzed, the rate should reflect the patient's entire needs. If the patient is very ill, one may wish to provide almost all breaths as mandatory breaths so that the work of triggering is removed. Rates up to 35 are generally acceptable unless the patient cannot fully exhale at such rapid rates (e.g., status asthmaticus). Slower rates should then be used even if hypercapnea occurs.
- **Tidal volume:** The use of tidal volumes of 6 cc/kg for ARDS patients has been shown to reduce mortality when compared with higher tidal volumes. Evidence also suggests that lower tidal volumes may reduce the risk of ventilator-induced lung injury.
- **FiO_2:** In general, start with 100% FiO_2. Attempts should be made to decrease O_2 to the lowest amount needed to keep arterial saturation > 90% or PaO_2 > 60 mmHg.
- **Flow rate:** Rates of 60 L/min are sufficient for most patients. Rates must often be increased in patients with ARF and COPD.
- **Sensitivity:** A sensitivity of −1 to −3 cm H_2O is often used. If the ventilator is too sensitive (a more positive number), breaths may be triggered simply by moving the patient or ventilator tubing. Flow triggering is also possible.
- **PEEP:** A small amount (5 cm H_2O) is typically used. Increased levels are used in patients with ARDS to improve oxygenation and possibly to prevent further lung injury. Higher levels of PEEP may also be used in patients with cardiogenic pulmonary edema to improve oxygenation as well as to decrease preload and afterload.
- **Plateau pressure:** Measured by occluding the expiratory port at end inspiration. Since flow is held at the end of a breath, this pressure reflects the static compliance of the lungs and chest wall. The peak-plateau difference helps determine what the source of the high pressure is.

$$\text{Static compliance} = V_T / (P_{PL} - \text{PEEP})$$

  where V_T = tidal volume and P_{PL} = plateau pressure.
- **Peak pressure:** Measured directly by the ventilator. Reflects pressure due to flow resistance (ventilator circuit, endotracheal tube, proximal aiways) and lung and chest wall compliance. Increases in peak pressure suggest either decreased lung/chest wall compliance or increased airway resistance. If the peak pressure is elevated, examine the patient and measure plateau pressure (see Table 4-4).
- **Auto-PEEP:** Measured by covering the expiratory port on the ventilator at end expiration. Caused by delayed emptying of the lungs and subsequent initiation of a new breath before the lungs have fully emptied. Common in mechanically ventilated patients with COPD and asthma.

> ***Ventilator settings–***
>
> **MTRIP**
>
> **M**ode
> **T**idal volume
> **R**ate
> **I**nspired O_2
> **P**EEP

SHOCK

A physiologic state characterized by reduced tissue perfusion and subsequent tissue hypoxia. Prolonged tissue hypoxia often leads to cell death, organ damage, multiple organ system failure, and eventual death.

TABLE 4-4. Algorithm for Increased Peak Pressure

Peak Pressure	Plateau Pressure	Causes	Management
↑	↑	Pneumothorax, ARDS, pulmonary edema, pneumonia.	Decompression, low V_T, diuretics, antibiotics.
↑	Normal or significantly lower than the peak inspiratory pressure (difference > 10 cm H_2O).	Occluded endotracheal tube; biting on endotracheal tube; bronchoconstriction.	Suctioning, sedation, β-agonists.

SYMPTOMS/EXAM

Most patients who present with shock are hypotensive. This decrease in blood pressure is due to a fall in cardiac output and/or a reduction in systemic vascular resistance (SVR). Regardless of the cause of shock, the majority of patients are also tachypneic and tachycardic and appear to be in distress. A narrowed pulse pressure, cool extremities, and delayed capillary refill suggest a cardiac cause with diminished cardiac output. By contrast, fever, a bounding pulse, warm extremities, and rapid capillary refill suggest an infectious cause with preserved or increased cardiac output and decreased SVR. Decreased JVP might suggest hypovolemia, and the presence of elevated JVP, pulsus paradoxus, and muffled heart sounds implies pericardial tamponade.

DIAGNOSIS

Shock can be categorized into four different types, as indicated in Table 4-5. If the type of shock cannot be determined after careful physical examination, additional information can be obtained using invasive monitoring devices.

TABLE 4-5. Categories of Shock

	Cardiac Output	SVR	PCOP	$S\bar{v}O_2$[a]	Examples
Distributive	↑	↓	↓	↔ or ↑	Sepsis, anaphylaxis.
Cardiogenic	↓	↑	↑ (except in RV infarct)	↓	Acute MI, CHF.
Hypovolemic	↓	↑	↓	↓	Trauma, bleeding.
Obstructive	↓	↑	↑ (tamponade) or ↓ (pulmonary embolism)	↓	Tamponade, pulmonary embolism, tension pneumothorax.

[a] $S\bar{v}O_2$ = mixed venous arterial saturation.

- **Central venous catheter:** Use in the superior vena cava can provide an estimate of right heart filling pressures.
- **Pulmonary artery catheter:** Can help measure cardiac output, pulmonary capillary occlusion pressure (PCOP), and $S\bar{v}O_2$ and help calculate SVR to differentiate the type of shock. However, controversy exists over the use of pulmonary artery catheters in this setting, as they have not been shown to improve patient outcomes.
- **Echocardiography:** Useful for distinguishing poor cardiac function from hypovolemia; can also confirm pericardial tamponade or significant pulmonary hypertension.

Treatment

Regardless of cause, treatment should focus on resuscitation and improving end-organ perfusion.

Adrenal insufficiency and severe hypothyroidism or hyperthyroidism may present clinically as shock.

- Aggressive IV fluid hydration should be given to patients with hypovolemic or distributive shock. Blood products should be given in cases of trauma or acute bleeding.
- Broad-spectrum antibiotics should be given empirically if infection is suspected. If a patient remains in shock despite restoration of intravascular volume, vasoactive drugs such as dopamine, norepinephrine, phenylephrine, and vasopressin should be considered.

SEPSIS

A clinical syndrome associated with severe infection that arises from systemic inflammation and uncontrolled release of proinflammatory mediators, leading to extensive tissue injury. Despite improvements in antibiotics and advances in critical care, mortality and morbidity remain high. Sepsis can be viewed as a spectrum of disease that includes systemic inflammatory response syndrome (SIRS), sepsis, severe sepsis, and septic shock. These conditions within the continuum of sepsis are defined in Table 4-6.

Symptoms/Exam

Patients in the early phases of sepsis are often anxious, febrile, tachycardic, and tachypneic. The physical exam is variable and may initially demonstrate

TABLE 4-6. Conditions Associated with Sepsis

Condition	Definition
SIRS	Clinical syndrome recognized by the presence of two or more of the following: ▪ Temperature > 38°C or < 36°C ▪ HR > 90 bpm ▪ RR > 20 breaths per minute or $Paco_2$ < 32 mmHg ▪ WBC > 12,000 cells/mm^3, < 4000 cells/mm^3, or > 10% bands
Sepsis	SIRS with definitive evidence of infection.
Severe sepsis	Sepsis with organ dysfunction and hypoperfusion.
Septic shock	Sepsis with hypotension despite adequate fluid resuscitation combined with altered mental status, oliguria, and/or lactic acidosis.

bounding pulses, warm extremities, and rapid capillary refill in the patient with SIRS. However, signs may progress to showing weak pulses, cool extremities, and slow capillary refill in patients with severe sepsis and septic shock.

DIFFERENTIAL

Cardiogenic, obstructive, or hypovolemic shock; fulminant hepatic failure; drug overdose; adrenal insufficiency; pancreatitis.

DIAGNOSIS/TREATMENT

- Always obtain appropriate cultures before initiating antibiotic therapy These should include the following:
  - At least two sets of blood cultures, with at least one drawn percutaneously.
  - Cultures of other sites, including urine, CSF, wounds, respiratory secretions, or other body fluids, as indicated by the clinical situation.
- IV antibiotic therapy should be initiated within the first hour of severe sepsis and should adhere to the following criteria:
  - Include at least one drug that penetrates into the suspected source of sepsis.
  - Be reassessed after 48–72 hours on the basis of clinical and microbiological information.
  - Continue for 7–10 days, guided by clinical response once a pathogen is identified.
  - Include combination therapy for *Pseudomonas* infection in neutropenic patients.
- Initial resuscitation should begin as soon as the syndrome is recognized. During the first six hours of resuscitation, goals should include the following:
  - **Central venous pressure (CVP):** 8–12 mmHg.
  - **Mean arterial pressure (MAP):** > 65 mmHg.
  - **Urine output:** ≥ 0.5 mL/kg/hour.
  - **Central venous or mixed venous saturation:** ≥ 70%.
- Start vasopressors if no sustained response is seen to fluid challenge.
  - Norepinephrine and dopamine are first-line agents.
  - Vasopressin may be considered after failure of fluids and conventional vasopressors.
  - Treatment should be guided by the placement of an arterial catheter in most patients.
  - Treatment should **not** include low-dose dopamine for renal protection.
- Recombinant human activated protein C is recommended for patients with a high risk of death and with no absolute contraindication related to bleeding.

FEVER IN THE ICU

Fever is a common problem in the ICU and is defined as a temperature of > 38.3°C (≥ 101°F). Accurate and reproducible measurements are necessary to detect disease. Mixed venous blood in the pulmonary artery is the ideal site for measuring core body temperature. Ear thermometry is reproducible and is usually only a few tenths of a degree below core body temperature. Oral and axillary measurements are not recommended. A systematic and comprehensive diagnostic approach is necessary, as both infectious and noninfectious sources are common causes of fever in the ICU.

Noninfectious causes of fever in the ICU—

PAID WOMAN

Pancreatitis/**P**ulmonary embolism
Adrenal insufficiency
Ischemic bowel
Drug reaction/**D**VT
Withdrawal
Other
Myocardial infarction
Acalculous cholecystitis
Neoplasm

Infectious causes of fever in the ICU—

VW CARS

Ventilator-associated pneumonia
Wound infection
C. *difficile* colitis
Abdominal abscess
Related to catheter
Sepsis/**S**inusitis

SYMPTOMS/EXAM

Patients in the ICU often cannot describe symptoms because of invasive devices and sedation. The patient's medical history and medications should thus be carefully reviewed. A thorough examination should follow, with particular attention paid to assessment of the sinuses, heart, lungs, skin, and intravascular device sites.

DIFFERENTIAL

The etiologies of fever in the ICU are given in the mnemonics **PAID WOMAN** and **VW CARS.**

DIAGNOSIS/TREATMENT

- Obtain blood cultures as well as other cultures (wound, urine, stool).
- If an obvious source of infection is identified, appropriate antibiotics should be started. If there is no obvious source of infection and fever is ≤ 39°C (≤ 102°F), evaluate for the noninfectious causes listed above. If fever > 39°C (> 102°F), remove old central lines and culture the catheter tip at the same time as a peripheral blood culture.
- An NG tube should be removed and replaced with an orogastric tube, and a CXR should be reviewed for any new infiltrates. Empiric antibiotics are warranted if fever persists.
- If fever continues despite empiric, broad-spectrum antibiotics, consider abdominal imaging and antifungal coverage.

CHAPTER 5

Dermatology

Siegrid Yu, MD

COMMON SKIN DISORDERS

Acne

Due to excess sebum, abnormal follicular keratinization, and proliferation of *Propionibacterium acnes.* Medications that exacerbate acne include glucocorticoids, anabolic steroids, lithium, some antiepileptics, OCPs with androgenic potential, and iodides. **Dietary factors do not play a significant role.**

Isotretinoin is teratogenic and is contraindicated in pregnancy. Side effects include dry skin, cheilitis, transaminase elevation, and hypertriglyceridemia. Depression has also been associated with isotretinoin use.

SYMPTOMS/EXAM

Noninflammatory comedones ("blackheads and whiteheads") and **inflammatory** papules, pustules, or nodules.

TREATMENT

Three-pronged treatment:

- **Decrease sebum:** Antiandrogens, spironolactone, isotretinoin.
- **Regulate follicular keratinization:** Topical retinoids.
- **Treatment of *P. acnes* and inflammation:** Antibiotics (topical and systemic) and benzoyl peroxide.

Rosacea

A chronic inflammatory **facial** disorder affecting middle-aged to older adults.

In recalcitrant cases of acne, signs such as hirsutism and irregular menses may point to possible endocrine disorders (congenital adrenal hyperplasia, polycystic ovarian syndrome, Cushing's disease).

SYMPTOMS

- Presents with episodic flushing and facial erythema.
- **Triggers** include hot liquids, spicy food, alcohol, sun, and heat.

EXAM

- **No comedones are seen.** Exam reveals erythematous papules and pustules and telangiectasias.
- Symmetric **central facial** involvement (malar cheeks, nose, chin, forehead).
- **Rhinophyma** is most often seen in men with long-standing disease (see Figure 5-1).
- Red eyes may result from blepharitis, keratitis, conjunctivitis, and episcleritis.

Facial steroid creams may cause a dermatitis that resembles rosacea.

TREATMENT

- Avoid triggers.
- **Topical** therapy (metronidazole gel or cream; sodium sulfacetamide lotion).
- Give **systemic antibiotics** when there is ocular involvement or if topical therapy is ineffective.
- Oral isotretinoin for severe disease.

Seborrheic Dermatitis

Disease associations include **AIDS, Parkinson's,** and **stroke.** Also seen in acutely ill patients. Inflammatory reaction to *Malassezia furfur* yeast.

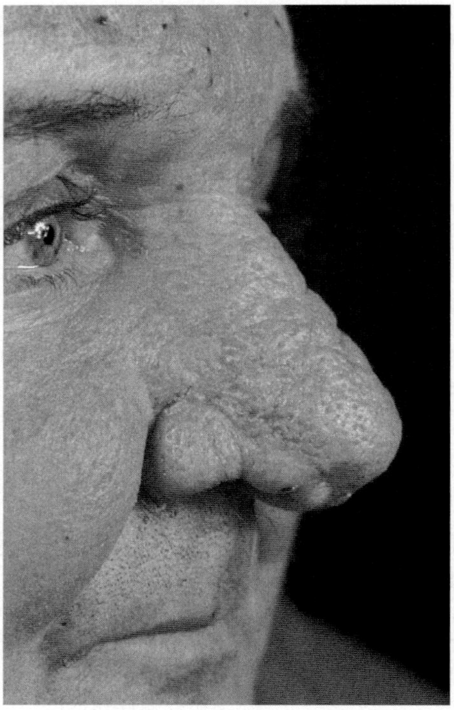

FIGURE 5-1. Rosacea with rhinophyma—erythema, edema, and telangiectasias on the nose.

(Reproduced, with permission, from Wolff K, Johnson RA, Suurmond D. *Fitzpatrick's Color Atlas and Synopsis of Clinical Dermatology*, 5th ed. New York: McGraw-Hill, 2005:11.)

SYMPTOMS/EXAM

- Exam reveals dry or "greasy," yellow, sharply demarcated scales on an erythematous base.
- Crusts and fissures with bacterial superinfection may be seen.
- Usually localized to the **scalp, postauricular region, central facial** (especially eyebrows and nasolabial folds), and flexural areas.

TREATMENT

- **Scalp:**
  - Shampoos containing tar, zinc pyrithione, or selenium.
  - Ketoconazole 2% shampoo lathered on the scalp, face, and back.
  - Topical steroids for more resistant disease.
- **Face:** Mild intermittent topical steroids +/– ketoconazole 2% cream.
- **Intertriginous areas:** Low-potency steroid lotions or creams +/– ketoconazole 2% cream.

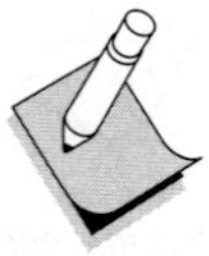

Severe, recalcitrant seborrheic dermatitis may be a clue pointing to underlying HIV infection. To prevent medication-related complications, high-potency topical steroids should not be used on the face or groin.

Psoriasis

An immune-mediated (possibly T-cell-based) inflammatory disease with a genetic predisposition and characterized by a bimodal peak incidence at 22 and 55 years of age. Has variable clinical presentations:

- **Localized plaque type:** Most common.
- **Guttate ("droplike"):** Occurs in young adults following strep throat.
- **Generalized pustular or erythrodermic:** Rare life-threatening variants.

Symptoms

- Usually asymptomatic, although **itching** may be present.
- **Koebner's phenomenon** may be seen when psoriatic lesions are induced at sites of injury or irritation to normal skin.
- **Triggers** include trauma, stress, and **medications** (lithium, β-blockers, prednisone taper, antimalarials, NSAIDs).
- A severe form is seen in **HIV** infection.

Exam

- Exam reveals sharply demarcated, erythematous plaques with **silvery-white scales** (see Figure 5-2).
- **Nail pitting** (fine "ice-pick" stippling) is also seen.
- Bilateral, often symmetric involvement of the extensor surfaces (elbows, knees), scalp, palms, and soles.
- The **inverse variant** involves the flexural surfaces (axillae, groin).

Diagnosis

- Diagnosed by clinical findings; biopsy is rarely performed.
- In guttate psoriasis, consider ASO titer and/or throat culture for group A β-hemolytic streptococcal infection.

Treatment

- **Limited disease (< 30% of body surface area):** Potent topical steroids, vitamin D analog (calcipotriene), topical retinoids, coal tar, anthralin.

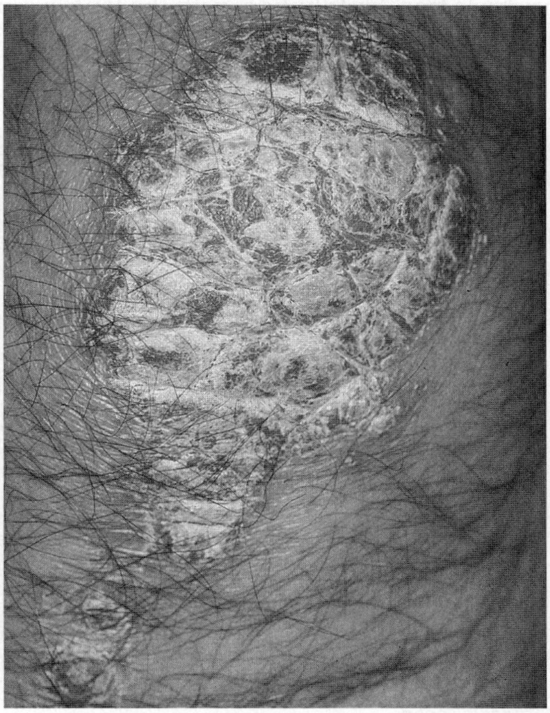

FIGURE 5-2. Psoriasis vulgaris (elbow).

A well-demarcated erythematous plaque is seen with a thick white scale. (Reproduced, with permission, from Wolff K, Johnson RA, Suurmond D. *Fitzpatrick's Color Atlas and Synopsis of Clinical Dermatology*, 5th ed. New York: McGraw-Hill, 2005:57.) (Also see Color Insert.)

Systemic steroids are contraindicated in the treatment of psoriasis owing to the risk of inducing pustular psoriasis and severe disease rebound upon withdrawal of medication.

- **Generalized disease (> 30% of body surface area):** UVB light, oral retinoids, PUVA (psoralen and UVA).
- **Refractory disease:** Methotrexate, cyclosporine, sulfasalazine, biologics (e.g., alefacept, efalizumab, etanercept).
- **Guttate psoriasis:** Penicillin VK or erythromycin to treat strep throat.
- Day treatment with crude coal tar and UVB is associated with disease remission in > 80% of cases.

COMPLICATIONS

Psoriatic arthritis (< 10%), especially affecting the **DIP joints** of the hands, and **sacroiliitis.**

Pityriasis Rosea

Occurs most often in young adult **females.** Human herpesvirus 7 (HHV-7) may be a causative agent.

SYMPTOMS

- Presents with mild pruritus.
- A larger **"herald patch"** often precedes the generalized trunk eruption by 1–2 weeks.

EXAM

- Exam reveals dull pink plaques (up to 2 cm in diameter) with a "cigarette paper" appearance, a silver **collarette of scale,** and a well-demarcated erythematous base (see Figure 5-3).
- Shows a **"Christmas tree"** distribution, with the long axis of lesions following lines of cleavage.

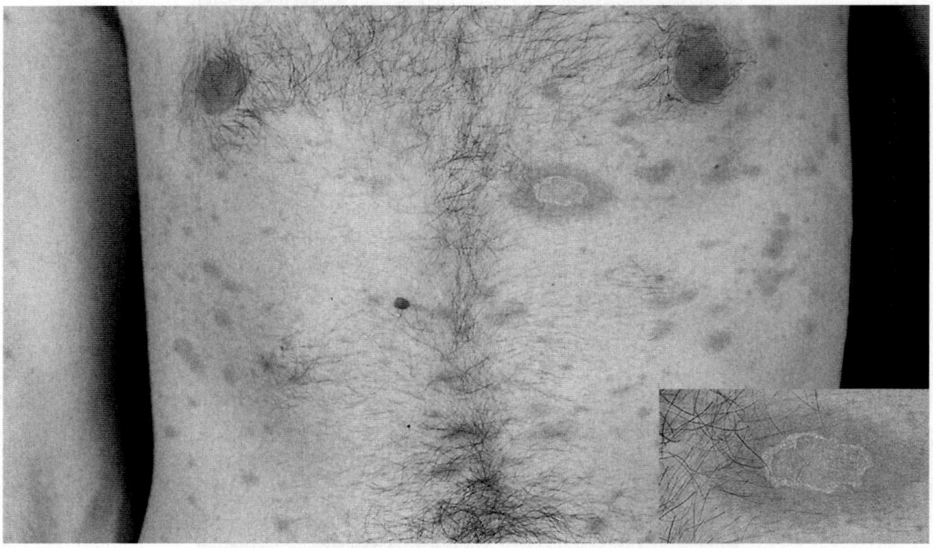

FIGURE 5-3. Pityriasis rosea.

Pink plaques with an oval configuration are seen that follow the lines of cleavage. Inset: Herald patch. The collarette of scale is more obvious on this magnification. (Reproduced, with permission, from Wolff K, Johnson RA, Suurmond D. *Fitzpatrick's Color Atlas and Synopsis of Clinical Dermatology,* 5th ed. New York: McGraw-Hill, 2005:119.) (Also see Color Insert.)

- Involves the trunk and proximal extremities; **spares the face.**
- An inverse pattern involving the axilla and groin may also be seen.

TREATMENT

A **self-limited** illness with spontaneous resolution within about two months.

CUTANEOUS INFECTIONS

Impetigo

A superficial infection of the epidermis that is **contagious** and **autoinoculable**; caused by *Staphylococcus*, group A streptococcus, or both. Infection may occur as a primary event or as a secondary superinfection of an underlying dermatitis.

SYMPTOMS/EXAM

- Primary lesions are vesicles or pustules, most often affecting the **face.**
- Vesicles or pustules rupture, forming erosions with an overlying **honey-colored crust.**

Bullous impetigo is usually caused by S. aureus.

DIAGNOSIS

Gram stain and culture can confirm clinical suspicion if the diagnosis is in doubt.

TREATMENT

- Mupirocin ointment for limited disease.
- Systemic antibiotics for more severe involvement.

Recurrent impetigo suggests S. aureus *nasal carriage. Treat with either oral rifampin in combination with another antistaphylococcal antibiotic or intranasal mupirocin.*

COMPLICATIONS

Most cases resolve without scarring. When left untreated, lesions can progress to deeper infections and even sepsis.

Erysipelas

Acute cellulitis usually affecting the **central face; due to** β-hemolytic streptococci. Elderly and immunocompromised patients are at greater risk than the general population.

SYMPTOMS

- Patients are **systemically ill** with fevers, chills, and malaise.
- Lesions are hot, painful, and **rapidly advancing.**

EXAM

Exam reveals **brightly erythematous,** smooth, indurated edematous plaques with raised, **sharply demarcated** margins.

TREATMENT

Prompt administration of **IV antibiotics** with activity against β-hemolytic streptococci.

COMPLICATIONS

If the condition is left untreated, bacteremia and sepsis may develop.

Anthrax

Caused by *Bacillus anthracis*, a gram-positive, spore-forming aerobic rod; transmitted through the skin or mucous membranes or by inhalation via contaminated soil, animals, animal products, or **biological warfare.** Some **95% of anthrax cases worldwide are cutaneous.**

Symptoms

- Three clinical manifestations—cutaneous, GI, and pulmonary (woolsorters' disease).
- A two- to seven-day incubation period is followed by the development of characteristically evolving lesions (see below).
- Presents with fever, malaise, headache, nausea, and vomiting.

Exam

- The primary lesion is a small, erythematous macule that evolves into a papule with **vesicles,** significant erythema, and **edema.**
- One to three days later, the papule ulcerates, leaving the characteristic **necrotic eschar.**
- **No pain or tenderness.**
- Suppurative regional adenopathy may develop.

Diagnosis

The causative organism is identified by smear (gram-positive encapsulated rods) or culture.

Treatment

- **IV penicillin G** is standard therapy.
- Oral tetracycline may be effective for mild, localized cutaneous disease.
- Aminoglycosides, macrolides, or quinolones are second-line agents in penicillin-allergic patients.
- Most cutaneous cases resolve spontaneously without significant sequelae, but 10–20% of untreated cutaneous cases may result in death.

Dermatophytid (id reaction) is a hypersensitivity reaction to a tinea infection on a distant body site (e.g., a patient with tinea pedis develops pruritic vesicles on the hands).

Dermatophytosis (Tinea) and Id Reaction

A superficial fungal infection of the skin, hair follicles, and nails that is transmitted from person to person via **fomites.** Scalp infection is seen mainly in children. Predisposing factors include atopic dermatitis, immunosuppression, sweating, and occlusion.

Symptoms/Exam

- **Tinea pedis:** Presents with dry scales, maceration, and/or fissuring of the web spaces; scaling in a "moccasin" or "ballet slipper" distribution; and vesicles and bullae.
- **Tinea cruris (groin):** Erythematous, well-demarcated plaques are seen with **clear centers** and active, advancing, scaly, **sharp borders.**

A tinea patient with pain suggests a secondary bacterial infection.

Diagnosis

KOH +/– fungal culture of skin scraping to identify hyphae.

TREATMENT

- Maintain good hygiene; keep affected areas dry.
- Topical antifungals; oral antifungals in refractory cases.
- **Topical therapy is usually ineffective for onychomycosis,** and the risk and benefits of oral antifungal therapy should be considered.
- Griseofulvin is the treatment of choice for tinea capitis.

COMPLICATIONS

Maceration and fissuring of skin may provide a portal of entry for bacteria, resulting in **cellulitis.**

Tinea pedis affecting the web spaces is the most common cause of cellulitis in otherwise healthy patients.

Tinea Versicolor

A mild infection caused by a nondermatophyte fungus (***Pityrosporum ovale***), facilitated by high humidity and sebum production.

SYMPTOMS/EXAM

- Exam reveals numerous round or oval, sharply demarcated macules that may be tan, brown, pink, or white.
- Scales are subtle.

DIAGNOSIS

KOH of skin scraping to identify hyphae and budding spores (**"spaghetti and meatballs"** appearance).

TREATMENT

- Selenium sulfide lotion or ketoconazole shampoo lathered on the scalp and affected areas of the trunk.
- **A single oral dose of ketoconazole 400 mg results in short-term cure in 90% of cases.**

Candidiasis

Risk factors include DM, obesity, sweating, heat, maceration, systemic and topical steroids, and chronic debilitation; antibiotics and OCP use may also be contributory.

SYMPTOMS/EXAM

- Favors moist intertriginous areas.
- Initial vesiculopustules enlarge and rupture, becoming eroded and confluent.
- **Brightly erythematous,** sharply demarcated plaques are seen with scalloped borders (see Figure 5-4).
- **Satellite lesions** (pustular lesions at the periphery) may coalesce and extend into larger lesions.

DIAGNOSIS

Usually a clinical diagnosis, supported by KOH with pseudohyphae and yeast forms or culture.

TREATMENT

- Keep affected areas dry.
- Topical antifungals are highly effective.

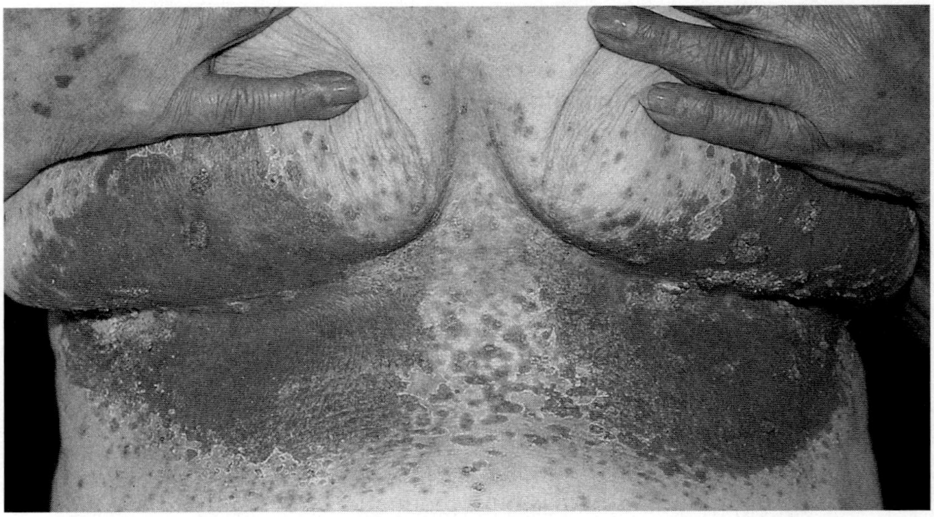

FIGURE 5-4. Cutaneous candidiasis—intertrigo.

Small peripheral satellite papules and pustules coalesce to create a large eroded area in the submammary region. (Reproduced, with permission, from Wolff K, Johnson RA, Suurmond D. *Fitzpatrick's Color Atlas and Synopsis of Clinical Dermatology*, 5th ed. New York: McGraw-Hill, 2005:719.) (Also see Color Insert.)

Herpes Simplex (HSV)

HSV-2 infection accounts for the majority of genital herpes lesions.

HSV-1 and HSV-2 are double-stranded DNA viruses with the ability to invade, remain latent, and then replicate within the nerve cell ganglia. Morbidity results from recurrent outbreaks. Transmission occurs through direct contact with mucosal surfaces. **Asymptomatic viral shedding** occurs in 60–80% of infected patients.

Symptoms/Exam

Presents with small, grouped vesicles on an erythematous base that crust, most commonly affecting the vermilion border of the lips, the genitals, and the buttocks.

The first outbreak of HSV is generally the most painful.

Diagnosis

Direct fluorescent antibody, viral culture, PCR, or evidence of viropathic changes on biopsy.

Treatment

Topical antivirals are ineffective in treating HSV infections.

- Lesions spontaneously heal within one week.
- Immediate treatment with oral antiviral agents may reduce the duration of the outbreak by 12–24 hours.
- Suppressive treatment should be considered in patients with frequent or severe outbreaks; such treatment can reduce outbreaks by 85% and viral shedding by 90%.
- Potent topical steroids reduce the pain, duration, and size of orolabial lesions.
- Immunosuppressed patients may require parenteral acyclovir.

Complications

- Disseminated cutaneous disease in patients with underlying dermatitis (**eczema herpeticum**).
- Immunosuppressed patients are at risk for potentially life-threatening **systemic disease** involving the lungs, liver, and CNS.

Patients with atopic dermatitis are at risk for eczema herpeticum, a diffuse HSV superinfection.

Herpes Zoster

Varicella-zoster virus (VZV) is the agent of the primary infection **varicella** (chickenpox) as well as for its reactivation in the form of **herpes zoster** (shingles). The risk of zoster increases with age and is also greater in immunosuppressed adults (HIV infection and malignancy).

Disseminated zoster or zoster in apparently healthy patients < 40 years of age should raise the suspicion of HIV disease.

Symptoms

Unilateral **dermatomal pain** followed by skin lesions.

The pain of zoster may precede skin lesions by several days and may mimic that of angina, pleurisy, cholecystitis, appendicitis, or hepatitis.

Exam

- Exam reveals clustered vesicular lesions, most commonly on the trunk or face (see Figure 5-5).
- The presence of > 25 lesions in noncontiguous dermatomes suggests disseminated zoster.
- Herpes zoster ophthalmicus accounts for approximately 7–10% of all zoster cases.

Vesicles on the nasal tip or side indicate nasociliary branch involvement (Hutchinson's sign) and should prompt referral to an ophthalmologist to exclude orbital involvement.

Diagnosis

Direct fluorescent antibody, viral culture, PCR, or evidence of viropathic changes on biopsy.

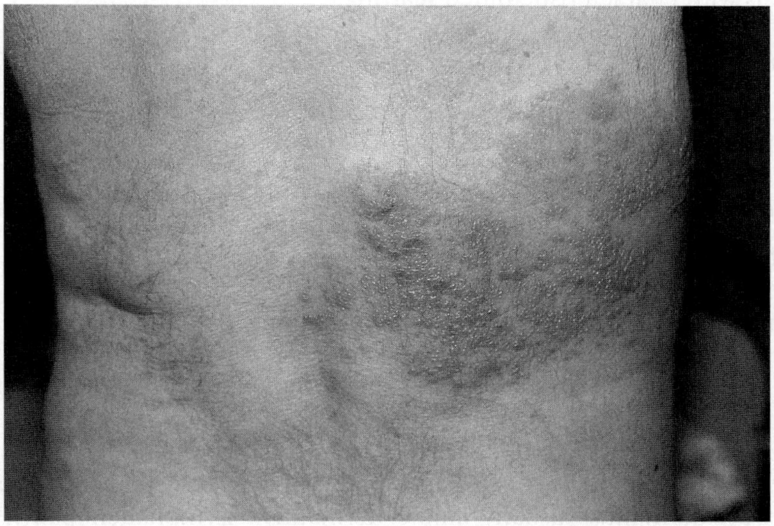

FIGURE 5-5. Varicella-zoster virus infection—herpes zoster in T8–T10 dermatomes.

Grouped vesicles and pustules are seen on a base of erythema and edema involving the posterior chest wall. (Reproduced, with permission, from Wolff K, Johnson RA, Suurmond D. *Fitzpatrick's Color Atlas and Synopsis of Clinical Dermatology*, 5th ed. New York: McGraw-Hill, 2005:823.)

Antiviral therapy within 72 hours may reduce the incidence and severity of PHN. This is especially important in the elderly, a population that is at increased risk for the development of this complication.

TREATMENT

- Antivirals (e.g., acyclovir) are most effective when started within 48 hours of onset.
- Treatment is always indicated in the presence of ocular involvement as well as for immunosuppressed and debilitated patients with extensive cutaneous involvement.

COMPLICATIONS

- **Postherpetic neuralgia (PHN):** Increased risk in the **elderly** and following **trigeminal** zoster.
- Treatment of shingles within 72 hours may reduce the incidence and severity of PHN.
- PHN treatment options include capsaicin, amitriptyline, gabapentin, and regional nerve blocks.

Smallpox

A DNA virus transmitted via viral implantation on the oropharyngeal or respiratory mucosa.

SYMPTOMS

- A 12-day incubation period is followed by the **sudden onset** of fever and malaise.
- A centrifugally spreading rash appears after the cessation of constitutional symptoms.

Patients with smallpox are infectious from the time of rash onset until all crusts have separated.

EXAM

- Erythematous macules evolve synchronously into vesicles and pustules.
- Lesions crust over in approximately two weeks, followed by separation of the crust.
- Heals with characteristic pitted scarring.

DIAGNOSIS

Electron microscopy (staining for poxvirus particles), PCR, IgM-specific antibody, or cell culture.

TREATMENT

- Antibiotics if secondary bacterial infection is suspected.
- **Vaccination is controversial.**
- Complications of **smallpox vaccination** include the following:
  - **Generalized vaccinia:** Infection with vaccinia virus 4–10 days after vaccination; characterized by disseminated papulovesicles that evolve into pustules. Can be due to autoinoculation upon contact with the vaccination site.
  - **Eczema vaccinatum:** Vaccinia virus superinfects the skin of patients with dermatitis (usually atopic dermatitis). Lymphadenopathy, fever, malaise, encephalitis, neurologic symptoms, and even death may occur on rare occasions.
- **High-risk conditions for vaccine-related complications** include **eczema** or exfoliative dermatitis, malignancies necessitating chemotherapy, HIV infection, hereditary immune deficiency disorders, and pregnancy.

- Vaccinia immune globulin may be used for the treatment of progressive vaccinia, eczema vaccinatum, severe generalized vaccinia, and periocular autoinoculation.

Smallpox patients become infectious as they develop dermatologic lesions. In smallpox, lesions are synchronous (all in the same stage), whereas in varicella, lesions are in various stages of development and healing.

COMPLICATIONS

- Corneal opacity and ulceration, arthritis and synovitis, pneumonitis, encephalitis.
- **The case fatality rate is 20–30%** and usually results from bacterial superinfection or severe inflammatory response.

Scabies

Skin infestation by the mite *Sarcoptes scabiei*. The female adult mite burrows and lays eggs in the stratum corneum. Highly **contagious;** spreads through prolonged contact with an infected host.

SYMPTOMS

- Presents with intense pruritus, especially at night.
- Itching and rash result from a delayed type IV hypersensitivity reaction to the mites, their eggs, or their feces, resulting in a two- to four-week delay between infection and onset of symptoms.
- Crusted (or "Norwegian") scabies occurs in immunocompromised and institutionalized patients.

EXAM

- Presents with small pruritic vesicles, pustules, and **burrows;** look in the **webbed spaces** of the fingers, volar wrists, elbows, **axillae,** belt line, feet, scrotum (in men), and areolae (in women).
- **The face is usually spared.**
- A generalized **hypersensitivity rash** may develop at distant sites.
- In crusted scabies, lesions are hyperkeratotic and crusted, covering large areas. Associated scalp lesions and nail dystrophy are also seen.

Itching and rash secondary to hypersensitivity reactions may persist for weeks or months despite effectively treated scabies infection.

DIAGNOSIS

Examine **skin scrapings** with light microscopy to identify mites, ova, or fecal pellets.

TREATMENT

- Apply **permethrin 5%** below the neck; leave on for eight hours and shower off. Treatment may be repeated in one week. Wash linens and clothing in hot water.
- **Ivermectin** may be needed to treat crusted scabies, conventional cases refractory to topical therapy, epidemics in institutions, or superinfected scabies.
- Other STDs should be excluded.

DERMATOLOGIC MANIFESTATIONS OF SYSTEMIC DISEASES

Cardiovascular

INFECTIVE ENDOCARDITIS

Dermatologic findings associated with infective endocarditis are outlined in Table 5-1.

TABLE 5-1. Dermatologic Manifestations of Infective Endocarditis

CLINICAL FINDINGS	CHARACTERISTICS
Petechiae	
Splinter hemorrhages	Subungual, dark red linear macules.
Roth's spots	Oval retinal hemorrhages with a clear, pale center.
Osler's nodes	Small, **tender,** violaceous papules on the pads of the digits (**O**sler = **O**uch).
Janeway lesions	Small, slightly papular, red/violaceous hemorrhages on the palmar and plantar surfaces. Most commonly seen in acute endocarditis.
Clubbing	
Peripheral emboli	

LIVEDO RETICULARIS

Obstruction of arteriolar flow from vasospasm, obstruction, hyperviscosity, or obstruction of venous outflow. May be **idiopathic** or due to numerous secondary causes; classic associations include atheroemboli (postangiography), hypercoagulable states including antiphospholipid antibody syndrome, SLE, and cryoglobulins.

SYMPTOMS/EXAM

- Symmetric; involves the extremities. More prominent with exposure to cold.
- Presents with mottled or **netlike bluish** (livid) discoloration of the skin (see Figure 5-6).

Livedo reticularis is a clinical reaction pattern resulting from vascular obstruction or hyperviscosity. Some cases are also drug induced.

DIAGNOSIS

Tests for underlying disease include CBC, cholesterol panel, coagulation studies, ANA, RF, and cryoglobulins.

TREATMENT

- Treat the underlying disease.
- Pentoxifylline 400 mg PO TID and low-dose aspirin may be helpful.

CHOLESTEROL EMBOLI

- The **kidneys and skin** are the most commonly affected organs.
- The **lower extremities** are more commonly affected than the upper extremities owing to atheroemboli from the abdominal aorta.
- Emboli may result from an intravascular procedure **(e.g., postangiography)** or may occur spontaneously.
- Skin findings include livedo reticularis, petechiae, purpura, and cyanotic digits.

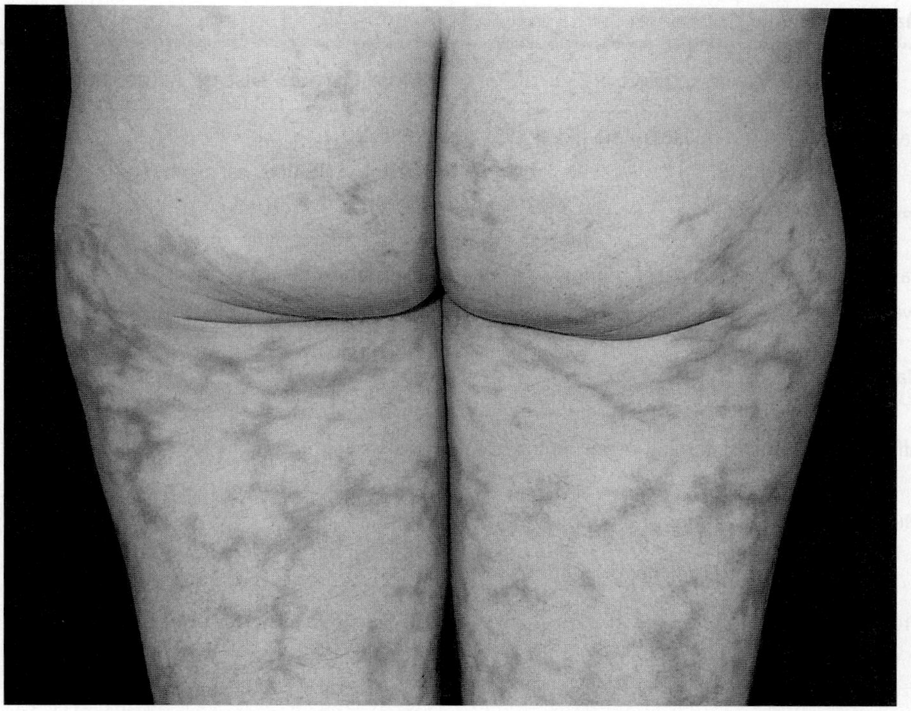

FIGURE 5-6. Symptomatic livedo reticularis.

A bluish, netlike, arborizing pattern is seen on the posterior thighs and buttocks and is defined by violaceous, erythematous streaks resembling lightning. (Reproduced, with permission, from Wolff K, Johnson RA, Suurmond D. *Fitzpatrick's Color Atlas and Synopsis of Clinical Dermatology*, 5th ed. New York: McGraw-Hill, 2005:381.) (Also see Color Insert.)

The prognosis of cryoglobulinemia is often guarded and is dependent on underlying disease.

Patients with oral lichen planus require regular follow-up, as the incidence of squamous cell carcinoma is increased by 5%.

Treatment for dermatitis herpetiformis consists of a gluten-free diet +/– dapsone.

Gastrointestinal

Table 5-2 outlines the dermatologic manifestations of common GI disorders, including porphyria cutanea tarda, cryoglobulinemia, lichen planus, and dermatitis herpetiformis.

Hematologic

Table 5-3 outlines the dermatologic manifestations of hematologic disorders.

Oncologic

Post-transplant Skin Malignancy

- Squamous cell carcinomas (SCCs) are more common than basal cell carcinomas (BCCs) in post-transplant patients.
- The incidence of malignancy increases with the duration of immunosuppressive therapy.

Transplant recipients should be regularly examined for skin cancers because such patients are at higher risk for such cancers.

Paraneoplastic Disease

Table 5-4 outlines the dermatologic manifestations of common paraneoplastic disorders.

TABLE 5-2. Dermatologic Manifestations of GI Disease

DISORDER	SKIN MANIFESTATIONS	MOST COMMON DISEASE ASSOCIATIONS
Porphyria cutanea tarda (see Figure 5-7)	Painless vesicles and bullae on the face and dorsa of the hands. Facial hypertrichosis.	HCV (85%). **Medications: NSAIDs, estrogens, tetracyclines.**
Cryoglobulinemia	Vasculitis of the skin (palpable purpura, livedo), kidneys, GI tract, and CNS.	**HCV, lymphoproliferative disorders (lymphoma, myeloma).**
Lichen planus (see Figure 5-8)	Flat-topped purple, polygonal, pruritic papules. Affect the flexor wrist, lumbar region, shins, and penis. Mucous membrane lesions are found in 40–50% of cases.	**Chronic HBV and HCV.** Primary biliary cirrhosis. Medications: streptomycin, tetracycline, NSAIDs, HCTZ, antimalarials.
Dermatitis herpetiformis (see Figure 5-9)	Pruritic, grouped blisters.	**Gluten-sensitive enteropathy, celiac disease.** Increased risk of GI lymphoma.
Pyoderma gangrenosum (see Figure 5-10)	Painful, rapidly advancing deep ulcer.	**Ulcerative colitis** > Crohn's disease.

TABLE 5-3. Dermatologic Manifestations of Hematologic Disease

DISORDER	SKIN MANIFESTATIONS	MOST COMMON DISEASE ASSOCIATIONS
Primary amyloidosis	**Blood vessel fragility leads to "raccoon eyes"** and **pinch purpura** (purpura due to mild trauma). **Macroglossia.**	**Multiple myeloma, Waldenström's macroglobulinemia.**
Secondary amyloidosis	Cutaneous signs are rare.	**Chronic inflammatory diseases:** ■ Rheumatoid arthritis (RA) ■ Leprosy, TB, osteomyelitis
Mastocytosis	Solitary **mastocytoma** or generalized urticaria. Positive **Darier's sign** (pruritus and wheal are elicited by stroking).	Symptoms include **urticaria, GI symptoms,** and **flushing.**

TABLE 5-4. Dermatologic Manifestations of Neoplastic Disease

DISORDER	SKIN MANIFESTATIONS	COMMONLY ASSOCIATED MALIGNANCY
Glucagonoma	Necrolytic migratory erythema; glossitis, angular cheilitis.	APUD cell tumors of the pancreas.
Dermatomyositis	Heliotrope rash, Gottron's papules (violaceous papules overlying finger joints); photodistributed eruption.	**Ovarian cancer; other solid tumors.**
Extramammary Paget's disease	Erythematous plaques with scales, erosion, and exudation. Affects the anogenital region.	Underlying vulvar or penile adenocarcinomas and regional internal malignancies.
Leukocytoclastic vasculitis	Small vessel vasculitis; palpable purpura.	Lymphoproliferative neoplasms; solid tumors.
Paraneoplastic pemphigus	Painful mucosal erosions. Pruritic; evolve into blisters.	**Non-Hodgkin's lymphoma.** Chronic lymphocytic leukemia.
Sign of Leser-Trélat	Abrupt eruption of numerous pruritic seborrheic keratoses.	**Adenocarcinomas** (60%), especially **gastric.**
Sweet's syndrome	Acute febrile **neutrophilic** dermatosis. Tender, rapidly expanding red plaque. Fever occurs in 50–80% of cases.	**Acute myeloid leukemia and lymphomas.** Also seen in RA.

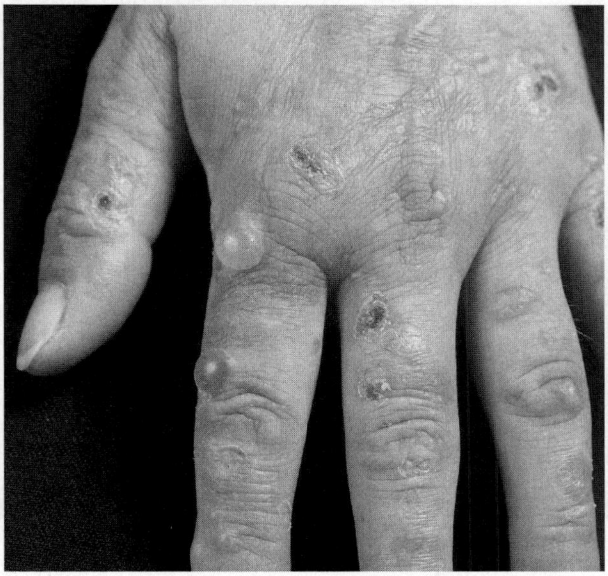

FIGURE 5-7. Porphyria cutanea tarda.

Bullae on the dorsum of the hand. (Reproduced, with permission, from Wolff K, Johnson RA, Suurmond D. *Fitzpatrick's Color Atlas and Synopsis of Clinical Dermatology*, 5th ed. New York: McGraw-Hill, 2005:247.) (Also see Color Insert.)

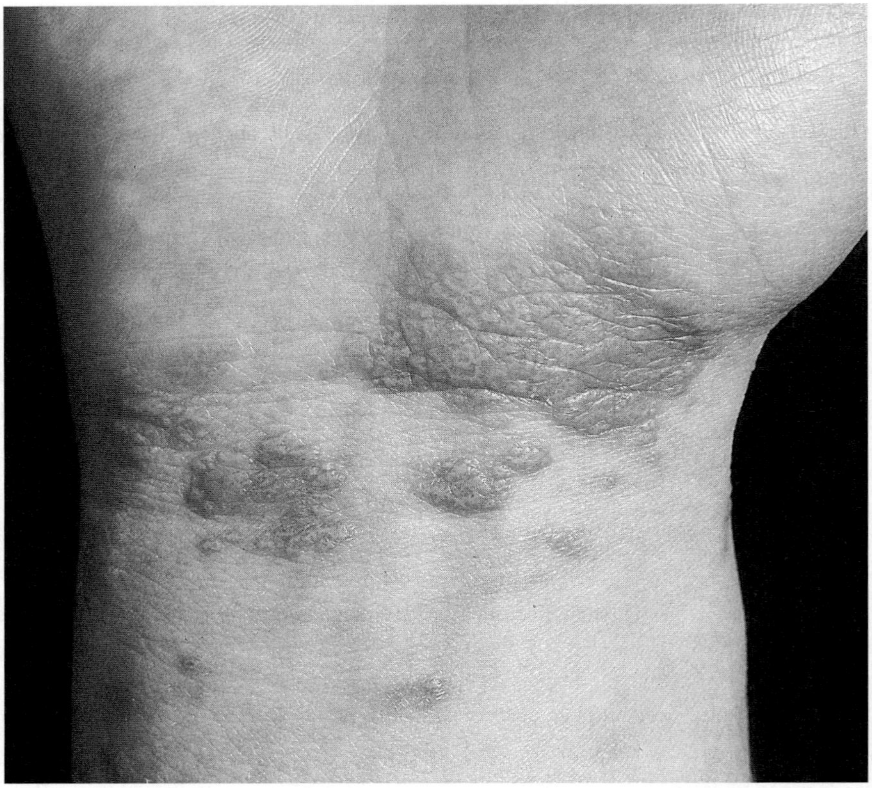

FIGURE 5-8. Lichen planus.

Flat-topped, polygonal, sharply defined, shiny violaceous papules. (Reproduced, with permission, from Wolff K, Johnson RA, Suurmond D. *Fitzpatrick's Color Atlas and Synopsis of Clinical Dermatology*, 5th ed. New York: McGraw-Hill, 2005:125.) (Also see Color Insert.)

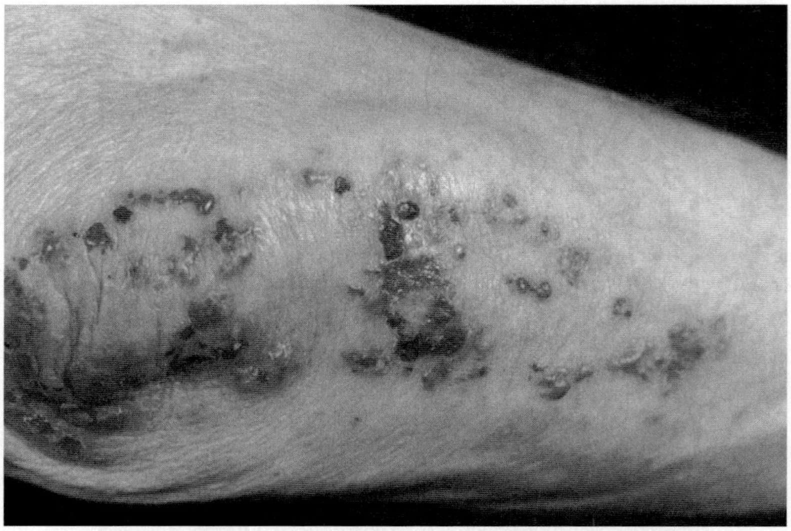

FIGURE 5-9. Dermatitis herpetiformis.

Grouped papules, crusts, and erosions primarily occurring on the elbows, knees, and sacral region. Primary lesions are often difficult to identify owing to intense pruritus and trauma from excoriation. (Reproduced, with permission, from Wolff K, Johnson RA, Suurmond D. *Fitzpatrick's Color Atlas and Synopsis of Clinical Dermatology*, 5th ed. New York: McGraw-Hill, 2005:111.)

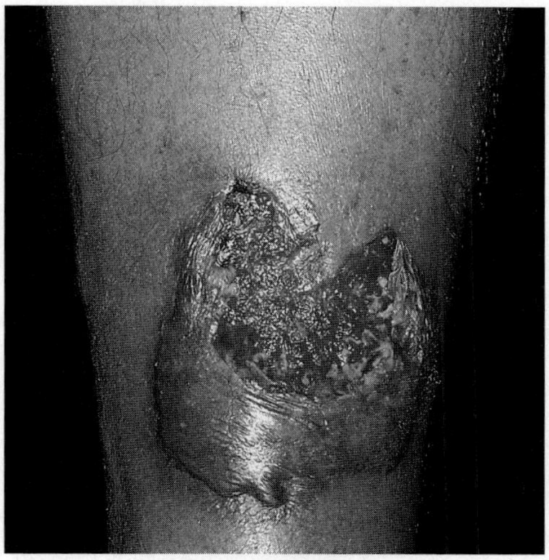

FIGURE 5-10. Pyoderma gangrenosum.

A painful ulcer with a dusky-red peripheral rim and an undermined border. (Reproduced, with permission, from Wolff K, Johnson RA, Suurmond D. *Fitzpatrick's Color Atlas and Synopsis of Clinical Dermatology*, 5th ed. New York: McGraw-Hill, 2005:153.) (Also see Color Insert.)

Endocrine and Metabolic

Table 5-5 outlines the dermatologic manifestations of endocrine and metabolic disorders.

Renal

Cutaneous signs associated with end-stage renal disease are as follows:

- Calcinosis cutis (metastatic)
- Calciphylaxis
- Ischemic ulcerations

TABLE 5-5. Dermatologic Manifestations of Endocrine and Metabolic Disease

Disorder	Skin Manifestations	Most Common Disease Associations
Acanthosis nigricans (see Figure 5-11)	Velvety, dirty hyperpigmentation; affects the axillae, groin, and neck. Insidious, asymptomatic.	**Insulin resistance:** DM, obesity, Cushing's disease. **Medications:** nicotinic acid, glucocorticoid therapy, OCPs, growth hormone therapy. **Paraneoplastic: gastric adenocarcinoma.**
Necrobiosis lipoidica	Waxy plaques with an elevated border. Affects the **lower legs** (> 80% pretibial). **Brownish**-red color; atrophic **yellow** center.	**DM.**
Xanthoma	Crops of small, discrete, **dome-shaped, yellow-orange papules.** Affects the eyelids and tendons (classically involving the Achilles tendon).	**Hyperlipidemia;** familial combined hypertriglyceridemia (triglyceride level > 1000 mg/dL).

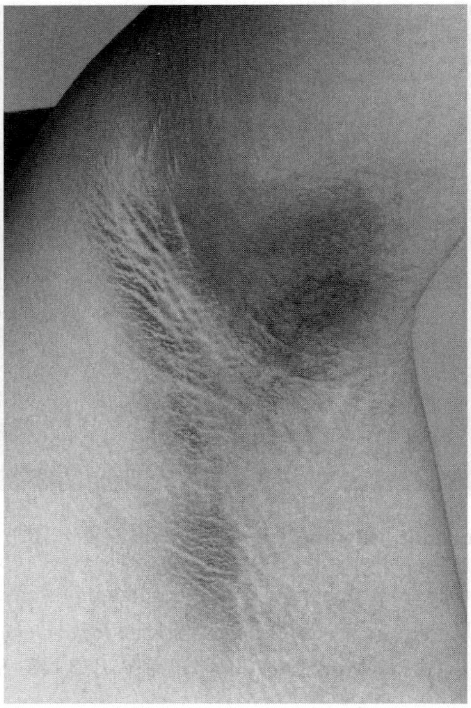

FIGURE 5-11. Acanthosis nigricans.

Velvety, dark-brown epidermal thickening of the neck. (Reproduced, with permission, from Wolff K, Johnson RA, Suurmond D. *Fitzpatrick's Color Atlas and Synopsis of Clinical Dermatology*, 5th ed. New York: McGraw-Hill, 2005:87.) (Also see Color Insert.)

- Lichen simplex chronicus
- Pigmentary alteration
- Porphyria cutanea tarda
- Prurigo nodularis
- Uremic frost
- Xanthomas
- Xerosis

HIV Disease

In HIV-infected patients, **seborrheic dermatitis** is the **most common** cutaneous condition, usually developing early and increasing in severity with decreasing CD4 count. Common skin disorders found in HIV-infected patients are listed in Table 5-6 and in the sections that follow. Table 5-7 outlines mucocutaneous findings commonly associated with HIV infection.

Kaposi's Sarcoma (KS)

A **vascular** neoplasm linked to infection with **HHV-8.** Often confused with skin lesions of *Bartonella* infection.

More than 90% of patients with pulmonary KS will have mucocutaneous KS. Inspect the skin and hard palate!

SYMPTOMS/EXAM

- Presents with asymptomatic mucocutaneous lesions that may bleed easily or ulcerate and cause pain.
- Less commonly involves the respiratory tract (nodules or hemoptysis) or the GI tract (GI bleed).

TABLE 5-6. Common Skin Disorders Found in HIV-Infected Patients

CD4 > 200	CD4 < 200	CD4 < 50
Seborrheic dermatitis Psoriasis Reiter's syndrome Atopic dermatitis Herpes zoster Acne rosacea Oral hairy leukoplakia (see Figure 5-12) Warts *S. aureus* folliculitis Mucocutaneous candidiasis KS	**Infection:** ■ Chronic HSV ■ Molluscum contagiosum ■ Bacillary angiomatosis ■ Systemic fungal infection ■ Mycobacterial infection ■ KS **Inflammatory:** ■ Eosinophilic folliculitis ■ Drug reactions ■ Photodermatitis ■ Prurigo nodularis	**Unusual opportunistic infections:** ■ Chronic HSV ■ Refractory molluscum contagiosum ■ Chronic VZV ■ Atypical mycobacteria ■ Crusted scabies ■ KS

DIAGNOSIS

Diagnose KS by skin biopsy.

TABLE 5-7. Mucocutaneous Findings Associated with HIV Infection

RISK FOR HIV INFECTION	MUCOCUTANEOUS FINDING
High—serotesting always indicated.	Acute retroviral syndrome KS Oral hairy leukoplakia Proximal subungual onychomycosis Bacillary angiomatosis Eosinophilic folliculitis Any STD Skin findings of injecting-drug use
Moderate—serotesting may be indicated.	Herpes zoster Molluscum contagiosum—multiple facial in an adult Candidiasis: oropharyngeal, esophageal, or recurrent vulvovaginal
Possible—serotesting may be indicated.	Generalized lymphadenopathy Seborrheic dermatitis Aphthous ulcers (recurrent, refractory to therapy)

Adapted, with permission, from Wolff K, Johnson RA, Suurmond D. *Fitzpatrick's Color Atlas and Synopsis of Clinical Dermatology,* 5th ed. New York: McGraw-Hill, 2005:937.

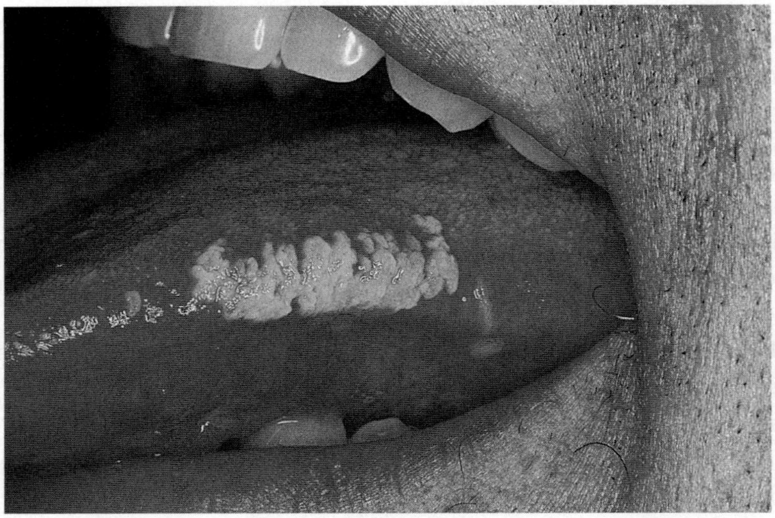

FIGURE 5-12. Oral hairy leukoplakia.

Corrugated white plaque on the lateral tongue. Essentially pathognomonic for HIV infection. (Reproduced, with permission, from Wolff K, Johnson RA, Suurmond D. *Fitzpatrick's Color Atlas and Synopsis of Clinical Dermatology*, 5th ed. New York: McGraw-Hill, 2005:943.) (Also see Color Insert.)

TREATMENT

- Highly active antiretroviral therapy (HAART).
- Local measures include intralesional chemotherapy, irradiation, laser surgery, and excision.

COMPLICATIONS

Larger or ulcerated lesions may bleed, cause functional disturbance, or obstruct lymphatic drainage.

Lipodystrophy is part of a metabolic syndrome that includes hyperlipidemia, insulin resistance, and type 2 DM.

HIV-ASSOCIATED LIPODYSTROPHY

Protease inhibitors are frequently implicated, most commonly **ritonavir/saquinavir,** followed by indinavir and nelfinavir. However, lipodystrophy can also occur in HIV-infected patients who are not on protease inhibitors.

SYMPTOMS/EXAM

- Facial and peripheral fat wasting (see Figure 5-13).
- Dorsothoracic fat pad hypertrophy (see Figure 5-14).
- Increased abdominal girth **(central adiposity)** secondary to accumulation of intra-abdominal fat.

Cutaneous signs of HIV-associated lipodystrophy should alert the physician to possible associated hyperlipidemia, insulin resistance, and type 2 DM.

TREATMENT

Substitution of a non–protease inhibitor may be beneficial.

COMPLICATIONS

Associated hyperlipidemia and impaired glucose tolerance lead to an increased risk of CAD.

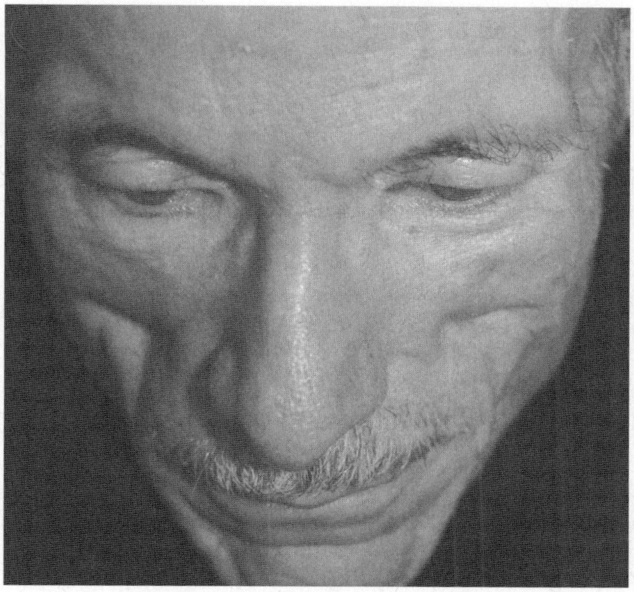

FIGURE 5-13. HIV-associated lipoatrophy.

Striking lipoatrophy of the midface. (Reproduced, with permission, from Wolff K, Johnson RA, Suurmond D. *Fitzpatrick's Color Atlas and Synopsis of Clinical Dermatology*, 5th ed. New York: McGraw-Hill, 2005:948.)

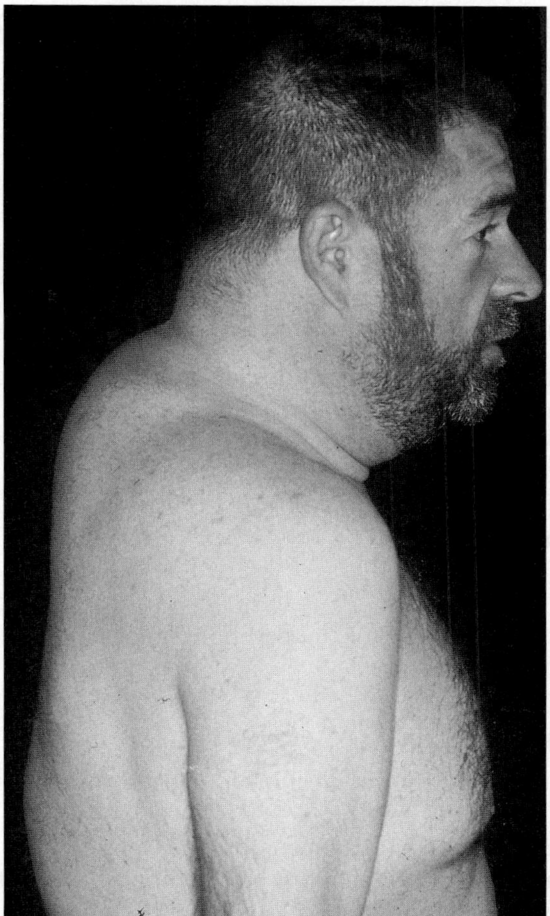

FIGURE 5-14. HIV-associated lipohypertrophy.

An increase in subcutaneous fat on the upper back creates a "buffalo hump." (Reproduced, with permission, from Wolff K, Johnson RA, Suurmond D. *Fitzpatrick's Color Atlas and Synopsis of Clinical Dermatology*, 5th ed. New York: McGraw-Hill, 2005:947.)

AUTOIMMUNE DISEASES WITH PROMINENT CUTANEOUS FEATURES

Table 5-8 lists the dermatologic manifestations of common autoimmune disorders, including SLE, dermatomyositis, and scleroderma.

Skin disease is the sole manifestation in 40% of cases of dermatomyositis.

CUTANEOUS REACTION PATTERNS

Table 5-9 outlines cutaneous reaction patterns, their signs and symptoms, and the diseases with which they are associated.

BLISTERING DISORDERS

Age-appropriate cancer screening and ovarian cancer screening are indicated for all adults with dermatomyositis.

Bullous pemphigoid and **pemphigus vulgaris** are **autoimmune blistering disorders** of the skin and mucous membranes resulting from the loss of epidermal cell-to-cell adhesion (see Table 5-10).

DIAGNOSIS

- Submit skin biopsy for histology and direct immunofluorescence.
- In bullous pemphigoid, indirect immunofluorescence reveals circulating anti–basement membrane antibodies in the sera of 70% of patients.

TREATMENT

Topical high-potency steroids for localized disease; prednisone +/– other immunosuppressants for diffuse disease.

CUTANEOUS DRUG REACTIONS

Dermatologic drug reactions include the following:

- **Hospital: Penicillins, sulfonamides,** and **blood products** account for nearly two-thirds of all cutaneous reactions.
- **Ambulatory setting: Antibiotics, NSAIDs, anticonvulsants.**
- Most frequent drug eruptions:
  - **Morbilliform** drug eruption (30–50% of cases).
  - **Fixed drug eruptions.**
  - **Urticaria** +/– angioedema.

See Tables 5-11 through 5-13 for the pathophysiology and clinical patterns of various drug eruptions.

DIAGNOSIS

- Clinical features favoring medication as a cause of drug reactions are as follows:
  - Previous experience with a given drug.
  - Lack of alternative explanations (worsening of preexisting disease, infection).

TABLE 5-8. Cutaneous Manifestations of Autoimmune Diseases

DISORDER	CUTANEOUS MANIFESTATIONS	SYSTEMIC ASSOCIATIONS
Systemic lupus erythematosus (SLE)	**Acute cutaneous** ■ Malar **("butterfly") rash** ■ Photodistribution **Other:** ■ Discoid plaques ■ Periungual telangiectasias ■ Alopecia ■ Lupus panniculitis	See Chapter 17 for details on the diagnosis and management of SLE.
Dermatomyositis (see Figure 5-15)	**Heliotrope rash** (violaceous rash over the eyelids) is nearly pathognomonic. **Gottron's papules** (flat-topped violaceous papules) over bony prominences, especially the MCP joints. **"Shawl sign"**: erythema over the upper back and chest.	**Increased risk of malignancy:** ■ Ovary ■ Other solid tumors: breast, lung, stomach, colon, uterus
Scleroderma (see Figures 5-16 and 5-17)	**Extremities:** ■ Raynaud's phenomenon ■ Sclerodactyly ■ Periungual telangiectasias ■ **Sclerosis** **Face:** ■ **Telangiectasias** ■ Masklike facies **Other:** ■ Cutaneous calcification	See Chapter 17 for a discussion of the systemic manifestations of scleroderma.
Morphea (localized scleroderma of unknown etiology)	Asymptomatic, with violaceous and then ivory-colored plaques.	Associated with *Borrelia burgdorferi* infection in Europe only and post–radiation therapy.

- **Timing:** Most drug reactions occur **within two weeks. Hypersensitivity reactions may be delayed up to eight weeks.**
- **Discontinuation:** Reaction should abate within three weeks.
- **Rechallenge:** Allows for a definitive diagnosis, although usually impractical.

■ **Drug levels:** Consider for dose-dependent reactions.
■ Skin biopsy is helpful in determining the reaction pattern but cannot identify the specific agent.
■ Peripheral **eosinophilia** is suggestive of drug sensitivity.

TABLE 5-9. Cutaneous Reaction Patterns and Their Associated Diseases

REACTION PATTERN	DEFINITION	SIGNS AND SYMPTOMS	ASSOCIATED DISEASES
Erythema nodosum	Inflammatory/immunologic reaction pattern of the panniculus.	**"Tender bumps on the anterior shins."** Appear as red, ill-defined erythemas but palpated as deep-seated nodules. Fever, malaise, arthralgias (50%).	**Infection:** ▪ Streptococcal ▪ TB ▪ Other bacteria, fungi, viruses **Medication:** ▪ Sulfonamides ▪ **OCPs** **Other:** ▪ **Sarcoidosis** (Lofgren's syndrome) ▪ Ulcerative colitis > Crohn's disease ▪ Leukemia ▪ Behçet's syndrome
Urticaria		Transient wheals, pruritus, dermatographism.	**Acute urticaria** (< 30 days): ▪ Arthropod bites ▪ Parasites ▪ **Medications** **Chronic urticaria** (> 30 days): ▪ **Idiopathic (80%)**
Erythema multiforme (EM) (see Figure 5-18)	Reaction pattern of dermal blood vessels and secondary epidermal changes.	**Target lesion:** ▪ Palms and soles, face, genitals ▪ Bilateral, symmetric **EM minor:** ▪ Little or no mucous membrane involvement ▪ No systemic symptoms **EM major:** ▪ Positive **Nikolsky's sign** ▪ Systemic: pulmonary, eyes	**Recurrent EM minor:** ▪ **HSV is the cause in 90% of cases** **EM major:** ▪ Medications: sulfonamides, NSAIDs, anticonvulsants (phenytoin) ▪ *Mycoplasma pneumoniae* **Idiopathic: 50%**

TABLE 5-10. Differential Diagnosis of Bullous Pemphigoid and Pemphigus Vulgaris

	BULLOUS PEMPHIGOID	PEMPHIGUS VULGARIS
Site of blistering	**Subepidermal.**	**Intraepidermal.**
Epidemiology	Age > 60. **Most common** autoimmune blistering disease.	Age 40–60.
Pruritus	Severe.	Not prominent.
Nikolsky's sign (superficial separation of skin with lateral pressure)	Negative.	Positive.
Oral mucosal lesions	Minority (< 30%).	Majority (> 50%).
Blisters and bullae	Intact, tense (see Figure 5-19).	Rupture easily; flaccid (see Figure 5-20)
Complications	Few.	Bacterial and viral **superinfection.** **High mortality if left untreated** owing to sepsis. Rare ocular involvement requires referral.
Systemic associations	None.	Rarely thymoma, myasthenia gravis.
Subtypes		**Drug induced** (penicillamine and ACEIs), **paraneoplastic.**

TREATMENT

The treatment of drug reactions is dependent on the cause.

CUTANEOUS ONCOLOGY

Atypical Nevi

Roughly 5–10% of individuals in the United States have one or more atypical nevi.

Patients with numerous atypical nevi (atypical nevus syndrome or dysplastic nevus syndrome) and two first-degree relatives with a history of melanoma have a lifetime risk of melanoma approaching 100%.

SYMPTOMS/EXAM

Lesions are > 6 mm with variegated hyperpigmentation and asymmetric, irregular, "fuzzy" borders (some with a "fried egg" appearance).

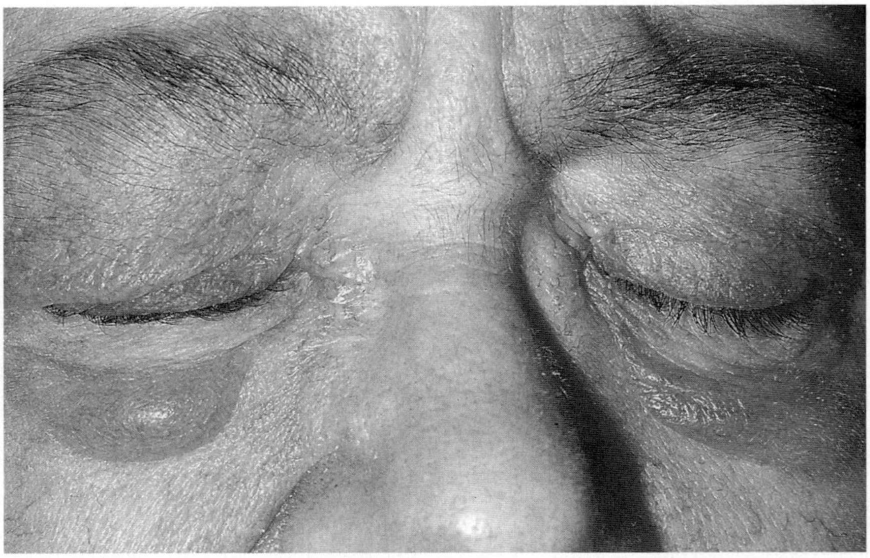

FIGURE 5-15. Dermatomyositis—heliotrope.

Violaceous (reddish-purple) rash and edema of the eyelids. (Reproduced, with permission, from Wolff K, Johnson RA, Suurmond D. *Fitzpatrick's Color Atlas and Synopsis of Clinical Dermatology*, 5th ed. New York: McGraw-Hill, 2005:373.) (Also see Color Insert.)

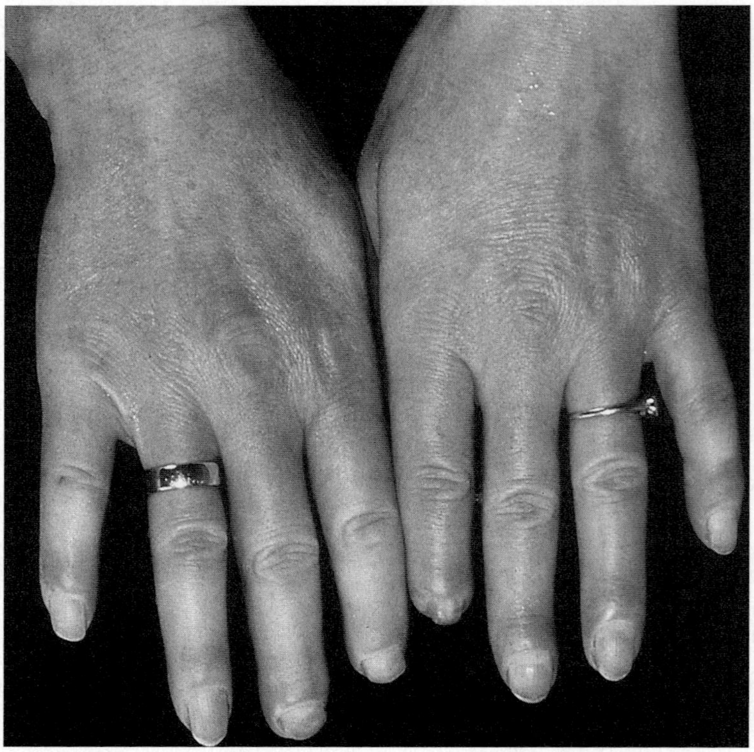

FIGURE 5-16. Scleroderma—Raynaud's phenomenon and acrosclerosis.

(Reproduced, with permission, from Wolff K, Johnson RA, Suurmond D. *Fitzpatrick's Color Atlas and Synopsis of Clinical Dermatology*, 5th ed. New York: McGraw-Hill, 2005:399.)

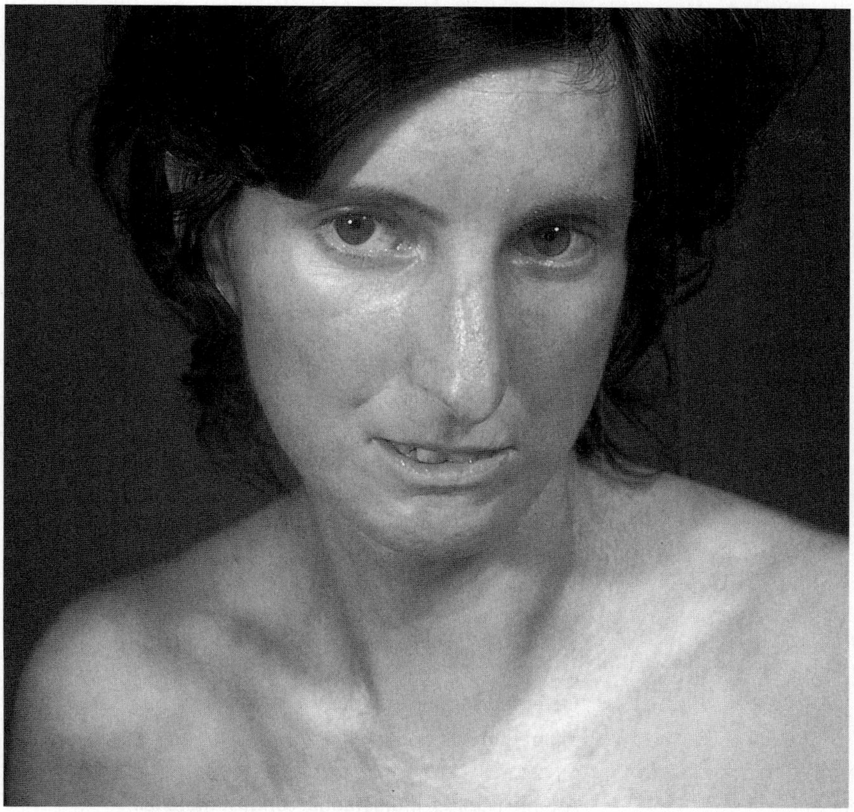

FIGURE 5-17. Scleroderma—masklike facies.

Stretched, shiny skin with loss of normal facial lines. (Reproduced, with permission, from Wolff K, Johnson RA, Suurmond D. *Fitzpatrick's Color Atlas and Synopsis of Clinical Dermatology*, 5th ed. New York: McGraw-Hill, 2005:400.) (Also see Color Insert.)

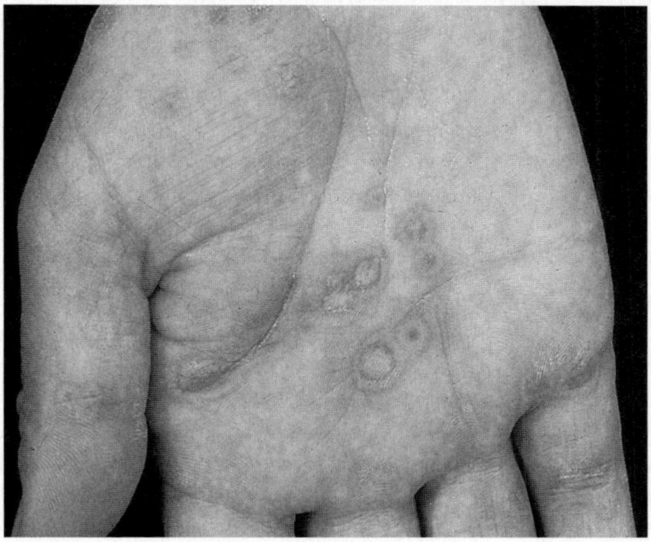

FIGURE 5-18. Erythema multiforme.

Targetoid lesions on the palms. (Reproduced, with permission, from Wolff K, Johnson RA, Suurmond D. *Fitzpatrick's Color Atlas and Synopsis of Clinical Dermatology*, 5th ed. New York: McGraw-Hill, 2005:141.) (Also see Color Insert.)

TABLE 5-11. Pathophysiologic Mechanisms of Drug Eruptions

Nonimmunologic Drug Reactions	
Mechanism	**Example**
Expected adverse effects	Chemotherapy-induced alopecia.
Ecologic disturbance	Candidiasis and antibiotics.
Overdosage	Warfarin purpura.
Drug interaction	Barbiturates and warfarin (purpura).
Cumulative	Argyria (silver nitrate), antimalarial pigmentation.
Idiosyncratic causes Altered metabolism Exacerbation of underlying disorder	Drug-induced lupus in response to procainamide in slow acetylators of *N*-acetyltransferase warfarin necrosis and lack of protein C. Lithium and psoriasis.
Phototoxic	Increased sensitivity to sun caused by toxic photoproducts of different drugs (tetracyclines).
Direct release of mast cell mediators	Aspirin, NSAIDs, radiographic contrast material.
Jarisch-Herxheimer phenomenon	Penicillin therapy for syphilis; antifungal therapy for dermatophyte.
Immunologic Drug Reactions	
Mechanism	**Example**
Type I: classic immediate hypersensitivity	Urticaria, angioedema, anaphylaxis.
Type III: immune complex	Leukocytoclastic vasculitis, serum sickness, urticaria, angioedema.
Type IV: delayed hypersensitivity	Contact dermatititis, exanthematous reactions, photoallergic reactions.
Systemic infection impairing immune response	Infectious mononucleosis: ampicillin-induced rash. HIV infection: sulfonamide-induced toxic epidermal necrolysis.
Unknown immunologic mechanisms	Lichenoid reactions, fixed drug eruption.

Adapted, with permission, from Kerdel FA, Jimenez-Acosta F. *Dermatology: Just the Facts.* New York: McGraw-Hill, 2003:36.

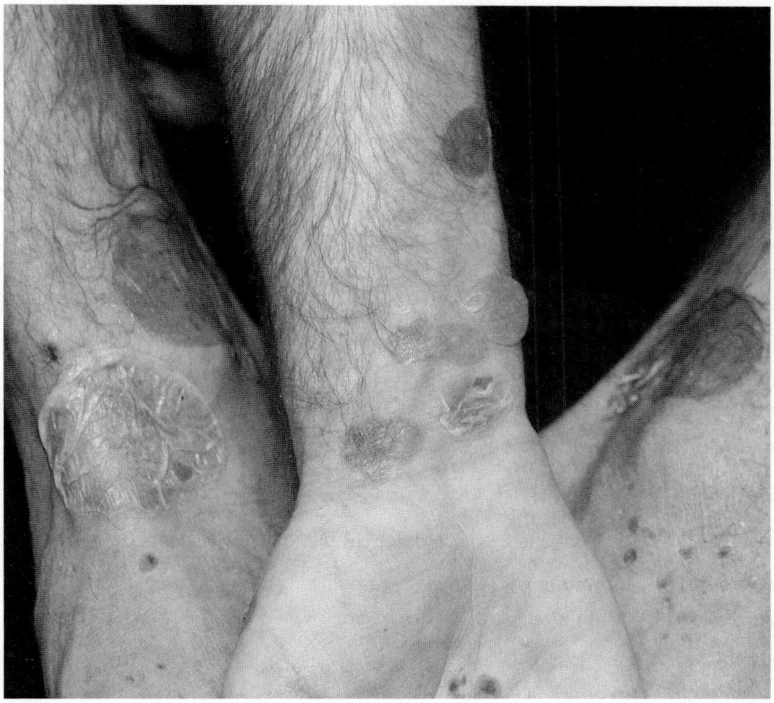

FIGURE 5-19. Bullous pemphigoid.

Tense bullae with serous fluid are seen in a patient with HIV infection. Postinflammatory pigmentary alteration is present at sites of prior lesions. (Reproduced, with permission, from Wolff K, Johnson RA, Suurmond D. *Fitzpatrick's Color Atlas and Synopsis of Clinical Dermatology*, 5th ed. New York: McGraw-Hill, 2005:108.) (Also see Color Insert.)

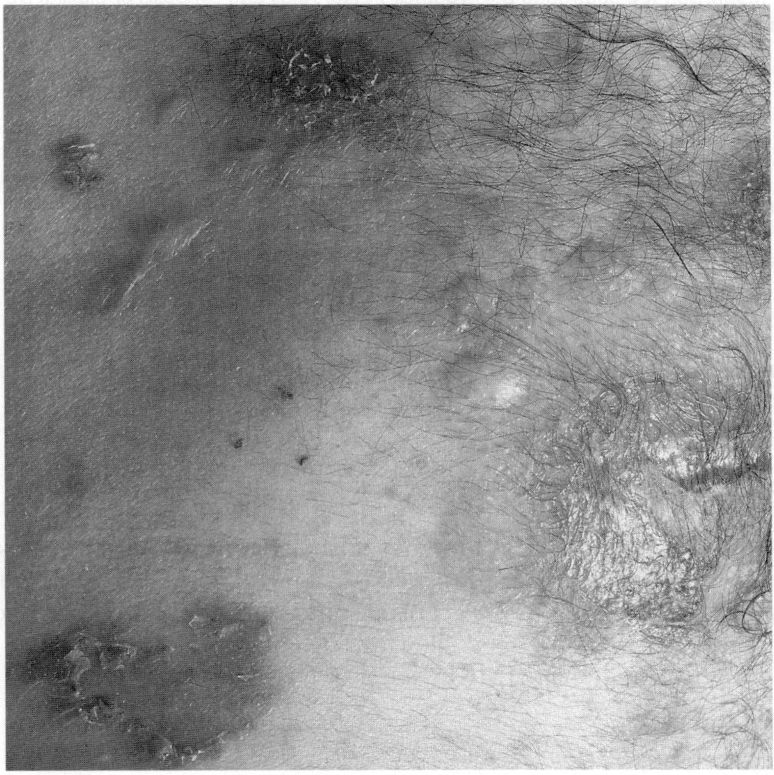

FIGURE 5-20. Pemphigus vulgaris.

Owing to the fragility of the blisters, pemphigus vulgaris presents as erosions. (Reproduced, with permission, from Wolff K, Johnson RA, Suurmond D. *Fitzpatrick's Color Atlas and Synopsis of Clinical Dermatology*, 5th ed. New York: McGraw-Hill, 2005:104.) (Also see Color Insert.)

TABLE 5-12. Immunologically Mediated Adverse Cutaneous Drug Reactions[a]

Type of Reaction	Pathogenesis	Examples of Causative Drug	Clinical Patterns
Type I	IgE mediated; immediate-type immunologic reactions.	Penicillin.	Urticaria/angioedema of skin/mucosa, edema of other organs, anaphylactic shock.
Type II	Drug + cytotoxic antibodies cause lysis of cells such as platelets or leukocytes.	Penicillin, sulfonamides, quinidine, isoniazid.	Petechiae due to thrombocytopenic purpura; drug-induced pemphigus.
Type III	IgG or IgM antibodies formed to drug; immune complexes deposited in small vessels activate complement and recruitment of granulocytes.	Immunoglobulins, antibiotics.	Vasculitis, urticaria, serum sickness.
Type IV	Cell-mediated immune reaction; sensitized lymphocytes react with drug, liberating cytokines, which trigger cutaneous inflammatory response.	Sulfamethoxazole, anticonvulsants, allopurinol.	Morbilliform exanthematous reactions, fixed drug eruption, lichenoid eruptions, Stevens-Johnson syndrome, toxic epidermal necrolysis.

[a] After the Gell and Coombs classification of immune reactions.

Reproduced, with permission, from Wolff K, Johnson RA, Suurmond D. *Fitzpatrick's Color Atlas and Synopsis of Clinical Dermatology,* 5th ed. New York: McGraw-Hill, 2005:543.

DIAGNOSIS

Excisional biopsy is warranted only when melanoma is suspected.

COMPLICATIONS

The incidence of melanoma is increased in patients with atypical nevi. A minority of melanomas arise from atypical nevi.

Melanoma

A malignancy of melanocytes that may occur on any skin or mucosal surface. It is the **seventh most common cancer** in the United States; the most prevalent cancer in women 25–29 years of age; and the second most common cancer in men 30–49 years of age, following testicular cancer. Risk factors are expressed in the mnemonic **MMRISK.**

> ***Malignant melanoma risk–***
>
> **MMRISK**
>
> **M**oles: atypical
> **M**oles: total number > 50
> **R**ed hair and freckling
> **I**nability to tan: skin phototypes I and II
> **S**evere sunburn, especially in childhood
> **K**indred: first-degree relative

TABLE 5-13. Clinical Features of Severe Cutaneous Reactions Often Induced by Drugs

Diagnosis	Mucosal Lesions	Typical Skin Lesions	Frequent Signs and Symptoms	Other Causes Not Related	Drugs Most Often Implicated
Stevens-Johnson syndrome (SJS) (see Figure 5-21)	Erosions usually at ≥ 2 sites.	Small blisters on dusky purpuric macules or atypical targets. Rare areas of confluence. Detachment of ≤ 10% of body surface area.	Some 10–30% present with fever.	Postinfectious EM major (HSV or *Mycoplasma*).	**Sulfa** drugs, amine **antiepileptics (phenytoin, carbamazepine), lamotrigine,** allopurinol, hydantoins.
Toxic epidermal necrolysis (see Figure 5-22)	Erosions usually at ≥ 2 sites.	Individual lesions are like those seen in SJS. Confluent erythema. Outer layer of epidermis readily separates from basal layer with lateral pressure (Nikolsky's sign). Large sheet of necrotic epidermis. Detachment of > 30% of body surface area.	Fever is nearly universal. "Acute skin failure," leukopenia.	Viral infections, immunization, chemicals, *Mycoplasma* pneumonia.	Same as above.
Anticonvulsant hypersensitivity syndrome	Infrequent.	Severe exanthem (may become purpuric). Exfoliative dermatitis.	**Some 30–50% of cases present with fever, lymphadenopathy, hepatitis, nephritis, carditis, eosinophilia, and atypical lymphocytes.**	Cutaneous lymphoma.	Anticonvulsants.
Serum sickness or reactions resembling serum sickness	Absent.	Morbilliform lesions, sometimes with urticaria.	Fever, arthralgias.	Infection.	
Anticoagulant-induced necrosis	Infrequent.	Erythema; then purpura and necrosis, especially of fatty areas.	Pain in affected areas.	DIC.	Warfarin, especially in the setting of low protein C or S.
Angioedema	Often involved.	Urticaria or swelling of the central part of the face.	Respiratory distress, cardiovascular collapse.	Insect stings, foods.	**NSAIDs, ACEIs,** penicillin.

Adapted, with permission, from Kasper DL et al (eds). *Harrison's Principles of Internal Medicine,* 16th ed. New York: McGraw-Hill, 2005:323. Data from Roujeau JC, Stern RS. Severe adverse cutaneous reactions to drugs. N Engl J Med 331:1272, 1994.

Symptoms

- **A changing mole.**
- **Superficial spreading** malignant melanomas are most common (responsible for 70% of all melanomas in Caucasians), arising on sun-exposed regions of older patients (see Figure 5-23).
- Other subtypes include nodular, lentigo maligna, and acral-lentiginous.

Exam

Physical findings are expressed in the mnemonic **ABCDEs.**

> ***Melanoma–***
>
> **The ABCDEs**
>
> **A**symmetry
> **B**orders: irregular
> **C**olor: variegated
> **D**iameter > 6 mm
> **E**volution: lesion changes over time

Diagnosis

- **Tumor thickness** (Breslow's classification) and lymph node status are the most important prognostic factors. Melanomas **< 1 mm** in thickness are considered **lower risk,** and **staging workup is not indicated in these cases.**
- Additional significant prognostic indicators include site, specific histologic features, and sex of the patient (men are at higher risk than women).

Treatment

Sentinel lymph node dissection is recommended for malignant melanomas > 1 mm thick and is also essential in medical decision making regarding adjuvant therapy. Further information on the workup and treatment of melanoma is given in Table 5-14.

Complications

Metastasis usually occurs in the following sequence: local recurrence, regional lymph nodes, distant metastasis (liver, lung, bone, brain). Five-year survival rates with lymph node involvement and distant metastasis are 30% and 10%, respectively.

The central face and ears are high-risk areas of increased recurrence and metastatic potential for BCCs.

Basal Cell Carcinoma (BCC)

Represent **80% of all skin cancers.** Occur in sun-exposed areas. The mean age at diagnosis is 62 years.

Symptoms/Exam

- **Head and neck:** Presents with papules or nodules with telangiectasias and a "pearly" or translucent quality. A central erosion or crust (noduloulcerative type) is often seen (see Figure 5-24).
- **Chest, back, and extremities:** A scaly erythematous plaque (superficial type) that may resemble a plaque of eczema.

Diagnosis

Shave biopsy.

Treatment

Treatment is dependent on individual tumor and patient characteristics. Both surgical and nonsurgical techniques are employed. Sun avoidance and patient education are key components of management.

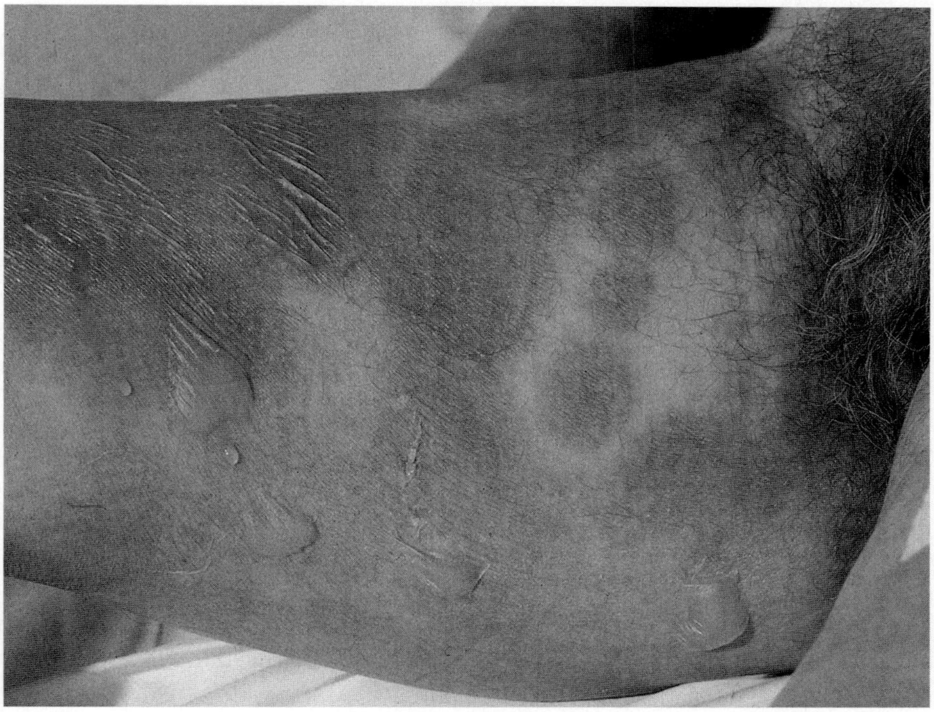

FIGURE 5-21. Stevens-Johnson syndrome.

Generalized eruption of initially targetlike lesions that become confluent, brightly erythematous, and bullous. (Reproduced, with permission, from Wolff K, Johnson RA, Suurmond D. *Fitzpatrick's Color Atlas and Synopsis of Clinical Dermatology*, 5th ed. New York: McGraw-Hill, 2005:145.) (Also see Color Insert.)

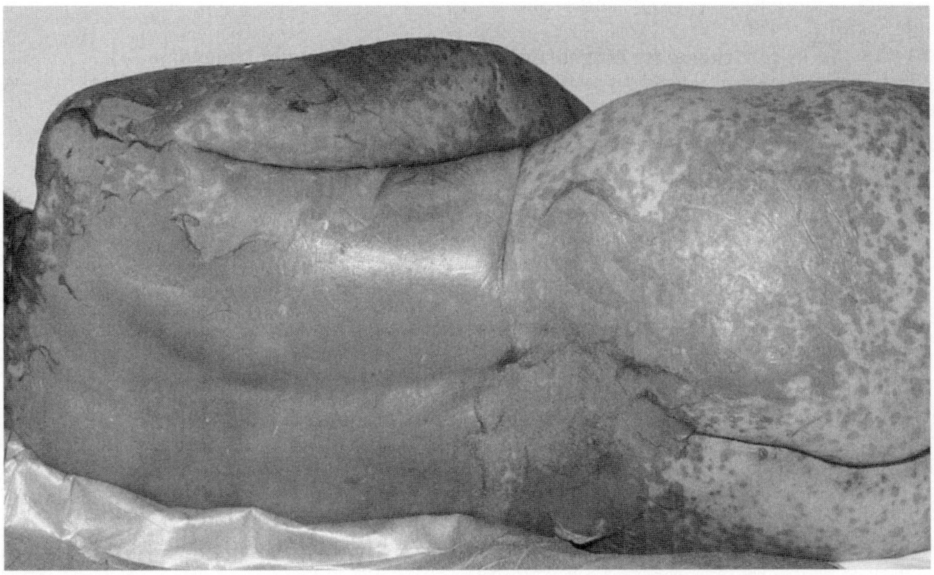

FIGURE 5-22. Toxic epidermal necrolysis.

Bulla formation with rapid desquamation revealing denuded, erosive areas. (Reproduced, with permission, from Wolff K, Johnson RA, Suurmond D. *Fitzpatrick's Color Atlas and Synopsis of Clinical Dermatology*, 5th ed. New York: McGraw-Hill, 2005:147.) (Also see Color Insert.)

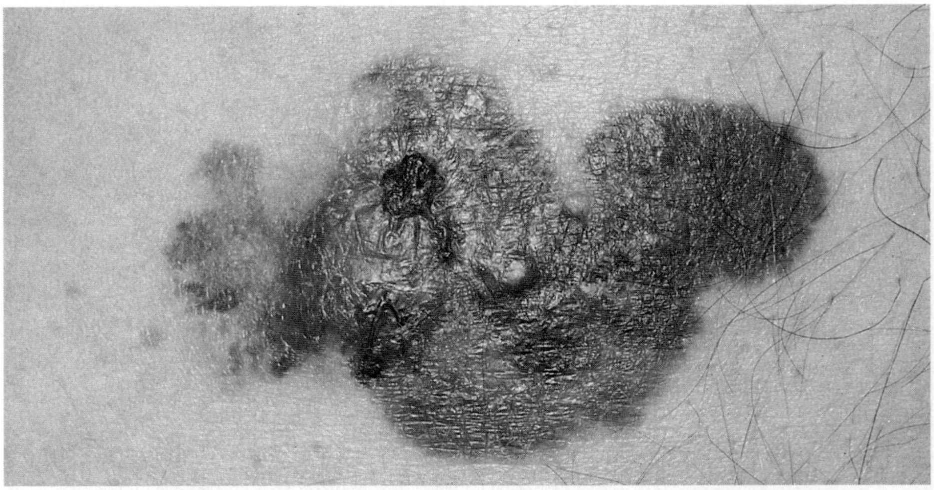

FIGURE 5-23. Superficial spreading melanoma.

A highly characteristic lesion with an irregular pigmentary pattern and scalloped borders. (Reproduced, with permission, from Wolff K, Johnson RA, Suurmond D. *Fitzpatrick's Color Atlas and Synopsis of Clinical Dermatology*, 5th ed. New York: McGraw-Hill, 2005:318.) (Also see Color Insert.)

TABLE 5-14. Scheme for Diagnostic Workup and Follow-up of Melanoma

	Follow-up	
Breslow Depth (mm)	**Physical Examination**	**CXR and Labs[a]**
Stage I	6 mo × 2 yr; 12 mo thereafter.	Initial.
Stage IIa	4 mo × 3 yr; 12 mo thereafter.	Yearly.
Stage IIb	4 mo × 3 yr; 6 mo × 2 yr; 12 mo thereafter.	Yearly.
Regional (Stage III) or distant (Stage IV) disease	3–4 mo × 5 yr; 12 mo thereafter.	Every other visit × 5 yr; yearly thereafter; initial CT scans of head/chest/abdomen/pelvis or PET if available.

[a] LFTs and LDH.

Adapted, with permission, from Kerdel FA, Jimenez-Acosta F. *Dermatology: Just the Facts.* New York: McGraw-Hill, 2003:271.

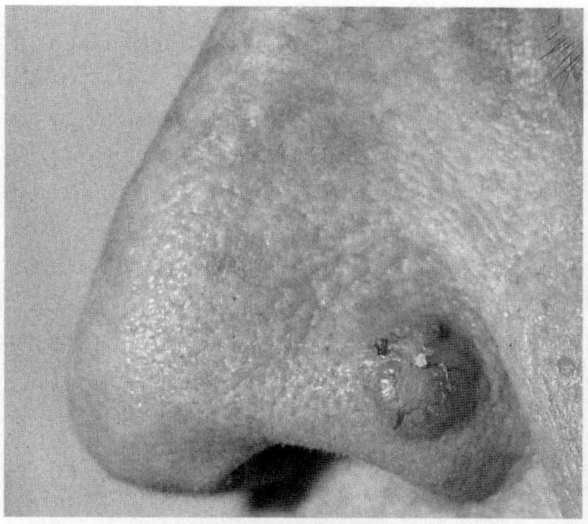

FIGURE 5-24. Nodular basal cell carcinoma.

A smooth, pearly nodule with telangiectasias. (Reproduced, with permission, from Wolff K, Johnson RA, Suurmond D. *Fitzpatrick's Color Atlas and Synopsis of Clinical Dermatology*, 5th ed. New York: McGraw-Hill, 2005:283.) (Also see Color Insert.)

COMPLICATIONS

Metastatic spread is uncommon (< 0.1%).

Squamous Cell Carcinoma (SCC)

Represent 20% of all skin cancers; typically affect patients > 55 years of age. Bowen's disease and erythroplasia (of Queyrat) are synonyms for SCC in situ. SCCs may arise within **actinic keratoses** or within HPV–induced lesions (see Figure 5-25).

SCC is more common and more aggressive in solid organ transplant recipients, chronically immunosuppressed patients, and HIV-infected patients.

DIAGNOSIS

Diagnosed by skin biopsy.

TREATMENT

- Because SCCs have a **higher metastatic and recurrence rate than BCCs,** treatment of invasive disease is primarily surgical.
- Prevention with sun avoidance and patient education are key components of disease management.

COMPLICATIONS

The overall five-year recurrence and metastatic rates are 8% and 5%, respectively.

In immunosuppressed patients, SCCs are more common than BCCs. These patients need to be followed more closely, as SCCs are more aggressive with higher metastatic potential.

Cutaneous T-Cell Lymphoma (CTCL)

Mycosis fungoides, an indolent malignancy of mature CD4+ helper T lymphocytes, is the most common form of CTCL. Average age at onset is 50 years (range 5–70); men are affected twice as often as women. Characterized by a long natural history.

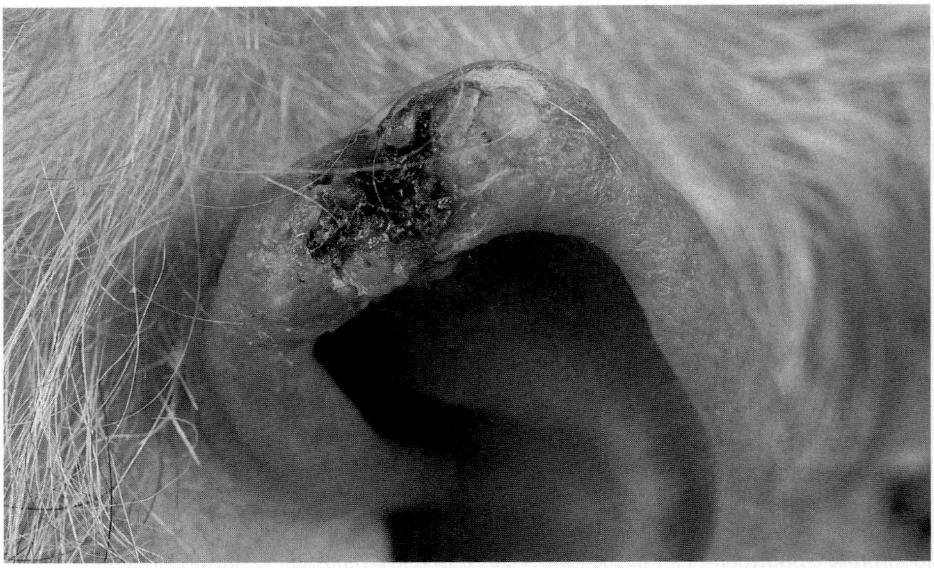

FIGURE 5-25. Squamous cell carcinoma.

A hyperkeratotic nodule with ulceration. (Reproduced, with permission, from Wolff K, Johnson RA, Suurmond D. *Fitzpatrick's Color Atlas and Synopsis of Clinical Dermatology*, 5th ed. New York: McGraw-Hill, 2005:279.)

SYMPTOMS/EXAM

- Presents with scaly, **pruritic, erythematous patches and plaques** (see Figure 5-26).
- Erythroderma with Sézary syndrome (rare).

COMPLICATIONS

Sézary syndrome is the leukemic form of CTCL and consists of erythroderma, lymphadenopathy, and circulating Sézary cells. Without therapy, its course is progressive, and patients succumb to opportunistic infections. Therapy includes treatment for CTCL as well as supportive measures for erythroderma.

Owing to the nondescript appearance of CTCL lesions, delay in diagnosis often approaches a decade. Survival is not affected in limited patch-stage disease.

MISCELLANEOUS

Photodermatitis

A group of inflammatory skin reactions attributable to the following:

- **UV radiation: Polymorphous light eruption** is a common photodermatitis, especially in Native Americans, and is due to **delayed-type hypersensitivity** to an antigen induced by UV radiation (especially UVA) (see Figure 5-27).
- **Medications: NSAIDs, antibiotics** (some tetracyclines), phenothiazines, sulfones, chlorothiazides, sulfonylureas.
- **Hereditary disorders:** Porphyrias, phenylketonuria, xeroderma pigmentosum.

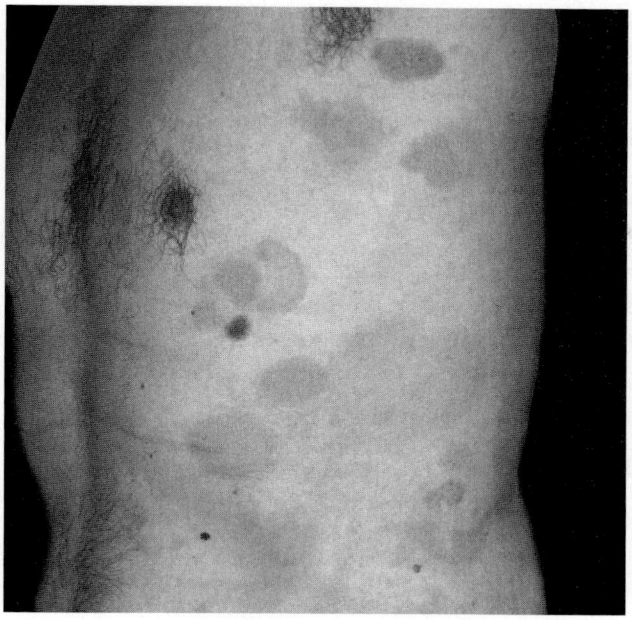

FIGURE 5-26. Cutaneous T-cell lymphoma/mycosis fungoides.

Erythematous plaques with scale are seen that mimic eczema, psoriasis, or dermatophytosis. (Reproduced, with permission, from Wolff K, Johnson RA, Suurmond D. *Fitzpatrick's Color Atlas and Synopsis of Clinical Dermatology*, 5th ed. New York: McGraw-Hill, 2005:529.)

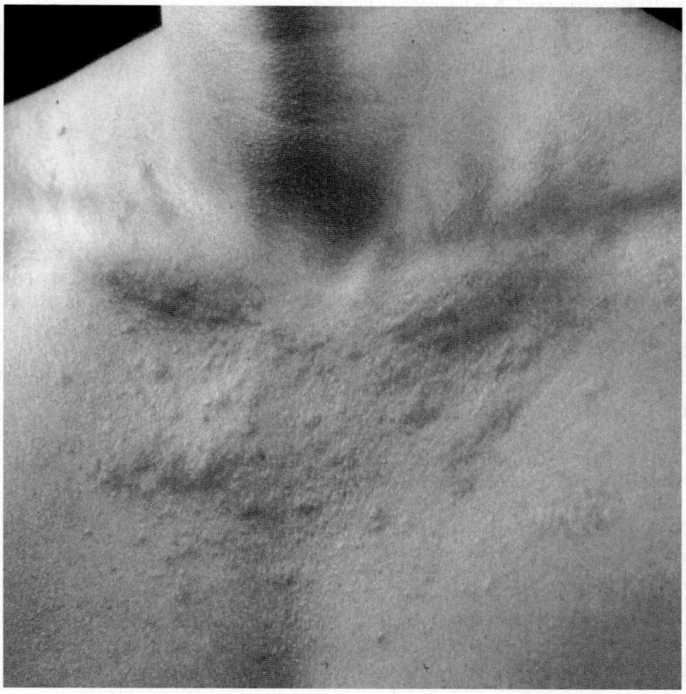

FIGURE 5-27. Polymorphous light eruption.

Extremely pruritic, clustered papules and vesicles are seen on sun-exposed areas. (Reproduced, with permission, from Wolff K, Johnson RA, Suurmond D. *Fitzpatrick's Color Atlas and Synopsis of Clinical Dermatology*, 5th ed. New York: McGraw-Hill, 2005:243.)

TABLE 5-15. Disorders of Hyperpigmentation

Disorder	Associated Diseases
Pigmented nevi, ephelides (freckles), lentigines	
Melasma	Estrogen effect; often seen in pregnancy.
Café-au-lait spots, axillary freckling	Neurofibromatosis.

In patients with recurrent photodistributed eruptions, consider diseases characterized by photosensitivity, including SLE.

Pigmentary Disorders

Tables 5-15 and 5-16 outline disorders associated with hyper- and hypopigmentation.

Verruca and Condyloma

Distinguished as follows:

- HPV causes clinical lesions that vary according to subtype. More than 150 types of HPV have been identified.
- **Verruca vulgaris,** the common wart (70% of all warts), occurs primarily on the extremities.
- **Condylomata acuminata,** warts in the **anogenital** region, are the most commonly diagnosed STD.
- Genital HPV types (**types 16 and 18**) play an important role in the malignant transformation of benign verrucae into **cervical and anogenital cancer.**
- Increased incidence and more widespread disease are seen in **immunocompromised** patients.

Treatment

- In immunocompetent patients, lesions usually **resolve spontaneously** over 1–2 years.
- Treatment modalities include mechanical destruction (cryotherapy, laser therapy) or stimulation of the immune system (topical imiquimod; application of sensitizing agents).

TABLE 5-16. Disorders of Hypopigmentation

Disorder	Associated Diseases
Vitiligo (melanocytes destroyed)	Hypothyroidism, hyperthyroidism, pernicious anemia, DM, Addison's disease.
Albinism	Eye and vision are often affected.
Piebaldism	Autosomal dominant; neurologic dysfunction.

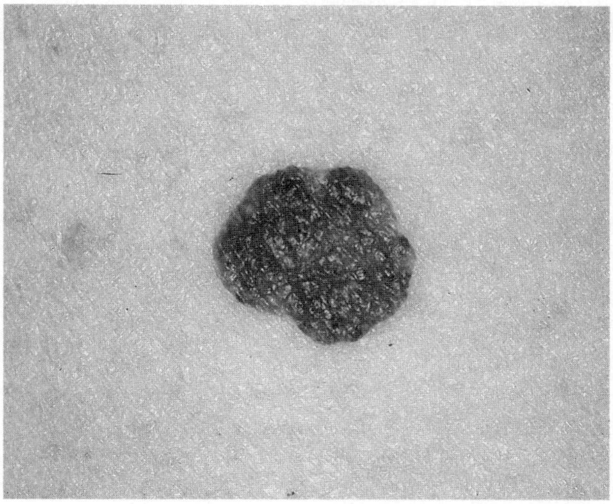

FIGURE 5-28. Seborrheic keratosis.

Brown, warty papules with a "stuck-on" appearance. (Reproduced, with permission, from Wolff K, Johnson RA, Suurmond D. *Fitzpatrick's Color Atlas and Synopsis of Clinical Dermatology*, 5th ed. New York: McGraw-Hill, 2005:206.)

COMPLICATIONS

Malignant transformation to SCC in certain subtypes.

Seborrheic Keratosis

- The most common benign epidermal growth; probably has an autosomal-dominant inheritance.
- Usually asymptomatic; rarely pruritic.
- Has a **"stuck-on"** appearance (see Figure 5-28).
- No treatment is necessary.

NOTES

CHAPTER 6

Endocrinology

Diana Antoniucci, MD
Karen Earle, MD

PITUITARY AND HYPOTHALAMUS

The hypothalamus produces oxytocin and ADH. The anterior pituitary produces and releases six hormones: ACTH, TSH, FSH, LH, GH, and prolactin. The posterior pituitary stores and releases ADH and oxytocin. Table 6-1 further describes the mechanisms of the various pituitary hormones. The subsections that follow describe disorders that stem from pituitary hormone deficiencies and related dysfunctions.

Diabetes Insipidus (DI)

Deficient ADH action, resulting in copious amounts of extremely dilute urine. Subtypes are as follows:

- **Central DI:** Caused by infection, tumors, cysts, hypophysectomy, histiocytosis X, granulomatous disease, vascular disruption, autoimmune disease, trauma, and familial factors.
- **Nephrogenic DI:** Caused by chronic renal disease, congenital and familial factors, hypercalcemia, hypokalemia, and **lithium.**

TABLE 6-1. Pituitary Hormones and Their Function

Hormone	Increased By	Decreased By	Excess	Deficiency	Notes
ADH	Thirst, high serum osmolality.	Low serum osmolality, low serum K^+.	SIADH.	DI.	
ACTH	CRH, stress.	High cortisol.	Cushing's syndrome.	Adrenal insufficiency.	Diurnal variation (peak at 3–4 A.M.).
TSH	TRH.	High T_4 and/or T_3.	Hyperthyroidism.	Hypothyroidism.	
LH/FSH	GnRH.	Gonadal sex steroids.		Hypogonadism.	In men, inhibin inhibits FSH.
GH	GHRH, hypoglycemia, dopamine.	Somatostatin.	**Childhood:** gigantism. **Adulthood:** acromegaly.	**Childhood:** short stature. **Adulthood:** poor sense of well-being.	
Prolactin	Pregnancy, nursing, TRH, stress.	Dopamine.	Galactorrhea, hypogonadism.	Inability to lactate.	Under tonic inhibition by hypothalamic dopamine.

SYMPTOMS/EXAM

- **Polyuria,** polydipsia.
- The hallmark is inappropriately **dilute urine** in the setting of **elevated serum osmolality.**
- **Hypernatremia** occurs if the patient lacks access to free water or if the thirst mechanism is inappropriate.

DIFFERENTIAL

Psychogenic polydipsia: Increased drinking, usually > 5 L of water per day, leading to dilution of extracellular fluid and water diuresis.

DIAGNOSIS

- **Plasma and urine osmolality** (see Table 6-2).
- **Water deprivation test:** The patient is denied access to water while serum and plasma osmolalities are checked regularly until serum osmolalities are elevated above normal.
- **DDAVP test** (synthetic vasopressin).

Keeping up with fluid losses from massive polyuria is a key component of DI treatment.

TREATMENT

- **Central DI:** Intranasal DDAVP administration.
- **Nephrogenic DI:** Treat the underlying disorder if possible. Thiazide diuretics and amiloride may be helpful.

COMPLICATIONS

Dehydration, hydronephrosis.

When a woman presents with amenorrhea, hyperprolactinemia, and a homogeneously enlarged pituitary gland (up to two times normal), the first thing to rule out is pregnancy!

Pituitary Tumors

Microadenomas are < 1 cm; macroadenomas are > 1 cm. Panhypopituitarism and visual loss increase in frequency with increasing tumor size.

SYMPTOMS/EXAM

- **Neurologic symptoms** (headache, visual field cuts, nerve palsies).
- **Hormonal excess or deficiency** (hypothyroidism, hypogonadism, hyperprolactinemia).
- **Incidental discovery on imaging study** (up to 10% of the general population have pituitary incidentalomas).

TABLE 6-2. Diagnosis of Central DI, Nephrogenic DI, and Psychogenic Polydipsia

TEST	CENTRAL DI	NEPHROGENIC DI	PSYCHOGENIC POLYDIPSIA
Random plasma osmolality	↑	↑	↓
Random urine osmolality	↓	↓	↓
Urine osmolality during water deprivation	No change	No change	↑
Urine osmolality after IV DDAVP	↑	No change	↑
Plasma ADH	↓	Normal to ↑	↓

DIFFERENTIAL

Table 6-3 outlines the differential diagnosis of sellar lesions.

DIAGNOSIS

- **Labs:** Once a tumor is identified, check TSH, free T_4, prolactin, ACTH, cortisol, LH, FSH, and testosterone in men to assess for hormonal excess or deficiency.
- **Pituitary imaging:** The best imaging of tumors is obtained with a **sellar-specific MRI. A regular MRI of the brain may miss these small tumors!**

TREATMENT

- **Surgical:** The **transsphenoidal** approach is successful in approximately 90% of patients with microadenomas.
- **Radiologic:** Gamma knife radiosurgery or conventional irradiation can be used.
- **Medical:** Some tumors shrink with hormonal manipulation.

TABLE 6-3. Differential Diagnosis of Sellar Lesions

- **Pituitary adenoma:**
  - Prolactinoma: Most common type of pituitary microadenoma
  - GH secreting
  - Nonfunctioning: One-third of all pituitary tumors; most common type of macroadenoma
  - ACTH secreting: Common cause of Cushing's disease
  - TSH secreting (rare; < 1% of pituitary tumors)
- **Physiologic enlargement of the pituitary gland:**
  - Lactotroph hyperplasia in pregnancy
  - Thyrotroph hyperplasia due to primary hypothyroidism
  - Gonadotroph hyperplasia due to primary hypogonadism
- **Craniopharyngioma**
- **Meningioma**
- **Primary malignancies:**
  - Germ cell tumors
  - Sarcomas
  - Chordomas
  - Lymphomas
  - Pituitary carcinomas
- **Metastases:**
  - Breast cancer
  - Lung cancer
- **Cysts:**
  - Rathke's cleft cyst
  - Arachnoid cyst
  - Dermoid cyst
- **Infections:**
  - Abscesses
  - Tuberculomas
- **Lymphocytic hypophysitis**

ENDOCRINOLOGY

COMPLICATIONS

- **Panhypopituitarism:** See the section on hypopituitarism below.
- **Apoplexy: Life-threatening;** see the discussion in the hypopituitarism section below.

Growth Hormone (GH) Excess

Etiologies of GH excess are as follows:

- **Benign pituitary adenoma:** In > 99% of cases, GH excess states are due to a GH-secreting pituitary adenoma. Typically macroadenomas (> 1 cm), as diagnosis is often delayed by as much as 10 years.
- **Iatrogenic:** Treatment of GH deficiency.
- **Ectopic GH or GHRH:** Extremely rare; seen with lung carcinoma and with carcinoid and pancreatic islet cell tumors.

SYMPTOMS/EXAM

In childhood, patients develop gigantism–delayed epiphyseal closure leading to extremely tall stature. In adulthood, patients develop acromegaly.

- **Cardiac:** Hypertension (25%), cardiac enlargement.
- **Endocrine: Glucose intolerance** (50%) or overt DM; hypercalciuria with nephrolithiasis (10%); hypogonadism (60% in females, 45% in males).
- **Constitutional:** Heat intolerance, weight gain, fatigue.
- **Neurologic:** Visual field cuts and headaches.
- **GI:** Increased colonic polyp frequency.
- **Other:** Soft tissue proliferation (enlargement of the hands and feet; **coarsening of facial features**); sweaty palms and soles; paresthesias (**carpal tunnel syndrome** is found in 70%); increase in shoe, ring, or glove size.

DIAGNOSIS

- **Laboratory:** Random GH is not helpful. **Elevated IGF-1 levels** are the hallmark.
- **Radiology:** MRI of the pituitary.

TREATMENT

- **Surgery:** Transsphenoidal resection is curative in 60–80% of cases.
- **Radiotherapy:** Second-line therapy.
- **Medical:** Used when surgical and/or radiation therapy are ineffective or not possible. Octreotide (a somatostatin analog) will decrease GH secretion. Pegvisomant, a GH receptor antagonist, will normalize IGF-1 levels in 80–90% of patients with acromegaly.

COMPLICATIONS

Panhypopituitarism and **cardiovascular** effects (hypertension, CHF, CAD).

Hyperprolactinemia

Most often caused by a **prolactinoma, the most common type of pituitary tumor.** The majority are microadenomas (< 1 cm). Can also be caused by many medications (see Table 6-4). Other etiologies are as follows:

- **Pregnancy:** Prolactin can reach 200 ng/mL in the second trimester.
- **Hypothalamic lesions; pituitary stalk compression or damage.**
- **Hypothyroidism:** TSH stimulates prolactin secretion.

Table 6-4. Medications That Cause Hyperprolactinemia

Amoxapine	Nicotine
Amphetamines	Phenothiazines
Anesthetic agents	Protease inhibitors
Butyrophenone	Progestins
Cimetidine and ranitidine	Reserpine
Estrogens	Risperidone
Hydroxyzine	SSRIs
Methyldopa	TCAs
Metoclopramide	Verapamil
Narcotics	

SYMPTOMS/EXAM

- **Women: Galactorrhea, amenorrhea,** oligomenorrhea with **anovulation** and infertility in 90%, hirsutism.
- **Men:** Impotence, decreased libido, galactorrhea (very rare).
- **Both:** Symptoms due to large tumor—headache, visual field cuts, and hypopituitarism.

Women typically present with prolactinomas earlier than men because of amenorrhea and galactorrhea. Therefore, women often have microprolactinomas (< 1 cm) at diagnosis, whereas men have macroprolactinomas.

DIAGNOSIS

- **Laboratory:** Elevated prolactin with normal TFTs and a **negative pregnancy test.**
- **Radiology:** Obtain an MRI if prolactin is elevated in the absence of pregnancy or the drugs listed above.

TREATMENT

- **Medical: Dopamine agonists** such as **bromocriptine** or **cabergoline.** Cabergoline is generally first-line therapy because it has fewer side effects.
- **Surgery:** Transsphenoidal resection is curative in 85–90% of patients.

Hypopituitarism

Diminished or absent secretion of one or more pituitary hormones.

SYMPTOMS/EXAM

Presentation depends on the particular hormone deficiency. In increasing order of importance, with **ACTH being preserved the longest,** pituitary hormones are lost as follows:

- **GH deficiency:** Usually asymptomatic in adults.
- **LH/FSH deficiency:** Hypogonadism. Manifested in men as lack of libido and impotence and in women as anovulatory cycles with irregular menses and amenorrhea.
- **TSH deficiency:** Hypothyroidism.
- **ACTH deficiency:** Adrenal insufficiency (weakness, nausea, vomiting, anorexia, weight loss, fever, and hypotension).

Note: ADH deficiency is seen only if the posterior pituitary is also involved.

In panhypopituitarism, ACTH is generally the last hormone to become deficient—and the most life-threatening.

DIFFERENTIAL

Remember the "**eight I's**": **I**nvasive, **I**nfiltrative, **I**nfarction, **I**njury, **I**mmunologic, **I**atrogenic, **I**nfectious, **I**diopathic.

- **Invasive causes:** Pituitary adenomas (usually nonproductive macroadenomas), craniopharyngioma, primary CNS tumors, metastatic tumors, anatomic malformations: (encephalocele and parasellar aneurysms).
- **Infiltrative causes:** Sarcoidosis, hemochromatosis, histiocytosis X.
- **Infarction:**
  - **Sheehan's syndrome:** Pituitary infarction associated with postpartum hemorrhage and vascular collapse. Typically presents with difficulty in lactation and failure to resume menses postpartum.
  - **Pituitary apoplexy:** Spontaneous hemorrhagic infarction of a preexisting pituitary tumor. Fulminant presentation with severe headache, visual field defects, ophthalmoplegia, and hypotension +/– meningismus. Constitutes an **emergency**; treat with corticosteroids +/– transsphenoidal decompression.

In a man with hypopituitarism and skin bronzing—think hemochromatosis.

- **Injury:** Severe head trauma can lead to anterior pituitary dysfunction and DI.
- **Immunologic causes: Lymphocytic hypophysitis.** During or just after pregnancy, 50% of patients have other autoimmune disease.
- **Iatrogenic:** Most likely after **radiation therapy.**
- **Infectious:** Rare; TB, syphilis, or fungi.
- **Idiopathic.**

DIAGNOSIS

Specific hormonal testing includes the following:

Tumors cause DI (by affecting posterior pituitary function) only when they are large and invade the suprasellar space. Primary pituitary tumors rarely cause DI.

- **ACTH/adrenal axis:** Abnormal ACTH, cortisol, and cosyntropin stimulation test.
- **Thyroid axis:** Low free T_4 (TSH levels are **not** reliable for this diagnosis, as levels may be low or normal).
- **Gonadotropins:** Low FSH/LH.
- **GH:** Low IGF-1.
- **ADH:** If DI is suspected, test as described in Table 6-2.

TREATMENT

Treat the underlying cause. Medical treatment consists of correcting hormone deficiencies:

- **ACTH:** Hydrocortisone 20–30 mg/day, two-thirds in the morning and one-third in the evening.
- **TSH:** Replace with levothyroxine, or LT_4 (adjust to a goal of normal free T_4).
- **GnRH:**
  - **Men:** Replace testosterone by injections or patches.
  - **Women:** If premenopausal, OCPs. If postmenopausal, consider low-dose estrogen.
- **GH:** HGH is available but controversial.
- **ADH:** Intranasal DDAVP 10 μg BID.

Seventy-five percent or more of the pituitary has to be destroyed before there is clinical evidence of hypopituitarism.

Empty Sella Syndrome

The subarachnoid space extends into the sella turcica, partially filling it with CSF and flattening the pituitary gland. Etiologies are as follows:

- **Primary:** Empty sella due to congenital incompetence of the diaphragma sellae. The **most common cause.**
- **Secondary:** Due to pituitary surgery, radiation therapy, or pituitary infarction.

Symptoms/Exam

- Partial or complete hypopituitarism.
- In primary empty sella, roughly 15% of patients have mild hyperprolactinemia.

Diagnosis

Sellar MRI may show herniation of the diaphragma sellae and CSF in the sella turcica.

Treatment

- Replace deficient hormones.
- If symptomatic hyperprolactinemia, treat with dopamine agonists.

THYROID

Tests and Imaging

Thyroid Function Tests (TFTs)

Table 6-5 outlines the role of TFTs in diagnosing thyroid disorders. Figure 6-1 illustrates the hypothalamic-pituitary-thyroid axis.

The single best screening test with which to evaluate thyroid function is TSH. Low levels most commonly represent hyperthyroidism; high levels suggest hypothyroidism.

TABLE 6-5. TFTs in Thyroid Disease

	TSH	Free T_4	T_3/Free T_3
Primary hypothyroidism	↑	↓	↓
Secondary (pituitary) hypothyroidism	↓	↓	↓
Tertiary (hypothalamic) hypothyroidism	↓	↓	↓
Primary hyperthyroidism	↓	↑	↑
Secondary hyperthyroidism	↑	↑	↑
Exogenous hyperthyroidism	↓	↑	Mild ↑
Euthyroid sick (acute)	Normal[a]	↑/normal	↓
Euthyroid sick (recovery)	↑	Normal	Normal

[a] Decreased if the patient is taking dopamine, glucocorticoids, narcotics, or NSAIDs.

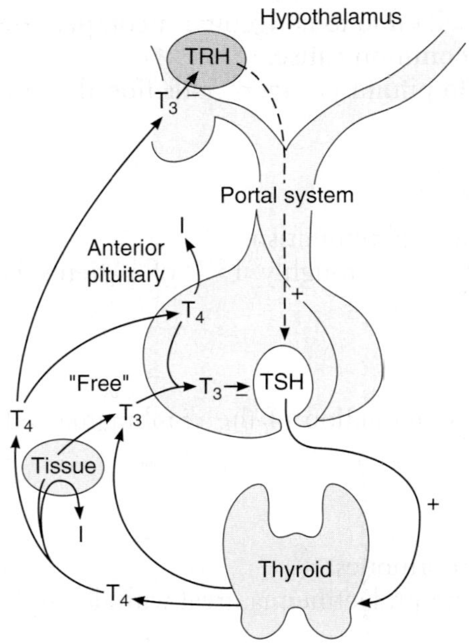

FIGURE 6-1. The hypothalamic-pituitary-thyroid axis.

TSH is produced by the pituitary in response to TRH. TSH stimulates the thyroid gland to secrete T_4 and low levels of T_3. T_4 is converted in the periphery by 5′ deiodinase to T_3, the active form of the hormone. Most T_4 is bound to TBG and is not accessible to conversion; therefore free T_4 provides a more accurate assessment of thyroid hormone level. (Reproduced, with permission, from Greenspan FS, Gardner DG. *Basic & Clinical Endocrinology*, 7th ed. New York: McGraw-Hill, 2004:232.)

Thyroid Antibodies

- **Thyroglobulin antibodies:** Found in 50–60% of patients with Graves' disease and in 90% of those with early Hashimoto's thyroiditis.
- **Thyroid peroxidase (TPO) antibodies:** Antibodies to a thyroid-specific enzyme (TPO); present in 50–80% of Graves' disease patients and in > 90% of those with Hashimoto's thyroiditis.
- **TSH receptor (TSHR) antibodies:** There are two types of this antibody:
  - **Thyroid-stimulating immunoglobulin (TSI):** Stimulates the receptor to produce more thyroid hormone; present in the serum of 80–95% of Graves' patients.
  - **TSHR-blocking antibodies:** Usually found in patients with autoimmune thyroiditis; rarely checked, and assays are somewhat variable.

Radionuclide Imaging of the Thyroid Gland

- ^{123}I is administered orally, and a scan of the thyroid is obtained at 8 and 24 hours.
- Used to gather information about the size and shape of the thyroid gland as well as the geographic distribution of its functional activity (i.e., to determine if hot or cold nodules are present). This part of the procedure is the **scan.**
  - A **hot** nodule implies overactivity of the nodule and is seen in toxic nodules.
  - A **cold** nodule implies no activity of the nodule and is seen in multinodular goiter and cancer.

- Also assesses overall activity of the gland, reported as **percent uptake** of the radiotracer (see Table 6-6). The uptake is also used to determine doses needed to ablate a gland with a high dose of ^{131}I.

Euthyroid Sick Syndrome

Seen in hospitalized or terminally ill patients, typically without symptoms. The **most common abnormality is a low T_3 level.** TSH levels vary, often rising during recovery phase; this should not be confused with hypothyroidism.

Thyroid medications are not indicated in euthyroid sick syndrome; treat the underlying illness.

Hypothyroidism

Affects 2% of adult women and 0.1–0.2% of adult men. Etiologies include the following:

- **Hashimoto's (autoimmune) thyroiditis:** The **most common cause in the United States.** Characterized by a small, firm gland.
- **Subacute thyroiditis:** See the thyroiditis section below.
- **Drugs:** Amiodarone, lithium, interferon, iodide (kelp, radiocontrast dyes).
- **Iatrogenic:** Postsurgical or post–radioactive iodine (RAI) treatment.
- **Iodine deficiency:** Rare in the United States but common worldwide. Often associated with a grossly enlarged gland.
- **Rare causes:** Secondary hypothyroidism due to hypopituitarism; tertiary hypothyroidism due to hypothalamic dysfunction; peripheral resistance to thyroid hormone.

Symptoms/Exam

- **Symptoms are nonspecific and include fatigue, weight gain, cold intolerance, dry skin, menstrual irregularities, and constipation.**
- On exam, the thyroid is often small but can also be enlarged.
- May also present with periorbital edema; rough, dry skin; peripheral edema; bradycardia; hoarse voice; coarse hair; shortened eyebrows; and delayed relaxation phase of DTRs.
- ECG may demonstrate low voltage.

Diagnosis

- **Labs:** The most common findings are an **elevated TSH** (> 10 mU/L) **and a decreased FT_4.** In Hashimoto's, there may be **positive antibodies** (TPO in 90–100% of patients; thyroglobulin antibody in 80–90% early on in the disease course).
- **Radiology:** RAI scan and ultrasound are not usually indicated.

TABLE 6-6. Thyroid Disease Differential Based on Radioactive Iodine Scans

Decreased Uptake	Diffusely Increased Uptake	Uneven Uptake	Normal
Thyroiditis Exogenous hyperthyroidism	Graves' disease	Multinodular goiter **(hot and cold)** Solitary toxic nodule **(hot)** Cancer **(cold)**	Euthyroid sick

Treatment

- **Thyroid hormone replacement:** Usually LT_4. The replacement dose is usually 1.6 μg/kg/day. In elderly patients or those with heart disease, start at 12.5–25.0 μg/day; then slowly increase the dose by 25-μg increments every month until euthyroid.
- Additional treatment may be required depending on the cause.

Autoimmune thyroid disease is often associated with other endocrine autoimmune disorders, most prominently pernicious anemia and adrenal insufficiency.

Complications

- **Myxedema coma:** Characterized by weakness, hypothermia, hypoventilation with hypercapnia, hypoglycemia, hyponatremia, water intoxication, shock, and death. Treatment is supportive therapy with rewarming, intubation, and IV LT_4. Often precipitated by infection or other stress. Consider glucocorticoids for adrenal insufficiency, which can coexist with thyroid disease.
- **Other complications:** Anemia (normocytic), CHF, depression, and lipid abnormalities (elevated LDL and TG).

Hyperthyroidism

Most commonly caused by **Graves' disease,** which affects females more often than males in a ratio of 5:1. Peak incidence is 20–40 years. Other etiologies are as follows (see also Table 6-7):

- **Solitary toxic nodule.**
- **Mutinodular goiter.**
- **Thyroiditis.**
- **Rare causes:** Exogenous thyroid hormone ingestion, struma ovarii (tumor produces FT_4 and FT_3), hydatidiform mole (hCG mimics TSH action), and productive follicular thyroid carcinoma.

Symptoms

Weight loss, anxiety, **palpitations,** fatigue, hyperdefecation, **heat intolerance,** sweating, amenorrhea.

Exam

Lid lag, tachycardia, increased pulse pressure, hyperreflexia. Other signs depend on the cause of hyperthyroidism and may include goiter (diffuse or multinodular), exophthalmos, dermopathy, and onycholysis (separation of the nail from the nail bed). Eye findings in Graves' disease (found in approximately 30–45% of patients) include ophthalmopathy (see Figure 6-2), proptosis, and periorbital edema. Graves' patients may also experience dermopathy (pretibial myxedema—looks like peau d'orange) and onycholysis (specific but found in < 10%).

Two physical findings are pathognomonic of Graves' disease: pretibial myxedema and exophthalmos.

Diagnosis

- **Labs:** TSH, FT_4, FT_3, thyroid antibodies (thyroglobulin and TPO antibodies in 50–90% of patients; TSHR antibodies in 80–95%).
- **Radiology:** RAI uptake and scan if the type of hyperthyroidism is in question or if RAI therapy is planned.

Treatment

- **Medications:** Methimazole (MMI) and propylthiouracil (PTU) can be used to decrease thyroid hormone production. **In pregnancy, PTU is the**

TABLE 6-7. Causes and Treatment of Hyperthyroidism

	THYROID EXAM	UNIQUE FINDINGS	RAI FINDINGS	TREATMENT
Graves' disease	Diffusely enlarged thyroid; bruit may be present.	TSI = TSH receptor antibody (positive in 80–95%); TPO (positive in 50–80% but low specificity).	Diffusely **increased** uptake.	Meds: MMI, PTU. RAI.
Solitary toxic nodule	Single palpable nodule.	Autoantibodies are usually absent.	Single focus of increased uptake.	Meds or RAI.
Multinodular goiter	"Lumpy-bumpy," enlarged thyroid.	Often have predominantly T_3 toxicosis.	Multiple hot and/or cold nodules.	Meds or RAI.
Subacute thyroiditis	Tender, enlarged thyroid.	Possibly associated with fever or viral illness. Elevated ESR; autoantibodies usually absent.	Diffusely **decreased** uptake.	NSAIDs, steroids if indicated.
Exogenous hyperthyroidism	Normal.	Patient may be taking weight loss medications or have psychiatric illness. Thyroglobulin levels are low.	Diffusely decreased uptake.	Discontinuation of thyroid hormone.

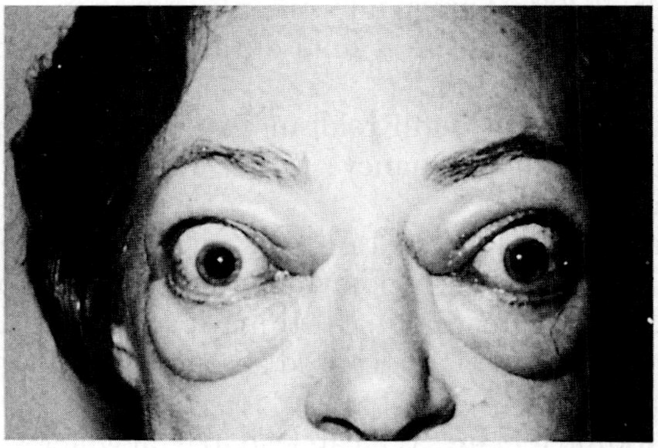

FIGURE 6-2. Graves' ophthalmopathy.

Characterized by periorbital edema, injection of corneal blood vessels, and proptosis. (Reproduced, with permission, from Greenspan FS, Gardner DG. *Basic & Clinical Endocrinology*, 7th ed. New York: McGraw-Hill, 2004:263.)

first choice (see the section on thyroid disease in pregnancy). In Graves', treatment for 18 months can lead to complete remission in 50% of cases. For thyroiditis, see the section below.

- PTU blocks both thyroid hormone formation and peripheral conversion; MMI blocks only hormone formation.
- β-blockers are used in the acute phase to control tachycardia if needed.

- **RAI:** The treatment of choice for toxic nodules. Avoid in pregnancy. Yields a 90% cure rate for Graves' with a single dose.
- **Surgery:** Indicated in uncontrolled disease during pregnancy, for extremely large goiter, or if patients object to RAI.

Elderly patients may present with apathetic hyperthyroidism, which is characterized by depression, slow AF, weight loss, and a small goiter.

Complications

- **Atrial fibrillation (AF):** Particularly common in the elderly population. Thyroid function should be checked in all cases of new AF. Associated with a higher risk of stroke than other causes of nonvalvular AF.
- **Ophthalmopathy:** Can lead to nerve or muscular entrapment (and thus to blindness or palsies). Can be precipitated or **worsened by RAI therapy,** especially in **smokers.** Treatment includes high-dose glucocorticoids and eye surgery.
- **Thyroid storm:** Characterized by **fever,** extreme tachycardia (HR > 120), delirium, agitation, diarrhea, vomiting, jaundice, and CHF. Treatment involves high-dose propranolol, PTU (600- to 1000-mg loading dose, then 200–250 mg q 4 h), glucocorticoids, and iodide (SSKI or Lugol's).

ENDOCRINOLOGY

Thyroiditis

Many different types; all **can present with hyper-, hypo-, and/or euthyroid states** (see Table 6-8).

In the United States, the most common effect of amiodarone on thyroid function is acute suppression of TSH.

Thyroid Disease in Pregnancy

There are three categories of thyroid changes in pregnancy:

1. **Normal changes of pregnancy:** Increased thyroid-binding globulin. This will increase total serum levels of T_4 and T_3, but free hormone levels should remain normal.
2. **Hyperthyroidism:**
   - Affects 0.05–0.20% of pregnant women.
   - In general, Graves' disease is mild during pregnancy but **flares in the early postpartum period.**
   - **Diagnosis:** As per hyperthyroidism in general, except **RAI is contraindicated during pregnancy.**
   - **Treatment:**
     - **Antithyroid medications:** All cross the placenta and have the potential to cause fetal hypothyroidism in the newborn. **PTU is the recommended treatment.** MMI may be used but can cause aplasia cutis, a rare congenital localized absence of skin that usually affects the scalp.
     - **Avoid iodine** therapy, as it can lead to fetal goiter.
     - **Propranolol** may be used transiently to control cardiovascular symptoms.
     - **Surgery:** Safe, especially during the second trimester.
   - **Complications if left untreated:** Spontaneous abortion (25%), premature delivery (45%), increased risk of a small-for-gestational-age (SGA) newborn.

TABLE 6-8. Clinical Features and Differential Diagnosis of Thyroiditis

TYPE	ETIOLOGY	CLINICAL FINDINGS	TESTS	TREATMENT
Subacute thyroiditis (de Quervain's)	Viral.	Hyperthyroid early, then hypothyroid. Tender, large thyroid; fever.	Elevated ESR; no antithyroid antibodies; low RAI uptake.	NSAIDs. Acetaminophen +/– steroids.
Hashimoto's thyroiditis	Autoimmune.	**Usually hypothyroid; painless** +/– goiter.	**95% have positive antibodies; anti-TPO most sensitive.**	Levothyroxine.
Suppurative thyroiditis	Bacteria > other infectious agents.	Fever, neck pain, tender thyroid.	TFTs normal. No uptake on RAI scan; positive cultures.	Antibiotics and drainage.
Amiodarone	Am**IOD**arone contains **IOD**ine.	Three changes due to amiodarone: 1. Asymptomatic TFT changes 2. Hypothyroidism 3. Hyperthyroidism	1. Increased FT_4 and total T_4; then low T_3 and high TSH. 2. High TSH; low FT_4 and T_3. 3. Low TSH; high FT_4 and T_3.	1. No treatment needed—will normalize eventually. 2. As for other hypothyroidism. 3. As for other hyperthyroidism +/– steroids.
Other medications	Lithium, α-interferon, interleukin-2.		Lithium typically causes hypothyroid profile.	Stop medication if possible.
Riedel's thyroiditis	Fibrosis; rare.	Compressive symptoms—stridor, dyspnea, SVC syndrome.	67% have positive antibodies.	Surgery.
Postpartum thyroiditis	Lymphocytic infiltration; seen after up to 10% of pregnancies.	Small, nontender thyroid.	May see hyper- or hypothyroidism. Antibodies often positive; RAI uptake low.	No treatment unless propranolol is needed for tachycardia.

3. **Hypothyroidism:**
   - New-onset hypothyroidism is rare during pregnancy. Always consider preexisting hypothyroidism, as most women need a higher dose of LT_4 replacement during pregnancy.
   - **Complications if left untreated:**
     - **Fetal complications:** Congenital anomalies, perinatal mortality, impaired mental and somatic development.
     - **Maternal complications:** Anemia, preeclampsia, placental abruption, postpartum hemorrhage.

ENDOCRINOLOGY

Thyroid Nodules and Cancer

The "90%" mnemonic applies:

- **90% of nodules are benign.**
- **90% of nodules are cold** on RAI uptake scan; 15–20% of these are malignant and 1% of hot nodules are malignant.
- **90% of thyroid malignancies present as a thyroid nodule or lump.**

SYMPTOMS/EXAM

Presents with a single, firm, palpable nodule.

DIFFERENTIAL

Thyroid nodules may be benign or one of four main types of cancer:

Primary thyroid cancer:

- **Papillary: Most common;** spreads lymphatically. **Excellent prognosis overall,** with a 98% 10-year survival for stage I or II disease (see Table 6-9).
- **Follicular:** More aggressive; spreads locally and hematogenously. Can metastasize to bone, lungs, and brain. Rarely produces thyroid hormone.
- **Medullary:** Tumor of parafollicular C cells. May secrete calcitonin. Fifteen percent are familial or associated with MEN 2A and MEN 2B.
- **Anaplastic:** Undifferentiated. **Poor prognosis;** usually in older patients.

Other: Metastases to thyroid (breast, kidney, melanoma, lung); lymphoma (primary or metastatic).

DIAGNOSIS

Always obtain TFTs. **All euthyroid and hypothyroid nodules should be biopsied with FNA.** Multinodular goiters are not biopsied unless there is a dominant nodule > 1 cm. Figure 6-3 outlines further criteria for the diagnosis of a thyroid mass.

TREATMENT

- **Nodules: See Figure 6-3.**

TABLE 6-9. Staging of Thyroid Cancer

STAGE	AGE < 45[a]	Age > 45	Five-Year Survival	Ten-Year Survival
I	Any T, any N, No M	T < 1 cm, no N, no M	99%	98%
II	Any T, any N, any M	T > 1 cm limited to thyroid, no N, no M	99%	85%
III		T beyond thyroid capsule, no N, no M; or any T, regional N, no M	95%	70%
IV		Any T, any N, any M	80%	61%

[a] Patients < 45 years of age can only be stage I or II.

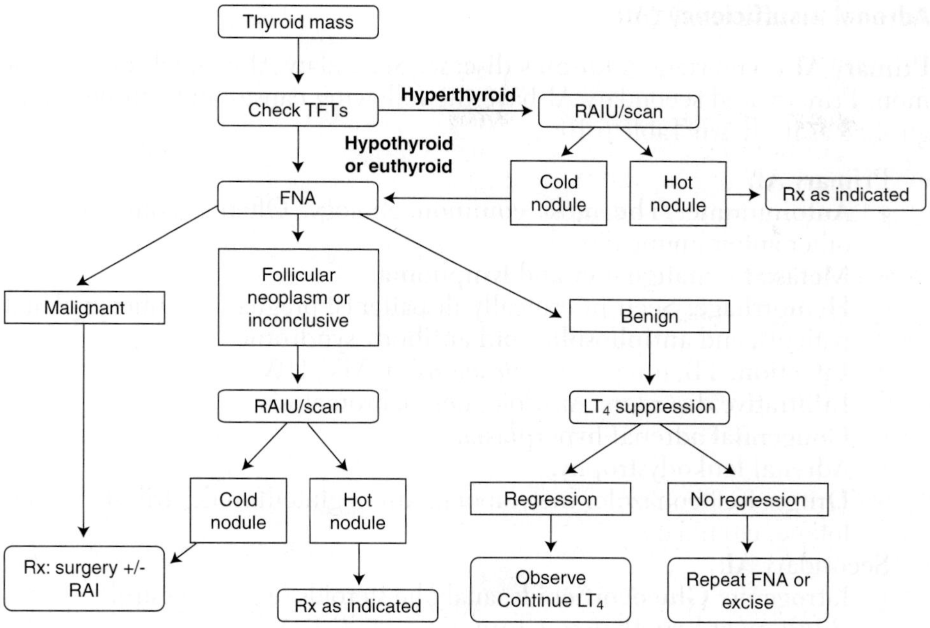

FIGURE 6-3. Evaluation of a thyroid mass.

- **Papillary/follicular cancer:**
  - **First:** Surgical thyroidectomy. **Second:** RAI ablation. **Third:** LT_4 to suppress TSH.
  - Thyroglobulin is a good marker for the presence of thyroid cancer tissue, so if elevated it can be used to follow patients.

ADRENAL GLAND

The adrenal gland has two main portions and is under control of the hypothalamus and pituitary (see Figure 6-4):

- **Medulla:** Produces catecholamines (epinephrine, norepinephrine, and dopamine).
- **Cortex:** Three further layers—remember as **GFR:**
  - Glomerulosa: Primary producer of mineralocorticoids (**aldosterone**).
  - Fasciculata: Primary producer of **cortisol** and androgens.
  - Reticularis: Produces androgens and cortisol.

ACTH and cortisol follow a circadian rhythm; levels are highest around 6:00 A.M.

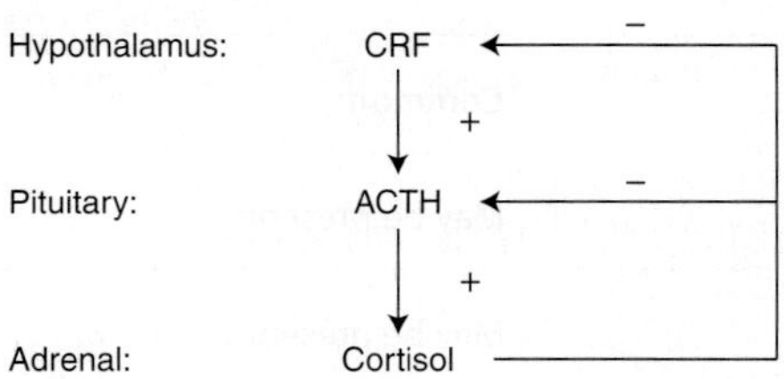

FIGURE 6-4. The hypothalamic-pituitary-adrenal axis.

Adrenal Insufficiency (AI)

The most common cause of AI is exogenous glucocorticoid use.

Primary AI is known as **Addison's disease.** Secondary AI is much more common. Primary and secondary AI have the following causes and can be distinguished as in shown Table 6-10:

- **Primary AI:**
  - **Autoimmune: The most common** etiology. Often accompanied by other autoimmune disorders.
  - **Metastatic malignancy** and **lymphoma.**
  - **Hemorrhage:** Seen in critically ill patients, pregnancy, anticoagulated patients, and **antiphospholipid antibody syndrome.**
  - **Infection:** TB, fungi (*Histoplasmosis*), CMV, HIV.
  - **Infiltrative disorders:** Amyloid, hemochromatosis.
  - **Congenital adrenal hyperplasia.**
  - **Adrenal leukodystrophy.**
  - **Drugs:** Ketoconazole, metyrapone, aminoglutethimide, trilostane, mitotane, etomidate.
- **Secondary AI:**
  - **Iatrogenic: Glucocorticoids,** anabolic steroids (e.g., megestrol).
  - **Pituitary or hypothalamic tumors.**

Hyperpigmentation indicates primary adrenal insufficiency (most notable in the oral mucosa, palmar creases, and recent scars).

SYMPTOMS/EXAM

Weakness, fatigue, anorexia, weight loss, nausea, vomiting, diarrhea, unexplained abdominal pain, postural lightheadedness. With primary AI, **hyperpigmentation** of the oral mucosa and palmar creases is also found. Exam reveals orthostatic **hypotension.**

A poststimulation cortisol level < 18 suggests AI.

DIAGNOSIS

- **Labs: Hyponatremia,** hyperkalemia, eosinophilia, azotemia due to volume depletion, mild metabolic acidosis and hypercalcemia.
- **Step 1—confirm the diagnosis of AI:**
  - **Random cortisol: Any random cortisol** $\geq$ 18 μg/dL rules out AI. However, a low or normal value is not useful.
  - **Cortrosyn stimulation test:**
    - Obtain baseline ACTH and cortisol.
    - Inject Cortrosyn (synthetic ACTH) 250 μg IM or IV.

Table 6-10. Primary vs. Secondary Adrenal Insufficiency

	PRIMARY	SECONDARY
ACTH	**High**	**Low**
Cortisol	Low	Low
Hyperkalemia	**Common**	No
Hyponatremia	May be present	May be present
Eosinophilia	May be present	Absent
Hyperpigmentation	May be present	**Absent**

- Check cortisol level 45–60 minutes later.
- Normal if poststimulation cortisol ≥ 18–20 μg/dL.
- Ancillary tests include metyrapone and insulin tolerance tests.

- **Step 2—distinguish primary from secondary AI. An elevated ACTH level in a patient with AI implies primary AI.**
- **Step 3—further evaluate the cause.** May include a CT of the adrenal glands (e.g., if infection, tumor, or hemorrhage is suspected) or a pituitary MRI (e.g., secondary AI without an obvious cause).

In acute secondary AI (e.g., pituitary apoplexy), a Cortrosyn stimulation test result is likely to be normal because the adrenal glands have not had time to atrophy. So if suspicion for AI is high, treat with steroids!

TREATMENT

- Hydrocortisone 20–30 mg/day, two-thirds in the morning and one-third in the evening (prednisone can also be used). Stress doses are as follows:
  - **Minor stress** (e.g., mild pneumonia): Double the usual dose.
  - **Major stress** (e.g., illness requiring hospitalization or surgery): 50 mg IV q 6–8 h; taper as illness improves.
- Fludrocortisone 0.05–0.10 mg/day. Note that this is needed **only in primary AI, not in secondary AI.**

COMPLICATIONS

Adrenal crisis—acute deficiency of cortisol, usually due to major stress in a patient with preexisting AI. Characterized by headache, nausea, vomiting, confusion, fever, and significant hypotension. The condition is **fatal** if not treated with immediate steroid therapy.

If a patient presents with acute bilateral adrenal hemorrhage, remember to test for antiphospholipid antibody syndrome.

Cushing's Syndrome

A syndrome due to excess cortisol. **Most cases are due to exogenous steroid use.** Cushing's disease (excess pituitary ACTH production) has a female-to-male ratio of 8:1. Etiologies are as follows:

- **Exogenous corticosteroids: The number one cause overall.**
- **Endogenous:**
  - **Cushing's disease** (70% of endogenous cases): Due to ACTH hypersecretion from a **pituitary** microadenoma.
  - **Ectopic ACTH** (15%): From nonpituitary neoplasms producing ACTH. Small cell lung carcinoma is the most common cause, but may also stem from bronchial carcinoids. Rapid increases in ACTH levels lead to marked hyperpigmentation, metabolic alkalosis, and hypokalemia without other cushingoid features.
  - **Adrenal** (15%): adenoma, carcinoma, or nodular adrenal hyperplasia.

SYMPTOMS/EXAM

Table 6-11 lists the clinical characteristics of Cushing's syndrome.

DIAGNOSIS

- **Lab abnormalities:** Metabolic alkalosis, hypokalemia, hypercalciuria, leucocytosis with relative lymphopenia, hyperglycemia, and glucose intolerance.
- Principles of evaluation (see Figure 6-5) are as follows:
  - Confirm excess cortisol production.
  - Determine if ACTH dependent or independent.
  - Use imaging to localize the source.

Table 6-11. Clinical Features of Cushing's Syndrome

General:	**Gonadal dysfunction:**
Obesity 90%	Menstrual disorders 70%
Hypertension 85%	Impotence, decreased libido 85%
Skin:	**Metabolic:**
Plethora 70%	Glucose intolerance 75%
Hirsutism 75%	Diabetes 20%
Striae 50%	Hyperlipidemia 70%
Acne 35%	Polyuria 30%
Bruising 35%	Kidney stones 15%
Musculoskeletal:	
Osteopenia 80%	
Weakness 65%	
Neuropsychiatric (85%):	
Emotional lability	
Euphoria	
Depression	
Psychosis	

Reproduced, with permission, from Greenspan FS, Gardner DG. *Basic & Clinical Endocrinology,* 7th ed. New York: McGraw-Hill, 2004:401.)

Treatment

- **Cushing's disease:** Transsphenoidal pituitary adenoma resection.
- **Ectopic ACTH:**
  - Treat the underlying neoplasm.
  - If the neoplasm is not identifiable or treatable:
    - Pharmacologic blockade of steroid synthesis (ketoconazole, metyrapone, aminoglutethimide).
    - Potassium replacement (consider spironolactone to aid potassium maintenance, as these patients require industrial doses of potassium replacement).
    - Bilateral adrenalectomy if all else fails.
- **Adrenal tumors:** Unilateral adrenalectomy.

Complications

Complications include all those associated with long-term glucocorticoid therapy—e.g., diabetes, hypertension, cardiovascular disease, obesity, and osteoporosis. Unusual, notable complications include:

- **Immune compromise:** Susceptibility to infections such as *Nocardia*, PCP, and other opportunistic pathogens.
- **Nelson's syndrome:** Seen in rare Cushing's disease patients who have been treated with bilateral adrenalectomy, in whom a previously microscopic pituitary adenoma grows rapidly, causing severe hyperpigmentation and the neurologic sequelae of a large sellar tumor.

Hyperaldosteronism

May account for 0.5–10.0% of patients with hypertension. Etiologies are as follows:

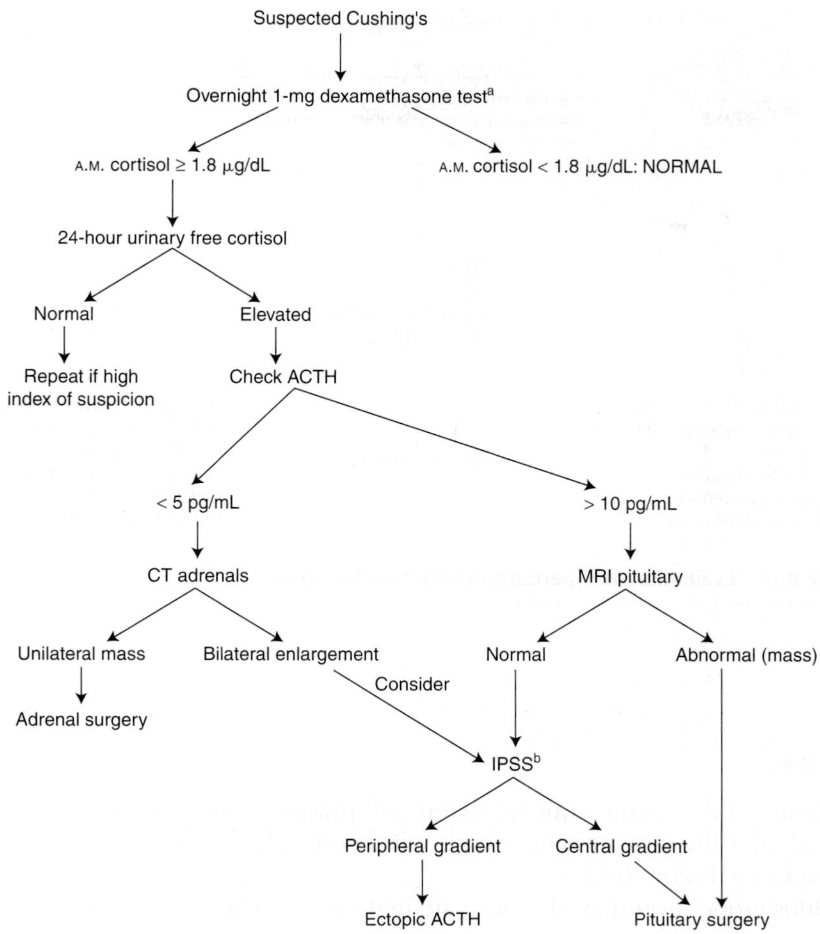

FIGURE 6-5. Evaluation and diagnosis of Cushing's syndrome.

[a] Overnight 1-mg dexamethasone test: Give patient 1 mg dexamethasone PO to be taken at 11:00 P.M. The following morning, check cortisol between 7:00 and 9:00. If cortisol < 1.8 μg/dL, normal; no Cushing's.

[b] IPSS = inferior petrosal sinus sampling. Catheters are used to measure levels of ACTH draining from the pituitary and periphery before and after CRH stimulation. If the gradient is greater from the pituitary, it suggests a central source. If greater from the periphery, the source is peripheral.

- **Aldosterone-producing adenoma (Conn's disease):** Accounts for 60% of primary aldosteronism (PA); three times more common in women.
- **Idiopathic hyperaldosteronism:** One-third of PA; normal-appearing adrenals or bilateral hyperplasia is seen on CT scan.
- **Glucocorticoid-suppressible aldosteronism:** A rare autosomal-dominant form.
- **Angiotensin II–responsive adenoma:** Accounts for 5% of PA.
- **Aldosterone-producing adrenocortical carcinoma:** Rare; < 1% of PA. **Hyperandrogenism** is a clue to the diagnosis.

SYMPTOMS/EXAM

Hypertension and hypokalemia are classic, although a low K^+ is not necessary for diagnosis. Most patients are asymptomatic, and there are no characteristic physical findings.

ENDOCRINOLOGY

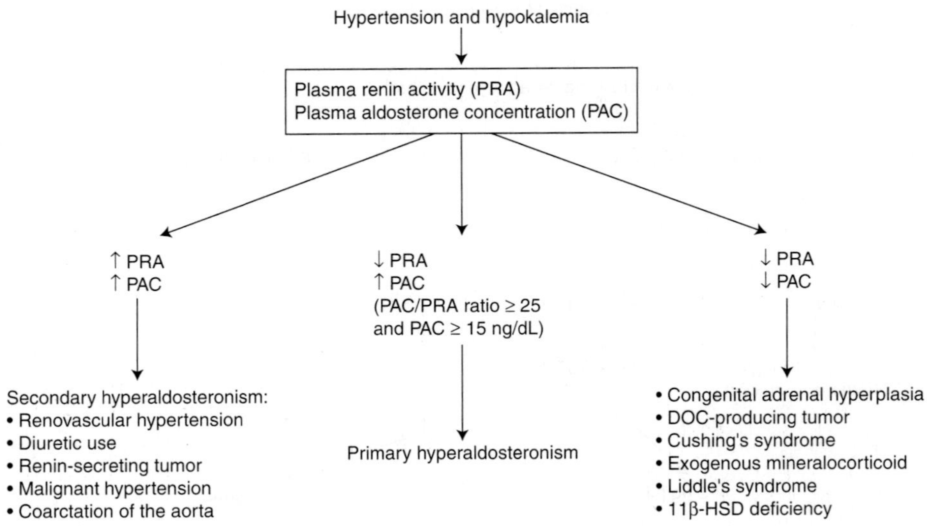

FIGURE 6-6. Evaluation of hypertension with hypokalemia.

Diagnosis

- **Plasma aldosterone concentration** and **plasma renin activity**: Best evaluated after the patient is on a high-salt diet or salt supplementation for one week (see Figure 6-6).
- Aldosterone level may also be evaluated with a 24-hour urine collection.

If primary hyperaldosteronism is diagnosed, obtain an **adrenal CT** to distinguish between Conn's and idiopathic hyperaldosteronism

Treatment

A PAC/PRA ratio ≥ 25 is characteristic of PA.

- **Spironolactone** (in high doses, up to 400 mg/day) or **eplerenone** blocks the mineralocorticoid receptor and usually normalizes K^+. In men, the **most common side effect is gynecomastia,** but other side effects may occur—e.g., rash, impotence, and epigastric discomfort.
- **Unilateral adrenalectomy** is recommended for patients with a single adenoma.

Pheochromocytoma

Pheochromocytoma rule of 10's:

10% are normotensive
10% occur in children
10% are familial
10% are bilateral
10% are malignant
10% are extra-adrenal (called paragangliomas)

Rare tumors (affecting < 0.1% of patients with hypertension and < 4% of patients with adrenal incidentalomas) that arise from chromaffin cells and **produce epinephrine and/or norepinephrine.**

Symptoms

- **Episodic attacks** of throbbing in the chest, trunk, and head, often precipitated by movements that compress the tumor.
- **Headaches, diaphoresis, palpitations,** tremor and anxiety, nausea, vomiting, fatigue, abdominal or chest pain, weight loss, cold hands and feet, and constipation.

Exam

Approximately 90–95% of patients have hypertension, but in 25% of cases, hypertension is episodic. Orthostasis is usually present.

Differential

Adrenal tumor (90% of pheochromocytomas) vs. extra-adrenal locations.

Diagnosis

- **Step 1**—make a biochemical diagnosis:
  - **24-hour urinary metanephrine and normetanephrines or plasma-free metanephrine and normetanephrines:** These levels are usually at least 2–3 times elevated in patients with pheochromocytomas.
- **Step 2**—localize the tumor:
  - **CT** or **MRI** of the adrenals is used to find adrenal pheochromocytomas.
  - If the adrenals appear normal, a ^{123}**I-MIBG** scan can localize extra-adrenal pheochromocytomas and metastases. They are approximately 85% sensitive but 99% specific.

Treatment

- **Prepare the patient for surgery:**
  - **Phenoxybenzamine:** Blocks catecholamines—a key first step.
  - **β-blockers:** Used to control heart rate, but only **after** BP is controlled and good β-blockade has been achieved.
- **Hydration:** It is essential that patients be well hydrated before surgery.
- **Surgical resection** by an experienced surgeon is the definitive treatment for these tumors. Associated with a **90% cure rate.**
- **Follow-up:** Should include 24-hour urine for metanephrines and normetanephrines two weeks postoperatively. If levels are normal, surgical resection can be considered complete. Patients should then undergo yearly biochemical evaluation for at least 10 years.

Complications

Hypertensive crises, MI, cerebrovascular accidents, arrhythmias, renal failure, dissecting aortic aneurysm.

Adrenal Incidentalomas

Adrenal lesions are found incidentally in approximately 2% of patients undergoing abdominal CT for unrelated reasons. Autopsy series indicate a prevalence of 6%.

Exam

Depends on whether the lesion is functioning or nonfunctioning. If functioning, refer to the discussions above.

Differential

- **Functioning adenoma:** Cushing's syndrome, pheochromocytoma, aldosteronoma.
- **Nonfunctioning adenoma:** Carcinoma, benign adenoma, metastatic lesion.

*Patients with pheochromocytoma are usually thin—"**F**at **Ph**eos are **F**ew and **F**ar between."*

Do not use β-blockers in patients with pheochromocytoma before adequate adrenergic blockade has been achieved, as unopposed β-blockade can lead to paroxysmal worsening of the hypertension.

When an adrenal incidentaloma is discovered, always rule out pheochromocytoma, as surgery in patients with untreated pheochromocytoma can be life-threatening.

If a patient has a history of malignancy, the probability that an adrenal lesion is a metastasis is 25–30%. This is the only instance in which to consider biopsy of the lesion (after pheochromocytoma is ruled out).

DIAGNOSIS/TREATMENT

- **Step 1**—rule out functioning tumor:
  - 24-hour urine to rule out pheochromocytoma (see above).
  - Dexamethasone suppression test to rule out subclinical Cushing's.
  - Plasma renin activity and aldosterone level to screen for aldosteronoma in hypertensive patients.
- **Step 2**—treatment is based on the size and functional status of the mass:
  - If the lesion is < 4 cm and nonfunctioning, repeat imaging at 6 and 12 months.
  - If the lesion is > 4 cm and nonfunctioning, resect.
  - If functioning, treat as you would for pheochromocytoma, Cushing's, or aldosteronoma.

DISORDERS OF LIPID AND CARBOHYDRATE METABOLISM

Diabetes Mellitus (DM)

Table 6-12 lists the criteria used by the American Diabetes Association (ADA) to diagnose DM. Three **autoantibodies** are commonly found in patients with type 1 DM:

- Anti-glutamic acid decarboxylase antibody.
- Anti-ICA 512 antibody.
- Anti-insulin antibody. Most people will develop anti-insulin antibodies with insulin treatment; therefore these antibodies are useful only in the first 1–2 weeks after insulin therapy is initiated.

Screening criteria are shown in Table 6-13.

SYMPTOMS/EXAM

- **Presents with the three "polys": polyuria, polydipsia, polyphagia.**
- **Other:** Rapid weight loss, dehydration, blurry vision, neuropathy, altered consciousness, acanthosis nigricans, vulvovaginitis.
- **Signs of DKA: Kussmaul respirations** (rapid deep breaths); **fruity breath odor** from acetone.

*Hemoglobin A_{1c} is used to monitor treatment and is **not** an accurate way to make the initial diagnosis of diabetes.*

DIFFERENTIAL

- **Type 1 DM:** Caused by autoimmune destruction of the pancreatic islet cells; associated with a genetic predisposition.
- **Type 2 DM:** Due to insulin resistance; accounts for roughly 90% of DM cases in the United States. Shows a strong polygenic predisposition.
- **Secondary causes of DM:** Insulin deficiency or resistance from many causes, such as CF, pancreatitis, Cushing's syndrome, and meds (gluco-

Table 6-12. Criteria for the Diagnosis of DM (ADA Guidelines, 2005)

The presence of any one of the following is diagnostic:
1. Symptoms of diabetes plus a **random** glucose concentration ≥ **200 mg/dL** (11.1 mmol/L).
2. **Fasting** plasma glucose ≥ **126 mg/dL** (7 mmol/L) on 2 separate occasions.
3. Two-hour postprandial glucose ≥ 200 mg/dL (11.1 mmol/L) during oral glucose tolerance test (with a 75-g glucose load).

TABLE 6-13. Diabetes Screening Criteria (ADA Guidelines, 2002)

1. Testing should be considered in all individuals ≥ 45 years of age and, if normal, repeated q 3 years.
2. Testing should be considered at a younger age and carried out more frequently in the following individuals:
■ Overweight (body mass index [BMI] ≥ 25 kg/m²).
■ First-degree relative with diabetes.
■ Members of high-risk ethnic groups (African-American, Hispanic, Native American, Asian-American, Pacific Islander).
■ Delivered a baby weighing > 9 lb or diagnosed with gestational diabetes.
■ Hypertension.
■ Have an HDL < 35 mg/dL and/or a TG level > 250 mg/dL.
■ Impaired glucose tolerance or impaired fasting glucose on previous testing.

corticoids, thiazides). Also due to genetic defects in beta-cell function (e.g., mature-onset diabetes of the young, or MODY).

- **Latent autoimmune diabetes in adults:** Generally considered a form of type 1 DM seen in adults. Patients have positive autoantibodies, but the course is less severe than that in children.

Age does not determine the type of DM; more children are being diagnosed with type 2 DM and more adults with type 1 DM.

TREATMENT

- **Routine diabetic care:** See Table 6-14.
- **Glycemic control:** For therapeutic goals, see Table 6-15.
  - **Oral medications for type 2 DM:** See Table 6-16. Treatment is usually initiated with a single agent (metformin or a sulfonylurea). Often, a second or third agent will be added as the disease progresses.
  - **Insulin:** For all type 1 DM and many type 2 DM patients (see Table 6-17); potential insulin regimens include **"basal-bolus"** (**basal** coverage with intermediate- to long-acting insulin, plus **bolus** short-acting before meals) and **continuous SQ insulin infusion** delivered via an SQ catheter.
- **Immunosuppression:** Experimental in newly diagnosed type 1 DM.
- **Pancreatic/islet cell transplant:** Experimental.

First-line treatment of type 2 DM in an obese patient with normal renal function (Cr < 1.5) is metformin.

COMPLICATIONS—ACUTE

Acute complications of DM can stem from ketoacidosis or from hyperosmolar coma (see Tables 6-18 and 6-19):

- **Ketoacidosis:** Can be the initial manifestation of type 1 DM but may occur in patients with type 1 or type 2 DM when a stressor is present (e.g., infection, infarction, surgery, medical noncompliance). Often presents with abdominal pain, vomiting, Kussmaul respirations, and a fruity breath odor. Mortality is just < 5%. Treat the precipitating event when possible.
  - The first goal is to close the anion gap with **insulin;** the glucose will decrease as the gap closes. Start IV insulin drip; once the anion gap has closed, the insulin may be switched to SQ. Start SQ insulin at least two hours before discontinuing the insulin drip.
  - **Fluids:** Start with NS; when corrected Na to < 150 mg/dL, switch to ½ NS or D5 ½ NS.

TABLE 6-14. Routine Diabetic Care

- **Diet and exercise:** Low-fat, low-carbohydrate diet with exercise four times per week or as tolerated.
- **Hemoglobin A_{1c} (HbA_{1c}):** Measure at least two times per year in stable patients, more frequently during medication changes.
- **BP control: Goal systolic BP < 130 mmHg.** First-line therapy is usually ACEIs or ARBs, but β-blockers and diuretics may also be used.
- **Lipids: Goal LDL < 100 mg/dL.**
- **Aspirin therapy:** 75–325 mg of aspirin per day in all adult patients with DM and macrovascular disease; consider use in patients ≥ 40 years of age with one or more risk factors.
- **Smoking cessation:** All patients should be advised not to smoke.
- **Nephropathy screening:** Annual microalbumin screen in type 1 DM patients five years after initial diagnosis and in all type 2 DM patients. **Treat microalbuminuria with ACEIs or ARBs.**
- **Foot care:** A comprehensive foot examination annually with visual inspection at each visit.
- **Retinopathy:** Type 1 DM patients should have an initial eye exam within 3–5 years of onset and then annually. Type 2 DM patients should have an initial exam soon after diagnosis and annually thereafter. Laser therapy can reduce the risk of vision loss.
- **Immunizations:** Annual influenza vaccine in patients > 6 months of age; at least one lifetime pneumococcal vaccine for adults.
- **Preconception care:** HbA_{1c} should be normal or as close as possible to normal before conception; oral antidiabetic agents and ARBs/ACEIs should be discontinued before pregnancy.

Continue an insulin drip until the anion gap closes even after the glucose has normalized.

  - **Potassium:** Usually falsely elevated due to acidosis, so when in the 4.0–4.5 range, start K^+ replacement (potassium levels will fall with treatment).
  - Bicarbonate, magnesium, and phosphate are usually not needed.
- **Hyperosmolar coma:** Characterized by significant hyperglycemia (often > 600 mg/dL), hyperosmolality, and dehydration without ketosis. Mortality is 40–50%, as this often occurs in elderly patients with many comorbidities. There is often a precipitating event (infection, infarction, intoxica-

TABLE 6-15. Treatment Goals for Nonpregnant DM Patients (both type 1 and type 2)

	NORMAL	GOAL	ADDITIONAL ACTION SUGGESTED
Plasma average preprandial glucose (mg/dL)	< 110	90–130	< 90 or > 150
Plasma average bedtime glucose	< 120	110–150	< 110 or > 180
Whole blood average preprandial glucose (mg/dL)	< 100	80–120	< 80 or > 140
Whole blood average bedtime glucose (mg/dL)	< 110	100–140	< 100 or > 160
HbA_{1c} (%)	< 6	< 7	> 8

TABLE 6-16. Medication Classes Used in Type 2 DM

CLASS	NAMES	DOSING	ADVERSE EFFECTS	COMMENTS
Sulfonylureas	Glimepiride, glipizide, glyburide, tolazamide, tolbutamide.	QD or BID.	Hypoglycemia.	Different medications have varying degrees of renal or liver metabolism.
Biguanides	Metformin.	BID or TID.	GI effects (nausea, diarrhea, decreased appetite).	Rare hypoglycemia; promotes weight loss. Lactic acidosis risk is increased in the presence of renal disease (Cr > 1.5), CHF, severe respiratory disease, and liver disease as well as in the elderly (> 80 years).
Meglitinides	Repaglinide, nateglinide.	Premeal (TID).	Hypoglycemia.	Short action for postprandial hyperglycemia.
Thiazolidinediones	Rosiglitazone, pioglitazone.	QD or BID.	Rare hypoglycemia, fluid retention and edema.	May cause liver disease; LFTs should be checked q 2 months for the first year of treatment and then periodically. Not to be used in patients with heart failure.
α-glucosidase inhibitors	Miglitol, acarbose.	TID.	Gas, bloating, diarrhea.	Start low and gradually increase the dose. Should not be used in people with GI problems.

tion, medical noncompliance). Presents with "polys," weakness, lethargy, and confusion (when osm > 310) or coma (osm > 330). Treatment is similar to that for DKA: treat the underlying stressor and give fluids, insulin drip, and electrolyte replacement.

- **Fluids:** Often need 6–10 L. Start with NS and then follow with ½ NS; add D5 when glucose < 250. Watch for pulmonary edema and volume overload in elderly patients.

TABLE 6-17. Summary of Insulin Characteristics

	INSULIN TYPE	ONSET	PEAK ACTION	DURATION
Ultra-short-acting	Lispro, insulin aspart.	5–15 minutes.	1.0–1.5 hours.	3–4 hours.
Short-acting	Regular.	15–30 minutes.	1–3 hours.	5–7 hours.
Intermediate-acting	Lente, NPH.	2–4 hours.	8–10 hours.	18–24 hours.
Long-acting	Ultralente, glargine.	4–5 hours.	8–14 hours (glargine has virtually no peak).	25–36 hours.

ENDOCRINOLOGY

TABLE 6-18. DKA vs. Hyperosmolar Coma

	DKA	Hyperosmolar Coma
Serum HCO_3	Low (< 15 mEq/L)	Normal or slightly low
pH	< 7.3	> 7.3
Blood glucose	< 800 mg/dL and can be normal	Often > 800 mg/dL
Serum ketones	> 5 mmol/L	< 5 mmol/L
Urine ketones	Large	Small

TABLE 6-19. Formulas to Guide DKA and Hyperosmolar Coma Management

- Anion gap = Na – Cl – CO_2 (normal: 8–20; use measured Na)
- Calculated osmolality = 2 × (Na + K) + glucose/18 + BUN/2.8.
- Corrected Na = measured Na + 1.5 (glucose – 150)/100

  OR

  Corrected Na = measured Na + [(glucose – 100) × 1.6] / 100

- **Insulin drip:** See the DKA section above.
- **Potassium:** See the DKA section above.

If a patient is in a coma and serum osmolality < 330, hyperosmolarity is probably not the cause of the coma; look for another etiology.

Complications—Chronic

- **Microvascular complications:**
  - **Retinopathy:** Occurs after DM has been present for 3–5 years. Prevent with yearly eye exam and photocoagulation therapy for retinal neovascularization.
  - **Nephropathy:** The first sign is usually microalbuminuria. Prevent with BP control, glucose control, ACEIs or ARBs.
  - **Neuropathy:** Often progressive, involving the distal feet and hands. Prevent with foot care, careful inspection, and podiatry as needed.
- **Macrovascular complications:** Increased risk for MI and stroke. Prevent with aspirin therapy in high-risk patients, low threshold for cardiac stress testing, and keep LDL < 100.
- **Hypoglycemia:** Most often occurs in patients taking insulin, although oral medications can also cause this condition. See the hypoglycemia section for details.
- Studies indicate that **tight glycemic control** can decrease the incidence of chronic complications, especially microvascular disease.

Gestational Diabetes (GDM)

Any degree of glucose intolerance with onset during pregnancy. Women should be screened for GDM during pregnancy; those at high risk should have a glucose tolerance test as soon as possible, and those with average risk should be tested between 24 and 28 weeks. Low-risk women do not need testing. Patients at low risk include the following:

- Women < 25 years of age.
- Those with a normal weight prior to pregnancy.
- Members of ethnic groups with a low prevalence of GDM.
- Those with no first-degree relatives with DM.
- Those with no history of abnormal glucose tolerance.
- Those with no prior poor obstetric outcome.

Pregnant women with neither type 1 nor type 2 DM are usually managed with insulin, as limited data are available on diabetic drugs during pregnancy. Drugs that are always contraindicated include ACEIs, ARBs, and metformin.

DIAGNOSIS

Either a 100-g or a 75-g glucose load can be used (see Table 6-20). Two or more elevated levels are needed for diagnosis.

TREATMENT

- Obese women should be put on a calorie-restricted diet.
- Insulin is recommended when nutrition therapy fails to maintain self-monitored glucose at the following levels:
  - Fasting glucose < 95 (whole blood) or < 105 (plasma).
  - One-hour postprandial < 140 (whole blood) or < 155 (plasma).
  - Two-hour postprandial < 120 (whole blood) or < 130 (plasma).
- Oral agents are not recommended, although there are some early data on the safety of the sulfonylureas.
- Fetal size should be monitored, and patients may be referred for cesarean section.

Metabolic Syndrome

Associated with insulin resistance, with the diagnosis based on the presence of any three of the following (Adult Treatment Panel III criteria):

- Abdominal obesity (waist circumference > 40 inches in men, > 35 inches in women).
- TG ≥ 150 mg/dL.
- HDL < 40 mg/dL in men, < 50 mg/dL in women.
- BP ≥ 130/≥ 85 mmHg.
- Fasting glucose ≥ 110 mg/dL.

Hypoglycemia

Although most hypoglycemic reactions occur in patients being treated with insulin, they may also occur in those on sulfonylureas, meglitinides, and, rarely, metformin.

TABLE 6-20. Diagnosis of Gestational Diabetes

	100-g LOAD	75-g LOAD
	Diagnose GDM if glucose (in mg/dL) ≥	Diagnose GDM if glucose (in mg/dL) ≥
Fasting	95	95
1 hour	180	180
2 hours	155	155
3 hours	140	N/A

Autonomic symptoms can be blunted in patients on β-blockers or in patients with lack of awareness of hypoglycemia after repeated hypoglycemic episodes.

Acute pancreatitis is a risk when TG > 1000 mg/dL. Episodes are often precipitated by alcohol binges or nonadherence to a low-fat diet.

Hypertriglyceridemia can cause milky-appearing serum when TG > 350 mg/dL.

HMG-CoA reductase inhibitors should not be used as single or first-line therapy for hypertriglyceridemia. Only atorvastatin and simvastatin at maximal doses effectively reduce TG.

TABLE 6-21. Diagnosis of Hypoglycemia

	Insulin	C-Peptide	Sulfonylurea Screen
Insulinoma[a]	High	High	–
Factitious insulin ingestion	High	Low	–
Sulfonylureas	High	High	+

[a] A **72-hour fast** is necessary to rule out insulinoma.

Symptoms/Exam

- **Neuroglycopenic symptoms** (low glucose delivery to the brain): Mental confusion, stupor, coma, focal neurologic findings mimicking stroke, death.
- **Autonomic symptoms:** Tachycardia, palpitations, sweating, tremulousness, nausea, hunger.

Differential

- **Insulin reaction:** Too much insulin, too little food, or too much exercise can cause hypoglycemia in patients on insulin.
- **Sulfonylurea overdose:** Especially problematic in elderly patients or in patients with renal failure causing decreased medication clearance.
- **Factitious hypoglycemia:** A surreptitious or inadvertent (incorrect medication dispensed) hypoglycemic agent use in a nondiabetic patient.
- **Insulinomas:** Rare tumors of the pancreatic islets cells that secrete insulin. Usually single, benign tumors that should be resected surgically.
- **Reactive hypoglycemia:** Hypoglycemia after a meal may be seen in patients with "dumping syndrome."
- **Autoimmune hypoglycemia:** A rare condition with anti-insulin antibodies that cause hypoglycemia.

Diagnosis

Diagnosis should proceed as follows (see also Table 6-21):

- **Step 1:** Check a glucose level at the time symptoms arise to confirm hypoglycemia.
- **Step 2:** Distinguish the causes of hypoglycemia in nondiabetic patients.

Treatment

- **Conscious patients:** Glucose tablets; orange juice or other sugar-containing beverages.
- **Unconscious patients:** Give 1 mg glucagon IM or 50% glucose solution IV. If these are not available, honey, syrup, or glucose gel may be rubbed into the buccal mucosa.

Familial Lipid Abnormalities

Table 6-22 outlines the presentation of various lipid abnormalities. All of these disorders should be treated with low-fat diets and weight reduction. Also

TABLE 6-22. Common Familial Lipid Abnormalities

Disease[a]	Cholesterol	TG	LDL	HDL	Signs/Symptoms	Treatment
ISOLATED HYPERTRIGLYCERIDEMIA					**Eruptive** cutaneous **xanthomas,** lipemia retinalis, acute pancreatitis.	
Lipoprotein lipase deficiency (AR)	Normal	2000–25,000	Normal	Low		
Apo C-II deficiency (AR)	Normal	2000–25,000	Low	Low	Childhood diagnosis. hepatosplenomegaly.	Dietary; meds not very effective.
Familial hypertriglyceridemia (AD)	Normal	200–500	Normal	Low	Obesity and insulin resistance are common.	Anti-TG meds.[b]
ISOLATED HYPERCHOLESTEROLEMIA					**Tendon xanthomas.**	
Familial hypercholesterolemia—deficiency or malfunction of LDL receptor (AD)	Heterozygous: 275–500 Homozygous: > 500	Normal	Very high	Normal	Premature CAD. Homozygous: CAD in first decade.	Statin + niacin.
Familial defective Apo B-100—impaired LDL binding	275–500	Normal	Very high	Normal	Premature CAD.	Statin + niacin.
COMBINED HYPERTRIGLYCERIDEMIA AND HYPERCHOLESTEROLEMIA						
Familial combined hyperlipidemia (AD)	250–500	250–750	High	Low	Premature CAD. Associated with metabolic syndromes.	Statin + niacin
Familial dysbetalipoproteinemia—APO E2 isoform (AR)	250–500	250–500	High	Normal	**Palmar** and tubular **xanthomas** and xanthelasmas.	Fibrates + niacin or statin.

[a]AR = autosomal recessive; AD = autosomal dominant.

[b]Anti-TG meds = gemfibrozil, fenofibrate, niacin, and clofibrate.

note that hypertriglyceridemia can be markedly worsened by secondary factors such as alcohol, hypothyroidism, estrogen therapy, and poor diabetes control.

Sodium can be falsely decreased when TG levels are elevated. To correct, add 1.6 mg/dL to Na^+ per 100 mg/dL TG over 100 mg/dL.

MINERAL METABOLISM AND METABOLIC BONE DISEASE

Calcium Metabolism

Figure 6-7 delineates the hormonal control of calcium metabolism. Figure 6-8 graphically depicts the mechanisms of vitamin D metabolism.

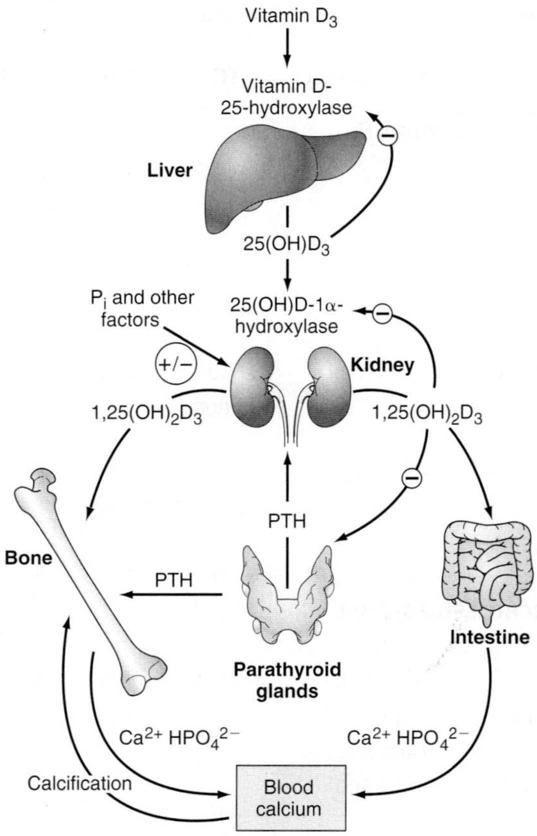

FIGURE 6-7. Schematic representation of the hormonal control loop for vitamin D metabolism and function.

Low serum calcium levels prompt a proportional increase in PTH concentration, which mobilizes calcium from the bone. PTH also increases the synthesis of $1,25(OH)_2$ vitamin D in the kidney, which in turn stimulates the mobilization of calcium from bone, increases absorption of calcium in the intestine, and downregulates PTH synthesis.(Reproduced, with permission, from Kasper DL et al. *Harrison's Principles of Internal Medicine,* 16th ed. New York: McGraw-Hill, 2005:2246.)

Hypercalcemia

Eighty percent of hospitalized hypercalcemia cases are due to malignancy. Eighty percent of outpatient hypercalcemia cases are due to primary hyperparathyroidism.

Most commonly presents as an incidentally discovered laboratory abnormality in an asymptomatic patient. Can be classified into PTH-mediated hypercalcemia (primary hyperparathyroidism) vs. other causes:

- **Primary hyperparathyroidism:** See the separate section below.
- **Malignancy-associated hypercalcemia:** Occurs in 10–15% of malignancies and portends a poor prognosis. In 98% of patients, the identity of the tumor is obvious at presentation. Has three mechanisms:
  - **Tumor release of PTH-related peptide (PTHrP)—most common:** Homologous to PTH, but **not** detected by intact PTH serum assay, and does not increase 1,25-DHD production. Seen with solid tumors (e.g., breast, lung, renal cell, ovarian, and bladder carcinoma).
  - **1,25-DHD production by tumor:** Associated with lymphomas.
  - **Local osteolysis from metastases or adjacent tumor mass:** Typically multiple myeloma and breast cancer.

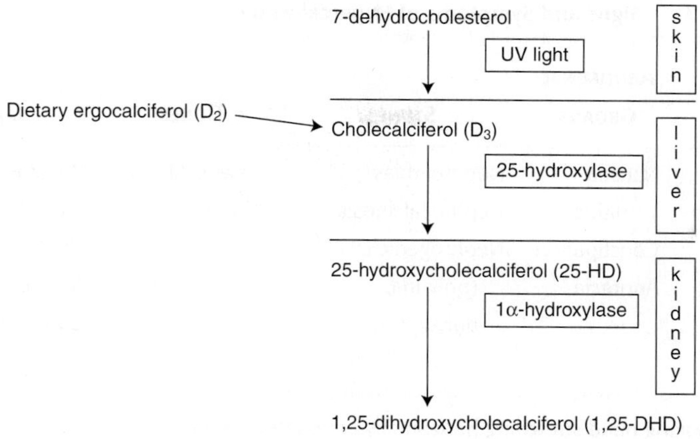

Figure 6-8. Vitamin D metabolism.

Vitamin D is derived when UV light from the sun hits the skin, converting 7-dehydrocholesterol into cholecalciferol (D_3), or when ergocalciferol (D_2) is ingested and then converted to D_3. D_3 is 25-hydroxylated to 25-hydroxycholecalciferol (25-HD) in the liver. 25-HD is the primary storage form. 25-HD is converted to 1,25-dihydroxycholecalciferol (1,25-DHD) in the kidney under PTH regulation. 1,25-DHD is the active form of the hormone.

- **Granulomatous disorders:**
  - Granulomas contain 25-HD 1-hydroxylase, which allows them to make **1,25-DHD.**
  - Treatment with glucocorticoids is uniquely effective, directly suppressing the 1-hydroxylase enzyme.
- **Endocrinopathies:**
  - Ten percent of **thyrotoxic** patients have mild hypercalcemia.
  - **Adrenal insufficiency.** Rare: pheochromocytoma, VIPoma.
- **Hypervitaminosis A and D:**
  - Vitamin A excess leads to bone resorption and associated hypercalcemia.
  - Vitamin D excess leads to elevated 25-HD levels, which stimulate increased intestinal absorption of calcium and decreased renal excretion.
- **Drug induced:** Thiazides, lithium, calcium-based antacids, estrogens, androgens, PTH 1-84.

Symptoms/Exam

Best remembered by the mnemonic **"psychic moans, abdominal groans, stones, and bones"** (see Table 6-23).

Diagnosis

- When an elevated serum calcium level is found, first correct for albumin level:

  $$\text{Corrected } Ca^{++} = \text{serum Ca (mg/dL)} + [0.8 \times (4.0 - \text{albumin (g/dL)})]$$

  i.e., for each 1.0-mg/dL decrease in albumin, add 0.8 to measured total serum calcium.

- Next, obtain a PTH. If elevated, the differential should include PTH-mediated causes of hypercalcemia; if suppressed, a PTHrP, 25-HD, and 1,25-DHD should be obtained (see Table 6-24).

ENDOCRINOLOGY

TABLE 6-23. Signs and Symptoms of Hypercalcemia

Psychic Moans	Abdominal Groans	Stones	Bones	Other
Lethargy	Nausea	Nephrolithiasis	Osteitis fibrosa	Weakness
Depression	Vomiting	Nephrocalcinosis	Arthritis	Hypertonia
Psychosis	Constipation	Nephrogenic DI (polyuria, polydipsia)		Bradycardia
Ataxia	Anorexia			Shortened QT
Stupor				Band keratopathy[a]
Coma		Uremia		

[a] A mottled-looking band stretching horizontally across the cornea.

TREATMENT

- **Hydration with normal saline is the essential element in treating acute hypercalcemia.** Often requires 2.5–4.0 L of NS per day; start at 300–500 cc NS per hour unless CHF.
- **Loop diuretics** are indicated **only after complete rehydration.**
- IV **bisphosphonates** (pamidronate or zoledronate):
  - The treatment of choice in suspected hypercalcemia of malignancy.
  - Its effect on serum calcium will be **delayed at least 24 hours,** and the calcium nadir will occur approximately 3–5 days after injection. Hypocalcemic effects will last 4–6 weeks.
  - Side effects include a mild increase in serum creatinine in approximately 15% of patients, transient fever and myalgia in 20% of patients, and hypophosphatemia.
- **Calcitonin** (SQ):
  - Use only in the presence of severe symptomatic hypercalcemia.
  - Works faster than bisphosphonates, but efficacy is lost after three days owing to tachyphylaxis.
- **Glucocorticoids:** First-line treatment in patients with vitamin D– or vitamin A–mediated hypercalcemia.

Primary Hyperparathyroidism

Incidence is 42 in 100,000. The female-to-male ratio is 2:1. **Eighty percent are due to a single parathyroid adenoma;** the rest are due to gland hyperplasia and cancer. Can be part of MEN 1, MEN 2A, and isolated familial hyperparathyroidism.

TABLE 6-24. Laboratory Findings Associated with Hypercalcemia

	Calcium	Phosphorus	PTH	PTHrP	Other
PTH mediated	↑	↓	↑	↓	
PTHrP mediated	↑	↓	↓	↑	
1,25-DHD mediated	↑	↑	↓	↓	↑ 1,25-DHD
Vitamin D intoxication	↑	↑	↓	↓	↑ 25-HD

Symptoms/Exam

- Like hypercalcemia—"**psychic moans, abdominal groans, stones, and bones.**"
- **Eighty-five percent of patients are asymptomatic and diagnosed on screening laboratories.**
- Osteoporosis.
- **Renal: Nephrolithiasis;** gradual onset of **renal insufficiency** from nephrocalcinosis and nephrogenic DI.
- **Osteitis fibrosa cystica:** Increased bone turnover, causing bone pain and pathologic fractures. Also elevated alkaline phosphatase. X-rays of phalanges and skull reveal subperiosteal resorption of cortical bone. Osteolytic lesions due to brown tumors (cystic bone lesions containing fibrous tissue) may also be apparent.

Differential

- **Familial benign hypocalciuric hypercalcemia (FBHH):** Autosomal dominant; lifelong asymptomatic mild hypercalcemia. Differentiated from primary hyperparathyroidism by normal PTH and marked **hypocalciuria.** This syndrome **requires no therapy.**
- **MEN syndromes:** See the section on MEN below.
- **Lithium therapy:** Lithium shifts the set point for PTH secretion, resulting in hypercalcemia.

Diagnosis

Made by laboratory tests **showing increased PTH, increased Ca^{++}, and decreased phosphorus.** Further evaluation should include the following:

- 24-hour urinary calcium and creatinine.
- Evaluation of renal function with creatinine.
- Bone mineral density (BMD) evaluation by dual-energy x-ray absorptiometry (DEXA).

Imaging studies of the parathyroid glands are rarely indicated or necessary.

If diagnosis is uncertain or the patient is asymptomatic, consider FBHH and check for hypercalciuria before sending the patient for a parathyroidectomy!

Treatment

Parathyroidectomy is the treatment of choice. The **cure rate is 95%,** and the complication rate (hypoparathyroidism, recurrent laryngeal nerve injury) is < 1%. **Surgery is recommended under the following conditions:**

- Age < 50.
- Serum calcium 1.0 mg/dL above the upper normal level.
- 24-hour urine calcium > 400 mg.
- Creatinine clearance reduced by 30%.
- BMD with T-score < –2.5 at any site.

Hyperparathyroidism causes the greatest osteopenia at the forearm, followed by the hip. The spine is least affected.

Complications

Nephrolithiasis, nephrocalcinosis with renal insufficiency, osteopenia, osteoporosis.

Hypocalcemia

Symptoms/Exam

- **Neuromuscular excitability:** Paresthesias, seizures, organic brain syndrome, or the hallmark, **tetany**—a state of spontaneous tonic muscular

contraction. Often heralded by numbness and tingling of the fingertips and perioral zone, its classic component is carpopedal spasm.
    - **Chvostek's sign:** Contraction of facial muscles in response to tapping of the facial nerve. Note that 25% of normal individuals have a positive Chvostek's sign all the time.
    - **Trousseau's sign:** Elicited by inflating a BP cuff to 20 mmHg above systolic pressure for three minutes. A positive response is carpal spasm (positive in 1–4% of normals).
- Soft tissue calcium deposition (cataract, calcification of basal ganglia).
- **Cardiac:** Prolonged QT interval.
- **Dermatologic:** Dry, flaky skin with brittle nails.

DIFFERENTIAL

- **Hypoparathyroidism:** Most often **postsurgical.** Also autoimmune, familial, infiltrative (hemochromatosis or Wilson's), or idiopathic. Treat with chronic oral calcitriol (1,25[OH]$_2$ vitamin D) and calcium.
- **Pseudohypoparathyroidism:** A heritable disorder of **target organ resistance to PTH.** Has two forms: **isolated PTH resistance** or that associated with abnormal phenotype—**Albright's hereditary osteodystrophy** (short stature, round face, short neck, brachydactyly). Treatment is the same as that for hypoparathyroidism.
- **Vitamin D deficiency:**
    - Risk factors include malabsorptive states (e.g., IBD, celiac sprue, post–gastric bypass surgery, chronic pancreatitis), lack of sun exposure, and dark skin.
    - Long-term deficiency in adults leads to **osteomalacia**—myopathy (proximal muscle pain and weakness) and poor bone mineralization with pseudofractures.
    - In children it leads to **rickets** (bony deformities—rachitic rosary, bowing of the lower extremities, frontal bossing).
    - **Diagnosis: Low 25-HD level** (< 20 ng/mL). Hypocalcemia, hypophosphatemia, secondary hyperparathyroidism, and increased alkaline phosphatase may also be seen.
    - **Treatment:** Oral vitamin D replacement at high doses; calcium.
- **Abnormal calcitriol metabolism:** Resistance or abnormal production—e.g., hereditary rickets.
- **Acute deposition or complex formation of calcium:**
    - Acute hyperphosphatemia: tumor lysis, parenteral phosphate administration, excessive oral phosphate.
    - Acute pancreatitis.
    - Blood transfusion (citrate buffer present in packed RBC precipitates with calcium).
    - Hungry bone syndrome.

Transfusion of multiple units of RBCs can lead to hypocalcemia due to precipitation of citrate buffer with calcium. Generally, only minimal temporary calcium replacement is needed, as total body calcium stores are normal.

DIAGNOSIS

First check calcium and correct for albumin; then check phosphorus, magnesium, and PTH (see Table 6-25). If PTH is elevated or normal, check 25-HD and renal function.

TREATMENT

- **Acutely:** If tetany, continuous IV calcium drip while starting oral calcium; calcitriol if needed.
- **Chronically:** Oral calcium and calcitriol if needed.

TABLE 6-25. Laboratory Findings Associated with Hypocalcemia

	Calcium	Phosphorus	PTH	Other
Hypoparathyroidism	↓	↑	↓	
PTH resistance	↓	↑	↑	
Vitamin D deficiency	↓	↓	↑	↓ 25-HD
1,25-DHD resistance	↓	↓	↑	↑ 1,25-DHD

Male and Secondary Osteoporosis

Secondary osteoporosis is defined as osteoporosis due to a treatable underlying disease.

Symptoms/Exam

Asymptomatic until a fracture occurs. Typical osteoporotic fractures are hip, vertebral compression, and Colles' fractures.

Diagnosis

BMD measurement by DEXA. The definition is based on World Health Organization (WHO) criteria, which use a T-score that is defined as the number of standard deviations below the average bone density for a young sex-matched cohort:

- **Osteopenia:** T-score < -1 and > -2.5.
- **Osteoporosis: T-score ≤ -2.5.**

Secondary osteoporosis should also be considered in women.

Further evaluation should include a search for secondary causes of osteoporosis based on clinical suspicion of any existing disorder that can cause or present as osteoporosis (see Table 6-26 for a full list):

- 25-HD level
- Serum calcium, phosphorus, and PTH
- 24-hour urinary calcium and creatinine
- SPEP/UPEP
- Testosterone level

Treatment

- **Bisphosphonates** (alendronate, risedronate) improve BMD and markedly reduce the risk of fracture.
- **Calcium 1500 mg/day with 800–1000 IU vitamin D per day** should be used in all patients with osteopenia or osteoporosis who do not have contraindications.
- **Teriparatide** (recombinant PTH) was recently approved for severe osteoporosis.
- **Calcitonin** is associated with minimal fracture prevention. Effective as an analgesic for acute vertebral fracture pain.

TABLE 6-26. Secondary Causes of Osteoporosis

- **Endocrine causes:**
  - Cushing's syndrome
  - Eating disorders
  - Hypogonadism (male or female)
  - Hyperprolactinemia (by inducing hypogonadism)
  - Hyperthyroidism
  - Hyperparathyroidism
  - Vitamin D deficiency
- **GI disorders:**
  - Liver disease
  - Malabsorptive conditions (mediated primarily via vitamin D deficiency):
    - Gastrectomy
    - Inflammatory bowel disorders
    - Gastric bypass
    - Pancreatic insufficiency
- **Marrow/hematologic disorders:**
  - Multiple myeloma
  - Leukemias/lymphomas
  - Systemic mastocytosis
  - Hemophilia
  - Thalassemia
- **Miscellaneous:**
  - Immobilization
  - Alcohol abuse
  - Tobacco use
  - Osteogenesis imperfecta
  - Rheumatoid arthritis
  - Ankylosing spondylitis

COMPLICATIONS

Fractures. Thirty percent of hip fractures lead to mortality in men. Vertebral fractures are associated with chronic pain and disability. This mortality rate is higher than that for hip fractures in women.

Paget's Disease

Accelerated bone turnover. Affects 4% of people > 40 years of age. **Most prevalent in northern Europe.**

The most common fractures in Paget's disease are vertebral crush fractures.

SYMPTOMS

Include pain, fractures, and deformity, most commonly in the **sacrum, spine, femur, skull, and pelvis.** Two-thirds of patients are asymptomatic.

EXAM

Depends on which bones are involved. Exam may reveal skull enlargement, frontal bossing, bowed legs, and cutaneous erythema, warmth, and tenderness over the affected site.

DIFFERENTIAL

Includes any localized bony tumor or cancer.

Immobilizing a patient with active Paget's can lead to hypercalcemia.

DIAGNOSIS

- **Laboratory tests: Increased alkaline phosphatase** and bone turnover markers (e.g., osteocalcin, urinary hydroxyproline, N-telopeptide). Normal Ca^{++} and phosphorus.
- **Imaging studies:**
  - **Plain radiography:** Involved bones are expanded and denser than normal. Erosions are seen in the skull (osteoporosis circumscripta). Affected weight-bearing bones may be bowed.
  - **Bone scan:** Increased uptake is seen in affected areas.

TABLE 6-27. Complications of Paget's Disease

- **Rheumatologic:**
  - Osteoarthritis
  - Gout
- **Neurologic:**
  - Deafness (from involvement of cranial nerves, with bony entrapment)
  - Spinal cord compression
  - Peripheral nerve entrapment (carpal and tarsal tunnel syndromes)
- **Cardiac:**
  - High-output CHF
- **Neoplastic** (in 1% of Paget's cases):
  - Osteosarcoma or chondrosarcoma
  - Giant cell tumor
- **Metabolic:**
  - Immobilization-induced hypercalcemia/hypercalciuria
  - Nephrolithiasis

TREATMENT

Bisphosphonates are the treatment of choice and lead to remission in most patients. Choices include IV pamidronate, oral alendronate, risedronate, or tiludronate

Paget's is one of the rare causes of high-output CHF due to hypervascularity of the bony lesions.

COMPLICATIONS

The complications of Paget's disease are outlined in Table 6-27.

MALE HYPOGONADISM

Testes are composed of seminiferous tubules, where sperm are produced (80–90% of testicular mass), and Leydig cells, which produce androgens.

SYMPTOMS/EXAM

- **Prepubertal androgen deficiency:** Poor secondary sexual development (small phallus and testes; sparse pubic, axillary, facial, chest, and back hair; high-pitched voice; low muscle mass), eunuchoid skeletal proportions.
- **Postpubertal androgen deficiency:** Decreased libido, erectile dysfunction, low energy. If prolonged, a decrease in facial and body hair may be seen.

DIFFERENTIAL

- **Hypothalamic/pituitary disorders:** Low testosterone with normal or low LH and FSH.
  - **Panhypopituitarism.**
  - **LH and FSH deficiency:** If associated with anosmia, **Kallmann's** syndrome.
- **Gonadal disorders:** Usually low testosterone, elevated LH and FSH.
  - **Klinefelter's syndrome:** The most common genetic cause of male hypogonadism (1/500). XXY karyotype. Can be associated with intellectual impairment.
  - **Adult seminiferous tubule failure:** Etiologies include mumps orchitis, leprosy, irradiation, alcoholism, uremia, cryptorchidism, lead poisoning, chemotherapeutic agents (e.g., cyclophosphamide, methotrexate), or idiopathic. Characterized by infertility, normal virilization, and normal testosterone levels.

If LH is low in the setting of a low testosterone level, an MRI is indicated to evaluate the pituitary gland.

TABLE 6-28. Diagnosis of Hypogonadism Based on Laboratory Tests

DISORDER	TESTOSTERONE	LH	FSH
Primary gonadal failure (Leydig cell failure)	↓	↑	↑
Seminiferous tubule failure	Normal	Normal	↑
Hypothalamic or pituitary dysfunction	↓	Normal or ↓	Normal or ↓
Partial androgen insensitivity	↑	↑	↑

  - **Adult Leydig cell failure (andropause):** A gradual decrease in testicular function after age 50, with declining testosterone levels.
  - **Bilateral anorchia (absence of testes):** At birth, normal male phenotype with cryptorchidism. Failed secondary sexual development.
  - Defects in androgen biosynthesis.
- **Defects in androgen action:**
  - **Complete androgen insensitivity:** Also known as **testicular feminization**—XY, with female phenotype, absence of uterus, absence of sexual hair, and infertility. Patients are usually raised as girls.
  - **Incomplete androgen insensitivity:** Phenotype varies with degree of insensitivity.

Androgen therapy in hypogonadal men can lead to gynecomastia.

DIAGNOSIS

Check testosterone first. If low, repeat testosterone with LH and FSH (see Table 6-28).

TREATMENT

- **Androgen replacement:** Can be done with IM testosterone injections, patches, or gel.
- If an underlying disorder is diagnosed (e.g., pituitary tumor), treat appropriately.

COMPLICATIONS

Infertility; osteoporosis can develop in the absence of androgens but can usually be prevented with appropriate testosterone replacement.

ENDOCRINE TUMORS

Multiple Endocrine Neoplasia (MEN)

A group of autosomal-dominant syndromes characterized by multiple endocrine tumors due to defective tumor suppressor genes (see Table 6-29).

*MEN 1 can be remembered as the **"3 P's"—Parathyroid, Pancreas, and Pituitary.***

DIAGNOSIS

Screening for MEN is as follows:

- **MEN 1:** Screen if there is a positive family history with serum calcium/PTH, serum gastrin, and serum prolactin.

TABLE 6-29. Characteristics of the MEN Syndromes

	MEN 1 WERMER'S	MEN 2A SIPPLE'S	MEN 2B
Hyperparathyroidism	**95%**	25%	Rare
Pancreatic tumors[a]	**30–80%**	N/A	N/A
Pituitary tumors	**20–25%**	N/A	N/A
Medullary thyroid cancer	N/A	**80–90%**	**100%**
Pheochromocytoma	N/A	**40%**	**50%**
Mucosal neuromas	N/A	N/A	**100%**
Ganglioneuromas of bowel	N/A	N/A	> 40%
Marfanoid habitus	N/A	N/A	**75%**
Carcinoid	20%	N/A	N/A
Adrenal adenomas	40%	N/A	N/A
Subcutaneous lipomas	30%	N/A	N/A
Genetics	MENIN gene	RET proto-oncogene	RET proto-oncogene

[a] Pancreatic tumors can be gastrinomas, associated with Zollinger-Ellison syndrome, insulinomas, glucagonomas, VIPomas, or nonfunctioning tumors.

- **MEN 2:** Screen if there is a positive history of MEN 2 or in any patient with medullary thyroid cancer or bilateral pheochromocytomas. Screen with RET proto-oncogene. If a RET proto-oncogene mutation is found, obtain basal stimulated calcitonin, plasma or urine metanephrines, serum calcium/PTH, serum gastrin, and serum prolactin.

Carcinoid Tumors and Syndrome

The most common neuroendocrine tumor of the gut, it may secrete **serotonin** or its precursors. Categorized as foregut (bronchus and stomach), midgut (small intestine and colon), or hindgut (rectum) in origin. Although carcinoid is often found incidentally and is asymptomatic, the classic carcinoid syndrome consists of episodic **flushing,** watery **diarrhea,** and **hypotension,** with or without asthma. Emotional stress, certain foods (tryptophan-containing foods), and straining with defecation can provoke symptoms. Diagnose with elevated serotonin metabolites in the urine (5-hydroxyindole acetic acid, or HIAA) and stage with CXR and an abdominal CT scan. Surgical resection is the first-line treatment; symptomatic relief may be obtained with octreotide.

Any medullary thyroid cancer patient needs to be considered for genetic screening with RET proto-oncogene, as 75% of these patients have a familial disorder.

Carcinoids cause the syndrome only when they are gut carcinoids, metastatic to the liver, or primary lesions draining into the systemic circulation.

Carcinoids of the bronchus can present as Cushing's syndrome because they can secrete ACTH in addition to serotonin precursors.

Zollinger-Ellison Syndrome

Caused by hypersecretion of gastric acid and **gastrin** by tumors of the pancreas or duodenum. Usually presents as refractory PUD despite *H. pylori* treatment or multiple ulcers in the duodenum and jejunum. Other causes of elevated gastrin should be considered (pernicious anemia, chronic atrophic gastritis, gastric carcinoma, and therapy with PPIs or H_2 blockers). Diagnosis is made by **elevated fasting serum gastrin levels** (in the absence of H_2 blocker or PPI therapy, as these can markedly elevate gastrin) in the presence of **refractory PUD.** Localize by abdominal imaging or octreotide scan. Surgical resection is recommended.

If a type 1 DM patient who has previously been well controlled on insulin regimen presents with new-onset hypoglycemia, consider ruling out Addison's, as type 1 DM patients are at increased risk for other autoimmune diseases.

AUTOIMMUNE POLYGLANDULAR SYNDROMES

Autoimmune, genetic syndromes leading to multiple glandular hypofunction (see Table 6-30).

TABLE 6-30. Autoimmune Polyglandular Syndromes Types I and II (APS I and II)

	APS I	**APS II**
Alternative name	APCED (autoimmune polyendocrinopathy-candidiasis-ectodermal dystrophy syndrome).	Schmidt's syndrome.
Genetics	Autosomal recessive—mutation in AIRE (autoimmune regulator gene).	Linked to HLA-DR3 or HLA-DR4. Female-to-male ratio = 3:1.
Endocrine manifestations	**Hypoparathyroidism**[a]—90%. **Hypoadrenalism**[a]—60%. Hypogonadism—45%. Hypothyroidism—12%.	Hypoadrenalism[b]—70%. Autoimmune thyroid disease[b] (hypo- or hyperthyroidism)—70%. Type 1 DM[b]—50%. Hypogonadism—5–50%.
Nonendocrine manifestations	**Mucocutaneous candidiasis**[a]—75%. Malabsorption—25%. Alopecia—20%. Pernicious anemia—15%. Autoimmune hepatitis—10%. Vitiligo—4%.	Pernicious anemia—15%. Vitiligo—4%. Celiac disease—3%. Autoimmune hepatitis.

[a] Diagnosis requires two of these three diseases.

[b] Diagnosis requires at least two of these three diseases.

CHAPTER 7

Gastroenterology and Hepatology

Scott W. Biggins, MD

Infectious Esophagitis

Most common in immunosuppressed patients (e.g., those with AIDS, leukemia, or lymphoma and those on chronic immunosuppressive agents). Common pathogens include *Candida albicans*, HSV, and CMV.

Symptoms/Exam

- Odynophagia, dysphagia, chest pain.
- Oral lesions are not reliable diagnostic indicators.
- *C. albicans* is the etiologic agent in < 75% of cases and CMV or HSV in < 50%.
- Shoddy cervical lymphadenopathy.

Differential

GERD, pill esophagitis, dyspepsia, esophageal stricture or mass lesion, esophageal motility disorders.

Diagnosis

- Monitor response to an empiric antifungal treatment trial.
- Upper endoscopy with biopsy and brushing for culture and histopathology if the empiric trial yields no response.
  - ***C. albicans:*** Yellow, white, linear, adherent plaques.
  - **CMV:** Few large, superficial ulcerations.
  - **HSV:** Numerous small, deep ulcerations.

Treatment

- Treat or adjust underlying immunosuppression.
- ***C. albicans:*** Treatment depends on host immune status.
  - **Immune-competent patients:** Topical therapy; nystatin swish and swallow five times a day × 7–14 days.
  - **Immunocompromised patients:** Oral therapy; initially fluconazole 100–200 mg/day. If unresponsive, consider increasing fluconazole or giving itraconazole, other azoles, caspofungin, or amphotericin.
- **CMV:** Ganciclovir 5 mg/kg IV BID × 3–6 weeks.
- **HSV:** Acyclovir 200 mg PO five times a day or valacyclovir 1000 g PO BID.

Pill Esophagitis

Variables include contact time, drug type, and pill characteristics. Most cases arise without preexisting swallowing problems. Pills can remain in a normal esophagus > 5 minutes or for much longer with stricture or dysmotility. Risk is higher if pills are large, round, lightweight, or extended-release formulations.

Symptoms/Exam

Odynophagia, dysphagia, chest pain.

Differential

Infectious esophagitis, GERD, dyspepsia, esophageal stricture or mass lesion, esophageal motility disorders.

DIAGNOSIS

- **Review medications.** The following are most frequently associated with pill esophagitis:
  - **NSAIDs:** Aspirin, naproxen, ibuprofen, indomethacin.
  - **Antibiotics:** Tetracyclines (especially doxycycline), clindamycin.
  - **Antivirals:** Foscarnet, AZT, ddC.
  - **Supplements:** Iron and potassium.
  - **Cardiac:** Quinidine, nifedipine, captopril, verapamil.
  - **Bisphosphonates:** Alendronate, pamidronate.
  - **Antiepileptics:** Phenytoin.
  - **Others:** Theophylline.
- **Upper endoscopy:** Evaluate for stricture or mass lesion.

TREATMENT

- Discontinue the suspected drug. Look for symptom relief within 1–6 weeks.
- Patients should drink eight ounces of water with each pill and remain upright at least 30 minutes afterward.
- Proton pump inhibitors (PPIs) may facilitate healing in the presence of concurrent GERD.

Achalasia

An idiopathic esophageal motility disorder with loss of peristalsis in the distal two-thirds of the esophagus. Age at onset is 25–60; incidence increases with age. **Indistinguishable from esophageal dysmotility caused by Chagas' disease.**

SYMPTOMS/EXAM

Gradual-onset dysphagia to solids and liquids; slow eating (**"last person at the table to finish meal"**). Regurgitation of undigested food; weight loss. Heartburn may result from fermentation of retained food.

DIFFERENTIAL

Chagas' disease, esophageal tumors (primary, metastatic), web, stricture, Zenker's diverticulum, oropharyngeal dysphagia (muscular dystrophies, myasthenia gravis, Parkinson's disease), spastic dysmotility disorders (diffuse esophageal spasm, nutcracker esophagus; see Table 7-1), esophageal hypomotility (scleroderma).

DIAGNOSIS

- **CXR:** Suggestive; shows air-fluid levels in a dilated esophagus.
- **Barium esophagography:** Can be diagnostic. May see a dilated esophagus with loss of peristalsis and poor emptying or a smooth, symmetrically tapered distal esophagus with a **"bird's-beak"** appearance.
- **Endoscopy:** Required to exclude esophageal stricture or tumor.
- **Esophageal manometry:** Used to confirm the diagnosis. Shows complete **absence of peristalsis** and simultaneous contraction waves with low-amplitude, incomplete LES relaxation.
- **Endoscopic ultrasound:** Occasionally used to exclude tumor in suspicious distal esophageal lesions.

TREATMENT

- **Nitrates and calcium channel antagonists:** Relax LES tone, but have only modest efficacy.
- **Botulinum toxin injection:** Injected into the LES. Performed endoscopically and associated with an 85% initial response, but > 50% of patients require repeated injection within 6–9 months. Ideal if the patient is a poor candidate for more invasive treatment.
- **Pneumatic dilation:** Of those treated, > 75% have a durable response. Perforation rate is < 3%. Does not compromise surgical therapy.
- **Surgical myotomy:** Modified Heller cardiomyotomy; cuts the LES. Can be performed laparoscopically. Of all cases, > 85% have a durable response, but > 20% have severe gastroesophageal reflux (an antireflux procedure is often performed at the same time).

Patients with achalasia often lift their arms over their heads or extend their necks to aid in swallowing.

Diffuse Esophageal Spasm and Nutcracker Esophagus

Spastic (hypercontractile) motility disorders of the esophagus. **Distinguished from achalasia in that some peristalsis is retained** (see Table 7-1). Shows a female predominance; onset is usually after age 40.

SYMPTOMS/EXAM

Presents with intermittent substernal chest pain with radiation to the back or neck; pain is nonexertional and worsens with meals. Also associated with gradual-onset dysphagia to both solids and liquids. Regurgitation is less common than in achalasia. Weight loss is rare.

TABLE 7-1. Differential Diagnosis of Esophagitis

	ACHALASIA	NUTCRACKER ESOPHAGUS	DIFFUSE ESOPHAGEAL SPASM	SCLERODERMA
Peristalsis	Absent.	Normal.	Intermittently normal or absent.	Absent.
LES tone	Normal to increased with incomplete relaxation.	Normal to increased.	Normal to increased.	Decreased.
Esophageal body tone (amplitude)	Low.	Focal increased (distal).	Normal to high.	Low.
Predominant symptom	Progressive dysphagia.	Chest pain.	Chest pain.	Heartburn and dysphagia.

Differential

Cardiac chest pain, GERD, achalasia, Chagas' disease, esophageal tumors, esophageal hypomotility (scleroderma), peptic stricture.

Unlike achalasia, diffuse esophageal spasm and nutcracker esophagus often present with chest pain rather than with dysphagia.

Diagnosis

Diagnose as follows (see also Table 7-1):

- **Barium esophagography:** Can be diagnostic. Peristalsis is present but with delayed transit; esophageal spasms are focal (in nutcracker esophagus) or at multiple sites (in diffuse esophageal spasm).
- **Endoscopy:** Required to exclude esophageal stricture or tumor.
- **Esophageal manometry:** Used to confirm the diagnosis.
- **Ambulatory esophageal pH:** Used to evaluate for gastroesophageal reflux.

Treatment

- **Nitrates and calcium channel antagonists:** Relax LES tone, but have only modest efficacy.
- PPIs.
- No clear benefit is derived from botulinum toxin injection, esophageal dilation, or surgical myotomy.

Esophageal Rings, Webs, and Strictures

Plummer-Vinson syndrome includes esophageal webs, dysphagia, and iron deficiency anemia.

Esophageal rings, webs, and strictures are distinguished as follows (see also Tables 7-2 and 7-3):

- **Lower esophageal (Schatzki) rings:** Common (found in 6–14% of upper GI exams); located in the distal esophagus. Often associated with hiatal hernia, congenital defects, or reflux.
- **Webs:** Less common; located in the proximal esophagus. Congenital.
- **Strictures:** Result from injury (reflux, caustic, other).

Symptoms/Exam

Dysphagia for solids is worse than for liquids.

Differential

Cardiac chest pain, GERD, achalasia, Chagas' disease, esophageal tumors, esophageal hypomotility (scleroderma), peptic stricture.

TABLE 7-2. Differential of Esophageal Rings, Webs, and Strictures

	Ring	Web	Stricture
Etiology	Congenital or peptic injury.	Congenital.	Peptic injury, caustic injury.
Esophageal location	Distal.	Proximal.	Mid-distal.
Treatment	Dilation.	Dilation.	Dilation.

TABLE 7-3. Causes of Esophageal Dysphagia

CAUSE	CLUES
Mechanical obstruction:	**Solid foods worse than liquids:**
Schatzki ring	Intermittent dysphagia; not progressive
Peptic stricture	Chronic heartburn; progressive dysphagia
Esophageal cancer	Progressive dysphagia; age over 50
Motility disorder:	**Solid and liquid foods:**
Achalasia	Progressive dysphagia
Diffuse esophageal spasm	Intermittent; not progressive; may have chest pain
Scleroderma	Chronic heartburn; Raynaud's phenomenon

Reproduced, with permission, from Tierney LM et al. *Current Medical Diagnosis & Treatment 2004,* 43rd ed. New York: McGraw-Hill, 2004.)

DIAGNOSIS

- **Barium esophagography:** Can be diagnostic. Normal peristalsis; luminal abnormality is seen.
- **Endoscopy:** Required to exclude esophageal stricture or tumor.

TREATMENT

Esophageal dilation; PPIs to decrease recurrence of peptic stricture.

Schatzki rings cause intermittent large-bolus solid-food dysphagia ("steakhouse syndrome").

Barrett's Esophagus

Replacement of normal esophageal squamous epithelium with metaplastic columnar epithelium and goblet cells ("specialized epithelium"). Some 5–10% of patients present with chronic GERD and incidence increases with GERD duration. Most common in Caucasian men > 55 years of age. The risk of adenocarcinoma is 0.5% per year, is greater in males than in females, and is higher among Caucasians.

Screen for Barrett's esophagus in patients with chronic GERD symptoms, especially in Caucasian men. If Barrett's is not present, there is no need for further screening.

DIAGNOSIS

- **Upper endoscopy:** Suggestive but not diagnostic. **Salmon-colored islands or "tongues"** are seen extending upward from the distal esophagus.
- **Biopsy:** Diagnostic.
  - Metaplastic **columnar epithelium** and **goblet cells** are seen.
  - **Specialized intestinal metaplasia on biopsy is associated with an increased risk of neoplasia.**

TREATMENT

- PPIs.
- Adenocarcinoma surveillance is necessary only if patients are candidates for esophagectomy.
- Upper endoscopy with four-quadrant biopsies every 2 cm of endoscopic lesions.
- Screening frequency is based on the presence of dysplasia after two consecutive annual exams:
  - **None:** Every 2–3 years.

- **Low grade:** Every 6–12 months.
- **High grade: Verify with a second expert pathologist.** Roughly 30–40% of cases progress to adenocarcinoma, but management is controversial. The standard of care is esophagectomy or, alternatively, endoscopic ablation with photodynamic therapy or argon plasma coagulative therapy.

Biopsies of Barrett's esophagus that show high-grade dysplasia necessitate verification with a second expert pathologist, since esophagectomy will be a consideration.

Dyspepsia

Localized pain or discomfort in the upper abdomen. Distinct from but can present with GERD (retrosternal burning). In the United States, the prevalence of dyspepsia is 25%, but only 25% of those affected seek care. Of these, **> 60% have nonulcerative dyspepsia and < 1% have gastric cancer.**

SYMPTOMS/EXAM

Upper abdominal pain or discomfort, fullness, bloating, early satiety, belching, nausea, retching or vomiting.

DIFFERENTIAL

Nonulcerative dyspepsia (> 60%), food intolerance (overeating, high-fat foods, alcohol, lactose intolerance), drug intolerance (NSAIDs, iron, narcotics, alendronate, theophylline, antibiotics), peptic ulcer disease (PUD) (10–25%), reflux esophagitis (15–20%), gastric cancer (< 1%), chronic pancreatitis, pancreatic cancer, biliary colic.

DIAGNOSIS/TREATMENT

Endoscopic biopsy, H. pylori *stool antigen, and urea breath test can assess active* H. pylori *infection and gauge treatment success.* H. pylori *serology measures only past exposure and cannot be used to confirm eradication.*

In patients < 50 years of age with no alarm features, gastric cancer is a rare etiology of dyspepsia, and direct endoscopy is not a cost-effective measure.

- **Alarm features:** Look for new-onset dyspepsia in patients > 50 years of age, weight loss of > 10%, melena, anemia, persistent vomiting, hematemesis, dysphagia, odynophagia, abdominal mass, a history of PUD, and a family history of gastric cancer.
  - **If any alarm features are present:** Prompt endoscopy.
  - **If no alarm features are present:** Dietary assessment and education; discontinue suspect medications. Consider a trial of empiric acid suppression; consider testing for and treating *H. pylori* (see below).
- **Determine the local prevalence of *H. pylori*.**
  - **If > 20%:** Test for *H. pylori* (serology, stool antigen, or breath test). If positive, institute *H. pylori* eradication therapy. If negative, initiate a trial of acid suppression for 6–8 weeks.
  - **If < 20%:** Institute a trial of acid suppression for 6–8 weeks.
- **For persistent symptoms:**
  - If the patient received *H. pylori* eradication therapy, test for eradication (with stool antigen or breath test, **not with serology**). If not eradicated, treat again with a different regimen. If eradicated, refer to endoscopy.
  - If the patient received a trial of PPIs, refer to endoscopy.
- **Endoscopy:**
  - **If unrevealing:** Diagnose with nonulcerative dysphagia and provide reassurance; consider a trial of low-dose TCAs (desipramine 10–25 mg QHS) and possible psychological therapy.
  - **If revealing:** Manage as indicated.
- Table 7-4 summarizes treatment options for PUD.

TABLE 7-4. Treatment Options for Peptic Ulcer Disease

- **Active *H. pylori*–associated ulcer:**
  1. Treat with anti–*H. pylori* regimen for 10–14 days. Treatment options:
     - PPI twice daily[a]
     - Clarithromycin 500 mg twice daily
     - Amoxicillin 1 g twice daily (or metronidazole 500 mg twice daily if penicillin allergic)

     - PPI twice daily
     - Bismuth subsalicylate two tablets four times daily
     - Tetracycline 500 mg four times daily
     - Metronidazole 250 mg four times daily

     - Ranitidine bismuth citrate 400 mg twice daily (not available in the United States)
     - Clarithromycin 500 mg twice daily
     - Amoxicillin 1 g or tetracycline 500 mg or metronidazole 500 mg twice daily

     - (PPIs are administered before meals. Avoid metronidazole regimens in areas of known high resistance or in patients who have failed a course of treatment that included metronidazole.)
  2. After completion of 10- to 14-day course of *H. pylori* eradication therapy, continue treatment with PPIs once daily or H_2 receptor antagonists (as below) for 4–8 weeks to promote healing.

- **Active ulcer not attributable to *H. pylori*:**
  1. **Consider other causes:** NSAIDs, Zollinger-Ellison syndrome, gastric malignancy. Treatment options:

     a. **PPIs:**
     - **Uncomplicated duodenal ulcer:** Treat for four weeks
     - **Uncomplicated gastric ulcer:** Treat for eight weeks

     b. **H_2 receptor antagonists:**
     - **Uncomplicated duodenal ulcer:** Cimetidine 800 mg, ranitidine or nizatidine 300 mg, famotidine 40 mg, once daily at bedtime for six weeks
     - **Uncomplicated gastric ulcer:** Cimetidine 400 mg, ranitidine or nizatidine 150 mg, famotidine 20 mg, twice daily for eight weeks
     - **Complicated ulcers:** PPIs are the preferred drugs

- **Prevention of ulcer relapse:**
  1. **NSAID-induced ulcer:** Prophylactic therapy for high-risk patients (prior ulcer disease or ulcer complications, use of corticosteroids or anticoagulants, age > 70 with serious comorbid illnesses). Treatment options:
     - PPI once daily
     - COX-2 selective NSAID (rofecoxib, celecoxib, valdecoxib)
     - In special circumstances, misoprostol 200 μg 3–4 times daily
  2. **Chronic "maintenance" therapy:** Indicated in patients with recurrent ulcers who either are *H. pylori* negative or have failed attempts at eradication therapy. Once-daily PPI or H_2 receptor antagonist at bedtime (cimetidine 400–800 mg, nizatidine or ranitidine 150–300 mg, famotidine 20–40 mg).

[a] PPIs: Omeprazole 20 mg, rabeprazole 20 mg, lansoprazole 30 mg, pantoprazole 40 mg, esomeprazole 40 mg. All PPIs are given twice daily except esomeprazole (once daily).

Reproduced, with permission, from Tierney LM et al. *Current Medical Diagnosis & Treatment 2004,* 43rd ed. New York: McGraw-Hill, 2004.

Gastroesophageal Reflux Disease (GERD)

In the United States, some 40% of adults report having GERD symptoms at least once per month, and 7% report having daily symptoms. The most common predisposing condition is pregnancy; 50–80% of pregnant women have

GERD. Although most have mild GERD, 40–50% develop esophagitis, 5% ulcerative esophagitis, 4–20% esophageal strictures, and 5–10% Barrett's esophagus. The risk of severe GERD is greater in men than in women and greatest in those > 40 years of age.

Symptoms

- Retrosternal burning sensation (heartburn) that begins in the epigastrium and radiates upward (typically within one hour of a meal, during exercise, or when lying recumbent) and is at least partially relieved by antacids.
- **Water brash** (excess salivation), **bitter taste,** globus (throat fullness), odynophagia, dysphagia, halitosis, otalgia.
- **"Atypical" symptoms (up to 50%):** Cough, hoarseness, noncardiac chest pain.

Exam

Poor dentition; wheezing. Exam is often normal.

Differential

Infectious esophagitis (CMV, HSV, *Candida*), pill esophagitis (alendronate [Fosamax], tetracycline), PUD, dyspepsia, biliary colic, CAD, esophageal motility disorders.

Diagnosis

- **Typical symptoms without alarm features (dysphagia, odynophagia, weight loss, bleeding, anemia):** Sufficient to make the diagnosis. Treat with an empiric trial of PPIs for 4–6 weeks.
- **If the patient is unresponsive to therapy trial or has atypical symptoms, dysphagia, or odynophagia:**
    - **Barium esophagography:** Has a limited role, but can identify strictures.
    - **Upper endoscopy with biopsy:** Normal in > 50% of patients with GERD (most have nonerosive reflux disease) or may reveal endoscopic esophagitis grades 1 (mild) to 4 (severe erosions, strictures, Barrett's esophagus). Strictures can be dilated.
    - **Ambulatory esophageal pH monitoring:** Gold standard, but often unnecessary. Indicated for correlating symptoms with pH parameters when endoscopy is normal and (1) symptoms are unresponsive to medical therapy, (2) antireflux surgery is being considered, or (3) there are atypical symptoms (e.g., chest pain, cough, wheezing).

For true GERD, PPIs are highly effective, with < 5% of patients unresponsive to twice-daily doses.

Treatment

- **Behavioral modification:** Elevate the head of the bed six inches; stop tobacco and alcohol use. Advise patients to eat smaller meals, reduce fat intake, lose weight, avoid recumbency after eating, and avoid certain foods (e.g., mint, chocolate, coffee, tea, carbonated drinks, citrus and tomato juice).
- **Antacids (calcium carbonate, aluminum hydroxide):** For mild GERD. Fast, but afford only short-term relief.
- **H_2 receptor antagonists (cimetidine, ranitidine, famotidine, nizatidine):** For mild GERD or as an adjunct for nocturnal GERD while the patient is on PPIs.

- **PPIs (omeprazole, lansoprazole, rabeprazole, pantoprazole, esomeprazole):** The mainstay of therapy for mild to severe GERD. Safe and effective, with few side effects. Of all patients, **10–20% are unresponsive to daily dosage and < 5% to twice-daily dosage.**
- **Surgical fundoplication (Nissen or Belsey wrap):**
  - Often performed laparoscopically. Indicated for patients who cannot tolerate medical therapy or who have persistent regurgitation without an esophageal motility disorder.
  - **Outcome:** Of those treated, > 50% require continued acid suppressive medication and > 20% develop new symptoms (dysphagia, bloating, dyspepsia).
- **Endoscopic antireflux procedures:** Investigational.

After surgical fundoplication for GERD, > 50% of patients still require continued acid suppressive medication, and > 20% develop new symptoms (dysphagia, bloating, dyspepsia).

COMPLICATIONS

- **Peptic strictures:** Affect 8–20% of GERD patients; present with dysphagia. Malignancies must be excluded via endoscopy and biopsy; then treat with endoscopic dilation followed by PPIs.
- **Posterior laryngitis:** Chronic hoarseness from vocal cord ulceration and granulomas.
- **Asthma:** Typically has an adult onset; non-atopic and unresponsive to traditional asthma interventions.
- **Cough:** Affects 10–40% of patients, most without typical GERD symptoms.
- **Noncardiac chest pain:** After full cardiac evaluation, consider an empiric trial of PPIs or ambulatory esophageal pH monitoring.
- Barrett's esophagus, adenocarcinoma.

Atypical symptoms (cough, wheezing, chest pain) often occur without typical heartburn symptoms.

Gastroparesis

Delayed gastric emptying in the absence of obstruction. Most commonly related to diabetes, viral infection, neuropsychiatric disease, or postsurgical complications.

SYMPTOMS

Postprandial fullness, bloating, abdominal distention, early satiety, nausea, vomiting of digested food.

EXAM

Normal. Mild to moderate upper abdominal tenderness during episodes. Occasionally succussion splash is heard.

DIFFERENTIAL

- Diabetes-associated symptoms, postsurgical **(postvagotomy or Roux-en-Y)**, nonulcer dyspepsia, medications (anticholinergics, opiates).
- Hypothyroidism, scleroderma, muscular dystrophies, paraneoplastic syndrome (small cell lung cancer).

DIAGNOSIS

- **Solid-phase nuclear medicine gastric emptying scan:** Following administration of a radiolabeled meal, normal gastric retention is < 90%, < 60%, and < 10% at 60, 120, and 240 minutes, respectively.
- **Labs:** Electrolytes, hemoglobin A_{1c}, ANA, TSH.
- **Endoscopy:** To rule out structural lesions and ulcers causing obstruction.
- **Gastroduodenal manometry:** Not widely available, but can often distinguish myopathic from neuropathic patterns.

Gastroparesis can be a sign of undiagnosed diabetes.

"Idiopathic" gastroparesis can result from viral infections in young, healthy patients and is often self-limited, remitting within a few months.

TREATMENT

- **Dietary:** Small, frequent meals; low-fat, low-fiber diet.
- Tight glycemic control in diabetics.
- Decrease or discontinue opiates and anticholinergics.
- **Medications:**
  - **Cisapride:** Most effective, but its use is restricted owing to **QT-interval prolongation.**
  - **Metoclopramide:** A dopamine antagonist used as an antiemetic. Decreased effectiveness and adverse effects (extrapyramidal symptoms) are seen with long-term use.
  - **Domperidone:** A dopamine antagonist that is not approved for use in the United States.
  - **Erythromycin:** IV use has short-term efficacy; PO use is less effective chronically.
  - **Tegaserod:** May be effective, but not approved in the United States for use in treating gastroparesis.
- **Jejunostomy tube:** For intractable, severe gastroparesis without small bowel dysmotility.
- **Total parenteral nutrition:** For intractable, severe gastroparesis with small bowel dysmotility.
- **Gastric pacing:** Investigational.

LOWER GI TRACT

Acute Diarrhea

Diarrhea of < **4 weeks'** duration. Usually infectious, mild, and self-limited; cases are managed on an outpatient basis. Diarrhea accounts for 1.5% of all hospitalizations in the United States. Increased morbidity is seen in children, the elderly, and the immunosuppressed. Etiologies are as follows:

- **Bacterial:** *E. coli, Campylobacter, Salmonella, Shigella, C. difficile, Aeromonas.*
- **Viral:** Adenovirus, rotavirus, Norwalk agent.
- **Parasites:** *Entamoeba histolytica, Giardia lamblia, Cryptosporidium, Microsporidium.*
- **Drugs:** Antibiotics, NSAIDs, quinidine, β-blockers, magnesium-base antacids, PPIs, colchicine, theophylline, acarbose.
- **Other:** Food allergies; initial presentation of chronic diarrhea.

SYMPTOMS

Diarrhea, urgency, tenesmus, abdominal bloating and pain.

EXAM

Tachycardia, orthostasis, decreased skin turgor with dehydration, abdominal pain, distention.

DIAGNOSIS

- **Alarm features:** Evaluation is indicated in the presence of alarm features—e.g., fever > 38.5°C, severe abdominal pain, bloody diarrhea, immune compromise, age > 70 years, or severe dehydration (see Figure 7-1 and Table 7-5).

- **No alarm features** (short duration, nonbloody diarrhea, nontoxic exam): Treat with oral rehydration and symptomatic therapy. If no improvement is seen, evaluation is indicated.
- **Blood tests:** CBC, electrolytes, BUN, creatinine, ESR, ameba serology.
- **Stool tests:** O&P, *Giardia* antigen, *C. difficile* toxin, leukocytes, culture.
- **Endoscopy:** Flexible sigmoidoscopy or colonoscopy with biopsy.

Acute diarrhea (< 4 weeks' duration) is usually infectious and self-limited.

TREATMENT

- **Mild diarrhea:**
  - Oral rehydration (Pedialyte, Gatorade).
  - BRAT diet (bananas, rice, applesauce, toast).
  - **Antidiarrheals:** Loperamide 4 mg initially and then 2 mg after each stool (maximum 8 mg/day).
- **Severe diarrhea:** Oral or IV rehydration.
- **Empiric antibiotics:**
  - Indicated only in the presence of fever > 38.5°C, tenesmus, bloody stools, and fecal leukocytes (awaiting culture).
  - Ciprofloxacin 500 mg PO or 400 mg IV BID × 3–5 days.
  - Antibiotics are **not** recommended for nontyphoidal *Salmonella, Campylobacter, Aeromonas, Yersinia,* or *E. coli* O157:H7.

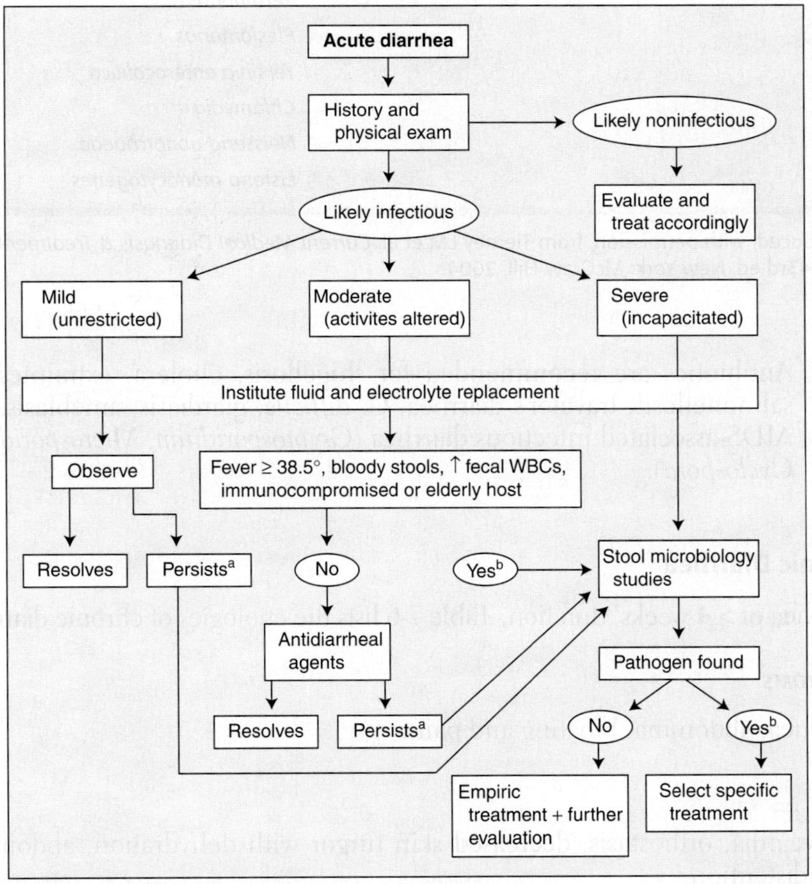

[a]Consider empiric treatment with metronidazole before evaluation.
[b]Consider empiric treatment with quinolone before evaluation.

FIGURE 7-1. Algorithm for the management of acute diarrhea.

(Reproduced, with permission, from Braunwald E et al. *Harrison's Principles of Internal Medicine,* 15th ed. New York: McGraw-Hill, 2001.)

TABLE 7-5. Causes of Acute Infectious Diarrhea

Noninflammatory Diarrhea	Inflammatory Diarrhea
Viral:	**Viral:**
Norwalk virus	CMV
Norwalk-like virus	**Protozoal:**
Rotavirus	*Entamoeba histolytica*
Protozoal:	**Bacterial:**
Giardia lamblia	1. **Cytotoxin production:**
Cryptosporidium	Enterohemorrhagic *E. coli*
Bacterial:	O157:H5 (EHEC)
1. **Preformed enterotoxin production**	*Vibrio parahaemolyticus*
S. aureus	*Clostridium difficile*
Bacillus cereus	2. **Mucosal invasion**
Clostridium perfringens	*Shigella*
2. **Enterotoxin production**	*Campylobacter jejuni*
Enterotoxigenic *E. coli* (ETEC)	*Salmonella*
Vibrio cholerae	Enteroinvasive *E. coli* (EIEC)
	Aeromonas
	Plesiomonas
	Yersinia enterocolitica
	Chlamydia
	Neisseria gonorrhoeae
	Listeria monocytogenes

Reproduced, with permission, from Tierney LM et al. *Current Medical Diagnosis & Treatment 2004,* 43rd ed. New York: McGraw-Hill, 2004.

- Antibiotics are recommended for shigellosis, cholera, extraintestinal salmonellosis, traveler's diarrhea, *C. difficile*, giardiasis, amebiasis, and AIDS-associated infectious diarrhea (*Cryptosporidium, Microsporidium, Cyclospora*).

Chronic Diarrhea

Diarrhea of > **4 weeks**' duration. Table 7-6 lists the etiologies of chronic diarrhea.

Symptoms

Diarrhea; abdominal bloating and pain.

Exam

Tachycardia, orthostasis, decreased skin turgor with dehydration, abdominal pain, distention.

Diagnosis

Diagnose as follows (see also Table 7-7):

- Exclude acute diarrhea, lactose intolerance, parasitic infection, ileal resection, medications, and systemic disease.

TABLE 7-6. Causes of Chronic Diarrhea

- **Osmotic diarrhea:**
  CLUES: Stool volume decreases with fasting; increased stool osmotic gap
  1. **Medications:** Antacids, lactulose, sorbitol
  2. **Disaccharidase deficiency:** Lactose intolerance
  3. **Factitious diarrhea:** Magnesium (antacids, laxatives)
- **Secretory diarrhea:**
  CLUES: Large volume (> 1 L/day); little change with fasting; normal stool osmotic gap.
  1. **Hormonally mediated:** VIPoma, carcinoid, medullary carcinoma of thyroid (calcitonin), Zollinger-Ellison syndrome (gastrin)
  2. Factitious diarrhea (laxative abuse); phenolphthalein, cascara, senna
  3. Villous adenoma
  4. Bile salt malabsorption (ileal resection; Crohn's ileitis; postcholecystectomy)
  5. Medications
- **Inflammatory conditions:**
  CLUES: Fever, hematochezia, abdominal pain.
  1. Ulcerative colitis
  2. Crohn's disease
  3. Microscopic colitis
  4. **Malignancy:** Lymphoma, adenocarcinoma (with obstruction and pseudodiarrhea)
  5. Radiation enteritis
- **Malabsorption syndromes:**
  CLUES: Weight loss, abnormal laboratory values; fecal fat > 10 g/24 h.
  1. **Small bowel mucosal disorders:** Celiac sprue, tropical sprue, Whipple's disease, eosinophilic gastroenteritis, small bowel resection (short bowel syndrome), Crohn's disease
  2. **Lymphatic obstruction:** Lymphoma, carcinoid, infectious (TB, *Mycobacterium avium–intracellulare*), Kaposi's sarcoma, sarcoidosis, retroperitoneal fibrosis
  3. **Pancreatic disease:** Chronic pancreatitis, pancreatic carcinoma
  4. **Bacterial overgrowth:** Motility disorders (diabetes, vagotomy), scleroderma, fistulas, small intestinal diverticula
- **Motility disorders:**
  CLUES: Systemic disease or prior abdominal surgery
  1. **Postsurgical:** Vagotomy, partial gastrectomy, blind loop with bacterial overgrowth
  2. **Systemic disorders:** Scleroderma, DM, hyperthyroidism
  3. IBS
- **Chronic infections:**
  1. **Parasites:** *Giardia lamblia, Entamoeba histolytica*
  2. **AIDS related:**
     Viral: CMV, HIV infection (?)
     Bacterial: *C. difficile, Mycobacterium avium* complex
     Protozoal: Microsporida (*Enterocytozoon bieneusi, Cryptosporidium, Isospora belli*)

- **Characterize diarrhea:** Watery, inflammatory, fatty/malabsorption.
- **Perform a focused initial evaluation:**
  - **Blood tests:** CBC, electrolytes, ESR, albumin.
  - **Blood test clues:**
    - **ESR:** Elevated if diarrhea is inflammatory.
    - **Iron deficiency anemia:** Points to malabsorption or inflammatory diarrhea.
    - **Antigliadin or antiendomysial antibodies:** Associated with celiac sprue.
    - **Neuroendocrine tumors:** VIP (VIPoma), calcitonin (medullary thyroid carcinoma), gastrin (Zollinger-Ellison syndrome), glucagon.
  - **Stool tests:** Electrolytes (calculate osmotic gap), 24-hour collection for weight and quantitative fat, standard cultures plus tests for *Aeromonas* and *Plesiomonas*, O&P.

TABLE 7-7. Differential Diagnosis of Chronic Diarrhea

	Osmotic	Secretory	Inflammatory	Fatty/Malabsorption
History	Stool volume decreases with fasting.	Large stool volume (> 1 L/day); no change with fasting.	Fever, abdominal pain, hematochezia.	Weight loss, greasy stools.
Exam	–	Severe dehydration.	Abdominal tenderness.	Glossitis.
Blood tests	–	Neuroendocrine peptides.	Leukocytosis, elevated ESR.	Anemia, hypoalbuminemia.
Stool tests	Osm gap > 125, Mg > 45, pH < 5.6.	24-hour stool Weight > 1000 g, osm < 50.	Leukocytes, fecal blood.	7-10 g fat/24 hours.
Differential	Laxative use, carbohydrate malabsorption.	Bacterial, viral, bile acid malabsorption, collagenous colitis, vasculitis, neuroendocrine, nonosmotic laxatives.	IBD, *C. difficile* colitis, invasive bacterial, viral, parasitic, ischemic, radiation, lymphoma, colon cancer.	Pancreatic exocrine insufficiency, celiac sprue, Whipple's disease, small bowel bacterial overgrowth, mesenteric ischemia.

- **Stool test clues:**
  - **Weight:** If the 24-hour stool weight > 1000 g, suspect secretory diarrhea; if < 250 g, suspect factitious diarrhea or IBS.
  - **Osmotic gap:** Calculated as 290 – 2 (stool Na + stool K). A gap of < 50 mOsm/kg implies secretory diarrhea; > 125 mOsm/kg implies osmotic diarrhea.
  - **pH:** A pH < 5.6 implies carbohydrate malabsorption.
  - **Fecal occult blood test (FOBT):** Suggests inflammatory diarrhea, but often positive with other types.
  - **Leukocytes:** Presence suggests inflammatory diarrhea.
  - **Fat:** Spot testing is not specific; a 24-hour fat > 7–10 g implies malabsorption.
  - **Laxative screen:** Elevated magnesium (> 45 mmol/L), phosphate, sulfate levels.
- **Urine tests.**
- **Urine test clues:** Neuroendocrine tumors—5-HIAA (carcinoid), VMA, metanephrines, histamine.
- **Endoscopy:** Flexible sigmoidoscopy or colonoscopy with biopsy; consider upper endoscopy.
- **Other:** Positive breath H_2 test suggests lactase deficiency. Give 25 g lactose challenge while fasting; test is positive if hydrogen is detected in exhaled breath.

Treatment

The treatment of chronic diarrhea is as follows (see also Figure 7-2):

- **Mild diarrhea:** See previous section.

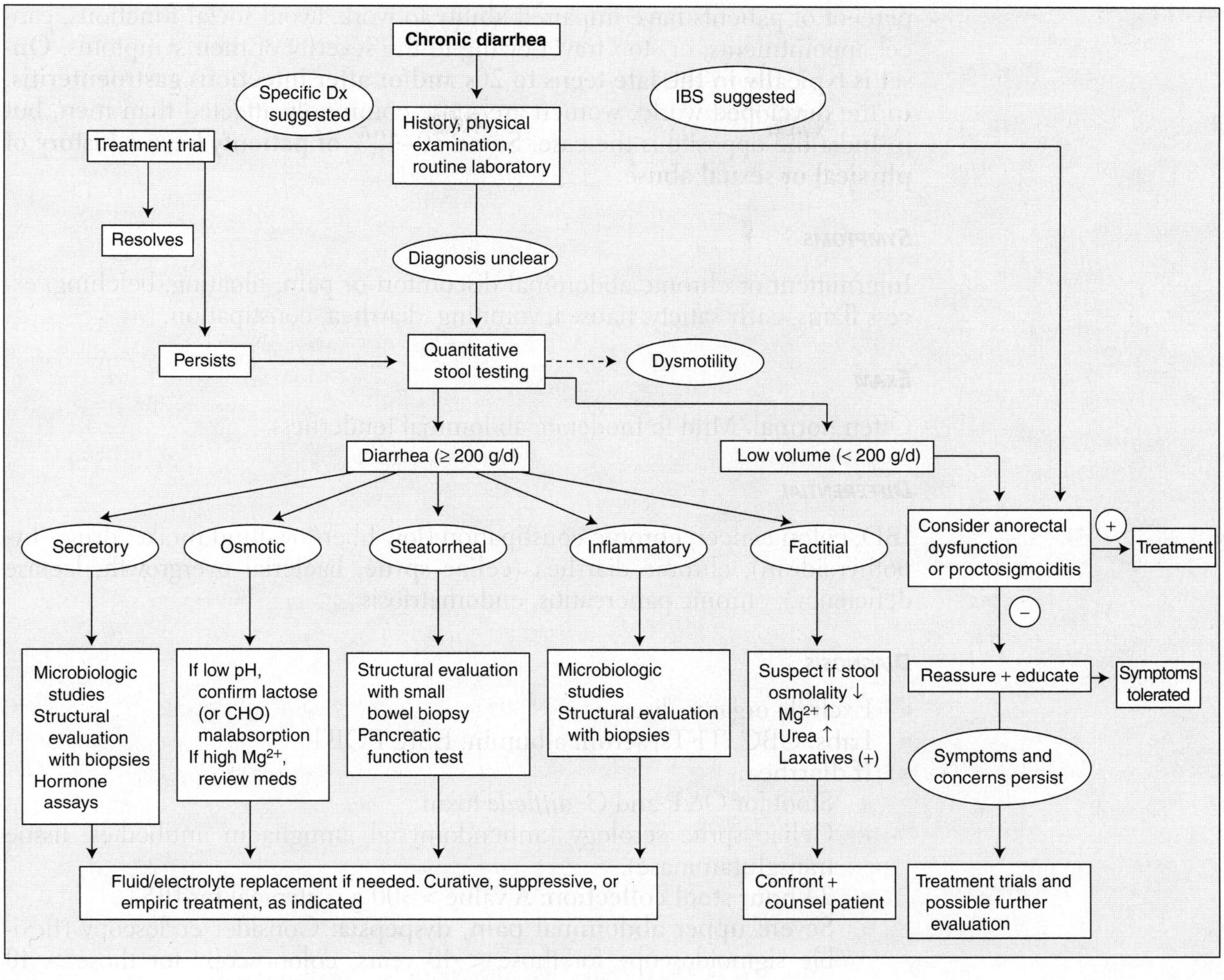

FIGURE 7-2. Algorithm for the management of chronic diarrhea.

(Reproduced, with permission, from Braunwald E et al. *Harrison's Principles of Internal Medicine*, 15th ed. New York: McGraw-Hill, 2001.)

- **Osmotic diarrhea:**
  - **Carbohydrate malabsorption (lactose, fructose, sorbitol):** Dietary modification, lactase supplements.
  - **Celiac sprue:** Gluten restriction.
  - **Whipple's disease/tropical sprue:** Antibiotics.
- **Secretory diarrhea:**
  - Clonidine 0.1–0.3 mg PO TID.
  - Octreotide 50–250 μg SQ TID.
  - Cholestyramine 4 g PO QD to QID.
- **Inflammatory diarrhea: IBD**—sulfasalazine, 5-ASA (mesalamine), corticosteroids, azathioprine, 6-mercaptopurine (6-MP).
- **Fatty diarrhea: Pancreatic exocrine insufficiency**—pancreatic enzyme supplements; empiric antibiotics for small bowel overgrowth.

In the United States, surreptitious laxative use accounts for 15% of referrals for chronic diarrhea and 25% of documented cases of secretory diarrhea.

Irritable Bowel Syndrome (IBS)

Abdominal **discomfort or pain** during the **prior three months** that is relieved by defecation and associated with a change in stool frequency or form. Forty percent of patients have impaired ability to work, avoid social functions, cancel appointments, or stop travel owing to the severity of their symptoms. **Onset is typically in the late teens to 20s and/or after infectious gastroenteritis.** In the developed world, women are more commonly affected than men, but in India the opposite is the case. Some **30–40% of patients have a history of physical or sexual abuse.**

SYMPTOMS

Intermittent or chronic abdominal discomfort or pain; bloating, belching, excess flatus, early satiety, nausea, vomiting, diarrhea, constipation.

EXAM

Often normal. Mild to moderate abdominal tenderness.

DIFFERENTIAL

IBD, colon cancer, chronic constipation (low-fiber/low-fluid intake, drugs, hypothyroidism), chronic diarrhea (**celiac sprue,** bacterial overgrowth, lactase deficiency), chronic pancreatitis, endometriosis.

DIAGNOSIS

- Exclude organic disease.
- **Labs:** CBC, TFTs, serum albumin, ESR, FOBT.
- **If diarrhea:**
  - Stool for O&P and *C. difficile* toxin.
  - Celiac sprue serology (antiendomysial, antigliadin antibodies, tissue transglutaminase).
  - **24-hour stool collection:** A value > 300 g is atypical for IBS.
  - **Severe upper abdominal pain, dyspepsia:** Consider endoscopy (flexible sigmoidoscopy for those < 40 years; colonoscopy for those > 40 years).

New-onset IBS often follows a diagnosis of infectious gastroenteritis.

TREATMENT

- Provide reassurance.
- Tactfully explain visceral hypersensitivity; validate symptoms.
- **Dietary trials:** Lactose-free, high-fiber diet.
- **Antispasmodics:** Dicyclomine, hyoscyamine, peppermint oil.
- **Antidepressants:** Desipramine, amitryptyline, fluoxetine, paroxetine.
- **Constipation-predominant type:**
  - Increase fluid intake.
  - Bowel habit training.
  - Tegaserod 6 mg BID (approved for women only).
  - Osmotic laxatives.
- **Diarrhea-predominant type:** Loperamide, cholestyramine.

Constipation

Normal bowel movement frequency is 3–12 per week. Constipation is defined as < 3 bowel movements per week or excessive difficulty and straining at defecation. Prevalence is high in the Western world and is **highest among children and the elderly.** Etiologies are as follows:

- **Dietary:** Low fiber, inadequate fluids.
- **Behavioral:** Short-term stress, travel, disrupted routine.

- **Structural:** Colonic mass or stricture, rectal prolapse, Hirschsprung's disease, solitary rectal ulcer syndrome.
- **Systemic:** Diabetes, **hypothyroidism, hypokalemia, hypercalcemia,** autonomic dysfunction.
- **Medications:** Narcotics, diuretics, calcium channel blockers, anticholinergics, psychotropics, clonidine.
- **Other:** Pelvic floor dysfunction, slow transit (pseudo-obstruction, psychogenic), IBS.

The first step in the evaluation of constipation is to understand the patient's true complaint.

Symptoms

Abdominal bloating or pain; nausea, anorexia.

Exam

Often normal, but may present with abdominal distention, tenderness, and/or mass; external hemorrhoids, anal fissures, and fecal impaction; or rectal prolapse with straining.

Normal bowel movement frequency ranges from 3 to 12 times per week.

Diagnosis/Treatment

- **Understand the complaint:**
  - Bowel movement frequency change, but in normal range.
  - Frequency of < 3 bowel movements per week.
  - Excessive difficulty and straining at defecation.
  - **Other:** Fecal incontinence, rectal prolapse, anal pain.
- **Initial evaluation:**
  - **Labs:** CBC, serum electrolytes **(especially potassium and calcium)**, TSH, FOBT.
  - **Age < 50 years and normal labs:** Trial of increased fiber (20–30 g/day), fluid intake.
  - **Age ≥ 50 or < 50 years and failed fiber/fluid trial or fecal occult blood or anemia:** Barium enema; flexible sigmoidoscopy or colonoscopy.
  - **No obstructive or medical disease:**
    - Decrease dose or discontinue suspect drugs.
    - Stepwise addition of (1) stool softeners (docusate), (2) osmotic laxatives (magnesium hydroxide, lactulose, sorbitol, polyethylene glycol), (3) enemas (tap water, mineral oil, soap suds, phosphate), and (4) colonic stimulants (bisacodyl, senna).
    - Consider tegaserod for women with constipation-predominant IBS.
    - Treat medical or obstructive disease.
  - **For refractory constipation:**
    - Consider colon transit and pelvic floor studies.
    - Consider psychological evaluation.
    - Consider surgical therapy in the absence of psychological abnormality along with documented slow transit or pelvic floor dysfunction.

Diverticulosis

Results from weakening of the colonic wall. In industrialized nations, has a 30–50% prevalence in patients > 50 years of age. Rates increase with low dietary fiber and advancing age. The sigmoid colon is most commonly affected (95%), followed by the left colon and right colon.

Symptoms

May be asymptomatic (85%) or present with mild intermittent abdominal pain, bloating, excessive flatulence, pellet-like stools, and irregular bowel habits.

EXAM

Normal; mild abdominal distention.

DIFFERENTIAL

Colorectal cancer, IBS.

DIAGNOSIS

- **Barium enema:** Accurate for diverticulosis, but insufficient to rule out colorectal cancer.
- **Colonoscopy:** The test of choice. Recommended for routine colorectal cancer screening in patients > 50 years of age.

TREATMENT

Dietary fiber 20–30 g/day; coarse bran or supplements (psyllium). Increases stool bulk; decreases colonic pressure and may prevent the formation of new diverticula.

COMPLICATIONS

- **Diverticular bleeding** affects 10–20% of patients with diverticulosis.
- Presents with painless rectal bleeding, usually from a single diverticulum (more frequently the sigmoid than other sites).
- Spontaneous cessation is common (80%), but approximately one-third of patients have recurrent bleeding.
- **Consider elective colonic resection after the second recurrence.**

Diverticulitis

Microperforations in the diverticula with associated inflammation. Occurs in 10–25% of those with diverticulosis; frequency increases with advancing age.

Diverticulitis is the most common cause of colovesical fistula.

SYMPTOMS

LLQ pain (93–100%); fever, nausea, vomiting, constipation, diarrhea, urinary frequency ("sympathetic cystitis").

EXAM

LLQ tenderness, localized involuntary guarding, percussion tenderness, tender LLQ fullness or mass.

DIFFERENTIAL

Appendicitis, IBD, perforated colon cancer, UTI, ischemic colitis, infectious colitis, sigmoid volvulus.

DIAGNOSIS

- **Labs:** Leukocytosis with PMN predominance.
- **UA:** Evaluate for UTI; consider colovesical fistula with pyuria and bacteriuria.
- **Flat and upright AXR:** A thickened colonic (sigmoid) wall is suggestive; free air suggests bowel perforation.

- **CT with IV and PO contrast:** The test of choice; has high accuracy. Look for a thickened bowel wall and pericolic fat stranding. Evaluate for complications (bowel perforation, abscess, fistula).
- **Colonoscopy:** Exclude malignancy eight weeks after presumed diverticulitis resolves.

Mild diverticulitis may be treated on an outpatient basis if there are no significant comorbidities, minimal symptoms, and no peritoneal signs.

TREATMENT

- May be treated on an outpatient basis if there are no significant comorbidities, minimal symptoms, and no peritoneal signs. Often requires hospitalization.
- IV fluids, bowel rest, NG suction for ileus or obstruction.
- **Broad-spectrum antibiotics:** Cover anaerobes, gram-negative bacilli, and gram-positive coliforms. Administer a 7- to 10-day course. IV ampicillin/sulbactam (Unasyn) or piperacillin/tazobactam (Zosyn); PO quinolones, amoxicillin/clavulanate (Augmentin).
- **Surgery:** For perforation, abscess, fistula, obstruction, or recurrent diverticulitis (> 2 episodes).

Consider elective "prophylactic" resection after the second attack of diverticulitis or diverticular bleeding.

COMPLICATIONS

- **Peritonitis:** Not excluded by the absence of free air. Associated with a high mortality (6–35%); **necessitates urgent surgical intervention.**
- **Abscess:** Pelvic abscess is most common. Percutaneous CT-guided drainage is often possible.
- **Fistula:** Colovesical fistulas (to the bladder) are found in men more often than in women. Other fistulas are to the vagina, small bowel, and uterus. Surgical intervention can often be postponed until the infection has been treated.

GI BLEEDING

Lower Gastrointestinal Bleeding (LGIB)

Defined as bleeding from a source distal to or lower than the ligament of Treitz, which divides the third and fourth portions of the duodenum. Of all cases, > 95% are from a colonic source and > 85% are self-limited. The hospitalization rate is 20 in 100,000 adults per year; risk increases 200-fold from the third to the ninth decade. Mortality is 3–5%. Etiologies include the following:

- Diverticulosis (40%).
- Vascular ectasia.
- Neoplasm, IBD, ischemic colitis, hemorrhoids, infectious, postpolypectomy.
- NSAID ulcers, radiation colitis, rectal varices, solitary rectal ulcer syndrome. Consider an upper GI source.

SYMPTOMS

Usually asymptomatic, but may present with abdominal cramps and, to a lesser extent, pain. Orthostasis is seen in severe cases.

EXAM

Hematochezia (bright red blood, maroon stools) or melena; pallor; abdominal distention with mild tenderness; hypotension, tachycardia.

Diagnosis

- **Demographics and history:**
  - Distinguish elderly, asymptomatic patients (diverticular, vascular ectasias) from young patients who present with pain (infectious, inflammatory).
  - **Description of first blood seen by patient:** Bright red blood indicates a distal or rapid proximal source; black or maroon blood points to a proximal source.
- Anoscopy to exclude an anal source; stool cultures if infection is suspected.
- **Mild to moderate LGIB**: Consider nasogastric lavage. Urgent colonic purge (over 4–6 hours); then colonoscopy.
- **Massive LGIB:**
  - Upper GI bleeding (UGIB) must be excluded with EGD. **Ten percent of UGIB cases present with hematochezia.**
  - **Technetium-labeled RBC scan and/or mesenteric angiography:** If > 6 units of blood are transfused, consider surgical investigation.
  - **Minimum bleeding rates: RBC scan, 1 PRBC unit every 2–4 hours;** mesenteric angiogram, 1 PRBC unit/hour.
- **Diagnostic colonoscopy:** Typically performed 12–48 hours after presentation and stabilization.

Treatment

Treatment is as follows (see also Figure 7-3):

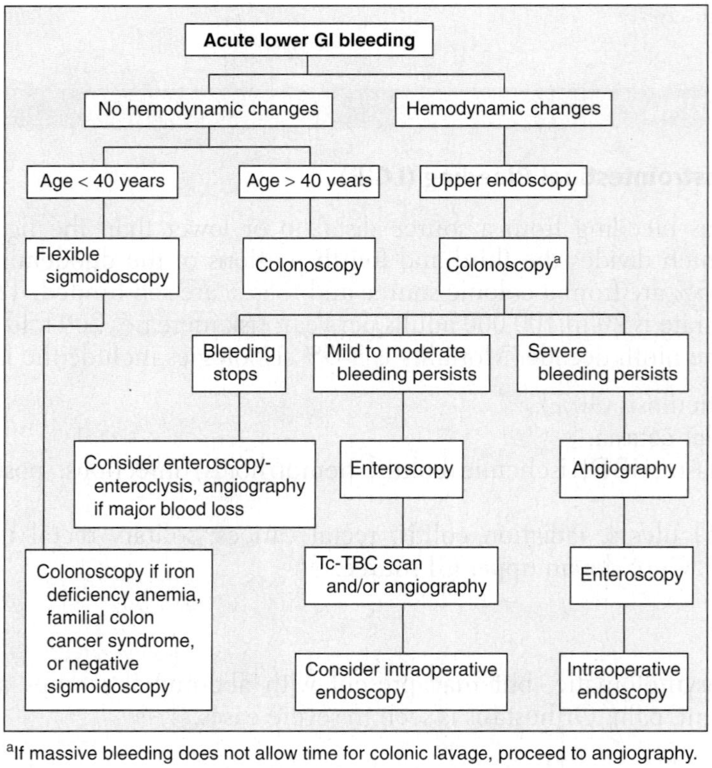

FIGURE 7-3. Suggested algorithm for patients with acute LGIB.

(Reproduced, with permission, from Braunwald E et al. *Harrison's Principles of Internal Medicine,* 15th ed. New York: McGraw-Hill, 2001.)

- **Stabilization:**
  - NPO; consider an NG tube and place two large-bore IVs.
  - **If there is no hemodynamic compromise, fluids/transfusions may be delayed.**
  - If the patient is in shock, treat with aggressive IV fluids and cross-matched blood with a **hematocrit goal of 25–30%.**
  - In the presence of active LGIB and platelets < 50,000/μL or if there is known impaired function (uremia, aspirin), transfuse platelets or desmopressin. With active LGIB and INR > 1.5, transfuse FFP.
- **Medical therapy:** H_2 receptor antagonists and PPIs have no role in the treatment of LGIB. Discontinue ASA and NSAIDs.
- **Urgent therapeutic colonoscopy:** Cautery or injection of saline or epinephrine. **Technically challenging with brisk LGIB** (urgent colonic purge requires sedation; often poor visualization).
- **Mesenteric angiography/embolization: The intervention of choice for brisk LGIB.** Associated with 80–90% cessation rates for those with a diverticular or vascular ectasia etiology, although 50% experience rebleeding.
- **Surgery: Indicated with active LGIB** involving > 4–6 units of blood in 24 hours or >10 units total. If the site is well localized, consider hemicolectomy; otherwise perform total abdominal colectomy.

Ten percent of UGIB patients present with hematochezia.

Acute Upper Gastrointestinal Bleeding (UGIB)

Incidence is 100 in 100,000 adults per year and increases with advancing age. Mortality is 10% and usually results from complications of underlying disease rather than from exsanguination. **Self-limited in 80% of cases.** The risk of rebleeding is low if bleeding occurred > 48 hours before presentation (see Table 7-8). Etiologies include the following:

- Peptic ulcer (55%).
- Gastroesophageal varices, vascular ectasia, Mallory-Weiss tear, erosive gastritis/esophagitis.
- **Other:** Dieulafoy's lesion, aortoenteric fistula, hemobilia.

TABLE 7-8. Risk Assessment in Patients with UGIB

	Low	Moderate	High
History	Age < 60.	Age < 60.	Age > 60, comorbidities, onset while in hospital.
Exam	SBP > 100, HR < 100.	SBP > 100, HR > 100.	SBP < 100, HR > 100.
EGD	Small, clean-based ulcer; erosions; no lesion found.	Ulcer with pigmented spot or adherent clot.	Active bleeding, varices, ulcer > 2 cm, visible vessel.
Rebleed risk	< 5%.	10–30%.	40–50%.
Triage	Ward/home.	Ward.	ICU.

Symptoms

Nausea, retching, hematemesis (bright red blood or "coffee ground" emesis), dyspepsia, abdominal pain, melena or hematochezia, orthostasis.

Exam

Melena or hematochezia, pallor, hypotension, tachycardia. Variceal bleeding may represent the stigmata of chronic liver disease.

Hematocrit is a poor early indicator of the amount of blood loss in UGIB.

Diagnosis

- **History:** Look for NSAID use (peptic ulcer), retching prior to hematemesis (Mallory-Weiss tear), alcohol abuse (erosions, Mallory-Weiss tear, varices), and prior abdominal aortic graft (aortoenteric fistula) (see Table 7-9).
- **NG tube lavage:** Useful if positive (red blood, coffee grounds); if negative (clear or bilious), does not exclude UGIB. **Ten percent of UGIB cases have negative lavage.**
- **EGD: Perform after stabilization and resuscitation** < 12 hours from admission. Diagnostic, prognostic, and therapeutic.
- *H. pylori* testing of all patients with peptic ulcers.

As little as 50 mL of blood in the GI tract can cause melena.

Treatment

- **Stabilization:** As with LGIB (see above).
- **Medical therapy:** H_2 receptor antagonists do not alter outcome. Continuous IV infusions of PPIs decrease rebleeding in documented PUD with high-risk stigmata. The efficacy of empiric use while awaiting endoscopy is unproven, but oral PPI administration is low risk and low cost. Give IV octreotide for suspected variceal UGIB; continue for three days if verified by EGD.
- **Endoscopy:** Of all patients with active UGIB at EGD, > 90% can be effectively treated with banding, sclerosant, epinephrine, and/or electrocautery.

TABLE 7-9. Sources of Bleeding in Patients Hospitalized for Acute UGIB

Source of Bleeding	Proportion of Patients (%)
Ulcers	35–62
Varices	4–31
Mallory-Weiss tears	4–13
Gastroduodenal erosions	3–11
Erosive esophagitis	2–8
Malignancy	1–4
No source identified	7–25

Reproduced, with permission, from Braunwald E et al. *Harrison's Principles of Internal Medicine,* 15th ed. New York: McGraw-Hill, 2001.)

- **Refractory UGIB:**
  - Esophageal balloon tamponade (Minnesota or Sengstaken-Blakemore tubes) for varices or as a bridge to TIPS or shunt.
  - Angiogram with intra-arterial embolization or surgery for refractory nonvariceal bleeding.
- ***H. pylori* eradication:** For all peptic ulcers causing UGIB with positive *H. pylori* testing.

Ten percent of documented UGIB cases have a negative NG tube lavage.

INFLAMMATORY BOWEL DISEASE (IBD)

Crohn's disease and ulcerative colitis are the primary chronic inflammatory diseases of the bowel. Table 7-10 summarizes the distinguishing features of both.

Crohn's Disease

A chronic, recurrent disease with patchy transmural inflammation of **any segment of the GI tract from the mouth to the anus.** Shows a propensity for the ileum and proximal colon; one-third involve only the terminal ileum, one-half the small bowel and colon, and one-fifth only the colon. Incidence is 4–8 in 100,000. More common among Ashkenazi Jews, those with a positive family history, and smokers; **smoking may exacerbate disease.** Shows a bimodal age of onset at 15–25 and 55–65 years. Clinical course is characterized by the development of fistulas and strictures.

Symptoms

RLQ or periumbilical pain, **nonbloody diarrhea,** low-grade fever, malaise, weight loss, anal pain, oral aphthous ulcers, postprandial bloating, abdominal cramping.

Exam

Abdominal tenderness, palpable tender abdominal mass, anal fissures, fistulas.

Differential

Ulcerative colitis, IBS, infectious enterocolitis (*Yersinia, Entamoeba histolytica,* TB, *Chlamydia*), mesenteric ischemia, intestinal lymphoma, celiac sprue.

Diagnosis

- **Labs:**
  - Anemia (chronic disease, iron deficiency, vitamin B_{12} deficiency), leukocytosis, low serum albumin, elevated CRP, elevated ESR.
  - **Poor correlation between lab results and disease severity.**
- **Stool studies:** Culture, O&P, *C. difficile* toxin.
- **Colonoscopy:** Evaluate the colon and terminal ileum for segmental (**"skip lesions"**), eccentric linear, and serpiginous ulcerations, strictures, and active ileal disease. Biopsy shows acute and chronic inflammation; **granulomas are seen < 25% of the time but are highly suggestive of Crohn's disease.**
- **Small bowel follow-through:** Evaluate for small bowel involvement.
- **CT scan:** Consider if there is clinical concern for abdominal abscess.
- **Immunologic markers:** Useful in indeterminate disease (Crohn's vs. ulcerative colitis, particularly if surgery is indicated). Markers used (see Table 7-11) include p-ANCA and ASCA.

TABLE 7-10. Distinguishing Features of IBD

Feature	Crohn's Disease	Ulcerative Colitis
Genetic predisposition	+	+
Worse with smoking	+	–
Age at onset	Bimodal: 15–25, 55–65 years.	Bimodal: 20–40, 60–70 years.
Abdominal pain	Sharp, focal.	Crampy; associated with bowel movement.
Bowel obstruction	Common.	Rare.
Gross hematochezia	Occasionally.	Common.
GI involvement	Mouth to anus; typically terminal ileum/proximal colon.	Colon only; rectum with progression proximally.
Pattern	Segmental, transmural, eccentric.	Continuous, nontransmural, circumferential.
Ulceration	Superficial to deep, linear, serpiginous.	Superficial.
Histology	Granulomas.	Crypt abscesses.
p-ANCA positive	20%.	70%.
ASCA positive	65%.	15%.
Fistula/stricture	Common.	Uncommon.
Extraintestinal manifestations	Uncommon.	Common.
Infliximab response	Often.	Occasionally.
Surgery curative	Never.	Often.

TABLE 7-11. Interpretation of p-ANCA and ASCA Values

Test	Result	Interpretation	Characteristics
p-ANCA ASCA	– +	Suggests Crohn's.	95% PPV, 92% specificity.
p-ANCA ASCA	+ –	Suggests ulcerative colitis.	88% PPV, 98% specificity.

TREATMENT

- **5-ASA agents:**
  - **Sulfasalazine:** Give 1.5–2.0 g BID. Released in the colon; **not active in the small bowel.** Used for induction and maintenance.
  - **Mesalamine (Pentasa, Asacol):** Give 4 g QID. **Released in the small bowel;** associated with > 40% remission in mild to moderate ileocecal Crohn's disease.
- **Antibiotics:**
  - **Useful even with no obvious infection.**
  - Metronidazole 10 mg/kg/day or ciprofloxacin 500 mg BID.
- **Corticosteroids:**
  - Suppress acute disease; useful in small and large bowel disease.
  - Prednisone 40–60 mg/day during acute flares with taper after response.
  - Significant long-term side effects include diabetes, hypertension, cataracts, metabolic bone disease, and psychosis.
  - Budesonide is an oral steroid with less systemic absorption; used for maintenance only.
- **Immunomodulatory drugs:**
  - Maintenance only; not for remission induction.
  - Used to minimize steroid exposure.
  - **Azathioprine (Imuran):** Give 2.0–2.5 mg/kg. Therapeutic effects are delayed 6–8 weeks; significant bone marrow suppression requires frequent initial monitoring.
  - **6-MP:** Give 1.0–1.5 mg/kg; similar to azathioprine.
  - **Methotrexate:** Second- or third-line maintenance therapy.
- **Infliximab (Remicade):** Recombinant anti-TNF, 5 mg/kg IV infusion. For moderate to severe fistulizing disease; **contraindicated for disease with strictures.** Repeat IV infusions every 2–4 weeks for three doses; then consider maintenance doses every eight weeks. **TB must be ruled out prior to use (PPD, CXR).** Long-term treatment is associated with waning efficacy and increased allergic reactions.
- **Surgery:** Some 50% of patients will require surgery for obstruction or abscess if refractory to medical therapy.

Of all IBD cases, > 10% cannot clearly be classified as ulcerative colitis or Crohn's disease.

TB exposure and active stricturing disease must be ruled out before infliximab is administered.

Crohn's colitis carries a risk of colon cancer similar to that of ulcerative colitis.

COMPLICATIONS

Strictures/obstruction, fistulas, abscess, colorectal cancer, malabsorption, nephrolithiasis, cholelithiasis.

Ulcerative Colitis

A chronic, recurrent disease with diffuse mucosal inflammation of the colon. Of all cases, > 50% are isolated to the rectum and sigmoid colon and < 20% involve the entire colon. Incidence is 3–15 in 100,000; age at onset is typically 20–40 years, but the disease also occurs in patients < 10 years of age and in the elderly. More common among Ashkenazi Jews, nonsmokers, and those with a family history; **smoking may attenuate disease.** Course is marked by repeated flares and remissions.

SYMPTOMS/EXAM

- Bloody diarrhea, crampy abdominal pain, fecal urgency, tenesmus.
- Abdominal tenderness; red blood on DRE.

DIFFERENTIAL

Infectious colitis (*Salmonella, Shigella, Campylobacter,* enteroinvasive *E. coli, C. difficile,* amebiasis), ischemic colitis, Crohn's colitis.

DIAGNOSIS

- **Labs:**
  - Anemia (chronic disease, iron deficiency, active hematochezia), leukocytosis, low serum albumin, elevated CRP, elevated ESR.
  - **Good correlation between labs (hematocrit, albumin, ESR) and disease severity.**
- **Stool studies:** Culture, O&P, *C. difficile* toxin.
- **Imaging:** For moderate and severe activity. AXR reveals loss of haustrations leading to **"lead pipe"** appearance and colonic dilation.
- **Colonoscopy:** Avoid if there is a severe flare. Evaluate the colon and terminal ileum. Look for rectal involvement (95–100%), **continuous circumferential ulcerations,** and **pseudopolyps.** The terminal ileum is occasionally inflamed from **"backwash ileitis."** Biopsies show acute and chronic inflammation, **crypt abscesses,** and **absence of granulomas.**

TREATMENT

Treatment depends on severity and on the location of active disease.

- **Distal disease:** Mesalamine or hydrocortisone by suppository or enema.
- **Distal and proximal disease:** Oral or IV agents.
- **Mild to moderate activity:**
  - Sulfasalazine 1.5–3.0 g PO BID.
  - Mesalamine 2.4–4.0 g PO QD.
  - Prednisone 40–60 mg PO QD if no response after 2–4 weeks.
- **Severe activity:**
  - Methylprednisolone 48–60 mg IV QD or hydrocortisone 300 mg IV QD.
  - Roughly 50–75% of patients achieve remission in 7–10 days.
  - **If no response is seen within 7–10 days, colectomy is usually indicated.**
  - Consider a trial of cyclosporine prior to colectomy.
- **Maintenance therapy:**
  - Sulfasalazine 1.0–1.5 g PO BID.
  - Mesalamine 800–1200 mg PO TID.
- **Surgery:**
  - Can be curative and can eliminate the risk of colon cancer.
  - Proctocolectomy with ileostomy is curative.
  - Proctocolectomy with ileoanal anastomosis is often curative, but 25% have "pouchitis," or inflammation of the neorectum.

NSAID use can induce a flare of ulcerative colitis or Crohn's disease.

COMPLICATIONS

Toxic megacolon, primary sclerosing cholangitis, colorectal cancer, extraintestinal manifestations (see Table 7-12).

The risk of colon cancer in those with ulcerative colitis > 10 years is 0.5–1.0% per year; colonoscopy is recommended every 1–2 years beginning eight years after diagnosis.

TABLE 7-12. Extraintestinal Manifestations of Ulcerative Colitis

RELATED	OFTEN RELATED	UNRELATED
Arthritis	Pyoderma gangrenosum	Ankylosing spondylitis
Erythema nodosum	Uveitis	Primary sclerosing cholangitis
Oral aphthous ulcers		
Episcleritis		

ISCHEMIC BOWEL DISEASE

Acute Mesenteric Ischemia

Most common in the elderly and in those with atherosclerotic or cardiovascular disease. In young patients, occurs with atrial fibrillation, vasculitis, hypercoagulative disorders (OCP use in young female smokers), and vasoconstrictor abuse. After infarction, mortality is 70–90%.

Symptoms

Acute-onset, severe abdominal pain (**"out of proportion to exam"**); sudden forceful bowel movement, often with maroon or bright red blood and nausea.

Exam

- **Early:** Agitation, writhing, soft abdomen with hyper- or hypoactive bowel sounds, positive fecal blood.
- **Later:** Distention, progressive tenderness, peritoneal signs, hypotension, fever.

Differential

Pancreatitis, diverticulitis, appendicitis, aortic dissection, perforated peptic ulcer, nephrolithiasis.

Diagnosis

- **High index of suspicion:** Maintain for patients > 50 years of age with CHF, cardiac arrhythmias, recent MI, or hypotension.
- **Labs:** Leukocytosis, metabolic acidemia (late finding only), **elevated serum amylase (with normal lipase)** and lactate.
- **AXR:** Can be normal or show air-fluid levels and **"thumbprinting" in the small bowel wall.**
- **CT:** Bowel wall thickening, luminal dilation, **gas in the bowel wall and portal vein,** necrotic bowel, vascular thrombosis.
- **Visceral angiogram:** Important diagnostically; may be therapeutic.

Early visceral angiography is critical in the diagnosis and management of acute mesenteric ischemia.

Treatment

- Correct hypotension, hypovolemia, and cardiac arrhythmias.
- Bowel rest; broad-spectrum IV antibiotics.
- Early selective angiography with papaverine infusion.
- Laparotomy, revascularization, bowel resection.
- Anticoagulation is postponed until > 48 hours after laparotomy.

Ischemic colitis typically affects the colonic "watershed" areas of the splenic flexure and rectosigmoid junction but spares the rectum.

Ischemic Colitis

Most common in the elderly and in patients with atherosclerotic or cardiovascular disease. Ranges from self-limited to life-threatening disease. **Watershed areas** (the splenic flexure and rectosigmoid junction of the colon) are the most common sites. Exsanguination and infarction are uncommon.

Symptoms/Exam

- Crampy left lower abdominal pain, hematochezia, nausea.
- Benign abdominal exam or mild LLQ tenderness.

Differential

IBD, infectious colitis, diverticulitis.

Diagnosis

- **Labs:** Leukocytosis.
- **AXR:** **"Thumbprinting"** on colon wall.
- **CT:** Bowel wall thickening, luminal dilation, pericolonic fat stranding. Vascular occlusion is uncommon.
- **Flexible sigmoidoscopy:** Contraindicated if peritoneal signs are present. Performed with minimal insufflation. Look for **segmental changes sparing the rectum** (due to preserved collateral circulation from hemorrhoidal plexus) and hemorrhagic nodules. Pale, dusky, ulcerative mucosa.

Treatment

- Correct hypotension, hypovolemia, and cardiac arrhythmias.
- Minimize vasopressors; give broad-spectrum IV antibiotics.
- Monitor for progression with serial exams and radiographs.
- If there are signs of infarction (tenderness, guarding, fever), laparotomy, revascularization, or bowel resection may be needed.

PANCREATIC DISORDERS

Acute Pancreatitis

Ascaris lumbricoides causes up to 20% of acute pancreatitis in Asia.

In the United States, > 80% of acute pancreatitis cases are from binge drinking or biliary stones; only 5% of heavy drinkers develop pancreatitis. Twenty percent of cases are complicated by necrotizing pancreatitis. Etiologies are as follows:

- EtOH and gallstones and, to a lesser extent, trauma.
- **Drugs:** Azathioprine, pentamidine, sulfonamides, thiazide diuretics.
- **Metabolic:** Hyperlipidemia or hypercalcemia.
- **Mechanical:** Pancreas divisum, sphincter of Oddi dysfunction, mass.
- **Infectious:** Viruses (e.g., mumps) and, to a lesser extent, bacteria and parasites (e.g., *Ascaris lumbricoides*).
- **Other:** Scorpion bite, hereditary pancreatitis, CF, pregnancy.

Gallstones and alcohol are the main causes of pancreatitis in the United States.

Symptoms

- Sudden-onset, persistent, deep epigastric pain, often with radiation to the back, that **worsens when patients are supine and improves when they sit or lean forward.**
- Severe nausea, vomiting, fever.

Exam

- Upper abdominal tenderness with guarding and rebound.
- **Severe cases:** Distention, ileus, hypotension, tachycardia.
- **Rare: Umbilical (Cullen's sign) or flank (Grey Turner's sign) ecchymosis.**
- **Other:** Mild jaundice with stones or xanthomata with hyperlipidemia.

DIFFERENTIAL

Biliary colic, cholecystitis, mesenteric ischemia, perforated hollow viscus, inferior MI, dissecting aortic aneurysm, ectopic pregnancy.

DIAGNOSIS

- **Labs:** Leukocytosis (10,000–30,000/μL); elevated amylase (more sensitive) and lipase (more specific). No clinical use for serial amylase or lipase (see Table 7-13). High serum glucose. **ALT > 3 times normal suggests biliary stones over EtOH; an AST:ALT ratio > 2 favors EtOH.** CRP declines with improvement.
- **Differential for elevated amylase:** Pancreatitis, pancreatic tumors, cholecystitis, perforation (esophagus, stomach, bowel), intestinal ischemia or infarction, appendicitis, ruptured ectopic pregnancy, mumps, ovarian cysts, lung cancer, macroamylasemia, renal insufficiency, HIV, DKA, head trauma. **Lipase is usually normal in nonpancreatic amylase elevations.**
- **AXR:** May show gallstones, "**sentinel loop**" (air-filled small bowel in the LUQ), and "**colon cutoff sign**" (abrupt ending of the transverse colon).
- **RUQ ultrasound:** Cholelithiasis without cholecystitis. Common duct stones are often missed or have passed.
- **CT:** Done initially to exclude abdominal catastrophes. At 48–72 hours, exclude necrotizing pancreatitis. **High risk of renal failure from contrast dye.**

CT is prognostic in severe pancreatitis and is used to evaluate for necrotizing pancreatitis as well as to assess the need for empiric antibiotics (imipenem).

TREATMENT

- NPO with nasojejunal tube feeds or total parenteral nutrition with severe disease and anticipated NPO status for > 3–5 days.
- Aggressive IV hydration.
- Pain control with narcotics; avoid morphine, as it increases sphincter of Oddi tone.
- Broad-spectrum IV antibiotics (imipenem) for severe necrotizing pancreatitis.

TABLE 7-13. Assessment of Pancreatitis Severity: Ranson's Criteria

24 HOURS: "GA LAW"	48 HOURS: "C HOBBS"
Glucose > 200 mg/dL	**C**a < 8 mg/dL
Age > 55	**H**ematocrit drop < 10%
LDH > 350 U/L	**O**$_2$, arterial PO$_2$ < 60 mmHg
AST > 250 U/L	**B**ase deficit > 4 mEq/L
WBC > 16,000 /μL	**B**UN rise > 5 mg/dL
	Sequestered fluid > 6 L

NUMBER OF CRITERIA	MORTALITY RATE
0–2	1%
3–4	16%
5–6	40%
7–8	100%

- **For gallstone pancreatitis (elevated serum bilirubin, signs of biliary sepsis):** ERCP for stone removal and cholecystectomy after recovery **but prior to discharge.**

For persistent pancreatitis (> 1 week), consider CT with FNA to rule out infected necrosis, which requires surgical debridement.

COMPLICATIONS

- **Necrotizing pancreatitis:**
  - Persistently elevated WBC count (7–10 days), high fever, organ failure.
  - If infected necrosis is suspected, perform percutaneous aspiration. If organisms are present on smear, surgical debridement is indicated.
- **Pancreatic pseudocyst:** Drainage is not required unless pseudocyst is present > 6–8 weeks and is enlarging and symptomatic.
- Renal failure, ARDS, splenic vein thrombosis (can cause isolated gastric varices).

Chronic Pancreatitis

Persistent inflammation of the pancreas with irreversible histologic changes, recurrent abdominal pain, and permanent loss of function. Characterized by the size of pancreatic ducts injured; "big duct" injury is from EtOH. Risk factors include EtOH (amount and duration) and smoking. Associated with an increased risk of pancreatic cancer (2% per year); 10- and 20-year survival rates are 70% and 45%, with deaths usually resulting from nonpancreatic causes. Etiologies are as follows:

- **EtOH (80%)** and, to a lesser extent, hereditary pancreatitis (CF, trypsinogen mutation).
- **Autoimmune:** Sjögren's, primary biliary cirrhosis.
- **Obstructive:** Pancreatic divisum, sphincter of Oddi dysfunction, mass.
- **Metabolic:** Malnutrition, hyperlipidemia, hyperparathyroid-associated hypercalcemia.

SYMPTOMS

Recurrent, deep epigastric and/or LUQ pain, often radiating to the back, that worsens with food intake and when patients lie supine and **improves when they sit or lean forward.** Episodes may last anywhere from hours to 2–3 weeks. Also presents with anorexia, fear of eating **(sitophobia),** nausea/vomiting, and, later, weight loss and steatorrhea.

EXAM

Normal. Mild to moderate upper abdominal tenderness during episodes. Rarely, there may be a palpable epigastric mass (pseudocyst) or spleen (from splenic vein thrombosis).

DIFFERENTIAL

Biliary colic, mesenteric ischemia, PUD, nonulcer dyspepsia, IBS, drug-seeking behavior.

DIAGNOSIS

Diagnosis is as follows (see also Table 7-14):

- No single test is adequate; routine labs are normal. Amylase and lipase are not always elevated during episodes.
- **Functional tests:**
  - Often normal in "small duct" chronic pancreatitis; not positive until 30–50% of the gland is destroyed.

TABLE 7-14. Diagnosis of Chronic Pancreatitis

	"BIG DUCT"	"SMALL DUCT"
Seen on ultrasound or CT	Yes	No
Seen on ERCP	Yes	Maybe
Etiology	EtOH	Non-EtOH >> EtOH
Loss of function (exocrine/endocrine)	Common	Less common
Responsive to decompression (stenting, surgery)	Often	Rarely

  - **72-hour fecal fat test on 100-g/day fat diet:** Positive if > 7 g fat in stool.
  - **Stool chymotrypsin and elastase:** Absent or low levels.
  - **Secretin test:** Most sensitive, but impractical. Give IV secretin and then measure pancreatic secretion via a nasobiliary tube.
- **Structural tests: Pancreatic calcifications on plain AXRs** (30%); "big duct" injury on ultrasound or CT. **Diagnosis with ERCP,** MRCP, and endoscopic ultrasound is increasing.
- **Histology:** Impractical gold standard; obtained by endoscopic ultrasound-guided biopsy. Fibrosis, mixed cellular inflammatory infiltrate, and architectural changes are seen.

Chronic pancreatitis of the "small duct" type may exhibit very subtle structural changes and is often associated with normal functional tests but marked symptoms.

TREATMENT

- Alcohol abstinence.
- Fat-soluble vitamins (vitamins A, D, E, and K), pancreatic enzymes.
- **Pain control:** Narcotics (avoid morphine), celiac plexus injection.
- ERCP with short-term pancreatic duct stenting and stone removal.
- **Surgical therapy for intractable pain and failure of medical therapy:** Puestow and Whipple procedures; less effective for "small duct" type.

COMPLICATIONS

- **Malabsorption:** Fat-soluble vitamins (A, D, E, and K), pancreatic enzymes.
- **Metabolic bone disease:** Osteopenia (33%) and osteoporosis (10%). Manage with calcium, vitamin D, bisphosphonates.
- Brittle DM, pancreatic pseudocyst, pancreatic cancer.

BILIARY DISEASE

Tables 7-15 and 7-16 classify diseases with jaundice and biliary tract disease.

Cholelithiasis (Gallstones) and Acute Cholecystitis

More common in women; incidence increases with age. In the United States, 10% of men and 20% of women > 65 years of age are affected; > 70% are cholesterol stones (see Table 7-17). Only 15% of patients become symptomatic by 10 years.

TABLE 7-15. Classification of Jaundice

TYPE OF HYPERBILIRUBINEMIA	LOCATION AND CAUSE
Unconjugated hyperbilirubinemia (predominant indirect-acting bilirubin)	Increased bilirubin production (e.g., hemolytic anemias, hemolytic reactions, hematoma, pulmonary infarction). Impaired bilirubin uptake and storage (e.g., posthepatitis hyperbilirubinemia, Gilbert's syndrome, Crigler-Najjar syndrome, drug reactions). **Hereditary cholestatic syndromes:** Faulty excretion of bilirubin conjugates (e.g., Dubin-Johnson syndrome, Rotor's syndrome).
Conjugated hyperbilirubinemia (predominant direct-acting bilirubin)	**Hepatocellular dysfunction:** ▪ Biliary epithelial damage (e.g., hepatitis, hepatic cirrhosis) ▪ Intrahepatic cholestasis (e.g., certain drugs, biliary cirrhosis, sepsis, postoperative jaundice) ▪ Hepatocellular damage or intrahepatic cholestasis resulting from miscellaneous causes (e.g., spirochetal infections, infectious mononucleosis, cholangitis, sarcoidosis, lymphomas, industrial toxins) **Biliary obstruction:** Choledocholithiasis, biliary atresia, carcinoma of the biliary duct, sclerosing cholangitis, choledochal cyst, external pressure on the common duct, pancreatitis, pancreatic neoplasms.

Reproduced, with permission, from Tierney LM et al. *Current Medical Diagnosis & Treatment 2004,* 43rd ed. New York: McGraw-Hill, 2004.

- **Cholecystitis associated with gallstones:** Seen in > 90% of cases, with stone impacted in the cystic duct. Spontaneous resolution is achieved in > 50% of cases within 7–10 days.
- **Acalculous cholecystitis (without gallstones):** Usually seen in critically ill patients with no oral intake or after major surgical procedures; occurs after ischemia-related chronic gallbladder distention.

Acalculous cholecystitis is generally seen in the critically ill with no oral intake or after major surgical procedures.

SYMPTOMS

- **Cholelithiasis:** Often asymptomatic or may present as follows:
  - **Common:** Biliary colic (crampy, wavelike RUQ pain), abdominal bloating, dyspepsia.
  - **Uncommon:** Nausea/vomiting (except in small bowel obstruction from **gallstone ileus**).
- **Cholecystitis:** Sudden-onset severe RUQ or epigastric pain that may radiate to the right shoulder; nausea/vomiting, fever. Jaundice suggests common bile duct stones (choledocholithiasis) or compression of the common bile duct by inflamed impacted cystic duct (**Mirizzi's syndrome**).

EXAM

- **Cholelithiasis:** Normal exam.
- **Cholecystitis:** RUQ tenderness and voluntary guarding, positive **Murphy's sign** (inspiratory arrest with palpation of RUQ), fever, jaundice < 25%.

TABLE 7-16. Diseases of the Biliary Tract

	Clinical Features	Laboratory Features	Diagnosis	Treatment
Asymptomatic gallstones	None.	Normal.	Ultrasound.	None.
Symptomatic gallstones	Biliary colic.	Normal.	Ultrasound.	Laparoscopic cholecystectomy.
Cholesterolosis of gallbladder	Usually asymptomatic.	Normal.	Oral cholecystography.	None.
Adenomyomatosis	May cause biliary colic.	Normal.	Oral cholecystography.	Laparoscopic cholecystectomy if symptomatic.
Porcelain gallbladder	Usually asymptomatic; high risk of gallbladder cancer.	Normal.	X-ray or CT.	Laparoscopic cholecystectomy.
Acute cholecystitis	Epigastric or RUQ pain, nausea, vomiting, fever, Murphy's sign.	Leukocytosis.	Ultrasound, HIDA scan.	Antibiotics, laparoscopic cholecystectomy.
Chronic cholecystitis	Biliary colic, constant epigastric or RUQ pain, nausea.	Normal. oral cholecystography	Ultrasound (stones), cholecystectomy. (nonfunctioning gallbladder).	Laparoscopic
Choledocholithiasis	Asymptomatic or biliary colic, jaundice, fever; gallstone pancreatitis.	Colestatic LFTs; leukocytosis and positive blood cultures in cholangitis; elevated amylase and lipase in pancreatitis.	Ultrasound (dilated ducts), ERCP.	Endoscopic sphincterotomy and stone extraction; antibiotics for cholangitis.

Reproduced, with permission, from Tierney LM et al. *Current Medical Diagnosis & Treatment 2004,* 43rd ed. New York: McGraw-Hill, 2004.

DIFFERENTIAL

- Choledocholithiasis, cholangitis, perforated peptic ulcer, acute pancreatitis.
- Appendicitis (with congenital high appendix or from pregnancy), hepatic abscess.
- Diverticulitis (hepatic flexure, transverse colon), right-sided pneumonia.

DIAGNOSIS

- **Cholelithiasis:** Often an incidental finding on abdominal ultrasound or CT.

TABLE 7-17. Types of Gallstones

	CHOLESTEROL	BLACK PIGMENTED	BROWN PIGMENTED
Regional/ethnic predictors	Western countries, Pima Indians, Caucasians >> blacks.	Africa, Asia.	Africa, Asia.
Risk factors	Age, female, pregnancy, estrogens, DM, obesity, rapid weight loss, elevated triglycerides, prolonged fasting, ileal disease **(Crohn's),** ileal resection, CF.	Chronic hemolysis **(sickle cell),** cirrhosis, high-protein diet.	Biliary infections, foreign bodies (stents, sutures), low-protein diet.

- Cholecystitis:
  - **Labs:** Leukocytosis with neutrophil predominance. Elevated total bilirubin (1–4 mg/dL) and transaminases (2–4 times normal) even without choledocholithiasis. Elevated alkaline phosphatase and amylase.
  - **RUQ ultrasound:** Less sensitive than HIDA scan but more readily available. Shows gallbladder wall thickening, pericholecystic fluid and inflammation, and localization of stones. **Radiographic Murphy's sign** (focal gallbladder tenderness under transducer) has 90% positive predictive value. Low sensitivity (50%) for choledocholithiasis.
  - **HIDA scan:** High sensitivity (95%) and specificity (90%). Assesses cystic duct patency; positive if nonvisualization of gallbladder with preserved excretion into the small bowel. **CCK stimulation assesses gallbladder contractility and aids in the diagnosis of acalculous cholecystitis.**

TREATMENT

- **Asymptomatic cholelithiasis:** No specific treatment is indicated (even in DM).
- **Symptomatic cholelithiasis:**
  - Consider prophylactic cholecystectomy.
  - Cholecystectomy can be postponed until recurrent symptoms are seen.
  - **The risk of recurrent symptoms is 30–50% per year; the risk of complications is 1–2% per year.**
- Cholecystitis:
  - **Antibiotics can be withheld if disease is mild and uncomplicated.**
  - **IV antibiotics:** Coverage of gram-negative enteric bacteria and enterococcus with antibiotics such as ampicillin and gentamicin or ampicillin/sulbactam if the patient is ill.
  - Bowel rest.
  - Cholecystectomy after symptom resolution but prior to discharge.

COMPLICATIONS

- **Gangrenous cholecystitis:** The most common complication (affects up to 20%), particularly in diabetics and the elderly. Patients appear septic.

- **Emphysematous cholecystitis:** Secondarily infected gallbladder with gas-forming organisms. More common in diabetics and the elderly; associated with high mortality. Gangrene and perforation may follow.
- **Cholecystenteric fistula:** Uncommon. Stone erodes through the gallbladder into the duodenum. Large stones > 2.5 cm can cause small bowel obstruction **(gallstone ileus).**
- **Mirizzi's syndrome:** Common bile duct obstruction by an inflamed impacted cystic duct. Uncommon.
- Gallbladder hydrops.
- **Porcelain gallbladder:** Intramural calcification. Increased risk of gallbladder cancer; cholecystectomy is indicated.

Choledocholithiasis and Cholangitis

Choledocholithiasis is defined as stones in the common bile duct. Cholangitis can be defined as biliary tree infection.

SYMPTOMS

- **Choledocholithiasis:** Similar to cholelithiasis, except **jaundice is more common in choledocholithiasis.** Other symptoms include biliary colic (crampy, wavelike RUQ pain), abdominal bloating, and dyspepsia. May also be asymptomatic.
- **Cholangitis:** Similar to cholecystitis but often more severe, with fever, jaundice, RUQ pain (Charcot's triad), and rigors.

EXAM

- **Choledocholithiasis:** Normal exam or mild RUQ tenderness; jaundice.
- **Cholangitis:**
  - Fever and RUQ tenderness with peritoneal signs (90%), jaundice (> 80%), hypotension, and altered mental status (15%).
  - **Charcot's triad (RUQ pain, jaundice, fever):** Present in only 70% of patients.
  - **Reynold's pentad (Charcot's triad plus hypotension and altered mental status):** Points to impending septic shock.

Charcot's triad = RUQ pain, jaundice, and fever/chills. Reynold's pentad = Charcot's triad plus hypotension and altered mental status.

DIFFERENTIAL

- **Choledocholithiasis:** Mass lesions (e.g., pancreatic and ampullary carcinoma, cholangiocarcinoma, bulky lymphadenopathy), parasitic infection (e.g., ascariasis), AIDS cholangiopathy, primary sclerosing cholangitis.
- **Cholangitis:** Perforated peptic ulcer, acute pancreatitis, appendicitis, hepatic abscess, diverticulitis, right-sided pneumonia.

DIAGNOSIS

- **Choledocholithiasis:**
  - **Labs:** No leukocytosis. Elevated total bilirubin (> 2 mg/dL), transaminases (2–4 times normal), and alkaline phosphatase.
  - **RUQ ultrasound:** Low sensitivity (< 50%).
  - **CT:** Higher sensitivity than RUQ ultrasound.
- **Cholangitis:**
  - **Labs:** Leukocytosis with neutrophil predominance; elevated total bilirubin (> 2 mg/dL), transaminases (> 2–4 times normal), alkaline phosphatase, and amylase; bacteremia.

- **RUQ ultrasound:** Dilation of the common bile duct and cholelithiasis are frequently seen.
- **ERCP:** Perform < 48 hours after presentation, ideally after IV antibiotics and fluids. Requires sedation. Diagnostic and therapeutic.
- **Percutaneous transhepatic cholangiography (PTHC):** An alternative if ERCP is unavailable, unsafe, or unsuccessful. Does not require sedation.

TREATMENT

- **Choledocholithiasis:** ERCP with sphincterotomy/stone removal **and** cholecystectomy.
- **Cholangitis:**
  - **Broad-spectrum IV antibiotics:** IV ampicillin/sulbactam (Unasyn) or ticarcillin/clavulanate (Timentin). If the patient is responsive to antibiotics, biliary decompression can be elective; otherwise it is indicated emergently.
  - **ERCP:** Biliary decompression and drainage (sphincterotomy, stone removal, biliary stenting).
  - **PTHC:** A temporary alternative to ERCP that allows biliary decompression (stenting and drainage).
  - Cholecystectomy after recovery if cholangitis forms biliary stones.

COMPLICATIONS

Gallstone pancreatitis, gram-negative sepsis, intrahepatic abscesses.

AIDS Cholangiopathy

An opportunistic biliary infection caused by CMV, *Cryptosporidium*, or *Microsporidium*. CD4 is usually < 200/mL.

SYMPTOMS/EXAM

RUQ pain/tenderness, fever, diarrhea. Jaundice is uncommon.

DIFFERENTIAL

Biliary stones, cholecystitis, primary sclerosing cholangitis.

DIAGNOSIS

- Elevated alkaline phosphatase.
- **ERCP:** Intra- and/or extrahepatic biliary stricturing; papillary stenosis.
- **Aspiration and culture of bile are key to diagnosis.**

TREATMENT

- ERCP with sphincterotomy and biliary stenting.
- IV antibiotics based on bile cultures.
- Treat underlying immunosuppression/HIV.

Primary Sclerosing Cholangitis

A chronic cholestatic disease characterized by fibrosing inflammation of the intrahepatic and extrahepatic biliary system **without an identifiable cause.** Most common among middle-aged males; median survival from the time of diagnosis is 12 years. Commonly associated with **IBD** (more frequently ulcerative colitis than Crohn's) and, to a lesser extent, with other autoimmune disorders (celiac sprue, sarcoidosis, Sjögren's syndrome, SLE, autoimmune hepatitis). Also associated with an increased risk of **cholangiocarcinoma.**

Symptoms

Gradual onset of fatigue and severe pruritus followed by jaundice and weight loss. Fever occurs with recurrent cholangitis.

Seventy-five percent of patients with primary sclerosing cholangitis have IBD, but the reverse is the case for only a small subset of IBD patients.

Exam

Jaundice, hepatosplenomegaly, hyperpigmentation, xanthomas, excoriations, stigmata of fat-soluble vitamin deficiency.

Differential

Secondary sclerosing cholangitis—biliary stones, congenital anomalies, infections, AIDS cholangiopathy.

Diagnosis

- Maintain a high clinical suspicion in patients with IBD, as the **diagnosis of IBD typically precedes that of primary sclerosing cholangitis.** Diagnosis is confirmed only by ERCP. Magnetic resonance cholangiography (MRC) is less sensitive and less specific.
- **Labs:** Look for **cholestatic pattern**—alkaline phosphatase > 1.5 times normal for six months; modest increase in bilirubin and transaminases.
- **Autoantibodies:** The sensitivity of **p-ANCA** is 70%; that of ANA is 25%.
- **Liver biopsy:** Look for pericholangitis and classic **"onion skin"** periductal fibrosis, focal proliferation and obliteration of bile ducts, cholestasis, and copper deposition.
- **ERCP:** Shows irregularity of the intra- and extrahepatic biliary tree, classically with **"beads on a string"** appearance. Secondary causes of sclerosing cholangitis usually have **only** extrahepatic bile duct involvement.

Primary sclerosing cholangitis is diagnosed by ERCP and shows a "beads on a string" appearance involving both intra- and extrahepatic bile ducts.

Treatment

- Focus on symptom control and on prevention and management of complications. Medical therapy to prevent or delay disease progression is largely ineffective.
- **Symptom control:** Treat pruritus (cholestyramine, ursodiol, phenobarbital, rifampin).
- **Prevention and treatment of complications:** Steatorrhea/fat-soluble vitamin deficiency (bile acids, digestive enzymes, and vitamins A, D, E, and K), metabolic bone disease (Ca^{++}, bisphosphonates), recurrent bacterial cholangitis and dominant strictures (antibiotics, biliary drainage), biliary stones, **cholangiocarcinoma,** portal hypertension, end-stage liver disease.
- **Medical therapy:** Immunosuppression (corticosteroids, cyclosporine, azathioprine, methotrexate), antifibrogenics (colchicine), others (penicillamine, ursodeoxycholic acid). **The natural history of primary sclerosing cholangitis is not significantly changed by current medical therapy.**
- **Liver transplantation:** The treatment of choice for end-stage liver failure; five-year survival is 75%.

Primary Biliary Cirrhosis

A chronic cholestatic disease that primarily affects **middle-aged women of all races.** Prevalence is 19–240 cases in one million; 90–95% are women. Age at onset is 30–70; often associated with autoimmune disorders such as Sjögren's, rheumatoid arthritis, thyroid disease, celiac sprue, and CREST syndrome.

Symptoms

May be asymptomatic (50–60% at the time of diagnosis) or present with fatigue, **severe and intractable pruritus prior to jaundice,** and nocturnal malabsorptive diarrhea.

Exam

- Hepatomegaly, splenomegaly, skin pigmentation, excoriations (from pruritus), xanthelasma and xanthomata, **Kayser-Fleischer rings** (from copper retention, as in Wilson's disease).
- Late findings include jaundice and the stigmata of cirrhosis.

Differential

Biliary obstruction (stones, benign or malignant mass), autoimmune hepatitis, primary and secondary sclerosing cholangitis, drug-induced hepatitis, infiltrative diseases (sarcoidosis, lymphoma, TB).

Diagnosis

- Suspect with unexplained cholestasis or elevated serum alkaline phosphatase.
- **Labs:**
  - **Cholestatic pattern:** Alkaline phosphatase > 3–4 times normal; elevated GGT; slight increase in transaminases. Serum bilirubin is normal early in disease but elevated in late disease.
  - **Serum autoantibodies: Antimitochondrial antibodies (AMA) are detected in 95%** of cases. Also ANA (35%), SMA (66%), RF (70%), and antithyroid antibodies (40%).
  - **Other: Increased serum IgM,** total cholesterol, HDL, ceruloplasmin and urinary copper.
- **Imaging:** Ultrasound is initially useful for excluding biliary tract obstruction. MRI/CT can show nonprogressive periportal adenopathy; signs of portal hypertension are usually absent at the time of diagnosis.
- **Liver biopsy:** Important for diagnosis, staging, and prognosis.
- **ERCP:** Needed only to exclude primary and secondary sclerosing cholangitis.

Antimitochondrial antibody (present in 95% of patients) and elevated serum IgM are the best laboratory diagnostic tools for primary biliary cirrhosis.

Treatment

- Disease-modifying therapy has limited efficacy. Symptom control and prevention/treatment of complications are most important in management.
- **Ursodeoxycholic acid (UDCA):** The only FDA-approved disease-modifying agent; promotes endogenous bile acid secretion and may have immunologic effects. Give 13–20 mg/kg/day.
- **Liver transplantation:** The most effective treatment for decompensated primary biliary cirrhosis. Five-year survival is 85%; rates of recurrent primary biliary cirrhosis at 3 and 10 years are 15% and 30%, respectively. The need for liver transplant can be predicted by the Mayo Clinic model (based on patient age, total bilirubin, PT, and serum albumin)

Complications

- **Malabsorption:** Treat with fat-soluble vitamins (A, D, E, and K) and pancreatic enzymes.

- **Metabolic bone disease:** Osteopenia (affects 33%) and osteoporosis (affects 10%). Manage with calcium, vitamin D, and bisphosphonates.
- **Cirrhosis:** Late ascites, encephalopathy, portal hypertension.

HEPATITIS

Hepatitis A (HAV) and Hepatitis E (HEV)

Spread by fecal-oral transmission; cause acute (**not chronic**) hepatitis. More common in developing countries. The annual incidence of HAV in the United States is 70,000, whereas **HEV is rare and limited to travelers of endemic regions** (Southeast and Central Asia, the Middle East, Northern Africa, and, to a lesser extent, Mexico). HAV is typically asymptomatic, benign, and self-limited in children but can range from mild to severe acute hepatitis in adults. The rate of fatal acute liver failure from HAV is < 4% in patients < 49 years of age but can be as high as 17% in those > 49 years of age. **Unlike HAV, HEV in pregnancy has a high mortality** (> 20%).

SYMPTOMS

- Flulike illness, malaise, anorexia, weakness, fever, RUQ pain, jaundice, pruritus. Children are typically asymptomatic.
- Atypical presentations include acute liver failure, cholestasis (prolonged, deep jaundice), and relapsing disease (2–18 weeks after initial presentation).
- Figure 7-4 illustrates the typical course of HAV.

EXAM

Jaundice, RUQ tenderness.

DIFFERENTIAL

Acute HBV or, less frequently, HCV; mononucleosis, CMV, HSV, drug-induced hepatitis, acute alcoholic hepatitis, autoimmune hepatitis.

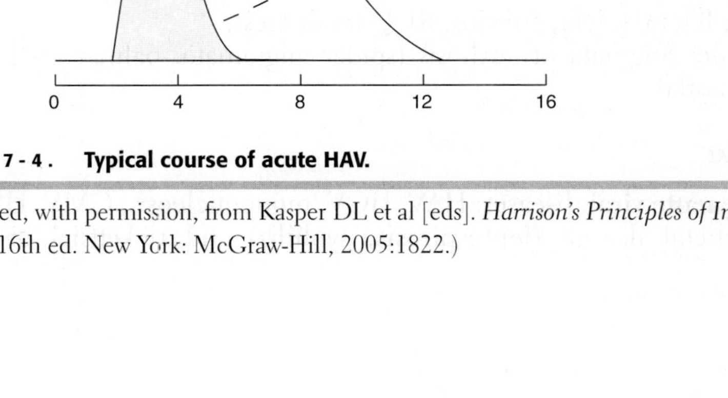

FIGURE 7-4. Typical course of acute HAV.

(Reproduced, with permission, from Kasper DL et al [eds]. *Harrison's Principles of Internal Medicine*, 16th ed. New York: McGraw-Hill, 2005:1822.)

DIAGNOSIS

- **History:** Inquire about ill contacts, substandard water supply, travel (HEV), and contaminated food **(shellfish, especially bivalve mollusks).**
- **Labs:**
  - **HAV:** Anti-HAV IgM (acute infection), anti-HAV IgG (prior exposure, vaccination), anti-HAV total measures IgM and IgG (acute infection, prior exposure, vaccination).
  - **HEV:** Anti-HEV IgM (acute infection), anti-HEV (prior exposure).

HAV and HEV cause variably severe acute hepatitis but do not cause chronic hepatitis.

TREATMENT

- No specific drug treatment is available for HAV or HEV.
- Supportive care.
- Consider early delivery for pregnant women with HEV (no proven benefit).

PREVENTION

- **Vaccination:** HAV vaccine is safe and effective, but no vaccine for HEV is currently available.
- **Indications for HAV vaccine:** Travelers to endemic regions, men who have sex with men, IV drug users, Native Americans, those with chronic liver disease **(all HCV positive)**, food handlers, day care center workers.
- **HAV immunoglobulin:** Effective for postexposure prophylaxis; supplement with first vaccine shot for those traveling immediately to endemic regions.

*Hepatocellular carcinoma can occur **before** cirrhosis from HBV, but this is not true of HCV.*

Hepatitis B (HBV) and Hepatitis D (HDV)

Some 400 million people worldwide have chronic HBV, including > 1 million in the United States. Transmission can be perinatal (most common worldwide), sexual, or percutaneous. Age at infection is **inversely related** to the risk of chronic infection. Of all patients with chronic HBV, 15–20% develop cirrhosis and 10–15% develop hepatocellular carcinoma. **HDV infection requires HBV coinfection.** In the United States, HDV is found primarily among IV drug users and hemophiliacs.

SYMPTOMS

- **Acute HBV:** Flulike illness, malaise, weakness, low-grade fever, serum sickness–like symptoms (arthritis, urticaria, angioedema), and RUQ pain; then jaundice (see Figure 7-5).
- **Chronic HBV:** Can be asymptomatic.
- **Extrahepatic manifestations:** Serum sickness, polyarteritis nodosa, glomerulonephritis.

EXAM

- **Acute:** Icteric sclera, arthritis, RUQ tenderness.
- **Chronic:** Stigmata of cirrhosis (spider angiomata, palmar erythema, gynecomastia).

DIFFERENTIAL

- **Other acute viral diseases:** HAV, HCV, mononucleosis, CMV, HSV.
- Spirochetal disease (**leptospirosis,** syphilis) and rickettsial disease (**Q fever).**

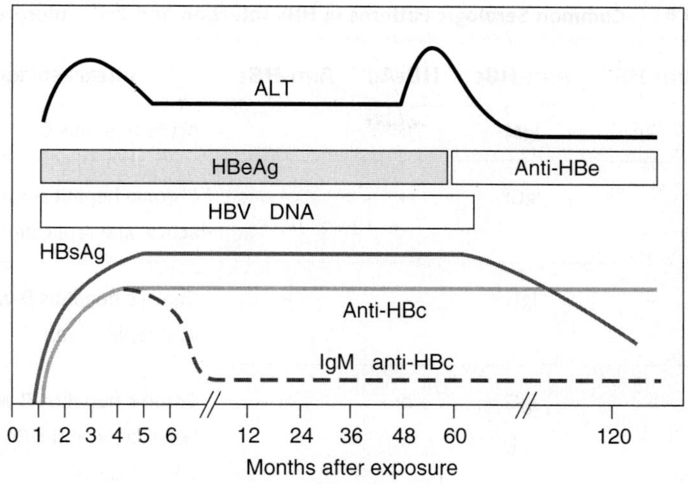

FIGURE 7-5. Typical course of acute HBV.

(Reproduced, with permission, from Kasper DL et al [eds]. *Harrison's Principles of Internal Medicine*, 16th ed. New York: McGraw-Hill, 2005:1825.)

- **Other chronic liver diseases:** Autoimmune disease, hemochromatosis, α_1-antitrypsin deficiency, Wilson's disease.

Diagnosis

- **HBsAg:** Surface antigen indicates **active** infection (see Table 7-18).
- **Anti-HBs:** Antibody to HBsAg; indicates past viral infection or immunization.
- **Anti-HBc:** IgM is an early marker of infection; IgG is the best marker for prior HBV exposure.
- **HBeAg:** Proportional to the quantity of intact virus and therefore infectivity. Some HBV variants (called **precore mutants**) cannot make HBeAg. Precore mutants have lower spontaneous remission, are less responsive to treatment, and are associated with a high risk of cirrhosis and hepatocellular carcinoma. Precore mutants are diagnosed by their high HBV DNA and negative HBeAg.
- **Anti-HDV:** Indicates past or present HDV infection. **Does not indicate immunity.**
- **HBV DNA:** Indicates active replication. A level of $> 10^5$ copies/mL is considered active; $> 10^2$ copies/mL are detectable by new assays.
- **Liver biopsy:** Not routinely needed prior to treatment. Indicated if diagnosis is in question or to evaluate for cirrhosis.

Treatment

- **Acute exposure/needlestick prophylaxis:** The CDC recommends that hepatitis B immune globulin (HBIG) be given **within 24 hours along with vaccine** if the patient was not previously immunized.
- Best responses to treatment are obtained with active hepatic inflammation (high ALT) and low HBV DNA levels.
- **Interferon-α:** Given SQ; associated with many side effects (e.g., psychiatric, bone marrow toxicity, hepatic decompensation). Contraindicated in cirrhosis.
- **Lamivudine:** Given PO; well tolerated, but resistance may develop.

TABLE 7-18. Common Serologic Patterns in HBV Infection and Their Interpretation

HBsAg	Anti-HBs	Anti-HBc	HBeAg	Anti-HBe	Interpretation
+	–	IgM	+	–	Acute hepatitis B.
+	–	IgG[a]	+	–	Chronic hepatitis B with active viral replication.
+	–	IgG	–	+	Chronic hepatitis B with low viral replication.
+	+	IgG	+ or –	+ or –	Chronic hepatitis B with heterotypic anti-HBs (about 10% of cases).
–	–	IgM	+ or –	–	Acute hepatitis B.
–	+	–	–	–	Vaccination (immunity).
–	–	IgG	–	–	False positive; less commonly, infection in remote past.

[a] Low levels of IgM anti-HBc may also be detected.

Reproduced, with permission, from Tierney LM et al. *Current Medical Diagnosis & Treatment 2004,* 43rd ed. New York: McGraw-Hill, 2004.

- **Adefovir:** Given PO; well tolerated and may be used to treat lamivudine-resistant virus; lower rates of resistance than laminvudine.
- Treat HDV by treating HBV.
- **Liver transplantation:** Treatment of choice for decompensated cirrhosis.

Needlestick transmission rates follow the rule of 3's: HBV 30%, HCV 3%, HIV 0.3%.

Hepatitis C (HCV)

Transmitted by percutaneous or mucosal blood exposure. Risk factors include blood transfusions received before 1992, IV drug use, and occupational exposure (needlesticks). Spontaneous resolution occurs in 15–45% of patients, with the highest rates of resolution in children and young women. Chronic infection occurs in 55–85% of those exposed. Cirrhosis occurs within 20–30 years in 20% of those with chronic infection. Risk of carcinoma is 1–4%/year after cirrhosis.

Symptoms

- **Acute HCV:** Flulike illness, malaise, weakness, low-grade fever, myalgias, and RUQ pain; then jaundice (only 30% are symptomatic in acute disease).
- **Chronic HCV:** Often asymptomatic, or may present with **cryoglobulinemia** associated with vasculitic skin rash **(leukocytoclastic vasculitis)**, arthralgias, sicca syndrome, and glomerulonephritis. In the presence of cirrhosis, presents with fatigue, muscle wasting, dependent edema, and easy bruising.

Both HCV and HBV can cause cryoglobulinemia and glomerulonephritis.

EXAM

- **Acute:** Icterus, RUQ tenderness.
- **Chronic:** Stigmata of cirrhosis (spider angiomata, palmar erythema, gynecomastia).

DIFFERENTIAL

- **Other acute viral diseases:** HAV, HBV, mononucleosis, CMV, HSV.
- Spirochetal disease (**leptospirosis,** syphilis) and rickettsial disease (**Q fever**).
- **Other chronic liver diseases:** HBV, hemochromatosis, α_1-antitrypsin deficiency, Wilson's disease, nonalcoholic fatty liver disease, autoimmune hepatitis.

DIAGNOSIS

- **Screening:** HCV antibody (4–6 weeks after infection), qualitative PCR (for acute infection; can be positive 2–3 weeks after infection). Screen in patients with risk factors or persistently elevated transaminases.
- **Confirmatory:** Qualitative PCR or recombinant immunoblot assay (RIBA).
- **Prognostic:** Liver biopsy.

TREATMENT

- **Regimen:** SQ interferon (pegylated or standard) and PO ribavirin × 24 weeks (non–genotype 1) or × 48 weeks (genotype 1).
- **Predictive:** Quantitative PCR (low viral load indicates a better treatment response), genotype (non–genotype 1 is associated with a better treatment response).
- **Indications:** Age 18–60, HCV viremia, elevated aminotransferase levels.
- **Contraindications:** Psychosis, severe depression, symptomatic coronary or cerebrovascular disease, **decompensated cirrhosis,** uncontrolled seizures, severe bone marrow insufficiency, pregnancy or inability to use birth control, retinopathy, autoimmune disease.
- **Acute infection/needlestick prophylaxis:** Currently not recommended.
- **Chronic HCV:** Treatment is curative in up to 75–80% of non–genotype 1 cases but in < 20–40% for other subgroups.

Autoimmune Hepatitis

Characterized by hypergammaglobulinemia, periportal hepatitis, and autoimmune markers. Typically chronic, but 25% are characterized by acute onset and rare fulminant hepatic failure. Prevalence depends on gender and ethnicity; women are affected three times more often than men. Incidence among Northern American and European Caucasians is 1 in 100,000. Less common in non-Caucasians; in Japan, incidence is 0.01 case in 100,000. The risk of cirrhosis is 17–82% at five years. The main prognostic factors are severity of inflammation/fibrosis on liver biopsy and HLA type. Associated with other autoimmune diseases.

SYMPTOMS

Fatigue (85%), jaundice, RUQ pain. **Pruritus suggests alternative diagnoses.**

EXAM

- Hepatomegaly, jaundice, splenomegaly (with or without cirrhosis).
- **Acute:** Icteric sclera, arthritis, RUQ tenderness.

- **Chronic:** Stigmata of cirrhosis (spider angiomata, palmar erythema, gynecomastia).

DIFFERENTIAL

Advanced liver disease is a poor prognostic sign for treatment response but not a contraindication to the treatment of autoimmune hepatitis.

Wilson's disease, viral hepatitis (HBV, HCV), α_1-antitrypsin deficiency, hemochromatosis, drug-induced hepatitis, nonalcoholic steatohepatitis.

DIAGNOSIS

- **International Autoimmune Hepatitis Group (IAHG) criteria:** A definite or probable diagnosis of autoimmune hepatitis is made according to the following criteria: (1) magnitude of hypergammaglobulinemia, (2) autoantibody expression, and (3) certainty of exclusion of other diagnoses.
- **Extrahepatic associations:** Present in 10–50% of cases.
  - **Frequent:** Autoimmune thyroid disease, ulcerative colitis, synovitis.
  - **Uncommon:** Rheumatoid arthritis, DM, CREST syndrome, vitiligo, alopecia.

TREATMENT

The decision to treat autoimmune hepatitis is dependent on the severity of hepatic inflammation, not hepatic dysfunction.

- **Treatment indications:** Active symptoms, biochemical markers (elevated ALT, AST, or gamma globulin), histologic markers (periportal hepatitis, bridging necrosis).
  - The best treatment responses are obtained if there is active hepatic inflammation (high ALT).
  - **Relative contraindications:** Asymptomatic patients with mild biochemical inflammation (AST < 3 times normal); cirrhosis without histologic necroinflammation.
- **Prednisone monotherapy:** Give 60 mg QD; then taper over 4–6 weeks.
- **Steroid-sparing therapy:** Lower-dose prednisone (30 mg QD); then taper over 4–6 weeks in combination with azathioprine 50–75 mg QD.
- **Treatment end points:** Defined at the end of steroid taper.
  - **Remission:** No symptoms; AST < 2 times normal; biopsy with minimal inflammation.
  - **Treatment failure:** Progressive symptoms; AST or bilirubin > 67% of pretreatment values.
- **Liver transplantation:** Should be considered in the presence of decompensated liver disease, severe inflammation, and necrosis on liver biopsy with treatment failure or no biochemical improvement during the first two weeks of therapy.

Autoimmune hepatitis is associated with a high rate of anti-HCV false positives, so the diagnosis must be confirmed by checking a PCR assay for HCV viremia.

Drug-Induced Hepatitis

Ranges from subclinical with abnormal LFTs to fulminant hepatic failure. Accounts for 40% of acute hepatitis cases in U.S. adults > 50 years of age; for 25% of cases of fulminanat hepatic failure; and for 5% of jaundice cases in hospitalized patients. Drug-induced hepatitis can be characterized as intrinsic (direct toxic effect) or idiosyncratic (immunologically mediated injury) and as necroinflammatory (hepatocellular), cholestatic, or mixed. Risk factors include advanced age, female gender, increased number of drugs prescribed, underlying liver disease, renal insufficiency, and poor nutrition.

SYMPTOMS/EXAM

Constitutional symptoms, jaundice, RUQ pain, pruritus. Often asymptomatic.

DIFFERENTIAL

Viral hepatitis, ischemic hepatitis, Wilson's disease, α_1-antitrypsin deficiency, hemochromatosis, nonalcoholic steatohepatitis.

DIAGNOSIS

Diagnose as follows (see also Table 7-19):

- **Exclude other causes:** Obtain liver ultrasound with duplex and hepatitis serologies.
- Take a detailed drug history that includes dosage, duration, and use of concurrent OTC, alternative, and recreational drugs.
- **Labs: Elevated serum LDH;** transaminases typically range from 2–4 times normal (subclinical) to 10–100 times normal.
- **Drug withdrawal:** Most drug-induced hepatitis will improve with discontinuation of the toxic agent.
- **Liver biopsy:** Most useful for **excluding** other etiologies. Eosinophilic inflammatory infiltrate suggests drug-induced hepatitis; histologic patterns can implicate drug classes.

Elevated serum LDH suggests drug-induced hepatitis over viral hepatitis.

When ALT > 1000, consider drug/toxic, ischemic, congestive, and viral hepatitis.

TREATMENT

- Discontinue the implicated drug.
- Supportive care.
- **Liver transplantation:** Drug-induced fulminant hepatic failure has a low likelihood of spontaneous recovery.

Acetaminophen Toxicity

The most common cause of drug-induced hepatitis and drug-induced fulminant hepatic failure. Toxic dose is 10–20 g in nonalcoholics and 5–10 g in alcoholics.

- **Diagnosis:** High clinical suspicion with marked elevation of transaminases; serum acetaminophen level.

TABLE 7-19. Characterization of Drug-Induced Hepatitis

	INTRINSIC	IDIOSYNCRATIC
Relation to dosage	Dose dependent.	Dose independent.
Frequency	More common.	Less common.
Onset	Hours to days after starting drug.	Weeks to months after starting drug.
Toxicity	Direct toxic effect.	Immune-mediated toxicity.
Prognosis	Good.	Poor.
Implicated drugs	Acetaminophen, carbon tetrachloride, alcohol, *Amanita phalloides,* aflatoxins.	NSAIDs, INH, sulfonamides, valproic acid, phenytoin, ketoconazole.

- **Prognostic factors predicting death or need for liver transplant:** Arterial blood pH < 7.3 **or** hepatic encephalopathy grade 3 **or** 4 with INR > 6.5 and serum creatinine > 3.4 mg/dL.
- **Treatment:** N-acetylcysteine 140 mg/kg PO; then 70 mg/kg q 4 h × 17 doses.
- Liver transplantation.

Acetaminophen in modest doses (e.g., < 2 g/day) is much safer then NSAIDs for patients with cirrhosis.

Alcoholic Liver Disease

Alcohol accounts for 100,000 deaths per year in the United States, and 20% of these deaths are related to alcoholic liver disease, which carries a risk of progressive liver disease. Patients at risk include those exceeding the critical intake threshold (80 g/day in men and 20 g/day in women), females, blacks, those with poor nutritional status, and those with HBV or HCV infection. The spectrum of disease includes fatty liver (steatosis), acute alcohol hepatitis, and alcoholic **(Laënnec's)** cirrhosis.

Symptoms

- **Steatosis:** Asymptomatic or mild RUQ pain.
- **Acute alcoholic hepatitis:** Fever, anorexia, RUQ pain, jaundice, nausea, vomiting.
- **Alcoholic cirrhosis:** Patients may be asymptomatic or may present with anorexia, fatigue, and decreased libido.

Alcoholic hepatitis is not a prerequisite to alcoholic cirrhosis.

Exam

- Hepatomegaly, splenomegaly, cachexia, jaundice, spider telangiectasias, **Dupuytren's contractures,** parotid gland enlargement, gynecomastia, testicular atrophy.
- No symptoms specific to alcoholic liver disease.

Differential

Nonalcoholic steatohepatitis, nonalcoholic fatty liver disease, autoimmune hepatitis, hemochromatosis, α_1-antitrypsin deficiency, Wilson's disease, viral hepatitis, toxic or drug-induced hepatitis.

Diagnosis

- **History of habitual alcohol consumption:** The **CAGE questionnaire** is sensitive for alcohol abuse.
- **Alcoholic steatosis:** Modest elevation of **AST > ALT in a 2:1 ratio;** liver biopsy shows small (microvesicular) and large (macrovesicular) fat droplets in the cytoplasm of hepatocytes.
- **Alcoholic hepatitis:** Marked leukocytosis, modest elevation of AST > ALT in a 2:1 ratio, and markedly elevated serum bilirubin. Liver biopsy shows steatosis, hepatocellular necrosis, **Mallory bodies** (eosinophilic hyaline deposits), ballooned hepatocytes, and **lobular PMN inflammatory infiltrate.**
- **Alcoholic cirrhosis:** Liver biopsy shows micro- or macronodular cirrhosis and perivenular fibrosis that is not usually seen in other types of cirrhosis.

Treatment

- Mainstays are alcohol abstinence and improved nutrition. Social support (e.g., AA) and medical therapy (e.g., disulfiram, naltrexone) can assist with abstinence.

- **Alcoholic steatosis:** Can resolve with abstinence and improved nutrition.
- **Alcoholic hepatitis:**
  - **Corticosteroids improve survival** when discriminant function (DF) > 32 **and** there are no contraindications (active GI bleeding, active infection, serum creatinine > 2.3).
  - **Other therapies under study: Medium-chain triglycerides** and **pentoxifylline.** Pentoxifylline has anti-TNF effects but is less effective than corticosteroids when DF > 32.
  - **Long-term therapy:** Antioxidants S-adenosyl-methionine (SAMe), silymarin, vitamins A and E.
- **Alcoholic cirrhosis:** Hepatic function can significantly improve with abstinence and improved nutrition.
- **Liver transplantation:** Often precluded by active or recent alcohol abuse or use. Recidivism rates are high. Most transplant centers require at least six months of documented abstinence prior to listing for liver transplant.

Discriminant function (DF) measures the severity of alcoholic hepatitis. A DF > 32 predicts one-month mortality as high as 50%. DF = [4.6 × (patient's PT – control PT)] + serum bilirubin.

Nonalcoholic Fatty Liver Disease

The spectrum of disease ranges from benign steatosis (fatty liver) to steatohepatitis (hepatic inflammation). Prevalence in the United States is 15–25%. Steatosis occurs in nearly all cases; steatohepatitis is found in 8–20% of morbidly obese individuals independent of age. Disease is generally benign and indolent but can progress to cirrhosis in 15–20% of cases. Risk factors for severe disease include age > 45 years, body mass index (BMI) > 30, AST:ALT > 1, and type 2 DM.

*Alcoholic hepatitis can be treated with corticosteroids when DF > 32 **and** there are no contraindications (active GI bleeding, active infection, serum creatinine > 2.3).*

Symptoms

Fatigue, malaise, and, to a lesser extent, RUQ fullness or pain. Asymptomatic in 48–100% of patients.

Exam

- Hepatomegaly is common, but examination may be limited in the obese.
- Stigmata of chronic liver disease.

Nonalcoholic fatty liver disease is the third most common cause of abnormal LFTs in adult outpatients after medication and alcohol.

Differential

- Alcoholic liver disease.
- **Nutrition:** Total parenteral nutrition, kwashiorkor, rapid weight loss.
- **Drugs:** Estrogens, corticosteroids, chloroquine.
- **Metabolic:** Wilson's disease, abetalipoproteinemia.
- **Iatrogenic:** Weight reduction surgery with jejunoileal bypass, gastroplasty, or small bowel resection.

Diagnosis

Diagnose as follows:

- Exclude causes of liver disease, specifically alcoholic liver disease.
- **Aminotransaminases:** Typically **ALT > AST (×2–4), unlike alcoholic liver diseases, where AST > ALT**; poor correlation with presence and extent of inflammation. **Normal AST and ALT cannot exclude nonalcoholic fatty liver disease.**
- BMI is an independent predictor of the degree of hepatocellular fatty infiltration.
- Ultrasound or CT scan.
- Liver biopsy is the gold standard. Grade of inflammation and stage of fibrosis predict disease course and response to therapeutic intervention.

Normal LFTs do not exclude nonalcoholic fatty liver disease.

TREATMENT

- Gradual weight loss. Rapid weight loss may **increase** inflammation and fibrosis.
- Treat hyperlipidemia and diabetes.
- No FDA-approved therapy is available.
- Therapeutic agents under study include metformin, rosiglitazone, URSO, and vitamin E.

METABOLIC LIVER DISEASE

Hereditary Hemochromatosis

An **autosomal-recessive** disease. Homozygote prevalence is 1 in 300 persons. The most common genetic disease in Northern Europeans; the Caucasian carrier rate is 1 in 10. Associated with a major mutation in chromosome 6, the **HFE gene.** Associated with a normal life expectancy if there is no cirrhosis and the patient is adherent to treatment; survival is lower if the patient has **cirrhosis at the time of diagnosis.** Cirrhosis with hereditary hemochromatosis carries a high risk of hepatocellular carcinoma (200 times control population).

SYMPTOMS

Arthritis (pseudogout), skin color change, RUQ pain, symptoms of chronic liver disease (fatigue, anorexia, muscle wasting), loss of libido, impotence and dysmenorrhea, dyspnea on exertion. Often asymptomatic (10–25%).

EXAM

Hepatomegaly, skin hyperpigmentation (bronze skin), stigmata of chronic liver disease, hypogonadism.

Suspect hemochromatosis with type 2 DM, degenerative arthritis, or unexplained hypogonadism, heart failure, or liver disease.

DIFFERENTIAL

- **Chronic liver diseases:** HBV, HCV, alcoholic liver disease, nonalcoholic fatty liver disease, Wilson's disease, α_1-antitrypsin deficiency, autoimmune hepatitis.
- **Secondary iron overload diseases:** Homozygous α-thalassemia; multiple previous blood transfusions.

DIAGNOSIS

Screen for hemochromatosis with fasting serum transferrin saturation (TS) and ferritin; TS > 45% with an elevated ferritin suggests but does not confirm the diagnosis.

- Suspect hereditary hemochromatosis with unexplained high serum ferritin or iron saturation **even with normal LFTs.**
- **Fasting serum transferrin saturation (TS) and ferritin:** If TS > 45% and ferritin is elevated, hereditary hemochromatosis is suggested; check HFE genotype. A TS < 45% and normal ferritin exclude hereditary hemochromatosis.
- **HFE genotyping:** Homozygote is diagnostic **only if** (1) age < 40 years, (2) ferritin < 1000, and (3) transaminases are normal. Otherwise, confirmation with liver biopsy is necessary.
- **Liver biopsy:** The best means of making a definitive diagnosis; a hepatic iron index > 1.9 is diagnostic. Also used for disease staging (influences prognosis; need for hepatocellular carcinoma screening if cirrhotic)

TREATMENT

- Alcohol abstinence.
- Avoid high-dose vitamin C.

- **Phlebotomy:** Weekly or biweekly until serum ferritin < 50 ng/mL; then 3–4 times/year indefinitely.
- Screen first-degree family members.
- If the patient is cirrhotic, screen for hepatocellular carcinoma.
- Liver transplant for decompensated liver disease.

COMPLICATIONS

DM, restrictive cardiomyopathy, joint disease (chondrocalcinosis, degenerative arthritis, pseudogout), hepatocellular carcinoma, increased incidence of bacterial infections (especially *Vibrio*, *Yersinia*, and *Listeria* spp).

α_1-Antitrypsin Deficiency

α_1-antitrypsin protects tissues from protease-related degradation. The deficiency is encoded on chromosome 14; **autosomal-codominant** transmission. The Z allele is the most common deficiency, particularly in those of **Northern European** descent. α_1-antitrypsin deficiency is severe when homozygous (e.g., PiZZ) and intermediate when heterozygous (e.g., PiMZ). Liver disease is often seen in the neonatal period. The incidence of liver disease at ages 20, 50, and > 50 are 2%, 5%, and 15%, respectively, with males affected more often than females. There is a high incidence of hepatocellular carcinoma in those with cirrhosis. A high prevalence of HBV and HCV markers suggests synergistic liver injury.

SYMPTOMS

Neonatal cholestasis, occult cirrhosis, shortness of breath/dyspnea on exertion, panniculitis.

EXAM

Signs of cirrhosis (spider angiomata, palmar erythema, gynecomastia) and emphysema (clubbing, barrel chest).

Consider α_1-antitrypsin deficiency in any adult who presents with chronic hepatitis or cirrhosis of unclear etiology.

DIFFERENTIAL

- **Other metabolic liver diseases with childhood presentation:** Hereditary tyrosinemia, Gaucher's disease, glycogen storage disease, CF.
- **Chronic liver diseases:** HBV, HCV, hemochromatosis, Wilson's disease, autoimmune hepatitis, nonalcoholic fatty liver disease, alcohol.

DIAGNOSIS

- **Extrahepatic manifestations:** Basilar emphysema, pancreatic fibrosis, panniculitis.
- **Serum α_1-antitrypsin concentration:** For screening; α_1-antitrypsin is an acute-phase reactant. False-positive tests may be obtained with inflammation (even if PiZZ).
- **Serum α_1-antitrypsin phenotyping:** The screening and diagnostic test of choice.
- **Liver biopsy:** Characteristic eosinophilic α_1-antitrypsin globules are seen in the endoplasmic reticulum of periportal hepatocytes.

α_1-antitrypsin deficiency is associated with bilateral basilar pulmonary emphysema.

TREATMENT

- **Avoid cigarette smoking and alcohol; weight loss if obese.**
- Liver transplantation.

Wilson's Disease

An uncommon **autosomal-recessive** disease. Usually presents between ages 3 and 40; associated with mutations in the WD gene on chromosome 13. Decreased biliary copper excretion results in toxic copper deposition in tissues.

SYMPTOMS

- Abnormal behavior, personality change, psychosis, tremor, dyskinesia, arthropathy (pseudogout), jaundice.
- Clinical presentation can be acute, subacute, or chronic.
- **Organ involvement** (in descending order of frequency): Hepatic, neurologic, psychiatric, hematologic, renal (Fanconi's syndrome), other (ophthalmologic, cardiac, skeletal, endocrinologic, dermatologic).
- Mean age of hepatic symptoms (8–12 years) than that associated with neurologic symptoms (15–30 years).

EXAM

- Kayser-Fleischer rings, icterus, slowed mentation, hypophonia, tremor.
- **Chronic:** Clinical stigmata of cirrhosis.

The classic biochemical pattern of Wilson's disease consists of low alkaline phosphatase, marked hyperbilirubinemia, and modest aminotransaminase elevation (AST > ALT).

DIFFERENTIAL

- **Infiltrative diseases:** Hemochromatosis.
- **Chronic liver diseases:** HBV, HCV, hemochromatosis, α_1-antitrypsin deficiency, autoimmune hepatitis.
- **Copper overload diseases:** Hereditary aceruloplasminemia, idiopathic copper toxicosis, Indian childhood cirrhosis.

DIAGNOSIS

- Suspect Wilson's disease in patients 3–40 years of age with unexplained LFTs or liver disease associated with neurologic or psychiatric changes, **Kayser-Fleischer rings,** hemolytic anemia, and a positive family history.
- **Liver biochemistry tests:** Characteristically low alkaline phosphatase, marked hyperbilirubinemia and modest aminotransaminase elevations, AST > ALT.
- **Ceruloplasmin (CP):** Typically **low in Wilson's disease,** but a low CP is both insensitive (15% of cases have normal CP, since CP is an acute-phase reactant) and nonspecific (CP also low in nephrotic syndrome, protein-losing enteropathy, and malabsorption).
- **Urinary copper excretion: High** if symptomatic (100–1000 μg/24 hours; level may indicate disease severity). Normal excretion is < 40 μg/24 hours.
- **Liver biopsy:** High hepatic copper concentration (> 250 μg/g); may also be seen in primary biliary cirrhosis, primary sclerosing cholangitis, fibrosis, or cirrhosis.
- **Other: Serum copper concentration, slit-lamp exam.**

Characteristics of Wilson's disease—ABCD

Asterixis
Basal ganglia deterioration
Ceruloplasmin decreased
Cirrhosis
Copper increased
Carcinoma (hepatocellular)
Choreiform movements
Dementia

TREATMENT

- **D-penicillamine:** Improvement lags 6–12 months following treatment; maintenance is typically required.
- **Other:** Trientine, zinc, ammonium.
- **Liver transplant:** For acute hepatic or medically refractory Wilson's disease; reverses metabolic defect and induces copper excretion.

ADVANCED LIVER DISEASE

Cirrhosis

The final common pathway of many liver diseases that cause hepatocellular injury and lead to fibrosis and nodular regeneration. Reversal may occur with treatment of some chronic liver diseases (e.g., HBV, HCV).

SYMPTOMS

- Fatigue, anorexia, muscle wasting, loss of libido, impotence, dysmenorrhea.
- Decompensation associated with GI bleeding, encephalopathy (sleep-wake reversal, decreased concentration), ascites.

EXAM

- **Stigmata of chronic liver disease:** Palmar erythema, spider telangiectasia.
- **Dupuytren's contractures,** gynecomastia, testicular atrophy, bilateral parotid enlargement, **Terry's nails** (white, obscure nails).
- **Portal hypertension: Caput medusae,** splenomegaly, ascites.
- **Hepatic encephalopathy: Fetor hepaticus** smell, asterixis, confusion.

DIFFERENTIAL

- HCV, HBV, alcohol.
- Hemochromatosis.
- Primary sclerosing cholangitis, primary biliary cirrhosis, Wilson's disease, α_1-antitrypsin deficiency, cryptogenic liver disease, nonalcoholic steatohepatitis, autoimmune hepatitis, vascular (Budd-Chiari, veno-occlusive, right heart failure).
- Drug toxicity (methotrexate, amiodarone, nitrofurantoin), other (sarcoidosis, schistosomiasis, hypervitaminosis A, CF, glycogen storage disease).

DIAGNOSIS

Diagnose as follows (see also Tables 7-20 and 7-21):

- **Liver biopsy:** Gold standard; also useful in assessing etiology.
- Physical exam.
- **Labs:** Thrombocytopenia (splenic sequestration); elevated INR and low albumin (decreased hepatic synthetic function); elevated alkaline phos-

TABLE 7-20. Child-Turcotte-Pugh (CTP) Scoring

	1 POINT	2 POINTS	3 POINTS
Ascites	Absent	Nontense	Tense
Encephalopathy	Absent	Grades 1–2	Grades 3–4
Bilirubin (mg/dL)	< 2.0	2–3	> 3.0
Albumin (mg/dL)	> 3.5	2.8–3.5	< 2.8
PT (seconds over normal)	1–3	4–6	> 6

TABLE 7-21. Child-Turcotte-Pugh Classification

CTP SCORE	CHILD-PUGH CLASS	THREE-YEAR SURVIVAL (%)
5–6	A	> 90
7–9	B	50–60
10–15	C	30

phatase, serum bilirubin, and GGT (cholestasis); normal or elevated transaminases.

- **Imaging:** Ultrasound with duplex (ascites, biliary dilation, hepatic masses, vascular patency), CT (more specific than ultrasound for cirrhosis and masses), MRI (excellent specificity for hepatic masses).

Vaccination for HAV is indicated in all patients with chronic liver disease, including cirrhotics.

TREATMENT

- Avoid alcohol, iron supplements (except in iron deficiency), NSAIDs, and benzodiazepines; minimize narcotics; acetaminophen < 2 g/day.
- Fluid restriction is unimportant (unless serum Na < 125), and protein restriction should not be recommended.
- Administer pneumococcal and influenza vaccines.
- **Primary prophylaxis:** HAV and HBV vaccination; nonselective β-blockers for documented esophageal varices.
- **Secondary prophylaxis:** Antibiotics for spontaneous bacterial peritonitis (SBP); esophageal variceal banding or nonselective β-blockers +/– long-acting nitrates.
- Treat underlying disease.
- Consider screening for hepatocellular carcinoma with ultrasound and serum AFP every six months.
- **Liver transplantation:** Refer to a transplant center if minimal listing criteria are met or if uncertainty exists about eligibility for transplant.
- Treat complications (see below).

Refer to a liver transplant center when minimal listing criteria are present.

COMPLICATIONS

Hepatic encephalopathy, varices, ascites/SBP, hepatorenal syndrome, hepatopulmonary syndrome, hepatocellular carcinoma; portopulmonary syndrome.

Varices

Esophageal variceal hemorrhage (EVH) accounts for one-third of all deaths in cirrhotics. **Mortality with each EVH episode is 30–50%.** Alcoholic cirrhotics have the highest risk.

- **Esophageal variceal bleeding prophylaxis:**
  - **Primary:** Nonselective β-blocker (nadolol, propranolol).
  - **Secondary:** Endoscopic ablation (banding or sclerotherapy), nonselective β-blocker +/– long-acting nitrate, portocaval shunt (TIPS or surgical).
- Gastric and rectal varices are not treatable endoscopically.
- Portal hypertensive gastropathy is a common source of bleeding.
- **Treatment:** Portocaval shunt (TIPS or surgical) or liver transplant.

Endoscopic variceal band ligation is the endoscopic treatment of choice for secondary prophylaxis of EVH.

Ascites and Spontaneous Bacterial Peritonitis (SBP)

In the United States, > 80% of ascites cases are due to chronic liver disease (cirrhosis or alcoholic hepatitis). Some **10–30% of cirrhotics with ascites develop SBP every year.** Infection-related mortality is 10%, but the **overall in-hospital mortality rate is 30%.**

SAAG ≥ 1.1 g/dL is 96% accurate in detecting portal hypertension.

SYMPTOMS/EXAM

Shifting dullness, fluid wave, bulging flanks (low sensitivity, moderate specificity). Imaging (ultrasound, CT) is superior to examination. **SBP is often asymptomatic,** but patients may have fever, abdominal pain, and sepsis.

DIFFERENTIAL

Serum-ascites albumin gradient (SAAG) is helpful (see Table 7-22).

For SBP treatment, the addition of IV albumin to IV antibiotics significantly decreases renal impairment and mortality.

DIAGNOSIS

- **Diagnostic paracentesis:** Indicated in the presence of new-onset ascites, ascites present at hospital admission, and ascites with symptoms or signs of infection.
- Analysis:
  - **Routine: Cell count, culture, albumin, total protein.**
  - **Optional:** Glucose, LDH, amylase, Gram stain, cytology.
  - **Not useful:** pH, lactate.
- **SBP diagnosis: Ascites PMN > 250 cells/mL or** single organism on culture. **Multiple organisms on ascites culture suggest secondary peritonitis.**

TREATMENT

- **Ascites:** Dietary sodium restriction (< 2 g/day), furosemide and spironolactone (doses in 4:10 ratio—e.g., 40 mg:100 mg, 80 mg:200 mg), fluid restriction only if serum Na < 125 mEq/dL, large-volume paracentesis, portocaval shunt (TIPS), liver transplant.
- **SBP prophylaxis:** Fluoroquinolone or TMP-SMX. Indicated for cirrhotics hospitalized with GI bleed (three days), ascites with total protein < 1.5 g/dL (while hospitalized), or prior SBP (if the patient has ascites).
- **SBP treatment: Do not wait for culture results to begin treatment.** Cefotaxime or ceftriaxone IV × 5 days **and IV albumin.**

Ninety percent of cirrhotics presenting with ascites will respond to sodium restriction of < 2 g/day along with furosemide with spironolactone (at maximum doses of 160 mg and 400 mg, respectively).

Hepatic Encephalopathy

Neuropsychiatric changes in the setting of liver disease constitute hepatic encephalopathy until proven otherwise. Look for precipitating factors, including

TABLE 7-22. Significance of SAAG Values

HIGH SAAG (≥ 1.1)	LOW SAAG (< 1.1)
Cirrhosis	Peritoneal carcinomatosis
Alcoholic hepatitis	TB
Cardiac	Pancreatic
Vascular	Nephrotic syndrome
Myxedema	Bowel infarction
Fulminant hepatitis	

infection, GI bleeding, dehydration, hypokalemia, constipation/ileus, hepatocellular carcinoma, dietary protein overload, CNS active drugs (narcotics, benzodiazepines, anticholinergics), uremia, hypoxia, hypoglycemia, and noncompliance with hepatic encephalopathy treatment.

SYMPTOMS/EXAM

Insomnia, sleep-wake reversal, personality change, confusion.

DIAGNOSIS

Clinical. **Blood ammonia levels are rarely helpful.**

Hepatic encephalopathy is a clinical diagnosis. Diagnosis and treatment should not be based on blood ammonia levels.

TREATMENT

- Correct precipitating factors and anticipate treatment-related adverse effects.
- Oral/NG tube or rectally administered lactulose (adverse effects—dehydration and hypokalemia), oral neomycin (adverse effects—ototoxicity and renal toxicity), oral metronidazole (adverse effect—neuropathy), zinc, short-term protein restriction, branched-chain amino acid–enriched diet.

Hepatorenal Syndrome

Prognosis is grave; **median survival is 10–14 days.** Two-month mortality is 90%.

DIFFERENTIAL

Acute tubular necrosis, drug-induced disorders (NSAIDs, antibiotics, radiographic contrast, diuretics), glomerulonephritis, vasculitis, prerenal azotemia.

DIAGNOSIS

Exclude other cause of renal failure. Discontinue diuretics and then perform a plasma volume expansion trial with 1.5 L IV normal saline or 5% IV albumin. If serum creatinine decreases, suspect another diagnosis.

TREATMENT

Identify and treat precipitants. Restrict sodium to < 2 g/day if serum Na < 125 mEq/L; then restrict fluids to < 1.5 L/day. Treat infection; liver transplant is often required. **Renal failure from hepatorenal syndrome reverses with liver transplant.**

Liver Transplantation

Liver transplantation is a standard operation with excellent survival rates (80–90% at one year and 60–80% at seven years). The scarcity of available cadaveric donor livers is reflected in high mortality rates (up to 20% per year) in those awaiting liver transplantation. In 2002, > 5300 liver transplants were performed in the United States; 17,000 patients were on the waiting list, with **typical waiting times of eight months to three years.** Living-donor liver transplants constitute a promising alternative but comprise < 3% of all liver transplants.

THE PROCESS

- Determine the presence of other viruses (HAV, HCV, mononucleosis/EBV, CMV, HSV).

- Refer to a transplant center (often the rate-limiting step).
- Assess minimal listing criteria, indications, and contraindications (see below)
- Psychosocial and financial evaluation.
- Present to selection committee, where a decision is made on whether to place patient on wait list.
- Priority is determined by the Model for End-stage Liver Disease (MELD) score, a function of INR, total bilirubin, and serum creatinine; the higher the score, the higher the priority. For hepatocarcinoma, a MELD score is assigned independent of the calculated MELD score.

Liver graft allocation in the United States is a "sickest-first" system that is based on the MELD score (serum creatinine, total bilirubin, INR).

MINIMAL LISTING CRITERIA

- Immediate need for liver transplantation (e.g., fulminant hepatic failure).
- Estimated survival without transplant at one year < 90%.
- Child-Turcotte-Pugh (CTP) Class B or C (e.g., a CTP score ≥ 7).
- Portal hypertension bleed independent of CTP score.
- SBP independent of CTP score.

INDICATIONS

- **Acute hepatic failure:** Acetaminophen, other.
- **Cirrhosis with decompensation** (in descending order): HCV, EtOH, cryptogenic, primary biliary cirrhosis, primary sclerosing cholangitis, HBC, autoimmune hepatitis.
- **Hepatic malignancies:** Hepatocellular carcinoma stage 3A or lower.
- **Metabolic liver disease:** Hemochromatosis, α_1-antitrypsin deficiency, Wilson's disease, tyrosinemia, glycogen storage diseases.
- **Extrahepatic metabolic disease:** Hemophilia A and B, urea cycle enzyme deficiency, hyperoxaluria.

CONTRAINDICATIONS

- Compensated cirrhosis without complications (too early).
- Extrahepatic malignancy.
- Hepatocellular carcinoma stage 3B or 4.
- Active substance abuse and alcohol abuse (generally defined as occurring within the last six months); some centers include active smoking.
- Active untreated sepsis.
- Advanced untreatable cardiopulmonary disease.
- Cholangiocarcinoma.

COMPLICATIONS

- **Operative:** Biliary complications (25%), wound infections, death.
- **Immunosuppression:** Opportunistic infections (CMV, HSV, fungal, PCP, others), drug-related effects (hypertension, renal insufficiency, DM, cytopenias, tremor, headaches, nausea/vomiting, seizures, others), malignancies (lymphoma, others).
- **Recurrent disease** (in descending order): HCV, **alcoholism,** HBV, primary sclerosing cholangitis, primary biliary cirrhosis, autoimmune hepatitis.
- Acute rejection (up to 30% within the first three months after transplant).

NOTES

GASTROENTEROLOGY & HEPATOLOGY

CHAPTER 8

Geriatrics

Param Dedhia, MD
Serge Lindner, MD

NUTRITIONAL RECOMMENDATIONS

Nutritional guidelines for the elderly, as outlined by the United States Preventive Services Task Force (USPSTF), are no different from those for the general population and include the following:

- Reduction of dietary fats.
- Increased consumption of fruits, vegetables, and grain products containing fiber.
- Patients > 75 years of age who are on restricted diets are at risk of protein-calorie malnutrition and inadequate intake of both vitamin B_{12} and vitamin D.

> ***Causes of unintentional weight loss—***
>
> ***DETERMINE***
>
> **D**isease
> **E**ating poorly
> **T**ooth loss/mouth pain
> **E**conomic hardship
> **R**educed social contact
> **M**ultiple medicines
> **I**nvoluntary weight loss/gain
> **N**eed for assistance in self-care
> **E**lder years (> 85 years of age)

WEIGHT LOSS

Unintended weight loss exceeding 5% in one month or 10% in six months is common in those > 85 years of age as well as among nursing home residents (up to 45%), hospitalized patients (10–30%), and depressed patients. Although the cause of unintended weight loss cannot be identified in 25% of cases, the following are known etiologic factors (see also the mnemonic **DETERMINE**):

- **Medical:** Chronic heart disease, chronic lung disease, dementia, poor dentition, dysphagia, mesenteric ischemia, cancer, diabetes, hyperthyroidism (note that hyper- and hypothyroidism can present typically or atypically).
- **Psychosocial:** Alcoholism, depression, social isolation, limited funds, problems with shopping or food preparation, inadequate assistance with feeding.
- **Pharmacologic:** NSAIDs, antiepileptics, digoxin, SSRIs.

Appetite stimulants may increase weight but do not improve mortality.

TREATMENT

- Identify treatable medical, psychological, and social causes.
- Consider age-appropriate cancer screening (e.g., PSA, fecal occult blood test, mammography).
- Discontinue any offending drugs.
- A serum albumin and/or prealbumin level < 3.0 and a cholesterol level < 150 are associated with poor treatment outcome.

Tube feeding has complications and seldom improves mortality.

COMPLICATIONS

Associated with high morbidity within two years of onset. Risk factors include falls, isolation, skin breakdown, and nursing home placement.

IMMUNIZATIONS/PROPHYLAXIS

Influenza Vaccine

- More than 90% of influenza-related deaths occur in those > 60 years of age.
- Among community dwellers in this age group, influenza vaccine is > 50% effective in reducing influenza-related illness.
- The rate of reduction is lower in those > 70 years of age owing to diminished immune response.
- Among those living in long-term care settings, immunization can reduce influenza by 30–40%, pneumonia and hospitalizations by 50–60%, and death by 80%.

- Immunizations should be administered annually, prior to the onset of influenza season (usually from mid-October to mid-November).

All those > 65 years of age should receive pneumococcal vaccination.

Pneumococcal Vaccine

- There are > 90 different types (serotypes) of pneumococcus.
- Most serious infections are caused by the 23 serotypes contained in the 23-valent polysaccharide vaccine.
- Pneumococcal infection is a common cause of bacteremia, pneumonia, and meningitis.
- Pneumococcal vaccine is 50–80% effective in preventing invasive bacteremia but has no significant effect on outpatient pneumonia and hospitalization for pneumonia.

Those vaccinated before 65 years of age should have a repeat vaccination five years after the initial one.

Tetanus Vaccine

- Clinical tetanus is rare in the United States and occurs primarily among older adults who are unvaccinated or underimmunized.
- Patients > 60 years of age typically account for 60% of all cases of tetanus.

If a patient has never received a primary tetanus series, three doses are required. Otherwise, give a booster dose of tetanus-diphtheria toxoid vaccine every 10 years.

Aspirin

Because most elderly patients have a heart disease risk exceeding 3%, aspirin prophylaxis is recommended to all those with a life expectancy of > 5 years.

Vitamin D

In addition to its effect on bone mineral density (BMD), vitamin D may reduce the risk of fracture by improving muscle function, thereby decreasing the risk of falls.

Vitamin E

Vitamin E may slow (but not prevent) disease progression in those with established Alzheimer's.

SENSORY IMPAIRMENT

- Vision screening should be conducted on elderly patients by Snellen chart. Consider referral to a ophthalmologist for further screening.
- Screening for hearing impairment should be conducted with otoscopic and audiometric testing for those who exhibit deficits.

SLEEP DISORDERS

Two sleep states have been identified: non–rapid eye movement (NREM) and rapid eye movement (REM). A typical night of sleep begins with NREM, with REM occurring after 80 minutes. Both sleep states then alternate, with REM periods increasing as the night progresses. NREM includes four stages:

- **Stages 1 and 2:** Classified as light sleep. Stage 1 is a transition from wakefulness to sleep.
- **Stages 3 and 4:** Classified as deep, restorative sleep.

Symptoms/Exam

Changes in sleep occur as a normal part of aging. Such changes may affect sleep pattern (the amount and timing of sleep), sleep structure (stages), or both. Specifically, stages 1 and 2 may increase, while stages 3 and 4 may decrease. Typical complaints from patients > 65 years of age may thus include the following:

- Difficulty falling asleep.
- Midsleep awakening and increased arousal during the night.
- Nonrestorative sleep (may be perceived as decreased sleep time).
- Earlier bedtime and earlier morning awakening.
- Daytime napping.

Differential

- **Psychiatric:** Stress, depression, bereavement, anxiety.
- **Pain related:** Neuropathic pain, rheumatologic conditions, malignancy syndromes.
- **Physiologic:** Dyspnea resulting from cardiac and pulmonary conditions, nocturia, GERD.
- **Medication related (10–15%):**
  - **Respiratory medications:** Theophylline, β-agonists.
  - **Cardiovascular medications:** Furosemide, quinidine.
  - **Antidepressants:** Desipramine, nortriptyline, imipramine.
  - **Other:** Corticosteroids, caffeine.

Diagnosis/Treatment

There is limited evidence supporting the benefit of specialized testing with polysomnography by a primary care physician. However, the following issues should be addressed by the primary physician:

- **Sleep apnea** should be diagnosed and treated.
- **Stressors and psychiatric conditions** should be identified and treated as well.
- The following **sleep hygiene measures** should be recommended:
  - Adherence to a regular morning rise time.
  - Limiting of daytime napping.
  - Exercise during the day but not at night.
  - Avoidance of caffeine, alcohol, and nicotine in the evening.
  - Limiting of nighttime fluid intake to diminish the urge to urinate during sleeping hours.
  - Adjusting the environment to patient preferences (e.g., controlling noise, light, and temperature).
- **Medications:** Whereas no medications are recommended in the treatment of insomnia for the older patient, the use of the following medications should be actively discouraged:
  - **Benzodiazepines:** Increase the likelihood of falls, leading to hip fracture and motor vehicle accidents. Tolerance has also been widely noted.
  - **Antihistamines (e.g., diphenhydramine):** Have anticholinergic effects; tolerance has been noted.
  - **Melatonin:** Deficiency is difficult to measure, and effects on sleep disorders have not been proven.

DEPRESSION

Depression is greatly underdiagnosed in older patients. Epidemiologic data indicate that depression affects 1% of elderly individuals in the general community; 10% of those seeking primary care or in the hospital; and 40% of those who are permanently institutionalized. Risk factors are as follows:

- A prior episode of depression
- A positive family history
- Lack of social support
- Use of alcohol or other substances
- Parkinson's disease
- Recent MI
- A history of CVAs
- Social isolation
- Loss of autonomy

DIFFERENTIAL

The differential diagnosis of depression includes the following:

Depression has a high prevalence in those with Parkinson's disease.

- **Mild cognitive impairment:** A precedent to dementia (patients are likely to have predominantly depressive symptoms).
- **Parkinson's disease:** The early presentation of Parkinson's may mimic depression. Note, however, that a high percentage of Parkinson's patients develop depression.
- Fatigue and weight loss resulting from diabetes, thyroid disease, malignancy, or anemia.
- Sleep disturbance with daytime fatigue and depressed mood as a result of pain, nocturia, and sleep apnea.
- Bereavement, delirium, substance abuse.

TREATMENT

Medications for the treatment of depression in the elderly include the following:

- **SSRIs and TCAs:** Equally efficacious in elderly patients.
- **Psychostimulants:** Drugs such as dextroamphetamine or methylphenidate are sometimes used in patients with predominantly vegetative symptoms but are commonly associated with tachycardia, insomnia, and agitation.
- **MAOIs and tertiary amine TCAs:** Rarely used owing to their side effect profiles and likelihood of drug interactions.
- **Fluoxetine:** Rarely used because of its long half-life and inhibition of cytochrome P-450.
- Newer agents: Mirtazapine and venlafaxine may be useful in selected patients due to other side effect profiles.

Treatment options include the following:

- **Pharmacotherapy:**
  - Drugs are typically chosen on the basis of their side effect profile (e.g., anxiety, insomnia, pain, weight loss).
  - Renal and hepatic function must also be considered and should be assessed before therapy is initiated.
  - Side effects typically last for four weeks, but weight gain and sexual dysfunction may last longer.
  - Individual side effect profiles include the following:
    - **TCAs:** Anticholinergic properties (dry mouth, orthostasis, and urinary retention) are most commonly seen, but TCAs are also associ-

        ated with conduction abnormalities (check an ECG). TCAs are lethal in overdose and should thus be avoided in those with suicidal ideation.
    - **SSRIs:** Nausea and sexual dysfunction are most common. Some SSRIs (e.g., paroxetine) also have anticholinergic effects and should be avoided in those with cognitive impairment.
    - **Venlafaxine:** May increase diastolic BP.
    - **Bupropion:** Lowers seizure threshold.
  - Although sexual dysfunction typically responds to sildenafil, consider switching to another agent or lowering the dose and augmenting with another agent.
- **Psychotherapy:** Cognitive-behavioral therapy, problem-solving therapy, and interpersonal psychotherapy are effective either alone or in combination with pharmacotherapy.
- **Electroconvulsive therapy (ECT):**
  - Associated with response rates of 60–70% in patients with refractory depression.
  - Side effects of confusion and anterograde memory impairment may persist for up to six months.
  - First-line therapy for patients who are severely depressed; those who are at high risk for suicide; and those who are not eligible for pharmacotherapy as a result of hepatic, renal, or cardiac disease.

CARDIOVASCULAR MEDICINE

Hypertension

- Patients between the ages of 60 and 80 should be screened and treated for both systolic and diastolic hypertension.
- The JNC 7 recommends an upper limit of 140 for systolic BP in the elderly.

In patients > 85 years of age with multiple comorbidities, hypertension should be treated with caution to prevent orthostatic hypotension, which can contribute to falls.

Hyperlipidemia

- Evidence exists to support the treatment of hyperlipidemia in elderly patients for secondary prevention of cardiovascular outcomes. Treating elders for primary prevention of cardiovascular disease, especially women and the very old, is more controversial. The goal for patients with CAD is LDL < 100 mg/dL (per the National Cholesterol Education Program).
- Dietary counseling must be based on the patient's overall nutrition status as well as on the risk of malnutrition.
- Statins are normally well tolerated. Rhabdomyolysis, the most serious side effect associated with statin use, is more commonly a result of drug interaction.
- Continued screening is recommended by the USPSTF, with consideration given to both life expectancy and overall risk factors.

URINARY INCONTINENCE

Defined as a complaint of involuntary leakage of urine, often resulting in unresolved physical, functional, and psychological morbidity as well as in diminished quality of life.

- May be partially or wholly attributable to remediable factors generally **outside of the lower urinary tract**—i.e., medical conditions, medications, and functional factors.

- **Lower urinary tract** causes of urinary incontinence include detrusor overactivity, impairment of urethral sphincter mechanisms, underactive detrusor, and bladder outlet obstruction (alone or in combination).
- Although a history, physical exam, and UA are often sufficient to provide a working diagnosis, a minority of patients require referral or specialized testing.

There are four primary classes of urinary incontinence—**urge, stress, overflow,** and **functional.**

Urge Incontinence

A complaint of involuntary leakage accompanied or immediately preceded by urgency. Characterized by abrupt urgency with moderate to large leakage as well as by urinary frequency and nocturia. Although the presumed cause is uninhibited bladder contractions/**detrusor overactivity,** this notion is controversial in that the latter may also be found in healthy, continent elderly individuals. This suggests that overactivity alone is not sufficient to cause incontinence. The following may lead to detrusor overactivity:

- Age-related changes.
- Interruption of CNS inhibitory pathways (e.g., by stroke or cervical stenosis).
- Bladder irritation caused by infection, bladder stones, inflammation, or neoplasms.
- In many cases, the disorder may be idiopathic.

Detrusor activity with impaired contractility (DHIC) is the most common cause of urge incontinence in frail older persons.

Most cases of urge incontinence arising in frail older persons are due to a combination of detrusor overactivity and impaired detrusor contractile function. Known as **detrusor hyperactivity with impaired contractility (DHIC),** this form of urge incontinence is characterized by urgency as well as by elevated postvoid residual in the absence of outlet obstruction.

- If the detrusor overactivity is triggered by a stress maneuver, the condition is often misdiagnosed as stress incontinence or as outlet obstruction and detrusor weakness.
- May promote urinary retention when bladder relaxants or other anticholinergic medications are used.

TREATMENT

- **Behavioral therapy:** Behavioral treatment for urge incontinence is based on two general principles: (1) frequent voluntary voiding to keep the bladder volume low, and (2) training of CNS and pelvic mechanisms to inhibit detrusor contractions. The option chosen depends on the patient's cognitive status.
  - **Cognitively intact patients:** Bladder training is used for patients with no cognitive impairments. It consists of timed voiding while awake (with initial frequency based on the smallest time interval between voids, obtained from the voiding record) and suppression of any intervening precipitant urgency using relaxation techniques.
  - **Cognitively impaired patients:** Scheduled voiding (timed voiding using an arbitrarily set interval, usually every 2–3 hours) is used for those with cognitive impairments.
- **Pharmacotherapy:** A bladder suppressant medication may be tried if behavioral methods are unsuccessful. These medications usually do not ablate detrusor overactivity but can nonetheless improve urinary incontinence. They include the following:

- Oxybutynin: Has direct antispasmodic effects by inhibiting the action of acetylcholine on smooth muscle. Shows the best demonstrated efficacy for urge incontinence.
- **Tolterodine:** Efficacy is similar to that of oxybutynin. Causes dry mouth less frequently than does oxybutynin, but more expensive.
- **Trospium:** A newly approved drug for the treatment of urge incontinence. Approximately 20% of patients experience dry mouth; 10% experience constipation.

Stress Incontinence

A complaint of involuntary leakage on effort or exertion or, alternatively, on sneezing or coughing. Characterized by stress leakage that occurs when increased intra-abdominal pressure overcomes sphincter closure mechanisms in the absence of a bladder contraction. Stress incontinence is the most common cause of urinary incontinence in younger women and the second most common cause of incontinence among older women. It may also occur in older men following transurethral or radical prostatectomy.

Stress incontinence is the most common cause of urinary incontinence in younger women.

TREATMENT

Treatment includes the following:

- **Pelvic muscle (Kegel) exercises:** Strengthen the muscular components of the urethral closure mechanism using principles of strength training (e.g., small numbers of isometric repetitions at maximal exertion). The considerable misinformation that exists about these exercises may adversely affect treatment outcomes.
- **Pessaries:** May benefit women with stress incontinence exacerbated by bladder or uterine prolapse.
- **Estrogen and α-adrenergic agonists:** Have yielded mixed results.
- **Surgery:** Offers the highest cure rates for stress incontinence in elderly women. Options include the following:
  - Bladder neck suspension procedures (transvaginal Burch colposuspension) to treat urethral hypermobility and genuine stress urinary incontinence.
  - Sling procedures using autologous or synthetic material to support the urethra.
- Effective treatment for men with postprostatectomy stress incontinence can be difficult.
  - Mild cases can be treated with pelvic muscle exercises and bulking injections.
  - Severe cases require supportive management with protective garments or catheters.

Overflow Incontinence

A complaint of involuntary dribbling and/or continuous leakage associated with incomplete bladder emptying due to **impaired detrusor contractility and/or obstruction.**

- Outlet obstruction is the second most common cause of urinary incontinence in older men (after detrusor overactivity resulting from BPH, prostate cancer, or urethral stricture), yet most obstructed men do not have urinary incontinence.

- Obstruction is uncommon in women but may result from corrective surgery for urinary incontinence or from a large, prolapsed cystocele that kinks the urethra during voiding.
- Patients with spinal cord injury may be obstructed by detrusor-sphincter dysregulation.

SYMPTOMS/EXAM

- Leakage is typically small in volume but continuous, often leading to significant wetting.
- Postvoid residual is elevated, and urinary stream is weak.
- Also characterized by intermittency, hesitancy, frequency, and nocturia.

TREATMENT

- Numerous medical and surgical alternatives are available for men with outflow obstruction due to BPH.
- Obstructed women with previous vaginal or urethral surgery may be treated with unilateral suture removal or remobilization of adhesions.
- Surgical correction or reduction by a pessary can treat a large prolapsed cystocele.
- For patients with detrusor underactivity, treatment is supportive. Drugs that impair detrusor contractility and increase urethral tone should be decreased or stopped and constipation should be treated.

Functional Incontinence

A complaint of inability to void in a commode without leakage as a result of poor mobility, dexterity, vision, or cognition. Characterized by physical and cognitive limitations.

EXAM/DIAGNOSIS

Evaluation should include the following:

- A genital exam should be performed in women to assess the vaginal mucosa for atrophy.
- Uncircumcised men should be checked for phimosis, paraphimosis, and balanitis.
- A rectal exam should be performed to look for masses or fecal impaction.
- In men, the rectal exam should also include examination of the prostate for consistency and symmetry.
- A neurologic exam should be conducted to evaluate sacral root integrity by testing perineal sensation, resting and volitional tone of the anal sphincter, and anal wink.
- Cognitive status and affect should be assessed along with motor strength and tone (especially with regard to mobility), and vibration and peripheral sensation should be evaluated for peripheral neuropathy.

Use catheters only as a last resort in functional incontinence.

TREATMENT

- Fluid management is important, especially decreasing evening fluid intake in older persons with urge incontinence.
- Pads and protective garments can be used, with the type of garment depending on patient gender and on the type and volume of urinary incontinence leakage.
- Catheters should be the treatment of last resort, as their use is associated with significant morbidity.

Mixed Incontinence

A complaint of involuntary leakage associated with urgency as well as with exertion, effort, sneezing, or coughing. It is likely due to a combination of detrusor overactivity and sphincter impairments associated with stress incontinence. The most common type of urinary incontinence in women. Other, rare etiologies of mixed incontinence are as follows:

- Extraurethral (from fistulas).
- Impaired detrusor compliance (an excessive pressure response to filling, usually due to spinal cord injury)

FECAL INCONTINENCE

Defined as continuous or recurrent uncontrolled passage of fecal material (> 10 mL) for at least one month in an individual > 3–4 years of age. Fecal incontinence is a devastating disability that adversely affects self-confidence and can lead to social isolation. It is the second leading cause of nursing home placement.

- Loss of continence can result from dysfunction of the anal sphincter, abnormal rectal compliance, decreased rectal sensation, or a combination of any of these abnormalities.
- Dysfunction of the levator ani muscle appears to have a strong association with the severity of incontinence.
- Fecal incontinence is usually multifactorial, since these derangements often coexist (see Table 8-1).

TABLE 8-1. Etiologies of Fecal Incontinence

Etiology	Characteristics
Vaginal delivery	Incontinence occurs either immediately or after years. The most common injuries are anal sphincter tears or trauma to the pudendal nerve.
Surgical trauma	Surgery on the anal sphincter or surrounding structures.
Diabetes mellitus (DM)	Reduces internal anal sphincter resting pressure. Diarrhea is secondary to autonomic neuropathy.
Decreased rectal compliance	Rectal filling fails to produce a sensation of rectal fullness and the urge to defecate.
Impaired rectal sensation	A number of conditions are associated, including DM, MS, dementia, meningomyelocele, and spinal cord injuries.
Fecal impaction	A common cause in the elderly. Produces constant inhibition of internal anal sphincter tone, permitting leakage of liquid stool around the impaction.

DIAGNOSIS

- The history and physical exam can provide insight into the etiology, allowing for focused diagnostic testing.
- Inspection of the distal colon and the anus with flexible sigmoidoscopy and anoscopy can exclude mucosal inflammation, masses, or similar pathology.
- Complaints of diarrhea should be assessed with stool studies and a full colonoscopy.

TREATMENT

Stool consistency can be improved by supplementing the diet with a bulking agent, but this may exacerbate incontinence in patients with decreased rectal compliance (e.g., those with radiation proctitis or a rectal stricture).

- **Medical therapy:** Antidiarrheal drugs, along with the elimination of medications that are known to cause diarrhea, may be of benefit.
  - The goal is to reduce stool frequency and improve stool consistency.
  - Formed stool is easier to control than liquid stool.
  - Loperamide is more effective than diphenoxylate for reducing urgency.
  - Anticholinergic agents taken before meals may be helpful in patients who tend to have leakage of stools after eating.
- **Biofeedback therapy:** A painless, noninvasive means of cognitively retraining the pelvic floor and the abdominal wall musculature. However, insufficient evidence exists supporting its efficacy.
- **Surgery:**
  - A number of surgical approaches have been used for the treatment of fecal incontinence, including direct sphincter repair, plication of the posterior part of the sphincter, anal encirclement, implantation of an artificial sphincter, and muscle transfer procedures with or without electrical stimulation.
  - Colostomy should be reserved for those with intractable symptoms who are not candidates for other therapies.
- **Nerve stimulation:** Electrical stimulation of the sacral nerve roots can restore continence in patients with structurally intact muscles.
- **Supportive measures:** Can be instituted in most patients. May include avoiding foods or activities known to worsen symptoms, ritualizing bowel habits, and improving perianal skin hygiene.
- **Bedside interventions:** Stool impactions should be corrected and a bowel regimen instituted to prevent recurrence. Incontinence related to mental dysfunction or physical debility may benefit from scheduled defecation.

SEXUAL DYSFUNCTION

Older men and women frequently remain interested in sex despite a decrease in overall sexual activity. In men, decreased activity may result from a variety of factors, including atherosclerosis, neurologic disorders, medications, psychological factors, endocrine problems, social issues, limited availability of partners, decreased libido, and erectile dysfunction. In women, additional factors include vaginal dryness or burning and vaginal atrophy.

SYMPTOMS

- **Men:** Symptoms in men include inadequate erections, decreased libido, and orgasmic failure.
- **Women:** Symptoms in women include vaginal dryness or burning (atrophy), dyspareunia, slower time to orgasm, a need for prolonged clitoral stimulation, and decreased libido.

DIFFERENTIAL

Medication effects, psychosocial factors, anatomical problems, Peyronie's disease in men.

DIAGNOSIS

- **Men and women:** Diagnosis should include the following:
  - Screen for depression.
  - Assess time spent in foreplay or in stimulation.
- **Labs:** For men, serum testosterone should be considered, although the yield will be low if the man is lacking other signs of hypogonadism. If serum testosterone levels are low or low normal, consider a bioavailable testosterone level. LH and prolactin are not routinely necessary, as the hypothalamic-pituitary axis tends to become less responsive with aging. Other lab tests should be dictated by the history and physical (e.g., glycosylated hemoglobin).
- Poor response to vasoactive intracavernous injection suggests a vascular cause.

Look for possible depression in older persons with sexual dysfunction.

TREATMENT

- **Men:** Treatment options are as follows:
  - **Sildenafil, tadalafil:** Often effective, and the most acceptable option for patients. Caution should be exercised in patients with CAD, as these drugs are contraindicated with nitrates.
  - **Testosterone:** Should be used only for true hypogonadism. Associated with multiple side effects and an increased risk of prostate disease.
  - **Penile injections or vacuum devices:** May be effective, but rarely acceptable to patients.
  - **Other options:** Constriction rings, counseling, surgery for Peyronie's disease, penile prostheses.
- **Women:** Treatment options include topical estrogen creams or rings (if there is no hepatic or cardiac disease), increased stimulation time before intercourse, and possibly counseling.

PALLIATIVE AND END-OF-LIFE CARE

In the United States, approximately 80% of people die in hospitals or in long-term care facilities. Generally accepted goals of end-of-life care include the following:

- To continue to treat potentially **reversible** disease.
- To help **alleviate suffering,** including physical, psychological, social, and spiritual distress.
- To help the patient **prepare for death.**

Ethical and Legal Issues

- **Unique ethical considerations** include the following:
  - The concept of futile medical interventions, which may lead to conflicts between provider, patient, or family. Can often be resolved through discussions.
  - The individual has the right to refuse or withdraw medical treatments.
  - The potential to hasten death is permissible if the primary intention is to provide comfort and dignity and to relieve suffering (i.e., it is appropriate to prescribe as much morphine as needed to relieve suffering if

congruent with patient goals of care). This is often termed the "ethical principle of **double effect**."

- **Advance directives:**
  - Defined as oral or written statements made by patients when they are competent with the purpose of guiding their care should they become incompetent.
  - Valid only for futile care or terminal illness.
- **Durable power of attorney for health care (DPOA-HC):**
  - The patient designates a surrogate decision maker.
  - The role of the surrogate is to offer "substituted judgment" such as that which would be offered if the **patient** could speak for himself.
- **"Do not resuscitate" (DNR) orders:**
  - Only 15% of all patients who undergo CPR in the hospital survive to hospital discharge.
  - Patients should be informed about likely mortality outcomes as well as the potential adverse consequences of CPR and resuscitation attempts (e.g., fractured ribs, neurologic disability, invasive procedures).

Hospice Care

- Focuses on the patient and family rather than the disease; stresses the provision of comfort and pain relief rather than treating illness or prolonging life.
- Increases patient satisfaction; reduces family anxiety.
- Requires a physician's estimate of < 6 months of life remaining.

Symptom Management

*The use of opiates for end-of-life care is **not** associated with the development of addiction or abuse.*

- **Pain:**
  - Very common, yet often undertreated.
  - Use a numeric or analog scale to assess.
  - Help the patient set pain management goals (strike a balance between sedation or "double effect" and total pain relief).
  - Treat chronic pain around the clock with long-acting drugs.
  - Increase drugs as needed (there is no ceiling for pure opiates).
  - Use caution when combining analgesics (e.g., acetaminophen and NSAIDs).
  - Sedation typically precedes significant respiratory depression.
- **Dyspnea:**
  - Present in up to 50% of dying patients.
  - Identify and treat the underlying cause where possible.
  - Nonspecific treatment with opioids is highly effective.
  - Nonpharmacologic measures include O_2 and fresh air.
  - Benzodiazepines treat the associated anxiety but not the dyspnea itself.
- **Nausea and vomiting:**
  - If opiate related, consider a sustained-release formulation, a different agent at an equianalgesic dose, or the addition of a dopamine-antagonist antiemetic.
  - If due to an intra-abdominal process such as constipation, gastroparesis, or gastric outlet obstruction, try small food portions, NG tube aspiration, laxative/bowel regimens, prokinetic agents, high-dose corticosteroids, or 5-HT3 antagonists (e.g., ondansetron).
  - If related to increased ICP, use corticosteroids or palliative cranial irradiation as indicated.

- If due to vestibular disturbance, treat with anticholinergic or antihistaminic agents.
  - Consider around-the-clock dosing of antiemetics.
  - Benzodiazepines and dronabinol may also be quite effective.
- **Constipation:**
  - Often opiate related.
  - Behavioral treatments increase activity and fluid/fiber intake.
  - Bowel regimen is required for patients on opiates. Start stool softeners and bowel stimulants prophylactically, and add enemas and other treatments as needed.
- **Delirium and agitation:**
  - Many patients experience confusion before death.
  - Consider the usual reversible causes of delirium, and treat if indicated.
  - Consider the psychoactive effects of current medications.
  - Haloperidol or risperidone may be used if reversible causes are not identified and behavioral management is unsuccessful.
  - It may be acceptable to do nothing if the delirium does not bother the patient and family.

Remember the adverse mental status effects of all symptom-relieving drugs.

Nutrition and Hydration

- For patients with irreversible conditions, tube feeding has not been shown to improve mortality and comfort but has been shown to lead to complications.
- Dying patients who have stopped eating or drinking rarely experience hunger or thirst.
- Dry mouth can be managed with swabs and good oral care.

Withdrawal of Support

- Requests for withdrawal of care must be respected when received from appropriately informed and competent patients or their surrogates.
- Clinicians may recommend discontinuation of inappropriate interventions.

Psychological, Social, and Spiritual Issues

- Patients and families rank emotional support as one of the most important aspects of good end-of-life care.
- Clinicians can provide listening, assurance, and support as well as coordination with psychotherapy and group support.
- Depression must be treated and distinguished from normal anticipatory grief.
- The patient's spiritual concerns often require only a clinician's attention.

BIOMEDICAL ETHICS

The following are required of training programs in the care of the terminally ill:

- Assume an obligation to provide appropriate and humane care to the terminally ill.
- Negotiate goals of care with the patient and family, taking into consideration both the individual's values and preferences and the physician's professional judgment.

- In evaluating an older patient, seek out and consider the observations and opinions of family members and other concerned individuals, and bear in mind that the primary obligation is always to the patient.
- Understand the function and importance of a multidisciplinary approach toward caring for older persons, including appropriate respect for other health professionals and paraprofessionals and their roles in the provision of services.
- Understand that maintenance of function and quality of life are more often goals of care than are cures of disease.

POLYPHARMACY

Remember to think "drug effect" when making the differential diagnosis list for any given illness in the older adult.

Polypharmacy is a significant cause of hospital admissions and should be on the differential of any presentation. Annually, at least 35% of community-dwelling older adults experience an adverse drug event. Changes in physiologic function and pharmokinetics in the older patient promote increased sensitivity to medications and hence increase the possibility of iatrogenic illness. Such factors include the following:

- **Distribution:**
  - Decreased cardiac output, tissue perfusion, and tissue volume.
  - Impaired drug metabolism due to decreased GFR and reduced hepatic clearance.
  - Reduced protein binding of some drugs (e.g., warfarin, phenytoin) owing to low serum albumin.
  - Water-soluble drugs become more concentrated, and fat-soluble drugs have longer half-lives (volume of distribution).
- **Metabolism:**
  - **Phase I:** Oxidization and reduction by cytochrome P-450. Hepatic enzyme activity is decreased, affecting the metabolism of drugs with high first-pass metabolism (e.g., propranolol).
  - **Phase II:** Conjugation by acetylation, glucuronidation, or sulfation (not affected by aging).
- **Excretion:**
  - Renal function decreases by as much as 50% by age 85.
  - Half-life is determined by the volume of distribution as well as the clearance of a drug.

To prevent polypharmacy, start low and go slow (but conduct an adequate trial).

SYMPTOMS/EXAM

- **Delirium** can result from many drugs, including OTC cold remedies, anticholinergics, and analgesics (common but often overlooked in the elderly).
- Other common symptoms include nausea, anorexia, weight loss, parkinsonism, hypotension, and acute renal failure.

TREATMENT

- Try **nonpharmacologic means** before drugs.
- Improve adherence by keeping the dosing schedule simple (once daily is best), the number of pills low, and medication changes infrequent.
- Continually review the drug list for potential discontinuations.

COMPLICATIONS

The consequences of overprescribing include adverse drug events, drug-drug interactions, duplication of drugs, decreased quality of life, and unnecessary costs.

OSTEOPOROSIS

Most common in the elderly. Risk factors include the following:

- Advanced age
- Female gender
- Postmenopausal status
- Caucasian ethnicity
- Northern European ancestry
- A positive family history
- Prolonged inactivity
- Low calcium or vitamin D intake
- Thin bone structure or build
- Prolonged glucocorticoid/steroid exposure
- Tobacco use
- Alcohol use
- Use of antiepileptics or anticonvulsants

Osteoporosis may also be secondary to Cushing's syndrome, hypogonadism, hyperparathyroidism, osteomalacia, and multiple myeloma.

T-score of −2.5 or worse diagnoses osteoporosis.

DIAGNOSIS

- **BMD measurement:** Methods of diagnosing loss of BMD include the following:
  - **Dual-energy x-ray absorptiometry (DEXA):** The preferred method; highly accurate as well as inexpensive.
  - Other methods include quantitative CT and dual photon absorptiometry.
- **Interpretation of BMD studies:**
  - **T-scores:** Compare normal and healthy young bone. A score of −1.0 translates into a BMD 1 SD less than normal. **A score of −2.5 diagnoses osteoporosis.**
  - **Z-scores:** Compare a patient's BMD with those of age- and sex-matched controls. Used to track accelerated osteoporosis and treatment response.
- **Other radiologic findings:** The most significant radiologic findings are vertebral compression fractures.

TREATMENT

- **Diet:**
  - An optimal diet for the treatment or prevention of osteoporosis is one that includes an adequate intake of calories, calcium, and vitamin D.
  - Postmenopausal women and older men should take supplemental elemental calcium in divided doses at mealtimes with a goal of 1500 mg/day along with 800 IU of vitamin D daily.
- **Exercise:** Patients with osteoporosis as well as those seeking prevention should follow a regular weight-bearing exercise regimen to facilitate long-term compliance.
- **Cessation of smoking:** Smoking cessation should be strongly recommended, as smoking cigarettes significantly accelerates bone loss. Smoking one pack per day throughout adult life has been associated with a 5–10% reduction in bone density.
- **Bisphosphonates (alendronate or risedronate):**
  - Increase bone mass and reduce the incidence of vertebral and nonvertebral fractures.
  - Effective even in women who already have fractures.
  - A good treatment option for women with established osteoporosis.

Bisphosphonates and raloxifene are first-line treatments for the prevention of osteoporosis.

- **Selective estrogen receptor modulators (SERMs):**
  - Raloxifene has been used for the prevention and treatment of osteoporosis and is considered a first-line drug for disease prevention.
  - Evidence of its efficacy for established osteoporosis is not as strong as that for bisphosphonates.
  - Increases BMD.
  - Reduces total and LDL cholesterol concentrations without stimulating endometrial hyperplasia or vaginal bleeding.
  - Decreases the incidence of vertebral fractures.
- **Estrogen/progestin therapy:**
  - No longer a first-line approach toward the treatment of osteoporosis in postmenopausal women.
  - Associated with an increased risk of breast cancer, stroke, venous thromboembolism, and possibly coronary disease.
  - May be indicated in postmenopausal women with persistent menopausal symptoms or in those with an indication for antiresorptive therapy who cannot tolerate other drugs.
- **PTH (teriparatide):**
  - Despite the deleterious effect of PTH on bone, intermittent administration of recombinant human PTH stimulates bone formation more than resorption.
  - Exogenous PTH administration reverses osteoporotic bone structural changes without compromising cortical bone structure or strength.
  - Teriparatide is approved for use for fracture in high-risk patients, including those with a previous osteoporotic fracture, multiple risk factors for fracture, or failed previous treatment.
  - Treatment should be reserved for such patients in light of the need for daily injection, the drug's high cost, and the risk of osteosarcoma.
  - Should **not** be used in patients with Paget's disease.
- **Calcitonin:**
  - A less popular choice for treatment of osteoporosis is intranasal calcitonin. Most patients are poorly compliant because of the route of administration and cost.
  - Has analgesic effects.
  - Constitutes first-line therapy in patients who have substantial pain from an acute osteoporotic fracture.
- **Isoflavones:** A type of phytoestrogen that consists of micronutrient substances with properties similar to estrogen. Mixed results have been achieved in association with reduction in bone resorption and increase in bone mass density.
- **Thiazide diuretics:** For postmenopausal women who also have hypertension, treatment with a thiazide diuretic modestly attenuates bone loss. This effect is thought to be mediated by the hypocalciuric effect of these drugs, thereby improving calcium balance.
- **Androgens:**
  - Since men have higher bone density than women, it has been suggested that treatment with androgens might benefit women with osteoporosis.
  - The effect of treatment with androgen plus estrogen on BMD does not appear superior to the effect of estrogen alone.
  - Androgens also have virilizing effects.

FALLS

Roughly 30% of all falls occur in individuals ≥ 65 years of age, and approximately 50% occur in those ≥ 80 years of age. Falls also occur more frequently in hospitals and immediate posthospital settings. Additional risk factors include the following:

- Less agile gait
- Decreased positional sense and reflexes
- Decreased sensorium/vision
- Orthostatic hypotension
- Incontinence
- Postural hypotension
- A prior history of a cerebrovascular event
- Parkinson's disease
- A history of syncope (possible etiologies include CAD and aortic stenosis)
- Alcohol use
- Medications

PREVENTION

Preventive measures include the following:

- Improved lighting and correction of visual deficits.
- Decreasing psychotropic or other known offending medications.
- Vitamin D replacement for those who are deficient (shown to decrease falls and improve body sway).
- Exercise (particularly strengthening and balance exercises such as tai chi).
- Safety measures such as handrails, removal of rugs, use of shower rails and seats, use of ramps, and first-floor setup (the placement of bed, commode, and bath on the same floor—preferably the main level of the residence).
- Use of assistive devices.

COMPLICATIONS

- Roughly 50% of falls result in injury, and 10% require hospitalization.
- A prolonged amount of time spent on the floor (as occurs in roughly 3% of all falls) can lead to rhabdomyolysis, dehydration, and hypothermia.
- Associated with nursing home placement and functional decline.

HIP FRACTURES

More than 300,000 people ≥ 65 years of age are hospitalized each year with hip fractures, and roughly 25% of these patients die within one year as a result of the fracture or related complications.

SYMPTOMS

Presents with hip or groin pain after a fall. Patients are often unable to bear weight.

EXAM

With the patient in bed, the leg is shortened and externally rotated. Pain is likely to be observed on palpation or internal/external rotation. Look for other fall-related trauma such as head injury.

DIFFERENTIAL

Soft tissue injury, dislocation, avascular necrosis (AVN).

DIAGNOSIS

X-ray studies generally establish the diagnosis, usually on AP pelvis or hip series. Rarely, an MRI is needed to diagnose a subtle fracture or to confirm AVN. Generally, a hip fracture is also diagnostic of osteoporosis, necessitating treatment.

Assess goals of care with the hip fracture patient and, if necessary, with the surrogate decision maker. Operative management may not always be consistent with a frail patient with preexisting immobility and shortened life expectancy.

TREATMENT

The major components of therapy are as follows (see also the mnemonic O-ROT):

- **Orthopedic management:** Usually required, with the exact procedure depending on the type of fracture. Most surgeons now recognize the importance of expediting operative repair (should occur within 24 hours of the fracture).
- **Postoperative rehabilitation:** Should begin immediately or as soon as allowed by surgical recommendations. Includes mobilization, pain management, prevention of complications, and functional adaptation.
- **Osteoporosis treatment:** May include medical therapy as well as hip protectors.
- **Tertiary prevention of falls** (see above).

COMPLICATIONS

Immobility, venous thromboembolism, functional decline and death.

> ***Treatment of hip fracture–***
>
> **O-ROT**
>
> **O**rthopedic management (to include prophylactic anticoagulation until increased mobility)
> **R**ehab
> **O**steoporosis treatment
> **T**ertiary fall prevention

PRESSURE ULCERS

A higher incidence of pressure ulcers is found in hospitals and nursing homes than in homes with family caregivers. Causes include the following:

- Sustained pressure, primarily over bony prominences (e.g., sacrum, ischium, heels, trochanters).
- Shearing forces.
- Infection, friction, or moisture.

DIAGNOSIS

Staging is as follows:

- **Stage I:** Nonblanching erythema with pressure.
- **Stage II:** Partial-thickness skin loss.
- **Stage III:** Full skin loss.
- **Stage IV:** Tissue loss down to the level of muscle, tendon, or bone.

TREATMENT

Treatment should include the provision of a pressure-relieving surface, frequent repositioning, adequate nursing care, and debridement of dead or infected tissue.

PREVENTION

Preventive measures include competent nursing care, good hygiene and hydration, and adequate nutrition.

DEMENTIA

Defined as an acquired syndrome that involves a decline in memory along with at least one other cognitive domain, such as language, visuospatial capacity, or executive function. This decreased capacity interferes with social or occupational functioning. Risk factors are as follows:

- **Strong risk factors:**
  - Age (particularly Alzheimer's type)
  - A family history in first-degree relatives
  - Apolipoprotein E ε4 genotype
  - DM
  - Hypercholesterolemia
  - Low and high blood pressure
- **Other risk factors:**
  - Head trauma with loss of consciousness
  - A history of depression
  - Low educational achievement
  - Female gender (for Alzheimer's dementia)
  - Gait impairment (for those with non-Alzheimer's dementia)

SYMPTOMS/EXAM

Dementia is characterized by an insidious, progressive course without waxing and waning.

Dementia is more often a complaint of the family than of the patient. Early dementia involves mild cognitive impairment (MCI)—e.g., a decrease in recent memory and difficulty with daily functions. Other clinical characteristics include the following:

- Insidious onset
- Progressive course
- No altered consciousness; no waxing and waning after history and observation
- Reduced coping skills
- Getting lost in familiar places
- Poor impulse control/behavioral disturbance
- Diminishment in simple problem-solving ability

DIFFERENTIAL

The presentation of dementia can be further broken down by type.

Alzheimer's dementia is characterized by early loss of short-term memory.

- **Alzheimer's:**
  - Involves early, prominent loss of short-term memory; progressive memory loss; personality changes; and functional impairment.
  - Late in the disease, patients become totally dependent on others for basic care.
- **Vascular (multi-infarct dementia):**
  - May be due to multiple small strokes or cognitive impairment associated with a single stroke.
  - Often has sudden onset and a stepwise decline.
  - Neurologic deficits on exam are correlated with previous stroke, with presentation varying according to the location of the brain injury.
  - Vascular disease is detected on radiologic exam.
  - Vascular risk factors and other cardiovascular disease are often present.
  - Commonly coexists with Alzheimer's dementia.
- **Dementia with Lewy bodies:**
  - Patient has parkinsonian symptoms without frank Parkinson's disease, with sensitivity to neuroleptic medications.
  - Lewy bodies are found in the brain stem and cortex.
  - Produces disabling cognitive impairment progressing to dementia.
  - Characterized by fluctuation in cognition and persistent visual hallucinations.

- **Parkinson's:** Dementia associated with Parkinson's is most commonly associated with later stages of illness (as opposed to dementia with Lewy bodies).
- **Frontal lobe dementia:**
  - Involves impaired executive function (initiating activity, planning), poor self-awareness of one's deficits, and disinhibited behavior.
  - Pick's disease is one type (Pick bodies are found in the neocortex and the hippocampus).
  - Language disturbances include the following:
    - **Palilalia:** Compulsive repetition of one's speech.
    - **Logorrhea:** Profuse, unfocused speech.
    - **Echolalia:** Spontaneous repetition of words or phrases.
- **Reversible dementia:** It is important to note that these dementias are **potentially reversible**—i.e., not all will improve once the disorder is recognized and addressed.
  - **Medication induced:** Substances can include analgesics, anticholinergics, antipsychotics, and sedatives.
  - **Alcohol withdrawal or intoxication.**
  - **Metabolic disorders:** Includes thyroid disease, vitamin B_{12} deficiency, hyponatremia, hypercalcemia, and hepatic and renal insufficiency.

Depression can present as pseudodementia.

- **Depression:**
  - Commonly noted as pseudodementia.
  - Depression must be ruled out or aggressively treated prior to diagnosing new dementia.
  - Depression presenting as dementia is more likely to progress on to dementia.
- **CNS disease:** Includes chronic subdural hematomas, chronic meningitis, and normal pressure hydrocephalus.
  - The presentation of normal pressure hydrocephalus is described in the mnemonic **W**et, **W**obbly, and **W**acky:
    - **W**et—urinary incontinence.
    - **W**obbly—gait disturbance.
    - **W**acky—cognitive dysfunction.
  - The Miller-Fisher test compares before-and-after gait following removal of 30 cc of spinal fluid to predict the benefit of ventriculoperitoneal shunt.
- **Creutzfeldt-Jakob disease:**
  - A rare, infectious, rapidly progressive dementia that is usually fatal within one year of onset.
  - Diagnosis is based on clinical suspicion upon noticing rapid cognitive impairment accompanied by motor deficits and seizures.
  - EEG may show slow and periodic complexes.
  - Brain biopsy on autopsy is the only reliable means of diagnosis.
  - The disease is not treatable but is potentially transmissible.

DIAGNOSIS

Screening guidelines as set forth by the USPSTF are as follows:

- Some screening test have good sensitivity but only fair specificity in detecting cognitive impairment and dementia.
- The Mini-Mental Status Exam is the best-studied instrument for screening dementia.
  - Accuracy depends on age as well as on highest obtained educational level.
  - Sensitivity and specificity vary with cutoff points that are selected.

- It is important to make the diagnosis early in the clinical course to assist in anticipating and adhering to recommendations.

Treatment

Pharmacologic treatment for dementia includes the following:

- **Acetylcholinesterase inhibitors (donepezil):** Have been studied in patients with mild to moderate Alzheimer's dementia. Benefits include improvement or stabilization on neuropsychiatric scales, but benefits appear to be modest at two years. They may also have some benefit for behavioral symptoms of dementia.
- **Gingko biloba:** Studies have shown mixed results.
- **Selegiline:** Has shown no significant difference when compared to a placebo.
- **Vitamin E:** Has shown mixed results with delayed institutionalization in one trial, but results were not robust.
- **Estrogen:** Has shown no clinical benefit.
- **Memantine:** May be beneficial in moderate to severe Alzheimer's dementia, with or without concomitant acetylcholinesterase use.

Delusions are more common than hallucinations in demented patients.

ELDER ABUSE

Many forms of elder abuse exist, and while such abuse is **widespread,** it often goes unreported. Victims tend to be women > 80 years of age who may be physically frail and/or confused. Characteristics of abusers include the following:

- Often relatives or spouses of the victims.
- Adult children are the largest category of abusers across all forms of abuse.
- Often abuse alcohol.
- Often dependent on the victim for money and housing.

Types of Abuse

Table 8-2 outlines types of elder abuse and their presentation.

Interview Techniques

- Initially, the patient should be interviewed alone.
- Inquire about perceived safety.
- Inquire about the patient's dependency on caregivers, friends, and family.
- Ask specific questions about abuse in reference to the items in the Table 8-2.

Management

- Whenever abuse is confirmed, the highest priority should be placed on protecting the safety of the elderly person while simultaneously respecting that person's autonomy.
- Two key management issues should be addressed:
  - First, does the patient accept or refuse intervention?
  - Second, does the patient have the capacity to accept or refuse intervention?
- If the patient **accepts intervention,** management options are as follows:
  - Implementing a safety plan for the patient who is in immediate danger.

TABLE 8-2. Types and Characteristics of Elder Abuse

TYPE	DESCRIPTION
Domestic	Maltreatment of an older adult living at home or in a caregiver's home.
Institutional	Maltreatment of an older adult living in a residential facility.
Self-neglect	Behavior of an older adult who lives alone that threatens his or her own health or safety.
Physical abuse	Intentional infliction of physical pain or injury.
Financial abuse	Improper or illegal use of the resources of an older person without his/her consent, benefiting a person other than the older adult.
Psychological abuse	Infliction of mental anguish (e.g., humiliating, intimidating, threatening).
Neglect	Failure to fulfill a caretaking obligation to provide goods or services (e.g., abandonment; denial of food or health-related services).
Abandonment	Desertion of an elderly person by someone who has assumed responsibility for providing care to that person.
Sexual abuse	Nonconsensual sexual contact of any kind.

- Providing assistance that addresses the causes of mistreatment (e.g., referral to drug or alcohol rehabilitation for addicted abusers; homemaker services for overwhelmed caregivers).
- Referring the patient or family members to appropriate services.

- If the patient **has the capacity to accept intervention but refuses,** the physician's options include the following:
  - Educating the patient about the incidence of mistreatment of the elderly and the tendency for mistreatment to increase in frequency and severity over time.
  - Providing written information about emergency-assistance numbers and appropriate referrals.
  - Developing and reviewing a safety plan.
  - Developing a follow-up plan.
- If the patient **does not have the capacity to accept intervention,** the physician should discuss with Adult Protective Services issues such as assistance with financial management, guardianship, and court proceedings.

Reporting Requirements

- All states have laws about domestic or institutional abuse of the elderly, but these laws vary in the following ways:
  - The age at which a victim is covered
  - The definition of elder abuse

- Classification of the abuse as criminal or civil
  - Types of abuse covered
  - Reporting requirements
  - Investigation procedures
  - Remedies
- In many states, the suspicion of abuse is grounds for reporting, and the physician does not need to prove anything. Often the reporter remains anonymous.

NOTES

CHAPTER 9

Hematology

Thomas Chen, MD, PhD

ANEMIA

Approach to Anemia

Defined as a hemoglobin < 14 g/dL in males and < 12 g/dL in females **or** a hematocrit < 40% in males and < 37% in females. Many cases have > 1 cause. The best first steps in evaluation are measurement of the **absolute reticulocyte count** (see Figure 9-1) and review of the **peripheral smear.** The reticulocyte count can be used to categorize anemias as follows:

- **Hypoproliferative anemias:** Underproduction of RBCs with a low reticulocyte count. Classically subdivided by the MCV into **micro-, macro-,** and **normocytic** causes (see Table 9-1).
- **Hyperproliferative anemias:** Increased destruction or loss of RBCs. **Reticulocyte count is elevated.**
  - The two most common causes are **bleeding** and **hemolysis** (covered in a subsequent section).
  - **MCV is not helpful in the evaluation of hyperproliferative anemias.**

Anemia of chronic disease may be either normocytic or microcytic!

Iron Deficiency Anemia

Daily iron loss from exfoliation of the skin and mucosa averages 1 mg/day under normal conditions. In menstruating, pregnant, or lactating females, however, the loss can approach 3–4 mg/day. Each milliliter of whole blood contains approximately 0.5 mg of iron. Thus, even a trivial GI bleed of 10 mL/day (below the threshold of detection for stool guaiac testing) will overwhelm the body's ability to absorb iron, resulting in iron deficiency.

SYMPTOMS/EXAM

- General findings of anemia are skin and conjunctival pallor.
- **Features associated with iron deficiency** are as follows:
  - **Pica: Craving for nonfood substances, especially dirt.**
  - **Pagophagia:** Craving for ice chips.
  - **Cheilosis:** Fissures at the corners of the mouth.
  - **Glossitis:** Smooth tongue.
  - **Koilonychia:** Spooning of the fingernails.
  - **Dysphagia:** Due to esophageal webs **(Plummer-Vinson syndrome).**

- Total body Iron 2-4 gm
  - 50mg/kg in ♂
  - 35mg/kg in ♀.
- 1ml PRBC - 1mg iron.
- Red cell vol - 30ml/kg ♂
  - 27ml/kg ♀

  So 70kg ♂ has 2100ml Red cell & same amount of iron in his circulating blood.
- Only 200-400mg iron present in myoglobin & non heme enzymes.
- Storage pool 0.5-2gm as Hemosiderin or ferritin
- Heme iron abs 10-20%. Non heme iron abs 1-5%. becoz of interference by PO4 tannins

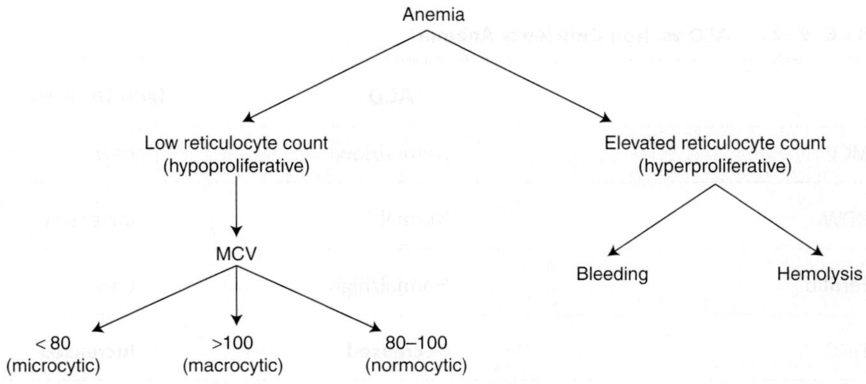

FIGURE 9-1. Algorithm for categorizing anemias.

TABLE 9-1. Classification of Hypoproliferative Anemias

Microcytic (MCV < 80)	Macrocytic (MCV > 100)	Normocytic (MCV 80–100)
"TAIL":	**Megaloblastic:**	ACD
Thalassemia trait	▪ B_{12} deficiency, folate deficiency	Aplastic anemia
Anemia of chronic disease (ACD)	▪ Myelodysplasia	Myelodysplasia
Iron deficiency	▪ Myeloma	Renal insufficiency
Lead toxicity	▪ Aplastic anemia	Mixed disorder
	▪ Pure red cell aplasia	Early disease process
	▪ Drug-induced bone marrow suppression	
	▪ Alcohol	
	Nonmegaloblastic:	
	▪ Liver disease	
	▪ Hypothyroidism	

Anemia from iron deficiency is rarely life-threatening, but the underlying cause of iron deficiency can be. Therefore, in any older patient with iron deficiency, evaluation of the GI tract for malignancy is usually indicated.

Differential

- Causes of iron deficiency include blood loss from menstruation, GI bleed, and frequent phlebotomy. Impaired iron ingestion or absorption is rare.
- **Anemia of chronic disease (ACD):** Table 9-2 distinguishes ACD from iron deficiency.
- **Lead poisoning:** Presents with elevated RBC protoporphyrin, basophilic stippling, and "lead lines" on the gums.

Diagnosis

- Classic findings are **microcytic, hypochromic** RBCs on peripheral smear with marked **anisocytosis** (see Figure 9-2). However, these findings are present in only a minority of patients.
- **Serum ferritin:** The most useful screen for iron deficiency. Values < 16 μg/L are diagnostic of iron deficiency, although normal values do not rule it out.
- Other iron indices are listed in Table 9-2.
- **Bone marrow biopsy** is rarely indicated.
- A **therapeutic trial of iron** may be diagnostic:
  - Reticulocytosis from iron typically begins 3–5 days after iron therapy.
  - Rise in hemoglobin lags behind by several days.

TABLE 9-2. ACD vs. Iron Deficiency Anemia

	ACD	Iron Deficiency
MCV	Normal/low	Low
RDW	Normal	Increased
Ferritin	Normal/high	**Low**
TIBC	**Decreased**	**Increased**
Soluble transferrin receptor	Normal	Increased

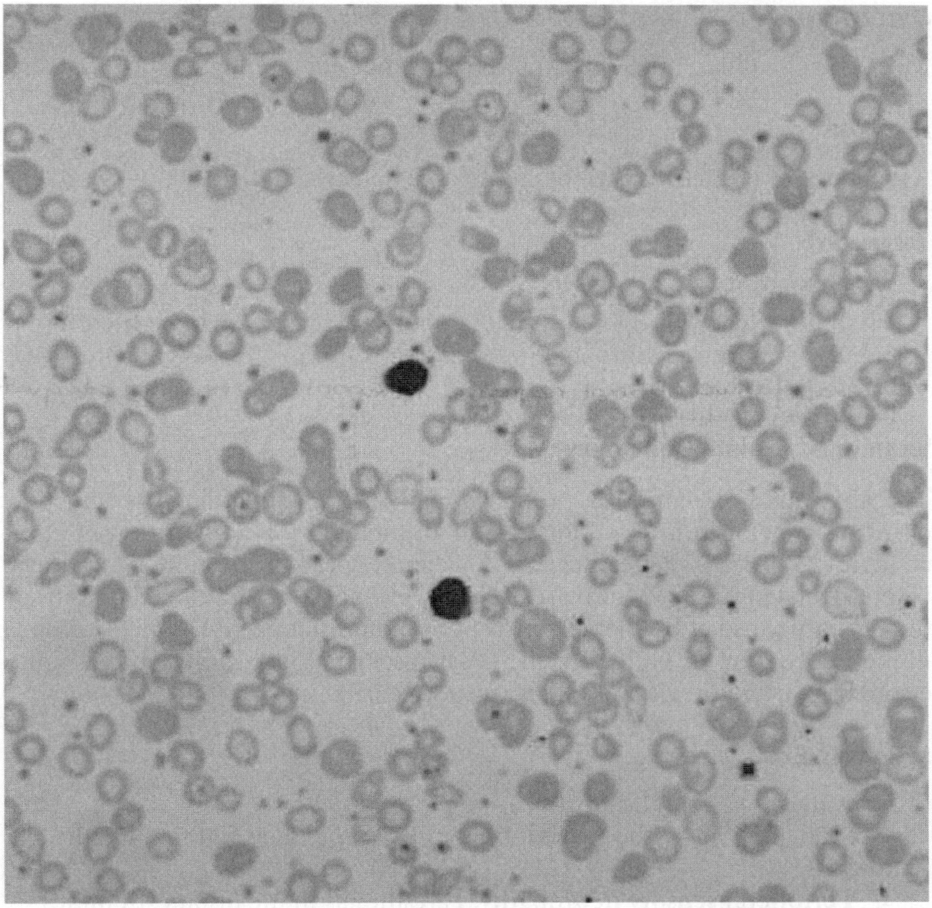

FIGURE 9-2. Iron deficiency anemia.

Note hypochromic cells (prominent central pallor) and microcytosis (RBCs smaller than the nucleus of the lymphocyte). There is also prominent thrombocytosis, a common associated finding with iron deficiency. (Also see Color Insert.)

TREATMENT

- **Oral iron replacement:** Goal is approximately 300 mg of elemental iron per day.
- **Parenteral iron:** Carries a risk of anaphylaxis; use only if the patient has a total inability to tolerate oral iron.
- Treat the underlying cause.

Anemia of Chronic Disease (ACD)

Caused by sequestration of iron in the reticuloendothelial system. The **most common cause of anemia in the elderly population;** often coexists with other causes.

SYMPTOMS/EXAM

Presents with symptoms of anemia and underlying disorders.

In ACD, the hematocrit is rarely < 25% unless renal failure or another cause of anemia coexists. Thus if hematocrit is < 25%, look for a cause of anemia other than ACD.

Differential

Must often be differentiated from iron deficiency anemia (see Table 9-2).

Diagnosis

A diagnosis of exclusion; peripheral smear is nonspecific.

Treatment

- Treat the underlying cause.
- High doses of erythropoietin (30,000–60,000 U/week) may be tried in patients with serum erythropoietin levels < 200 IU/L.
- In renal failure optimal responce to epoetin requires adequate intensity of dialysis.

Vitamin B_{12}/Folate Deficiency

The absorption of vitamin B_{12} requires many factors, including the secretion of intrinsic factor from the stomach and an intact terminal ileum. Vegans are at high risk for B_{12} deficiency, as B_{12} comes solely from animal products, whereas folate is derived from green, leafy vegetables. In developed countries, the primary cause of B_{12} deficiency is **pernicious anemia (PA)** due to autoimmune destruction of parietal cells. PA is associated with other autoimmune disorders (thyroiditis, vitiligo, Addison's disease).

Symptoms/Exam

- Glossitis and atrophic gastritis (in PA).
- Neurologic findings are present only in B_{12} deficiency and include the following:
  - **Peripheral sensory neuropathy:** Paresthesias in the distal extremities.
  - **Posterior column findings:** Loss of vibratory sensation and proprioception; gait instability.
  - Dementia or more subtle personality changes may occur at any time ("megaloblastic madness").
  - Neurologic changes are not always reversible with B_{12} replacement.
- Mild icterus due to ineffective erythropoiesis, causing intramedullary hemolysis.

Differential

The causes of B_{12} and folate deficiency are further outlined in Table 9-3.

TABLE 9-3. Causes of B_{12}/Folate Deficiency

B_{12} Deficiency	Folate Deficiency
Dietary deficiencies—very rare; typically in **strict vegans**	**Inadequate intake:**
Decreased intrinsic factor—the **most common cause;**	▪ Malnutrition
typically from **pernicious anemia** (autoimmune destruction	▪ Alcoholism
of parietal cells)	▪ Malabsorption (e.g., tropical sprue)
Gastrectomy	**Increased demand:**
Ileal resection	▪ Pregnancy
Crohn's disease	▪ Hemodialysis (folate lost in dialysate)
Tapeworm infestation (*D. latum*)	▪ Chronic hemolytic anemia
Bacterial overgrowth of terminal ileum	▪ Psoriasis

DIAGNOSIS

- **Labs:**
  - Low serum B_{12} level or RBC folate level.
  - Anemia with **MCV > 100** (may see one without the other).
  - Mild elevations in LDH and indirect bilirubin.
  - Pancytopenia in severe cases.
  - Elevated levels of homocysteine or methylmalonic acid may be seen.
- **Smear:** Macro-ovalocytes, **hypersegmented neutrophils** (any neutrophil with ≥ 6 lobes or the majority with ≥ 4 lobes); see Figure 9-3.
- **Bone marrow:** Megaloblastic (hypercellular, decreased myeloid/erythroid ratio, enlarged RBC precursors with relatively immature nuclei); **may mimic the blastic appearance of acute leukemia.**
- **Schilling test** establishes the **cause** of B_{12} deficiency. Stages I and II may be combined by using different radioactive labels for each step (see Figure 9-4).
- Anti–parietal cell antibodies can be measured to confirm PA as the cause of B_{12} deficiency.

Anemia or macrocytosis need not be present in clinically significant B_{12} deficiency. RBC folate is superior to serum folate level in detecting folate deficiency.

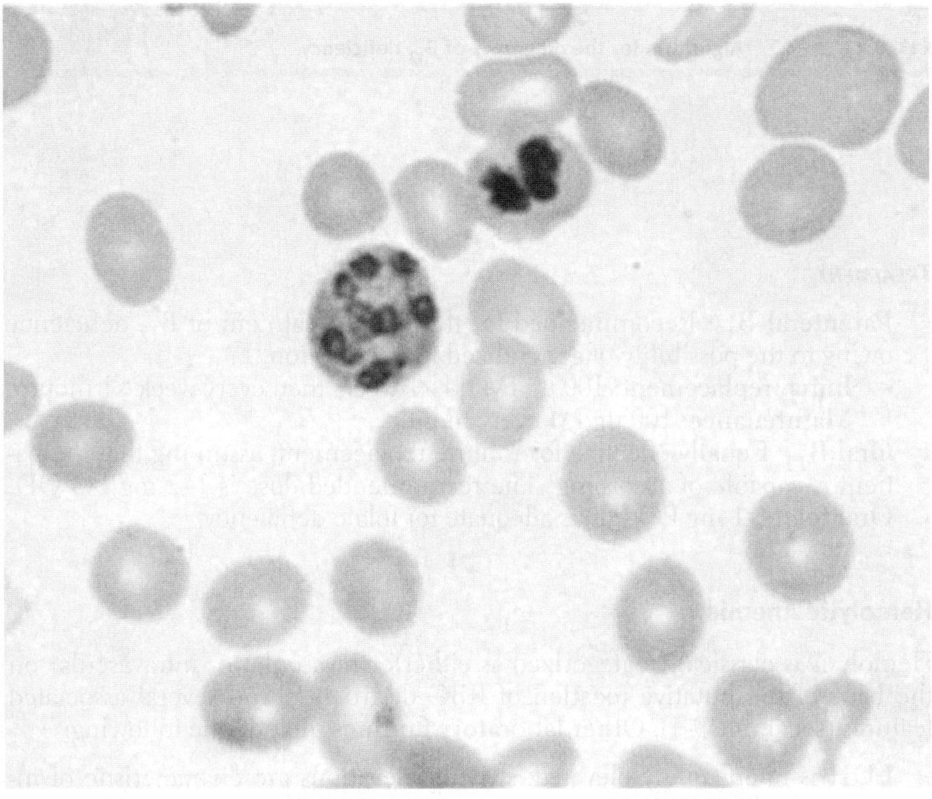

FIGURE 9-3. Megaloblastic anemia.

Note macro-ovalocytes and prominent hypersegmented neutrophil. (Reproduced, with permission, from Babior BM, Bunn HF. Megaloblastic anemias. In Kasper DL et al [eds]. *Harrison's Principles of Internal Medicine*, 16th ed. New York: McGraw-Hill, 2005.) (Also see Color Insert.)

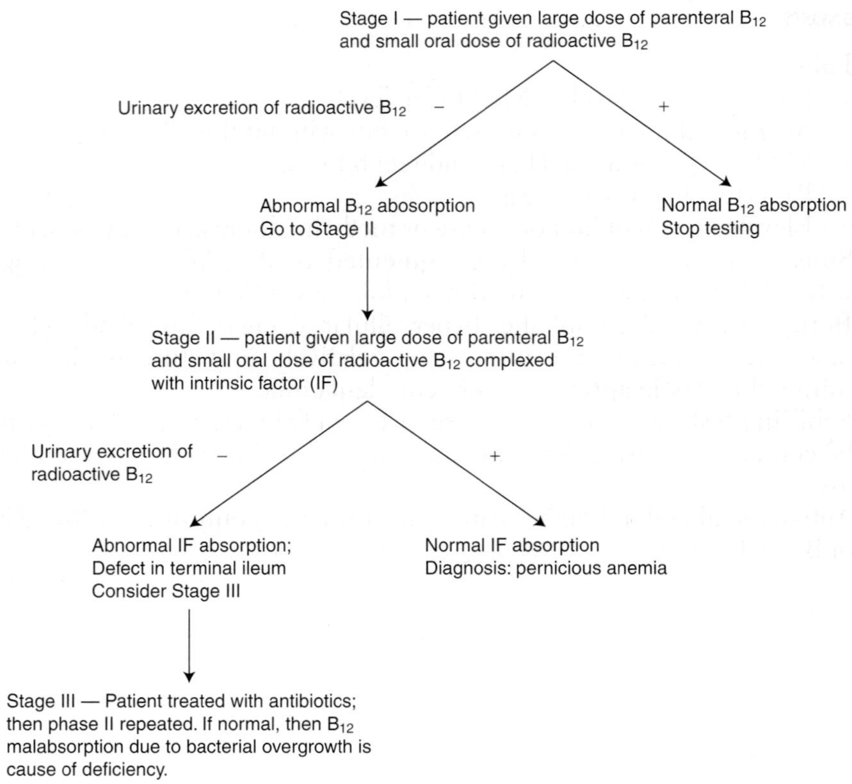

FIGURE 9-4. Algorithm for the diagnosis of B_{12} deficiency.

Before treating folate deficiency, exclude concomitant B_{12} deficiency in order to prevent acute exacerbation of neurologic symptoms in patients who receive folate but are B_{12} deficient.

TREATMENT

- **Parenteral B_{12}:** Recommended for the initial treatment of B_{12} deficiency owing to the possibility of generalized malabsorption.
  - **Initial replacement:** 100 μg IM qd ×1 week, then every week ×1 month.
  - **Maintenance:** 100 μg IM every month.
- **Oral B_{12}:** Equally effective for routine replacement, assuming that the patient is capable of absorbing. The recommended dose is 1–2 mg PO QD.
- **Oral folate:** 1 mg PO QD is adequate for folate deficiency.

Hemolytic Anemia

Hemolysis is classically categorized as either extravascular or intravascular on the basis of the putative location of RBC destruction and several associated features (see Table 9-4). **Other laboratory findings** include the following:

- **LDH** is often mildly elevated; striking elevations are characteristic of intravascular hemolysis.
- Indirect hyperbilirubinemia may occur up to 4 mg/dL; higher values usually indicate concomitant liver dysfunction.
- Chronic intravascular hemolysis may result in chronic hemoglobinuria, leading to iron deficiency.

TABLE 9-4. Extravascular vs. Intravascular Hemolytic Anemia

FEATURE	EXTRAVASCULAR	INTRAVASCULAR
Site of RBC destruction	Spleen	Bloodstream, liver
Peripheral smear findings	**Spherocytes** (see Figure 9-6)	**Schistocytes** (see Figure 9-7)
Serum haptoglobin	Normal or mildly decreased	Markedly decreased
Urine hemosiderin	Unchanged	Increased
Examples	Warm antibody immune hemolysis Hypersplenism Delayed transfusion reaction	Cold antibody immune hemolysis Acute transfusion reaction Microangiopathic hemolysis Oxidative hemolytic anemia PNH Hemoglobinopathies (sickle cell anemia) Infection-related (malaria, *Clostridium, Babesia*)

DIFFERENTIAL

- **Immune hemolysis:** Divided into **warm** or **cold** antibodies, referring to the temperature at which the responsible autoantibody will bind erythrocytes and thus predict several other characteristics (see Table 9-5).
- **Microangiopathic hemolytic anemias (MAHAs):** Characterized by **schistocytes** and a **negative Coombs'** test. Usually caused by fibrin strands in damaged microvasculature, resulting in sheared RBCs. Almost all are associated with thrombocytopenia.
- **Oxidative hemolytic anemia:** A classic example is **G6PD deficiency,** in which erythrocytes have a decreased ability to withstand oxidative stress.
  - **Any oxidative stress may precipitate hemolysis,** including viral infections, drugs (e.g., dapsone, sulfonamides, antimalarials, and nitrofurantoin), and dietary factors (e.g., fava beans).

TABLE 9-5. Immune Hemolysis Categories

	WARM ANTIBODY	COLD ANTIBODY
Autoantibody	IgG	IgM
Direct antiglobulin test	Positive for IgG	Positive for complement
Peripheral smear	**Spherocytes**	**Schistocytes**
Site of RBC destruction	Spleen	Liver
Associated conditions	Autoimmune diseases; CLL, lymphoma; α-methyldopa	*Mycoplasma* infection, EBV; CLL, lymphoma
Treatment	Steroids, splenectomy, immunosuppression	Warming extremities, plasmapheresis, alkylator medications

    - **Peripheral smear** shows bite cells (see Figure 9-5), spherocytes, and Heinz bodies (requires a special stain to see).
    - **Lab tests:** Elevated LDH, elevated indirect bilirubin during acute hemolysis; G6PD activity (remember that measuring this during an acute hemolytic episode will result in a false-negative test).
- **Paroxysmal nocturnal hemoglobinuria (PNH):**
    - A rare clonal stem cell disorder caused by defective expression of RBC membrane proteins (CD55 and CD59).
    - Characterized by episodic complement-mediated intravascular hemolysis.
    - Previously diagnosed by Ham's test (acidified serum hemolysis) or sucrose hemolysis test. Currently the **best test is flow cytometry for CD55 and CD59.**
    - Associated with several hematologic complications, including **pancytopenia, venous thromboses** (especially Budd-Chiari), and progression to myelodysplasia, aplastic anemia, or AML.
- **Sickle cell anemia:** This subtype is covered in the hemoglobinopathy section below.

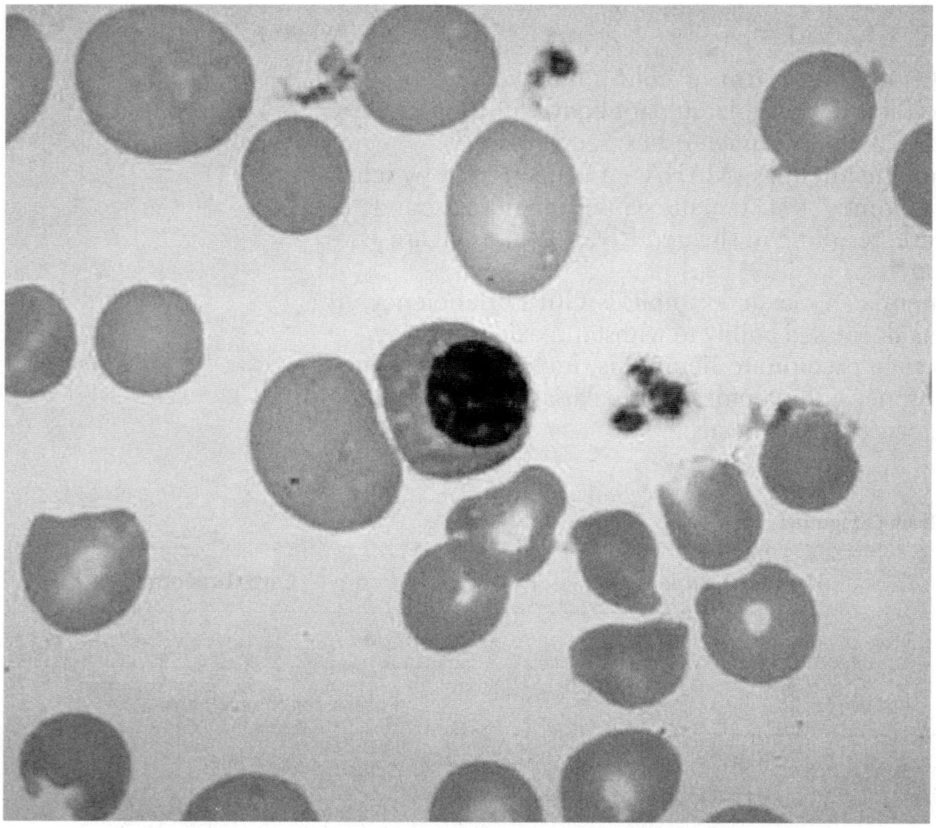

FIGURE 9-5. Bite cells.

Several characteristic bite cells are present in this patient with G6PD deficiency with acute oxidative hemolysis. (Courtesy of L Damon. Reproduced, with permission, from Linker CA. Hematology. In Tierney LM et al [eds]. *Current Medical Diagnosis & Treatment 2005*, 44th ed. New York: McGraw-Hill, 2005.) (Also see Color Insert.)

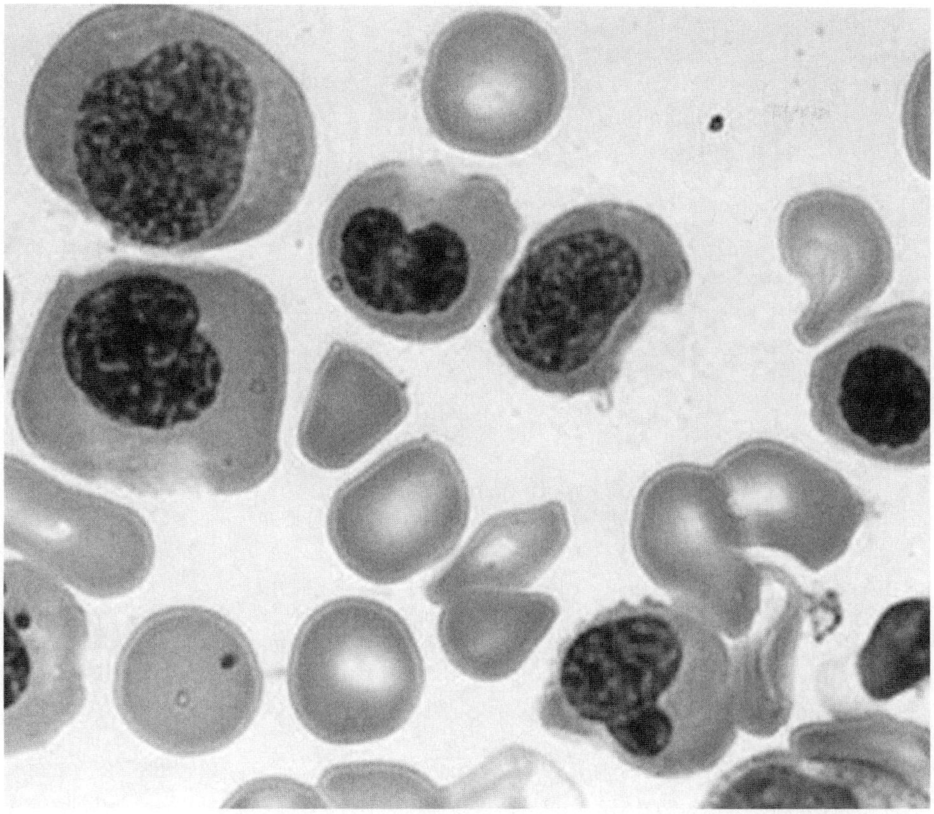

FIGURE 9-6. Spherocytes.

Characteristic spherocytes (small, round RBCs without central pallor) are present in addition to signs of markedly increased RBC synthesis (polychromasia, nucleated RBCs) in a patient with extravascular immune hemolysis. (Reproduced, with permission, from RS Hillman, MD, and KA Ault, MD, courtesy of the American Society of Hematology Slide Bank.) (Also see Color Insert.)

MICROANGIOPATHIES

Table 9-6 outlines the distinguishing features and treatment of microangiopathies.

Thrombotic Thrombocytopenic Purpura (TTP)

A rare disorder of unknown etiology that is characterized by microangiopathy, **elevated LDH,** and neurologic changes tempered by appropriate clinical suspicion. The **classic pentad**—fever, anemia, thrombocytopenia, neurologic changes, and renal failure—is seen in **< 10% of cases.**

SYMPTOMS/EXAM

- Patients usually present with anemia, bleeding, or neurologic abnormalities.
- Neurologic changes can be subtle and may include personality changes, headache, confusion, lethargy, or coma.

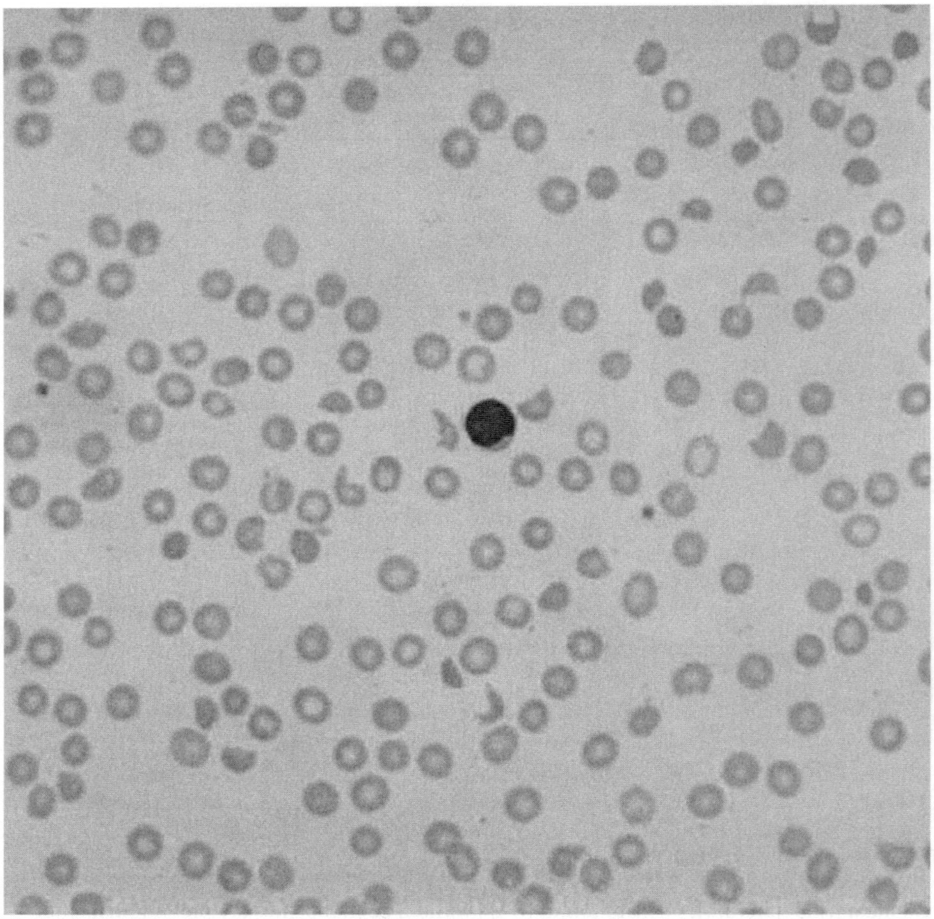

FIGURE 9-7. Schistocytes.

A large number of fragmented RBCs is characteristic of microangiopathic or intravascular hemolysis. In this case, the patient had HUS. (Courtesy of L Damon. Reproduced, with permission, from Linker CA. Hematology. In Tierney LM et al [eds]. *Current Medical Diagnosis & Treatment 2005*, 44th ed. New York: McGraw-Hill, 2005.) (Also see Color Insert.)

Differential

Associated conditions include the following:

- Medications (cyclosporin, tacrolimus, quinine, ticlopidine, clopidogrel, mitomycin C, estrogens).
- Pregnancy (overlaps with eclampsia and HELLP).
- Autoimmune disorders (SLE, antiphospholipid antibody syndrome, scleroderma, vasculitis).
- HIV.
- Bone marrow transplantation (autologous or allogeneic).

Diagnosis

- Peripheral smear shows evidence of thrombocytopenia with microangiopathy (i.e., **schistocytes**); **PT/PTT should be normal** unless DIC is also present.
- No standardized lab test exists for TTP.

TABLE 9-6. Differential and Treatment of Microangiopathies.

CAUSES OF MICROANGIOPATHY	DISTINGUISHING FEATURES	TREATMENT
DIC	Associated with severe infection, sepsis, and intravascular thrombus. Consumptive coagulopathy. **Elevated PT and PTT;** low fibrinogen.	Treat the underlying condition; cryoprecipitate (if indicated).
TTP	Elevated LDH, neurologic symptoms, **normal coagulation tests.**	Plasmapheresis with FFP, steroids, no platelet transfusions.
HUS	Elevated LDH, renal insufficiency, **normal coagulation tests.**	Hemodialysis if necessary; may be self-limiting.
Preeclampsia	Peripartum period; hypertension.	Early delivery; diuretics, antihypertensives.
HELLP syndrome	Peripartum period; elevated liver enzymes; probably a variant of eclampsia.	Early delivery.
Malignant hypertension	Hypertension.	Antihypertensives.
Vasculitis	Features of specific vasculitis.	Treat the underlying condition.
Miscellaneous (metastatic cancer, mechanical heart valve, severe burns)		Treat the underlying condition.

TREATMENT

- **Plasmapheresis:** Plasma exchange using FFP has a high response rate. It must be continued daily until neurologic symptoms resolve.
- If the patient is in a facility that lacks the capability for plasmapheresis, can be temporized with steroids and FFP infusion.
- Splenectomy is also used for relapsing cases.

Hemolytic-Uremic Syndrome (HUS)

Similar to TTP, but **without neurologic changes.** Characterized by microangiopathy, elevated LDH, and **renal failure**; associated with the same medications and conditions as TTP. Mostly a self-limited disease in children that is **associated with diarrheal illnesses** (e.g., ***E. coli*** **O157:H7**, *Shigella*, *Campylobacter*). Treat with supportive care and renal replacement therapy as needed for uremic symptoms. In adults, it usually progresses to renal failure unless actively treated with plasma exchange.

HEMOGLOBINOPATHIES

Thalassemias

Adult hemoglobin (HbA) is **primarily (97–99%) composed of two α chains plus two β chains ($\alpha_2\beta_2$)** in normal patients. In **thalassemia,** there is a decreased amount of either α or β chain (so HbA is reduced, while there is an increase in variant forms of hemoglobin such as HbA_2 and HbF). By contrast, **sickle cell anemia** is caused by specific **β-chain mutations.** There are **two general types of thalassemias: α and β.**

- **α-thalassemias** are seen in patients from **Southeast Asia and China** and are rarely seen in blacks.
- **β-thalassemias** are seen in patients from the **Mediterranean** and are rarely seen in Asians or blacks.
- Peripheral smear typically shows microcytosis, hypochromia, and basophilic stippling (β-thalassemia only). With increasing severity, increased nucleated RBCs and target cells are seen (see Figure 9-8).
- The severity of α-thalassemia depends on the number of α-globin genes functioning (see Table 9-7).
- β-thalassemia can be further subdivided into three types: β-thalassemia major, minor, and intermedia (see Table 9-8).

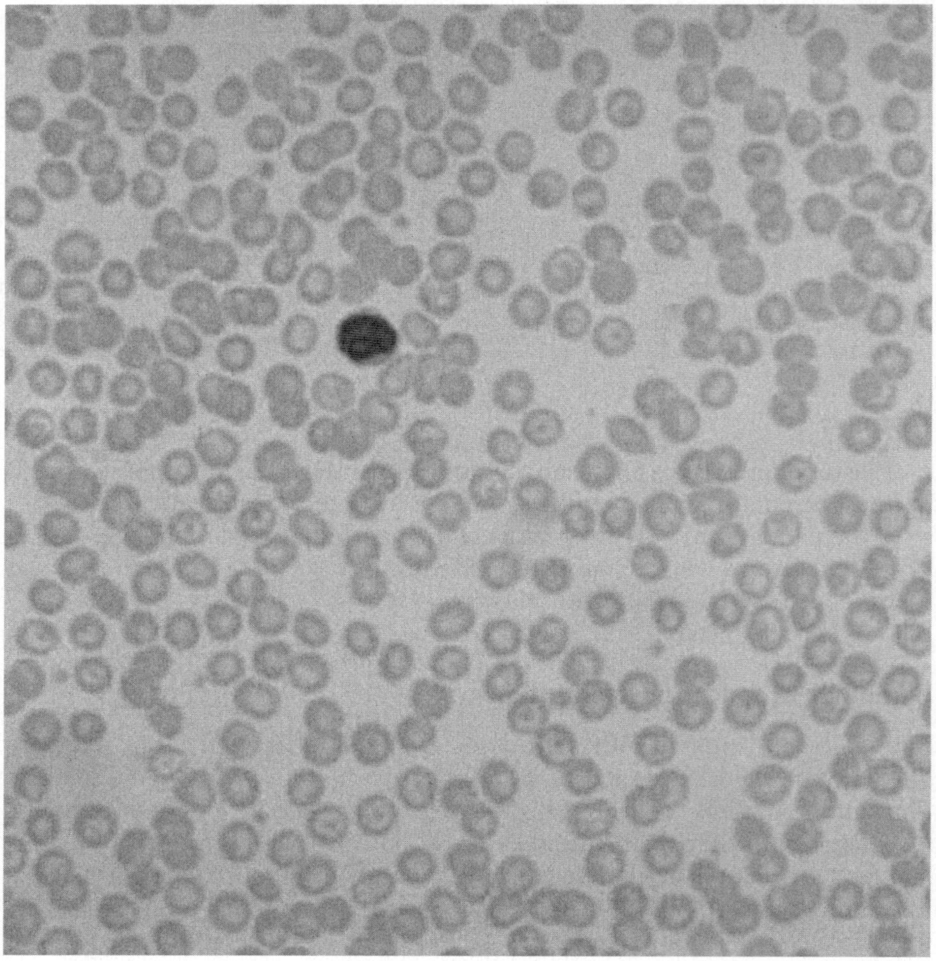

FIGURE 9-8. β-thalassemia major.

Note microcytic, hypochromic cells, target cells, and nucleated RBCs. (Courtesy of L Damon. Reproduced, with permission, from Linker CA. Hematology. In Tierney LM et al [eds]. *Current Medical Diagnosis & Treatment 2005*, 44th ed. New York: McGraw-Hill, 2005.) (Also see Color Insert.)

HEMATOLOGY

TABLE 9-7. Differential Diagnosis of α-Thalassemias

	α–THALASSEMIA TRAIT	HEMOGLOBIN H DISEASE	HYDROPS FETALIS
α-globin chains	2–3	1	0
Hematocrit	28–40%	22–32%	N/A
Hemoglobin electrophoresis	Normal	10–40% HbH	N/A
Clinical course	Normal life span	Chronic hemolytic anemia, exacerbated by stress	**Universally lethal as neonate**

Sickle Cell Anemia

Characterized by a homozygous defect in the β-globin gene that produces HbS. Heterozygotes have the sickle cell trait and are clinically normal except under extreme stress. Sickling is **increased** by **dehydration, acidosis, or hypoxia. Peripheral smear** shows target cells, Howell-Jolly bodies, and classic **sickle cells** (see Figure 9-9).

SYMPTOMS/EXAM

The clinical manifestations of sickle cell anemia are due to unstable sickle cells that hemolyze and aggregate to cause vaso-occlusion. **Acute vaso-**

TABLE 9-8. Differential Diagnosis of β-Thalassemias

	β–THALASSEMIA MAJOR (COOLEY'S ANEMIA)	β–THALASSEMIA MINOR	β–THALASSEMIA INTERMEDIA
β-globin synthesis	Almost complete absence	Near normal (heterozygous)	Moderately decreased
Hematocrit	< 10% without transfusions	28–40%	Variably low
HbA	0%	80–95%	0–30%
HbA_2	4–10%	4–8%	0–10%
HbF	90–96%	1–5%	90–100%
Life span	20–30 years	Normal	Adult
Transfusion-dependent	Yes	No	Variable
Clinical notes	Bony anomalies, hepatosplenomegaly, jaundice, transfusional iron overload	**Asymptomatic;** mild microcytic anemia	Mild bony anomalies; mild hepatosplenomegaly

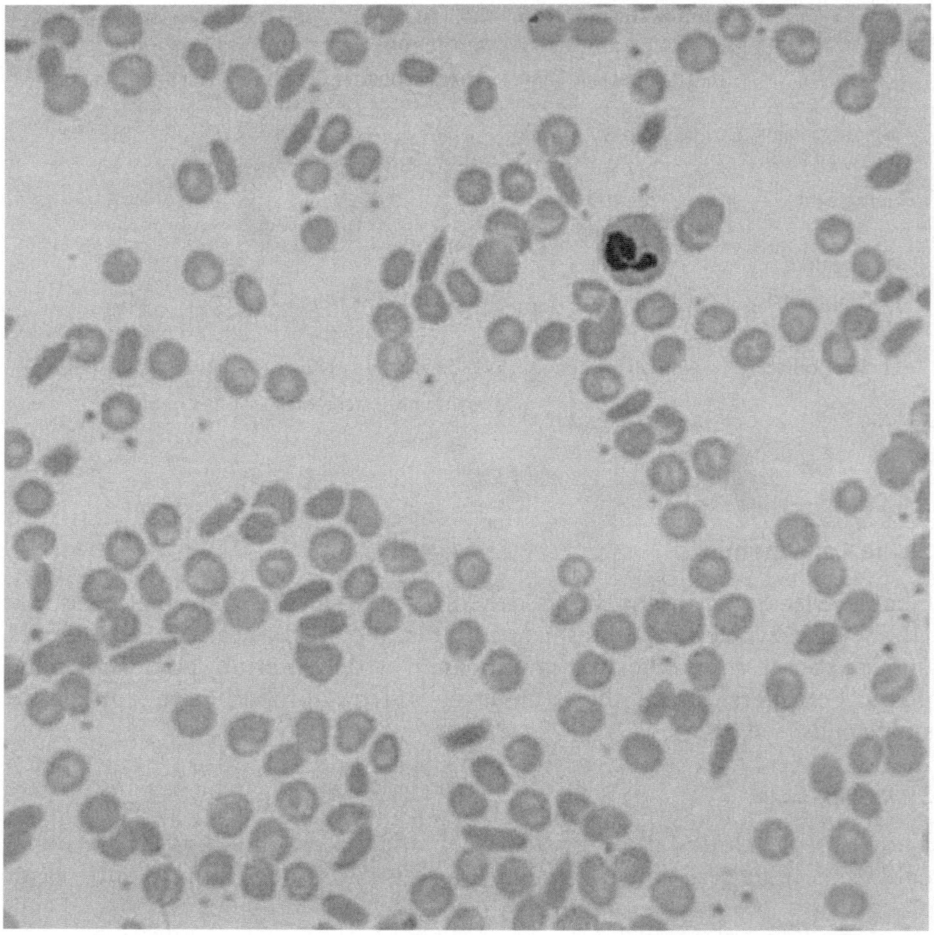

FIGURE 9-9. Sickle cell anemia.

Multiple sickle forms are characteristic. (Courtesy of L Damon. Reproduced, with permission, from Linker CA. Hematology. In Tierney LM et al [eds]. *Current Medical Diagnosis & Treatment 2005*, 44th ed. New York: McGraw-Hill, 2005.) (Also see Color Insert.)

occlusion manifests as pain crises, acute chest syndrome, priapism, stroke, and splenic sequestration. **Chronic vaso-occlusion** presents as renal papillary necrosis, avascular necrosis, autosplenectomy, and retinal hemorrhage. **Chronic hemolytic anemia** presents as jaundice, pigment gallstones, splenomegaly, and aplastic crisis.

- **Pain crises** can result from vaso-occlusion in any organ or tissue, typically in bones.
  - Triggered by factors that promote sickling.
  - Commonly manifest as pain in the back and long bones lasting for hours to days.
- **Acute chest syndrome** results from vaso-occlusion of the lung and **increases mortality.**
  - Characterized by **chest pain, hypoxia, fever, pulmonary infarcts, or infiltrates on CXR.**
  - May be impossible to differentiate from PE and pneumonia.

- Repeated episodes can lead to pulmonary hypertension and cor pulmonale.
- May require ICU admission and transfusions.

TREATMENT

- **Maintenance:**
  - Although not universally accepted, folate supplementation may be required.
  - Pneumococcal vaccination.
  - Screen yearly for retinal disease and renal dysfunction.
  - Consider hydroxyurea in patients with > 3 pain crises per year requiring hospitalization or in those with repeated episodes of acute chest syndrome.
- **Acute episodes:**
  - Treat pain crises with aggressive hydration, analgesics, supplemental O_2, and incentive spirometry.
  - Transfusions should be avoided given the risk of alloimmunization and iron overload. However, transfusions are indicated for severe vaso-occlusive emergencies (acute chest syndrome, priapism, stroke). Transfuse until HbS < 30%; exchange transfusion if necessary to keep hematocrit < 40%.

*Under stress, any clinical feature seen in sickle cell **anemia** homozygotes may be seen in heterozygotic patients with sickle cell **trait**.*

OTHER CBC ABNORMALITIES

Erythrocytosis

Defined as a hematocrit > 54% in males and > 51% in females. Categorized mainly as primary (polycythemia rubra vera) or secondary (reactive). The causes of **secondary** erythrocytosis are listed in Table 9-9.

DIAGNOSIS

- Repeat CBC or obtain historical records to ensure accuracy.
- If hematocrit is > 60% in males or > 56% in females, it is by definition an elevated RBC mass, and measurement of RBC mass is unnecessary.
- Exclude obvious causes of secondary erythrocytosis (see Table 9-9).
- Take a careful history, review a peripheral smear, and order appropriate labs and imaging studies (see Table 9-10).
- In nonsmokers, pulse oximetry is sufficient to measure arterial O_2 saturation. An O_2 saturation < 92% is low enough to cause erythrocytosis.
- In smokers, an ABG with carboxyhemoglobin level is necessary.
- Low ferritin and high B_{12}/folate levels are associated with polycythemia vera and not with secondary erythrocytosis.
- Low erythropoietin levels are suggestive of polycythemia vera but are not perfectly sensitive or specific.

Factors favoring polycythemia vera over secondary erythrocytosis include normal O_2 saturation, low ferritin and erythropoietin, and high B_{12} and folate.

TREATMENT

No specific management of secondary erythrocytosis is necessary. The treatment of polycythemia vera is covered in a separate section.

Thrombocytopenia

Defined as a platelet count < 150×10^9/L. Its causes are outlined in Table 9-11.

TABLE 9-9. Causes of Secondary Erythrocytosis

TYPE	ETIOLOGY
Congenital	High-affinity hemoglobin Congenitally low 2,3-DPG Autonomous high erythropoietin
Arterial hypoxemia	High altitude Cyanotic heart disease COPD Sleep apnea
Renal lesions	Renal tumors Renal cysts Hydronephrosis Renal artery stenosis
Liver lesions	Hepatoma Hepatitis
Tumors	Adrenal adenoma Carcinoid Uterine fibroids Cerebellar hemangioblastoma
Medications	Androgens

DIAGNOSIS

- Examine a peripheral smear.
  - Rule out platelet clumping.
  - Look for evidence of microangiopathy (i.e., schistocytes), marrow suppression (megaloblastic changes, dysplastic changes), and immature platelets (giant platelets) suggesting increased platelet turnover.
- Take a careful drug history.
  - Acetaminophen, H_2 blockers, sulfa drugs, furosemide, captopril, digoxin, and β-lactam antibiotics are all associated with thrombocytopenia.
  - Never forget **heparin-induced thrombocytopenia** (see the discussion of clotting disorders below).

TABLE 9-10. Evaluation of Erythrocytosis

LABS	IMAGING
Arterial O_2 saturation Ferritin, B_{12}, folate, creatinine, LFTs, uric acid Serum erythropoietin	RBC mass Abdominal ultrasound or CT scan

TABLE 9-11. Causes of Thrombocytopenia

INCREASED DESTRUCTION	DECREASED PRODUCTION	OTHER
Immune thrombocytopenia: ▪ Primary: autoimmune (i.e., ITP) ▪ Secondary: lymphoid malignancies, HIV, SLE, alloimmunization from prior platelet transfusions ▪ Drug induced: gold, abciximab, ticlopidine, quinine ▪ Heparin induced ▪ Post-transfusion purpura **Microangiopathies:** ▪ TTP, HUS, eclampsia ▪ DIC, sepsis ▪ Severe hypertension **Mechanical:** ▪ Artificial heart valves ▪ Hemangiomas ▪ Central venous catheters **Hypersplenism**	Essentially any cause of marrow suppression can cause thrombocytopenia in isolation. See the pancytopenia discussion below. **Probably the most important is drug-induced thrombocytopenia.**	Dilutional: from massive blood transfusions, fluid resuscitation. Pseudothrombocytopenia: from platelet clumping.

- Consider bone marrow biopsy if other findings suggest marrow dysfunction.
- Platelet-associated antibody tests are **not** useful.
- ITP is a diagnosis of exclusion.

TREATMENT

- Treat the underlying cause.
- Platelet transfusions in the absence of bleeding are usually unnecessary. Specific guidelines are given in the discussion of transfusion medicine below. Platelet transfusions are **contraindicated** in TTP/HUS and heparin-induced thrombocytopenia.

Inspect the med list. *Often the key diagnostic step lies in recognizing common medication causes of thrombocytopenia. Bone marrow biopsy is not always necessary to diagnose the majority of the disorders in Table 9-11.*

Thrombocytosis

Defined as a platelet count > 450 × 10^9/L. The main distinction is **reactive thrombocytosis** vs. **myeloproliferative syndrome.** The steps involved in the evaluation of thrombocytosis are outlined in Table 9-12.

Neutrophilia

Defined as an absolute neutrophil count > 10 × 10^9/L. The main distinction is between myeloproliferative disorder **(typically CML)** and reactive neutrophilia. Reactive neutrophilia is readily apparent from the history (inflammation, infection, severe burns, glucocorticoid, epinephrine) and from examination of a peripheral smear (Döhle bodies, toxic granulations).

TABLE 9-12. Evaluation of Thrombocytosis

EVALUATION	NOTES
Repeat CBC and examine peripheral smear.	Elevated platelet count may be spurious or transient. Clues to reactive thrombocytosis may be present.
Stratify by degree of thrombocytosis.	A platelet count < 600k is unlikely to be essential thrombocythemia. A platelet count > 1000k is less likely to be reactive thrombocytosis, but **many "platelet millionaires" still have reactive thrombocytosis.**
Identify causes of reactive thrombocytosis.	Iron deficiency anemia, rheumatoid arthritis, IBD, infection or inflammatory states, postsplenectomy, active malignancy, myelodysplasia with $5q^-$, sideroblastic anemia.
Rule out other myeloproliferative syndromes.	BCR-ABL by PCR in CML. Elevated RBC mass in polycythemia. Characteristic peripheral smear and splenomegaly in myelofibrosis.
Consider a bone marrow biopsy.	Megakaryocyte morphology can suggest essential thrombocythemia. Examination for myelodysplasia, sideroblasts.

*Elevated platelets from **reactive** thrombocytosis **does not** confer an increased risk of thrombosis. Therefore, if reactive thrombocytosis is suspected, no antithrombotic prophylaxis is warranted regardless of the platelet count!*

Eosinophilia

Defined as an absolute eosinophil count > 0.5×10^9/L. May be primary (idiopathic) or secondary.

- **Idiopathic hypereosinophilia syndrome:**
  - Extremely rare and heterogeneous.
  - A prolonged eosinophilia of unknown cause with the potential to affect multiple organs by eosinophil infiltration.
  - Almost all cases have bone marrow infiltration, but heart, lung, and CNS involvement predicts a worse outcome.
  - Some cases are treatable with imatinib mesylate (Gleevec).
- **Secondary eosinophilia:** Remember the mnemonic **NAACP.**
- Note that several drugs (nitrofurantoin, penicillin, phenytoin, ranitidine, sulfonamides) and toxins (Spanish toxic oil, tryptophan) have been reported to cause eosinophilia.

Causes of secondary eosinophilia—

NAACP

Neoplasm (especially myeloproliferative diseases)
Allergy, **A**topy, or **A**sthma
Addison's disease
Collagen vascular disease
Parasites

Neutropenia and Neutropenic Fever

Neutropenia is defined as an absolute neutrophil count (ANC) < 1.5×10^9/L (< 1.2 in blacks). Its causes are outlined in Table 9-13. **Gram-positive organisms account for 60–70% of cases of neutropenic fever.** Table 9-14 delineates factors affecting the risk of severe infection.

DIAGNOSIS

- Conduct a careful history and physical; don't forget mouth, perianal, groin, skin, and IV catheters.
- Directed studies include the following:
  - CBC with differential, renal and liver function, UA, O_2 saturation.
  - Obtain a CXR.
  - Two sets of blood cultures.

TABLE 9-13. Causes of Neutropenia

Impaired Production[a]	Increased Destruction
Cytotoxic chemotherapy and other drugs	Autoimmune neutropenia
Aplastic anemia and other marrow failure	Felty's syndrome
Congenital	Sepsis
Cyclic neutropenia	HIV
	Acute viral illness

[a] By far the most common cause.

- Culture other sites (nares, oropharynx, rectum, urine, stool) only if infection is suspected at those sites.
- If diarrhea is present, remember *C. difficile*.

Treatment

- Treat with **empiric antimicrobials.**
- **Broad-spectrum antibiotics** cover both gram-positive organisms and *Pseudomonas.*
- There are two accepted strategies—**monotherapy** (e.g., antipseudomonal cephalosporin) and **dual therapy** (e.g., aminoglycoside plus antipseudomonal penicillin).
- Consider **vancomycin** in the presence of the following:
  - A central venous catheter.
  - Substantial mucosal damage.
  - Positive blood cultures for a gram-positive organism.
  - Known colonization with methicillin-resistant *S. aureus.*
  - Hypotension or sepsis with no identified organism.
- **Reassess in 3–5 days:**
  - If the clinical picture has not worsened, continue the same treatment.
  - If cultures are negative, stop vancomycin.

TABLE 9-14. Risk of Severe Infection in Neutropenic Fever

	Low Risk	High Risk
Expected duration of neutropenia	≤ 7 days	> 7 days
Neutrophil nadir	> 100	≤ 100
Hepatic and renal function	Normal	Abnormal
Feature of malignancy	Remission	Uncontrolled
Bone marrow transplant	No	Yes
Comorbidities (e.g., inpatient, age > 60, COPD, prior fungal infection)	Absent	Present
Clinical distress (e.g., dehydration, hypotension, altered mental status)	Absent	Present

In febrile neutropenia, G-CSF reduces the duration of neutropenia by 1–2 days but does not reduce mortality.

  - If still febrile, consider adding antifungal coverage.
  - If the clinical picture has worsened, change antimicrobials.
- **Duration of antimicrobial therapy:**
  - Generally, continue antimicrobials until ANC > 500 and the patient is afebrile for 48 hours.
  - If low risk, stop antimicrobials regardless of ANC if the patient is afebrile for 5–7 days.
  - If the patient is persistently febrile but ANC ≥ 500, consider stopping antimicrobials after 4–5 days and evaluate for other sources of fever.
- **G-CSF and GM-CSF (filgrastim and sargramostim):**
  - Use is accepted in febrile neutropenia.
  - **Not** indicated in afebrile neutropenia or to **prevent** febrile neutropenia **unless the patient is high risk** (e.g., elderly, HIV, prior chemotherapy, active infection).

Pancytopenia

Almost always represents decreased bone marrow activity. Differentiated as follows:

- **Intrinsic bone marrow failure:**
  - Aplastic anemia
  - Myelodysplasia
  - Acute leukemia
  - Myeloma
  - Drugs—chemotherapy, chloramphenicol, sulfonamides, antibiotics
- **Infectious:**
  - HIV
  - Post-hepatitis
  - Parvovirus B19
- **Marrow infiltration:**
  - TB
  - Disseminated fungal infection (especially coccidioidomycosis, histoplasmosis)
  - Metastatic malignancy

Peripheral smear morphology is often helpful in diagnosis (see Tables 9-15 and 9-16).

TABLE 9-15. Summary of Peripheral Smear Morphology—RBCs

RBC Form	Associated Conditions
Schistocytes	Microangiopathy, intravascular hemolysis
Spherocytes	Extravascular hemolysis, hereditary spherocytosis
Target cell	Liver disease, hemoglobinopathy
Teardrop cell	Myelofibrosis, thalassemia
Burr cell (echinocyte)	Uremia
Spur cell (acanthocyte)	Liver disease
Howell-Jolly body	Postsplenectomy, functional asplenia

TABLE 9-16. Summary of Peripheral Smear Morphology—WBCs

WBC Form	Associated Conditions
Atypical lymphocyte	Mononucleosis, toxoplasma, CMV, HIV
Döhle body, toxic granulations	Infections, sepsis
Hypersegmented neutrophil	B_{12} deficiency
Auer rods	AML (especially M3)
Pelger-Huët anomaly	Myelodysplasia, congenital

BONE MARROW FAILURE SYNDROMES

Aplastic Anemia

Marrow failure with hypocellular bone marrow and no dysplasia. Typically seen in young adults or the elderly. Subtypes are as follows:

- **Autoimmune (primary):** The **most common type.** Assumed when secondary causes are ruled out.
- Secondary aplastic anemia is caused by multiple factors:
  - **Toxins:** Benzene, toluene, insecticides.
  - **Drugs:** Gold, chloramphenicol, clozapine, sulfonamides, tolbutamide, phenytoin, carbamazepine, and many others.
  - Post-chemotherapy or radiation.
  - **Viral:** Post-hepatitis, parvovirus B19, HIV, CMV, EBV.
  - PNH.
  - Pregnancy.

Symptoms/Exam

- Presents with symptoms of pancytopenia (fatigue, bleeding, infections).
- Adenopathy and splenomegaly **are not seen.**

Diagnosis

- **Labs: Pancytopenia** and **markedly decreased reticulocytes** are classically seen.
- **Peripheral smear:** Pancytopenia without dysplastic changes.
- **Bone marrow:** Hypocellular without dysplasia.

Treatment

- Supportive care as necessary (transfusions, antibiotics).
- Primary aplastic anemia:
  - Definitive treatment is allogeneic bone marrow transplant.
  - Remissions can sometimes be induced with antithymocyte globulin and cyclosporin.
- Treat secondary aplastic anemia by correcting the underlying disorder.

Pure Red Cell Aplasia (PRCA)

Marrow failure in erythroid lineage only.

Symptoms/Exam

Symptoms are related to anemia.

Differential

After other causes of isolated anemia have been excluded, distinguish autoimmune PRCA from that stemming from abnormal erythropoiesis.

- **Autoimmune:**
  - **Thymoma**
  - Lymphoma, CLL
  - HIV
  - SLE
  - Parvovirus B19
- **Abnormal erythropoiesis:**
  - Hereditary spherocytosis
  - Sickle cell anemia
  - Drugs (phenytoin, chloramphenicol)

Diagnosis

- **CBC:** Presents with anemia that is often profound, but WBC and platelet counts are normal. Markedly decreased reticulocytes.
- **Peripheral smear:** No dysplastic changes.
- **Bone marrow biopsy:** Abnormal erythroid maturation and characteristic giant pronormoblasts seen in parvovirus B19 infection.
- Parvovirus B19 serology or PCR.

Treatment

- IVIG may be helpful in cases due to parvovirus.
- Remove thymoma if present.
- Immunosuppression with antithymocyte globulin and cyclosporin.

Myelodysplastic Syndrome (MDS)

A clonal stem cell disorder that is characterized by dysplasia resulting in ineffective hematopoiesis, and that exists on a continuum with acute leukemia. Eighty percent of patients are > 60 years of age. MDS is associated with myelotoxic drugs and ionizing radiation and carries the risk of transforming to AML (but almost never to ALL). Its prognosis is related to the percentage of blasts, cytogenetics, and the number of cytopenias (see Table 9-17).

Symptoms/Exam

Symptoms are related to those of cytopenias.

Differential

Dysplasia can occur with vitamin B_{12} deficiency, viral infections (including HIV), and exposure to marrow toxins, so these factors must be ruled out before a diagnosis of MDS is made.

TABLE 9-17. Classification of Myelodysplastic Syndromes

SUBTYPE	CYTOPENIA	BLASTS	OTHER
Refractory anemia (RA)	At least one lineage.	< 1% in peripheral blood, < 5% in bone marrow.	
Refractory anemia with ringed sideroblasts (RARS)	At least one lineage.	< 1% in peripheral blood, < 5% in bone marrow.	> 15% ringed sideroblasts in marrow.
Refractory anemia with excess blasts (RAEB)	Two or more lineages.	< 5% in peripheral blood, 5–20% in bone marrow.	
Chronic myelomonocytic leukemia (CMML)		< 5% in peripheral blood, < 20% in bone marrow.	Peripheral blood monocytosis (> 1×10^9/L).
Refractory anemia with excess blasts in transformation (RAEB-T)			No longer used.

DIAGNOSIS

- Peripheral smear shows **dysplasia** (see Figure 9-10).
  - **RBCs:** Macrocytosis, macro-ovalocytes.
  - **WBCs:** Hypogranularity, hypolobulation (pseudo–Pelger-Huët).
  - **Platelets:** Giant or hypogranular.
- **Bone marrow:** Dysplasia and typically hypercellular.

TREATMENT

- Supportive care with transfusions, growth factors (generally associated with a poor response).
- Bone marrow transplantation is occasionally performed in younger patients.

MYELOPROLIFERATIVE SYNDROMES

A group of syndromes characterized by **clonal increase of bone marrow RBCs, WBCs, platelets, or fibroblasts.** Each is defined by the cell lineages predominantly affected. Syndromes have **considerable clinical overlap,** and occasionally it is difficult to distinguish between them (see Table 9-18).

Polycythemia Vera

Defined as an abnormal increase in all blood cells, predominantly RBCs. The most common of myeloproliferative disorders, it shows no clear age predominance.

SYMPTOMS/EXAM

- **Splenomegaly** is common.
- Symptoms are related to higher blood viscosity and expanded blood volume and include dizziness, headache, tinnitus, blurred vision, and plethora.

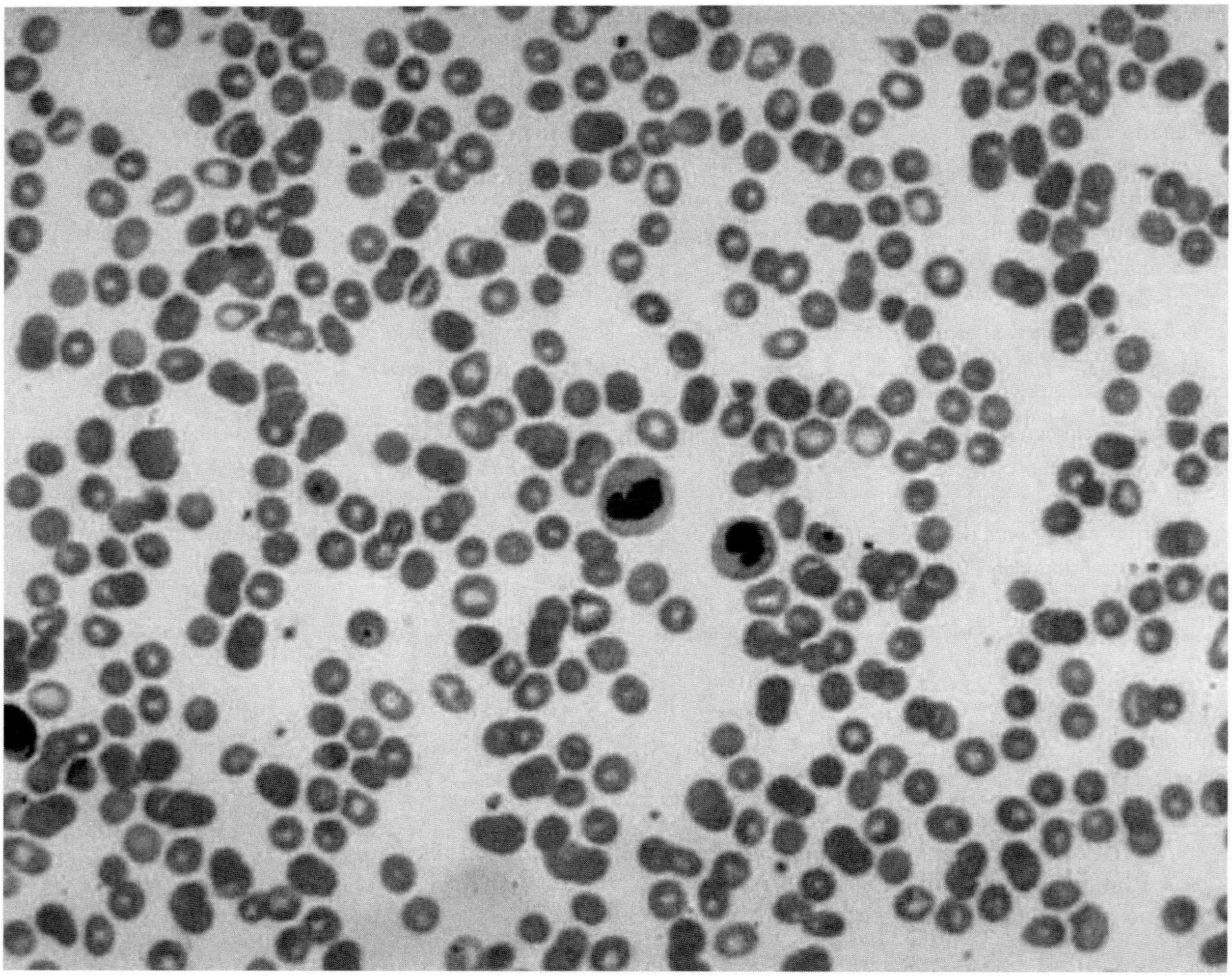

FIGURE 9-10. Myelodysplasia.

Both neutrophils in this slide demonstrate hypogranulation and hypolobation (pseudo–Pelger-Huët anomaly), suggesting myelodysplasia. (Courtesy of L Damon. Reproduced, with permission, from Linker CA. Hematology. In Tierney LM et al [eds]. *Current Medical Diagnosis & Treatment 2005*, 44th ed. New York: McGraw-Hill, 2005.) (Also see Color Insert.)

TABLE 9-18. Differentiation of Myeloproliferative Syndromes

	WBC	Hematocrit	Platelets	RBC Morphology
Polycythemia vera	Normal or increased	**Increased**	Normal or increased	Normal
CML	**Increased**	Normal or decreased	Normal	Normal
Myelofibrosis	Variable	Usually decreased	Variable	**Abnormal**
Essential thrombocythemia	Normal or increased	Normal	**Increased**	Normal

- **Erythromelalgia** is frequently associated with polycythemia vera and is characterized by erythema, warmth, and pain in the distal extremities. May progress to digital ischemia.
- Other findings include generalized pruritus, epistaxis, hyperuricemia, and iron deficiency from chronic GI bleeding.

DIAGNOSIS

- Exclude secondary erythrocytosis.
- Bone marrow aspirate and biopsy with cytogenetics.
- **Diagnostic criteria from the Polycythemia Vera Study Group** are outlined in Table 9-19.

Up to 20% of PV patients have thrombosis as presenting event.

TREATMENT

- **No treatment clearly affects the natural history of the disease,** so treatment should be aimed at controlling symptoms.
- **Phlebotomy** to keep hematocrit < 45% treats viscosity symptoms.
- Helpful medications include the following:
  - Hydroxyurea or anagrelide to keep platelet count < 400,000; prevents thromboses.
  - Allopurinol if uric acid is elevated.
  - The current standard is to recommend **low-dose aspirin** in patients with erythromelalgia or other microvascular manifestations. **Avoid aspirin in patients with a history of GI bleeding.**

COMPLICATIONS

Predisposes to both clotting and bleeding; may progress to myelofibrosis or acute leukemia.

Chronic Myelogenous Leukemia (CML)

An excessive accumulation of neutrophils that can transform to an acute process. It is defined by chromosomal translocation t(9;22), the **Philadelphia chromosome.**

SYMPTOMS/EXAM

- Hepatosplenomegaly is variable.
- Pruritus, flushing, diarrhea, fatigue, night sweats.
- **Leukostasis symptoms** (visual disturbances, headache, dyspnea, MI, TIA/CVA, priapism) typically occur when **WBC > 500,000.**

TABLE 9-19. Polycythemia Vera Study Group Criteria[a]

A1: Raised RBC mass or hematocrit ≥ 60% in males, 56% in females	**B1:** Platelet count > 400,000
A2: Absence of cause of secondary erythrocytosis	**B2:** Neutrophil count > 10,000 (> 12,500 in smokers)
A3: Palpable splenomegaly	**B3:** Splenomegaly by imaging
A4: Abnormal marrow karyotype	**B4:** Characteristic bone marrow colony growth (almost never used) or **low serum erythropoietin**

[a]A1 + A2 + A3 or A4 = polycythemia vera; A1 + A2 + any two B = polycythemia vera.

Diagnosis

- Markedly elevated neutrophil count.
- May see basophilia, eosinophilia, and thrombocytosis (see Figure 9-11).
- Leukocyte alkaline phosphatase (LAP) is low but rarely needed.
- The disease has three phases based on the percentage of blasts in peripheral blood:
  - **Chronic phase:** Bone marrow and circulating blasts < 10%.
  - **Accelerated phase:** Bone marrow or circulating blasts 10–20%.
  - **Blast crisis:** Bone marrow or circulating blasts ≥ 20%.
- The **Philadelphia chromosome is present in 90–95% of cases.** Detectable by cytogenetics or by PCR for the **BCR-ABL** fusion gene, performed on peripheral WBCs.
- Bone marrow biopsy is not necessary for diagnosis but is often done to determine the prognosis.

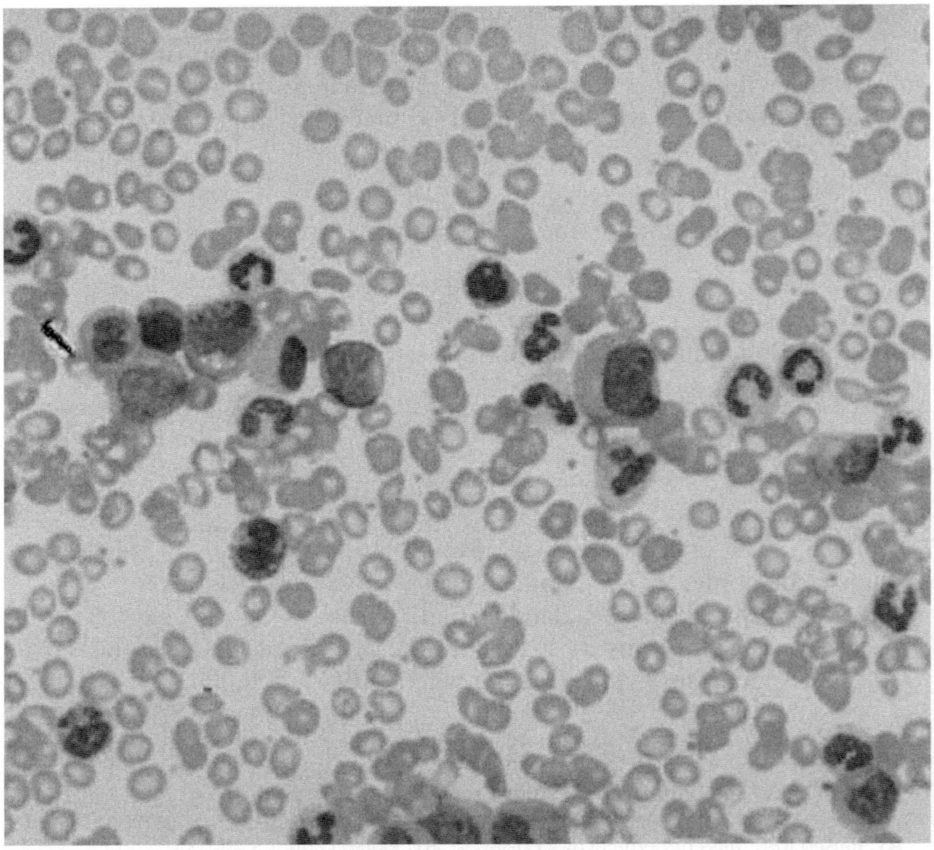

FIGURE 9-11. Chronic myelogenous leukemia.

Note the large number of immature myeloid forms in the peripheral blood, including metamyelocytes, myelocytes, and promyelocytes, as well as a large number of eosinophils and basophils. (Courtesy of L Damon. Reproduced, with permission, from Linker CA. Hematology. In Tierney LM et al [eds]. *Current Medical Diagnosis & Treatment 2005*, 44th ed. New York: McGraw-Hill, 2005.) (Also see Color Insert.)

TREATMENT

- The only curative therapy remains allogeneic bone marrow transplantation.
- Major remissions can virtually always be achieved with **imatinib mesylate (Gleevec).** However, the durability of these responses remains uncertain.
- Palliative therapies to reduce WBC counts include hydroxyurea, α-interferon, and low-dose cytarabine.

COMPLICATIONS

The natural history is progression from the chronic phase to the accelerated phase (median 3–4 years) and then to blast crisis.

Myelofibrosis (Agnogenic Myeloid Metaplasia)

Fibrosis of bone marrow leading to **extramedullary hematopoiesis** (marked splenomegaly, bizarre peripheral blood smear). Affects adults > 50 years of age and can be secondary to marrow insults, including other myeloproliferative disorders, radiation, toxins, and metastatic malignancies.

SYMPTOMS/EXAM

- Characterized by symptoms of cytopenias. Fatigue and bleeding are especially common.
- Abdominal fullness due to marked splenomegaly; hepatomegaly.

DIAGNOSIS

- **CBC:** Individual cytopenias or **pancytopenia.**
- **Abnormal peripheral smear: Teardrops,** immature WBCs, nucleated RBCs, giant degranulated platelets (see Figure 9-12).
- Bone marrow aspirate is usually **dry tap;** biopsy shows marked fibrosis.

TREATMENT

- Treatment is mostly supportive.
- Transfusions as necessary, but may be difficult with hypersplenism.
- Splenectomy or splenic irradiation if the spleen is painful or if transfusion requirements are unacceptably high.
- α-interferon or thalidomide is occasionally helpful.
- Allogeneic bone marrow transplantation for appropriate patients.

COMPLICATIONS

May evolve into AML with an extremely poor prognosis.

Essential Thrombocythemia

A clonal disorder with elevated platelet counts and a tendency toward thrombosis and bleeding. Has an indolent course with a **median survival > 15 years** from diagnosis.

SYMPTOMS/EXAM

- Patients are usually asymptomatic at presentation.
- Occasionally presents with erythromelalgia, pruritus, and thrombosis (at risk for both arterial and venous clots).

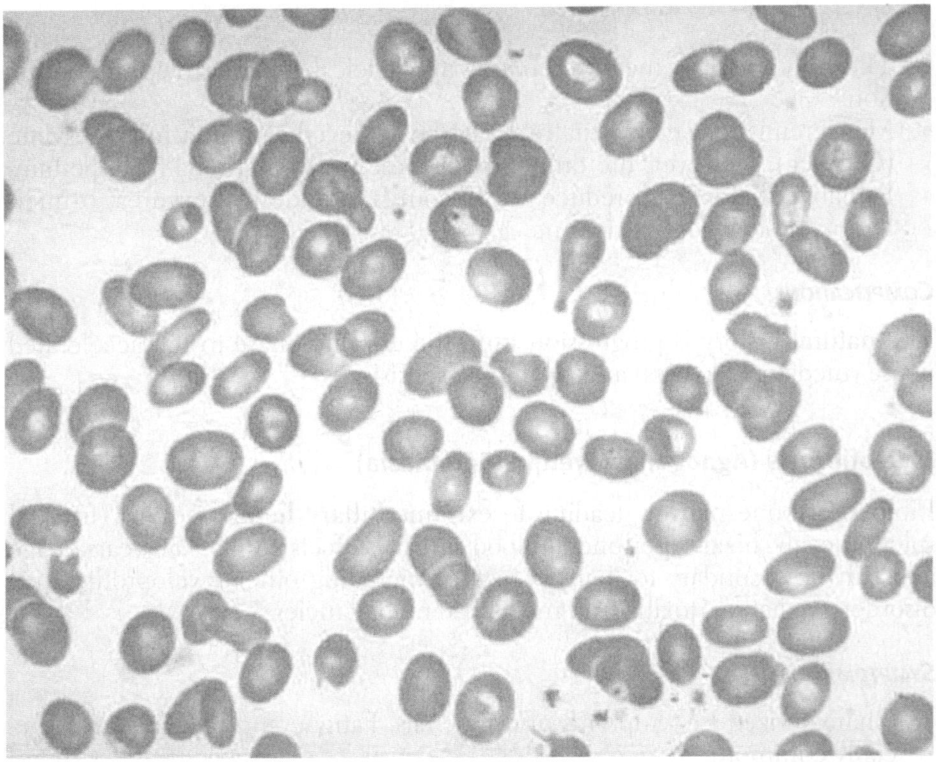

FIGURE 9-12. Myelofibrosis.

Note the large number of teardrop cells suggestive of bone marrow infiltrative disease.(Courtesy of L Damon. Reproduced, with permission, from Linker CA. Hematology. In Tierney LM et al [eds]. *Current Medical Diagnosis & Treatment 2005*, 44th ed. New York: McGraw-Hill, 2005.) (Also see Color Insert.)

Diagnosis

- Primarily a **diagnosis of exclusion.** The first step is to rule out secondary causes of thrombocytosis (see separate section).
- Diagnosed by a persistent platelet count > 600,000 with no other cause of thrombocytosis.

Treatment

- No treatment is needed if there is no evidence of thrombotic phenomena and platelet count < 500,000.
- Control platelet count with hydroxyurea, α-interferon, or anagrelide.
- Consider platelet pheresis for elevated platelets with severe bleeding or clotting.

Complications

The risk of converting to acute leukemia is approximately 5% over a patient's lifetime.

PLASMA CELL DYSCRASIAS

A group of disorders characterized by abnormal production of a paraprotein and often due to a monoclonal proliferation of plasma cells.

Amyloidosis

A rare disorder characterized by the deposition of amyloid material throughout the body. Amyloid is composed of amyloid P protein and a fibrillar component. **The most common are AA and AL amyloid** (see Table 9-20).

SYMPTOMS/EXAM

The characteristics of amyloidosis are somewhat dependent on the type of amyloid and organs involved:

- **Renal:** Proteinuria, nephrotic syndrome, renal failure.
- **Cardiac:** Infiltrative cardiomyopathy, conduction block, arrhythmia, low-voltage ECG, hypertrophy, and a **"speckled" pattern on echocardiography.**
- **GI tract:** Dysmotility, obstruction, malabsorption.
- **Soft tissues: Macroglossia, carpal tunnel syndrome,** "shoulder pad sign," "raccoon eyes."
- **Nervous system:** Peripheral neuropathy.
- **Hematopoietic:** Anemia, dysfibrinogenemia, factor X deficiency, bleeding.
- **Respiratory:** Hypoxia, nodules.

DIAGNOSIS

- **Tissue biopsy:** Amyloid yields the characteristic **apple-green birefringence** with Congo red stain.
- The choice of biopsy site depends on the clinical situation:
  - Biopsy of involved tissue has the highest yield.
  - Fat pad aspirate or rectal biopsies are generally low yield but minimally invasive.
- Once amyloid has been identified, investigate whether major organs are involved:
  - Check ECG and 24-hour urinary protein.
  - SPEP to screen for plasma cell dysplasia.
  - Consider malabsorption studies and echocardiography.

TABLE 9-20. Amyloid Types and Fibrillar Components

TYPE	FIBRILLAR COMPONENT	ASSOCIATION
AA	Acute-phase apolipoproteins	Chronic inflammation (TB, osteomyelitis, leprosy, familial Mediterranean fever)
AL	Immunoglobulin light chain	Plasma cell dyscrasia (e.g., multiple myeloma)
ATTR	Transthyretin	Familial
AM	β_2-microglobulin	Hemodialysis

TREATMENT

- **Amyloid due to familial Mediterranean fever:** Colchicine.
- **AL amyloid:** Treat as for myeloma.

COMPLICATIONS

Cardiac involvement associated with an extremely poor prognosis.

Multiple Myeloma

A malignancy of plasma cells that is often seen in older adults (> 60 years of age) and is almost always characterized by elevated IgG or IgA paraprotein **(M spike)** in serum or urine.

SYMPTOMS/EXAM

Due to two aspects of myeloma:

- **Plasma cell infiltration: Lytic bone lesions,** osteoporosis, **hypercalcemia, anemia,** plasmacytomas.
- **Paraprotein:** Depression of normal immunoglobulins leads to **infections;** excess protein may cause **renal tubular disease, amyloidosis,** or **narrowed anion gap** (due to positively charged paraproteins).

DIFFERENTIAL

The differential diagnosis of paraproteinemias is as follows (see Table 9-21):

- Amyloidosis.
- **Monoclonal gammopathy of undetermined significance (MGUS):**
  - Presence of M spike without other criteria for myeloma.
  - One percent per year convert to myeloma, so monitor regularly for the development of myeloma.
- **Waldenström's macroglobulinemia:**
  - A low-grade B-cell neoplasm characterized by **IgM** paraprotein.
  - **Elevated serum viscosity** (blurry vision, headaches, bleeding).

Table 9-21. Distinguishing Features of Various Monoclonal Paraproteinemias

	Myeloma	MGUS	Waldenström's Macroglobulinemia	Amyloidosis
Abnormal cell	Plasma cell	Plasma cell	Lymphoplasmacytes	Plasma cell
Lytic bone lesions	Present	Absent	Absent	Absent
Paraprotein	> 3.5 g IgG or > 2 g IgA	Less than myeloma	Any IgM	Any
Bone marrow	> 10% plasma cells	< 10% plasma cells	Lymphoplasmacytes	Amyloid deposition
Tissue involvement	Plasmacytomas	None	None	Amyloid deposition
Splenomegaly or adenopathy	Absent	Absent	Present	Absent

- Characterized by an indolent clinical course; treat as for low-grade non-Hodgkin's lymphoma.

DIAGNOSIS

The diagnostic criteria for multiple myeloma are delineated below and summarized in Table 9-22.

- CBC, creatinine, calcium, β_2-microglobulin, LDH.
- **SPEP with immunofixation electrophoresis (IFE), 24-hour UPEP:** To identify the M spike. Not all serum paraproteins are detectable in urine and vice versa.
- Bone marrow aspirate and biopsy.
- **Skeletal bone plain film survey: Lytic lesions** are seen in 60–90% of patients.
- Myeloma is a purely osteolytic lesion, so **bone scan is negative and alkaline phosphatase is normal.**

*Features **not** seen in myeloma include elevated alkaline phosphatase, positive bone scan, and splenomegaly. M spike may not be seen on UPEP or SPEP—obtain IFE if you still suspect myeloma.*

TREATMENT

- **Myeloma is incurable** except in rare patients who can receive allogeneic stem cell transplantation.
- Methods for reducing symptoms and preventing complications are listed in Table 9-23.

COMPLICATIONS

Infection, renal failure, pathologic bony fractures, hypercalcemia, anemia.

BLEEDING DISORDERS

Approach to Abnormal Bleeding

Excessive bleeding due to a defect in one of three variables: **blood vessels, coagulation factors,** and **platelets.**

BLOOD VESSEL DISORDERS

- A rare cause of abnormal bleeding.
- Weakness of the vessel wall may be **hereditary** (e.g., Ehlers-Danlos, Marfan's) or **acquired** (e.g., vitamin C deficiency or "scurvy," trauma, vasculitis).
- Bleeding is typically **petechial or purpuric,** occurring around areas of trauma or pressure (e.g., BP cuffs, collars, belt lines).

TABLE 9-22. Diagnostic Criteria for Multiple Myeloma[a]

MAJOR CRITERIA	MINOR CRITERIA
Bone marrow with > 30% plasma cells.	Bone marrow plasmacytosis 10–30%.
Monoclonal spike on SPEP > 3.5 g/dL for IgG or 2 g/dL for IgA, or ≥ 1 g/24 hours of light chain on UPEP in the presence of amyloidosis.	Monoclonal globulin spike less than levels in column 1.
	Lytic bone lesions.
Plasmacytoma on tissue biopsy.	Residual normal IgM < 50 mg/dL, IgA < 100 mg/dL, or IgG < 600 mg/dL.

[a] Diagnosis is established with one major and one minor criterion **or** with three minor criteria.

TABLE 9-23. Treatment of Multiple Myeloma

GOAL	TREATMENT
Reduce paraprotein	High-dose chemotherapy with autologous stem cell rescue (standard of care, but limited to patients with good functional status). Allogeneic bone marrow transplantation (experimental). Steroid and alkylator combination chemotherapy. Biological molecules (thalidomide, bortezomib).
Prevent skeletal complications	IV bisphosphonate if any evidence of skeletal compromise (bony lesions, osteopenia, hypercalcemia). No data for oral bisphosphonates. Radiation therapy and/or orthopedic surgery for impending pathologic fractures in weight-bearing bones.
Prevent infections	Pneumococcal and *Haemophilus* vaccines if not already immune. Reduce paraprotein. All fevers should be presumed infectious until proven otherwise.
Alleviate anemia	Reduce paraprotein. Consider erythropoietin or transfusion if severely symptomatic.
Prevent renal failure	Reduce paraprotein. Prevent hypercalcemia, dehydration.

COAGULATION FACTOR DISORDERS

- Significant bleeding risk only when clotting factor activity falls below 10%.
- More likely to see **hemarthroses** or deep tissue bleeds.
- Clotting factor disorders are either inherited or acquired.
  - **Inherited** (see separate sections):
    - **Hemophilia A:** Deficiency in factor **VIII.**
    - **Hemophilia B:** Deficiency in factor **IX.**
    - von Willebrand's disease (vWD).
  - **Acquired:**
    - **Factor inhibitors:** Elderly patients or patients with autoimmune diseases may acquire inhibitor, usually against factor VIII or factor VII.
    - Warfarin or heparin.
    - **Amyloid:** Associated with absorption of factor X in amyloid protein.
    - **Dysfibrinogenemia:** Seen in liver disease, HIV, lymphoma, and DIC.

*Remember the two causes of prolonged PTT that are **not** associated with bleeding: **lupus anticoagulant** (associated with clotting) and **factor XII deficiency** (no associated bleeding tendency).*

The differential diagnosis of clotting factor disorders is further outlined in Tables 9-24 and 9-25.

PLATELET DISORDERS

- Cause **petechiae,** mucosal bleeding, and menorrhagia; **exacerbated by aspirin.**
- Bleeding time is usually not necessary to determine.

TABLE 9-24. Diagnosis of Clotting Factor Disorders

CONDITION	PT	PTT	MIXING STUDY
Factor VII deficiency, warfarin use, vitamin K deficiency	Elevated	Normal	Corrects
Hemophilia	Normal	Elevated	Corrects
Heparin	Normal	Elevated	No correction unless heparin-adsorbed
Factor VIII inhibitor	Normal	Elevated	No correction
Lupus anticoagulant	Normal	Elevated	No correction (test with Russell viper venom)
DIC	Elevated	Elevated	Minimal correction
Liver disease	Elevated	Elevated	Corrects
Dysfibrinogenemia	Elevated	Elevated	Variable correction (test with reptilase time)

- Defects may be **quantitative** (see the thrombocytopenia section) **or qualitative.**
- **Qualitative platelet disorders:**
  - The **most common inherited defect is von Willebrand's factor (vWF) deficiency** (see separate section).
  - **Others:** Meds (aspirin, NSAIDs, IIB/IIIA inhibitors), uremia, and rare inherited defects (Glanzmann's, Bernard-Soulier).

Hemophilia

Hemophilias are **X-linked** deficiencies in clotting factors, so almost all patients are **male.**

- **Hemophilia A** = factor VIII deficiency (**"A eight"**).
- **Hemophilia B** = factor IX deficiency (**"B nine"**).

SYMPTOMS/EXAM

- Spontaneous bleeding in deep tissues, GI tract, and joints (hemarthroses).
- Variable severity, in part due to percent factor activity.
- Normal PT, prolonged PTT, mixing study corrects defect (unless inhibitor is present).
- Factor VIII or factor IX activity is low (0–10%).

Table 9-25. Review of Special Coagulation Tests

- **Mixing study:** To distinguish factor deficiency from inhibitor
- **Reptilase time:** To test for dysfibrinogenemia
- **Russell viper venom test:** To test for lupus anticoagulant
- **Ristocetin cofactor assay:** To test for vWF activity

TREATMENT

- There are two options for factor replacement:
  - **Recombinant factor:** Associated with less danger of HIV and HCV transmission than purified factor, but expensive.
  - **Purified factor concentrates:** Currently much safer than previous concentrates.
- Patients should be taught to self-administer factor in the event of spontaneous bleeding.
- Prophylaxis before procedures is as follows:
  - **Minor procedures:** For hemophilia A, DDAVP can be used if baseline factor VIII is 5–10%. Otherwise, replace with factor concentrates to 50–100% activity.
  - **Major procedures:** Replace with factor concentrate to 100% activity for the duration of the procedure and for 10–14 days.
- Acute bleeding:
  - **Minor bleeding:** Replace with factor concentrate to 25–50% activity.
  - **Major bleeding** (hemarthroses, deep tissue bleeding): Replace to 50% activity for 2–3 days.

von Willebrand's Disease (vWD)

The **most common inherited bleeding disorder.** In vWD, vWF complexes with factor VIII to induce platelet aggregation.

Aspirin is a common trigger of bleeding in patients with vWD and should be avoided.

SYMPTOMS/EXAM

- Exhibits a bleeding pattern similar to that of a platelet disorder (**petechiae,** mucosal bleeding/epistaxis, heavy menses, **exacerbated by aspirin**).
- Bleeding is almost always provoked (e.g., by aspirin, trauma, surgery).

DIAGNOSIS

- There are three basic types; type I is the most common (see Table 9-26).
- **Workup complex: Bleeding time** with aspirin provocation is often used as a screening tool; more specific tests are then added (ristocetin cofactor activity, von Willebrand multimers).

TREATMENT

- Avoid NSAIDs.

TABLE 9-26. Diagnosis of von Willebrand's Disease

Type	Factor VIII Antigen	vWF Activity (Ristocetin Cofactor)	vWF Multimers	DDAVP OK
I	Low/normal	Low (< 30%)	Normal	Yes
IIA	Low/normal	Absent	Abnormal	Yes
IIB	Low/normal	Low/normal	Abnormal	No
III	Low	Absent	Absent	Yes

- Prophylaxis before procedures includes the following:
  - DDAVP is acceptable for minor procedures **except** in type IIB.
  - Purified factor VIII for major procedures.

Disseminated Intravascular Coagulation (DIC)

Consumptive coagulopathy is characterized by **thrombocytopenia, elevated PT and PTT,** and **schistocytes** on peripheral smear in association with serious illness. Acute DIC is often a catastrophic event. In contrast, chronic DIC shows milder features and is associated with chronic illness (disseminated malignancy, intravascular thrombus).

Symptoms/Exam

- **Bleeding:** Oozing from venipuncture sites or wounds, spontaneous tissue bleeding, mucosal bleeding.
- **Clotting:** Digital gangrene, renal cortical necrosis, **underlying serious illness** (typically sepsis, trauma, or malignancy).

Diagnosis

- Low fibrinogen, platelets.
- Prolonged PT; variably prolonged PTT.
- The presence of microangiopathy (e.g., **schistocytes**) and elevated D-dimers is characteristic.

Lab tests in liver disease can mimic DIC (high D-dimers, prolonged PT and PTT, low platelets and fibrinogen). Schistocytes and the presence of an underlying disease associated with DIC make DIC more probable.

Treatment

- Treat the underlying cause.
- If there is no serious bleeding or clotting, no specific therapy is needed.
- Adjuncts include the following:
  - Cryoprecipitate to achieve fibrinogen > 150 mg/dL.
  - FFP if antithrombin III levels are low.
  - Platelet transfusions if severe bleeding and platelet count < 50.
  - Heparin at 500–750 U/hour can treat thrombotic complications, but titrate to a high normal PTT to prevent excessive bleeding

Idiopathic Thrombocytopenic Purpura (ITP)

A disorder of reduced platelet survival, typically by immune destruction in the spleen. ITP commonly occurs in childhood with viral illnesses but may also affect young adults. Subtypes are as follows:

- **Primary:** No identifiable cause.
- **Secondary:** Medications (gold, quinine, β-lactam antibiotics), CLL, SLE.

Symptoms/Exam

- Typically presents with petechiae, **purpura, mucosal bleeding,** and **menorrhagia.**
- **Spleen size is usually normal.**

Diagnosis

- Diagnosis is made by excluding other causes of thrombocytopenia.
- Antiplatelet antibodies, platelet survival times, degree of increase in platelet count after platelet transfusion, and bone marrow biopsy are **not** needed for diagnosis.

TREATMENT

Consensus guidelines are that treatment is not necessary if platelet counts > 50 and there is no bleeding. In the presence of acute bleeding, platelets can be transfused. Further treatment guidelines are given in Table 9-27.

CLOTTING DISORDERS

An extensive workup for thrombophilia is generally not indicated after a first DVT. Looking for extremely rare genetic conditions to explain a common problem is not cost-effective, and finding a genetic mutation does not always help the patient.

Approach to Thrombophilia

Venous thromboembolism (VTE) is **common,** affecting 1–3 in 1000 persons per year. Risk factors include pregnancy, surgery, smoking, prolonged immobilization, hospitalization for any cause, and active malignancy. In patients with a prior clot, recurrence rates are approximately 0.5% per year even when fully anticoagulated, with the highest risk occurring in the first year. An inherited thrombophilic state may be suspected in the following conditions:

- An unprovoked clot occurring in a young person (< 50 years of age).
- A clot in an unusual location (e.g., mesenteric vein, sagittal sinus).
- An unusually extensive clot.
- Arterial and venous clots.
- Strong family history.

DIFFERENTIAL

Look for a pattern of clots (see Table 9-28).

DIAGNOSIS

- Diagnostic testing during an **acute** thrombotic episode includes the following:
  - A **targeted history and physical exam** to screen for the disorders outlined in Table 9-28.
  - **CBC and peripheral smear** to screen for myeloproliferative syndrome.
  - **Baseline PTT** to screen for antiphospholipid antibody syndrome. If prolonged before anticoagulation, evaluate with Russell viper venom test.

TABLE 9-27. Treatment of ITP

TREATMENT	DOSE	EFFICACY	NOTES
Prednisone	1 mg/kg/day × 4–6 weeks	60% response rate	Time to remission 1–3 weeks.
IVIG	1 g/kg ×1 or 0.4 g/kg/day ×2	80–90% response rate	Rapid remission, but short-lived. Used for acute bleeding risk.
Splenectomy	N/A	70% remission rate	May require looking for accessory spleen.
Danazol	600 mg/day	10–80% response rate	Usually second line.
Anti-RhD	50 μg/kg ×1	80–90% response rate	Induces hemolytic anemia; works only with Rh^+ patients.

TABLE 9-28. Differential Diagnosis of Clotting Disorders

CLOT LOCATION	DIFFERENTIAL DIAGNOSIS
Arterial and venous	Malignancy Heparin-induced thrombocytopenia (HIT) syndrome Hyperhomocysteinemia PNH Myeloproliferative diseases Antiphospholipid antibody syndrome
Venous only	Factor V Leiden Prothrombin 20210 mutation Protein C or S deficiency Antithrombin III deficiency Oral estrogens Postsurgical, pregnancy, immobilization
Arterial only	Atherosclerosis Vasculitis

- Diagnostic testing in a **nonacute setting** proceeds as follows:
  - Best done when considering whether to stop or prolong anticoagulation:
    - Stop warfarin for two weeks (warfarin interferes with many of the tests).
    - Anticoagulation may be continued if desired with low-molecular-weight heparin (LMWH).
  - A typical "hypercoagulable panel" for venous thrombophilia includes the following:
    - Factor V Leiden
    - Prothrombin 20210 mutation
    - Resistance to activated protein C
    - Tests for antiphospholipid antibody
    - Homocysteine level
  - If there is a high probability of inherited thrombophilia, then add proteins C and S, and antithrombin III activity.

Of the specific tests for rare thrombophilic states, many are unreliable in the acute illness; only antiphospholipid antibody testing is indicated.

Factor V Leiden

Characterized by a gene frequency of 5% in unselected Caucasian populations and 0.05% in Asians and Africans. In unselected patients with DVT or PE, the incidence is 20%, and in patients with a high likelihood of inherited thrombophilia (young age, family history) it is 50%. Heterozygotes have a three- to eightfold increase in the risk of venous thrombosis; homozygotes have a 50- to 80-fold increased risk. In those with **venous clots only,** there is no increase in the risk of arterial clots.

DIAGNOSIS

The issue of whom to test for factor V Leiden is controversial. Table 9-29 outlines guidelines for making such a determination.

TABLE 9-29. Testing for Factor V Leiden

PROBABLY TEST	UNCLEAR WHETHER TO TEST	TESTING NOT RECOMMENDED
Unprovoked clot at young age (< 50 years).	All patients with unprovoked clots.	General population.
Clot in an unusual location or of unusual severity.	Clot after surgery or pregnancy despite prophylaxis.	All pregnant women.
Positive family history.		Women considering OCPs.
Recurrent thrombosis.		Presurgical screening.
Thrombosis provoked by pregnancy or OCPs.		

TREATMENT

The duration of anticoagulation after the first event should be as follows:

- **Heterozygous:** Same as for patients without the mutation.
- **Homozygous:** Extended anticoagulation is generally recommended.

PREVENTION

Guidelines for prophylaxis are as follows:

- Routine prophylaxis is generally not recommended if there is no history of clotting.
- Standard prophylaxis for surgical procedures.
- Recommend against smoking and OCPs.
- Prophylaxis during air travel is controversial.

Prothrombin 20210 Mutation

Characterized by a gene frequency of 2–3% in the general population, with a Caucasian predominance. The mutation causes a higher level of prothrombin, leading to a hypercoagulable state. In unselected patients with DVT or PE, 7% have the mutation. Heterozygotes have a threefold increased risk of thrombosis. Homozygous patients probably have a higher risk, but it is not well quantified. The disorder is not as well studied as factor V Leiden, but the approach and recommendations are similar.

Protein C and S Deficiency/Antithrombin III Deficiency

Rarer, but higher risk than factor V Leiden or prothrombin mutations. Given the rarity of these deficiencies, **testing is extremely low yield** in the absence of strong evidence of familial thrombophilia.

Hyperhomocysteinemia

Can be **genetic** (caused by a mutation in genes for cystathionine β-synthase or methylenetetrahydrofolate reductase) or **acquired** (due to a deficiency in B_6, B_{12}, or folate or to smoking, older age, or renal insufficiency). Associated with a twofold increased risk of venous thrombosis. Screen with fasting serum homocysteine level and treat with folate supplementation. Most authorities also recommend vitamins B_6 and B_{12}.

Antiphospholipid Antibody Syndrome (APLAS)

A syndrome of **vascular thrombi** or **recurrent spontaneous abortions** associated with laboratory evidence of autoantibody against phospholipids. Antiphospholipid antibodies are present in up to 5% of the general population, but the vast majority are transient and clinically insignificant.

Diagnosis

Diagnosis requires a clinical event **and** antiphospholipid antibody. Clinical characteristics are as follows:

- Venous and/or arterial thrombi.
- Thrombocytopenia.
- Livedo reticularis.
- Recurrent spontaneous abortions.
- **Antiphospholipid antibody:** Can include a variety of autoantibodies, but only one need be present.
  - **Lupus anticoagulant:** A clue to this may be prolonged PTT; confirm with a mixing study and Russell viper venom test.
  - **Anticardiolipin antibody.**
  - **Others:** Anti-phosphatidylserine, anti-β_2 glycoprotein I, **false positive VDRL.**

TABLE 9-30. Guide to Anticoagulant Medications

Medication	Pros	Cons	Tests Used to Monitor
UFH	Short half-life; can turn off quickly if patient bleeds. Although falling out of favor, still appropriate for acute coronary syndromes, cardiopulmonary bypass, acute thrombotic events, mechanical heart valves, and anticoagulation in renal failure.	Requires continuous IV infusion. Long-term use associated with osteoporosis. Risk of HIT.	Need to monitor PTT at least daily along with platelet count (for HIT). Reversible with protamine.
LMWH	**No need to monitor PTT—dosing is weight based.**	**Excretion is impaired in renal failure.** Not reversible with protamine. Requires injection.	**Will not prolong PTT;** if monitoring is required, measure factor Xa activity.
Warfarin	Oral.	Slow to reach therapeutic effect; requires adding UFH or LMWH when starting for acute clot. Teratogenic. Many drug interactions. Warfarin skin necrosis (rare).	**Monitor with INR;** appropriate INR and duration vary by clinical situation (see Table 9-31). Reversible with FFP or vitamin K.
Direct thrombin inhibitors (lepirudin or argatroban)	Used for anticoagulation in patients with HIT.	**Irreversible** thrombin inhibitors; require continuous IV infusion.	Monitor with PTT.

TREATMENT

Treatment is as follows (see also Table 9-30):

- **Acute thrombi:** Anticoagulate with LMWH, since PTT cannot be used to monitor unfractionated heparin (UFH).
- Long-term anticoagulation with warfarin. Target INR is controversial (see Table 9-31).
- Most authorities recommend **lifelong anticoagulation,** so it is important to verify the persistence of antiphospholipid.

Heparin-Induced Thrombocytopenia (HIT)

There are two types of HIT, as outlined in Table 9-32.

SYMPTOMS/EXAM

Type II HIT presents as follows:

- A decrease in platelet count after 4–7 days of exposure to heparin.
- May cause **arterial or venous clots.**
- Less common with LMWH than with UFH.
- Exposure to any dose of heparin (heparin flushes, heparin-coated catheters, minidose SQ heparin) can cause this syndrome.

DIAGNOSIS

- Type II HIT requires a high degree of clinical suspicion.
- Lab testing includes the following:
  - **Antibody against PF4** (platelet factor 4).
  - **Functional assay:** Detects abnormal platelet activation in response to heparin (heparin-induced platelet activation [HIPA], serotonin release).

TABLE 9-31. Guidelines for INR: Range and Duration of Anticoagulation

CONDITION	INR	DURATION
Provoked DVT/PE	2–3	6–18 weeks after offending condition resolved
Non-life-threatening DVT/PE	2–3	3–6 months
Life-threatening or severe DVT/PE	2–3	6–12 months vs. indefinite
Hereditary thrombophilia	2–3	6–12 months vs. indefinite
Atrial fibrillation (even paroxysmal)	2–3	Indefinite
Mitral stenosis with evidence of thrombosis or atrial fibrillation	2–3	Indefinite
Antiphospholipid antibody syndrome	2.5–4.0 (controversial)	Indefinite
Mechanical heart valve	3–4	Indefinite

TABLE 9-32. Types of HIT

Type	Dose-Dependent	Severity of Thrombocytopenia	Timing of Thrombocytopenia	Clinically Significant	Etiology
I	Yes	Mild	Immediate	No	Heparin-induced platelet clumping
II	No	Moderate/severe	4–7 days after exposure	**Yes**	Antibody against heparin-platelet complex

Treatment

- If any suspicion, immediately stop all heparin; do not wait for lab tests, as catastrophic clotting and/or bleeding can occur.
- If high suspicion, **treat with direct thrombin inhibitors** (lepirudin, argatroban) until platelet count recovers.
- Warfarin monotherapy is contraindicated in acute HIT with clots given the risk of skin necrosis.

Prevention

- Preferential use of LMWH given the lower incidence of HIT.
- If the patient has a history of HIT, do not use any heparin until 3–6 months have elapsed and lab tests are negative for HIT.

TRANSFUSION MEDICINE

Pretransfusion Testing

Pretransfusion tests include the following:

- **Type and cross:** Use when transfusion is **probable** (e.g., in an acutely bleeding patient). Test recipient plasma for reactivity against RBC from the donor—i.e., indirect Coombs' test on **donor** RBCs.
- **Type and screen** (aka "type and hold"): Use when transfusion is possible (e.g., in preoperative evaluation). Screen recipient plasma for antibody against a standardized RBC panel—i.e., indirect Coombs' test on **reference** RBCs.
- Consider the risks of transfusions (see Table 9-33).

*In noncardiac patients, aggressive transfusion strategies are associated with **worse** outcomes in ICU patients.*

Management of Transfusion Reactions

- Stop the transfusion immediately.
- Contact the blood bank immediately to start double-checking paperwork.
- Draw CBC, direct antiglobulin test, LDH, haptoglobin, indirect bilirubin, free hemoglobin, PT/PTT, UA, and urine hemoglobin.
- Repeat type and screen and draw blood culture.
- Send all untransfused blood with attached tubing back to the blood bank.

Transfusion Products

Table 9-34 lists common types of transfusion products and their applications.

TABLE 9-33. Risks of Transfusion Therapy

	RISK	CLINICAL FEATURES	TREATMENT	CAUSE	COMMENTS
Febrile nonhemolytic reactions	1–4 in 1000	Chills, rigors within 12 hours of transfusion.	Acetaminophen, diphenhydramine.	WBC or bacterial contaminant, or cytokines.	**Most common reaction.**
Allergic reaction	1–4 in 1000	Urticaria or bronchospasm.	As usual for urticaria or bronchospasm.	Allergic reaction to plasma contaminant.	Seen in **IgA deficiency;** prevented by using washed RBCs.
Delayed hemolysis	1 in 1000	Extravascular hemolysis 5–10 days after transfusion: jaundice, drop in hematocrit, positive Coombs' test, microspherocytes in peripheral smear.	Supportive care; send sample to blood bank to work up new alloantibody.	Low-titer antibodies against minor blood antigens.	Multiparous women or multiply transfused patients may be at greater risk.
Tranfusion-related acute lung injury (TRALI)	1 in 5000	**Noncardiogenic pulmonary edema,** usually **within six hours** of transfusion.	Supportive care.	Donor antibodies binding to recipient leukocytes in pulmonary capillaries.	Most cases resolve after 96 hours.
Acute hemolytic transfusion reaction	1 in 12,000	Chills, fever, backache, headache, hypotension, tachypnea, tachycardia. DIC may occur in severe cases.	Vigorous hydration to prevent acute tubular necrosis; if hemolysis is severe, consider forced diuresis with mannitol, urinary alkalinization.	**Severe** intravascular hemolysis due to preexisting antibody against donor RBC (typically ABO).	Usually due to a clerical error.
HBV	1 in 66,000				
HCV	1 in 103,000				
HIV	1 in 676,000				

Platelet Transfusion Threshold

The criteria for determining the platelet transfusion threshold are controversial but are as follows:

- A bleeding patient with a platelet count < 50,000.
- CNS bleeding with a platelet count < 100,000.

TABLE 9-34. Types of Transfusion Products

PRODUCT	DISTINGUISHING FEATURE	USE
Whole blood	Contains RBC and plasma.	Provides oxygen-carrying capacity and plasma volume expansion. For patients with massive blood loss (e.g., trauma).
Packed RBCs	RBC concentrated from donor unit.	Standard RBC product. Each unit raises hemoglobin 1 g/dL.
Washed RBCs	RBCs with plasma removed.	Prevent allergic reactions.
Irradiated RBCs	Irradiation.	Prevent graft-versus-host disease.
Leukocyte-depleted RBCs	Deplete donor leukocytes with WBC filter.	Prevent alloimmunization, febrile reactions, CMV transmission.
Random donor platelets	Pooled platelets from six donors.	Each "six pack" should raise platelet count by ~50,000.
Single-donor platelets	Platelets extracted from a single donor by apheresis.	Use if the patient is alloimmunized; each unit should bump platelets by 50,000.
FFP	All clotting factors, but high fluid volume.	To correct coagulopathy of liver disease or excess warfarin.
Cryoprecipitate	Factor VIII, fibrinogen, and vWF.	Use in **DIC** if fibrinogen < 100. Associated with a **high risk for transmitting infection** because not heat inactivated.

- Major surgery with a platelet count < 50,000.
- Asymptomatic but a platelet count < 10,000.

MISCELLANEOUS HEMATOLOGY

Lymphadenopathy

The primary goal is to distinguish **malignant** from **reactive** adenopathy (see Table 9-35).

DIFFERENTIAL

The differential diagnosis of lymphadenopathy is not exhaustive (see Table 9-36).

Porphyrias

A variety of disorders that have in common genetic **defects in heme synthesis.** Two types may present in adults: acute intermittent porphyria and porphyria cutanea tarda.

TABLE 9-35. Malignant vs. Reactive Adenopathy

	FAVORS MALIGNANT	FAVORS REACTIVE
Patient characteristics	Smoker; older age.	Age < 40.
Size	Larger.	< 1 cm almost always benign.
Consistency	Hard, matted, nontender, fixed.	Rubbery, mobile, tender.
Location	Supraclavicular (Virchow's node); periumbilical (Sister Mary Joseph's nodule).	Inguinal nodes up to 2 cm are normal.

ACUTE INTERMITTENT PORPHYRIA

Caused by a defect in **porphobilinogen deaminase. Autosomal dominant,** but most common in women in their 20s.

SYMPTOMS/EXAM

- Attacks of severe **abdominal pain.**
- Peripheral **neuropathy,** seizures, **psychosis,** basal ganglia syndromes.
- SIADH.
- Many factors and medications can trigger attacks, including alcohol, barbiturates, phenytoin, sulfonamides, caffeine, estrogens, food additives, and starvation.

TABLE 9-36. Causes of Lymphadenopathy

	GENERALIZED	REGIONAL
Infectious	Mononucleosis Hepatitis Acute HIV *Brucella* Syphilis Fungal diseases Scrub typhus Toxoplasmosis	Keratoconjunctivitis Cat-scratch disease Tularemia *Yersinia pestis* Chancroid Lymphogranuloma venereum Trachoma Scrofula
Neoplastic	Lymphoma CLL Post-transplant lymphoproliferation	Metastatic malignancy Histologic transformation
Other	Collagen vascular disease Angioimmunoblastic lymphadenopathy Phenytoin Serum sickness	Castleman's disease Kawasaki's disease Kikuchi's disease Sarcoidosis

Diagnosis

Look for excess aminolevulinic acid or porphobilinogen in the urine.

Treatment

Treatment consists of a high-carbohydrate diet and avoidance of precipitants.

Porphyria Cutanea Tarda

Associated with liver disease. May be acquired or hereditary.

Symptoms/Exam

- **Painless blistering** and fragility on the **dorsum of the hands;** increased facial hair.
- Attacks are precipitated by sun exposure and medications (tetracyclines, NSAIDs).

Diagnosis

- **Clinical:** Characteristic rash and risk factor.
- **Lab:** Elevated urine uroporphyrins.

Treatment

Avoid precipitants and treat the underlying disease.

Hemochromatosis

A disorder of excessive iron accumulation in multiple tissues. The liver is the primary organ affected. Eighty-five percent of cases are caused by a homozygous **mutation in the HFE gene** (7% of Caucasians carry this gene). Constitutes a risk factor for cirrhosis and hepatocellular carcinoma.

Consider hemochromatosis in a bronze, diabetic Caucasian with abnormal transaminases.

Symptoms/Exam

- Hepatomegaly, splenomegaly, ascites. GI bleeding from varices may be a late finding.
- Symptoms of liver, heart, pancreatic, adrenal, or testicular dysfunction.
- Other findings include arthropathy (usually due to pseudogout) and bronze skin coloration.

Diagnosis

- Transferrin saturation, ferritin, and serum iron are all high.
- **Liver biopsy:** Most accurate, but probably not needed if there is no clinical evidence of cirrhosis, ferritin < 1000, and transaminases are normal.
- HFE gene mutation.
- Identify organ dysfunction (liver panel, fasting glucose, ECG, testosterone, cosyntropin stimulation test, TSH).

Treatment

- **Decrease iron stores:**
  - Phlebotomy (can reverse early organ dysfunction).
  - Deferoxamine in patients who cannot tolerate phlebotomy.
  - Avoid iron supplementation (e.g., standard multivitamins), red meat.
- Genetic testing and counseling if homozygous for the HFE gene mutation.

TABLE 9-37. Common Vitamin Deficiencies

VITAMIN	DEFICIENCY	CLINICAL SYMPTOMS
A (retinol)		**Night blindness,** conjunctival xerosis, **Bitot's spots** (white spots on conjunctiva), keratomalacia.
B_1 (thiamine)	Dry beriberi Wet beriberi	Peripheral neuropathy, **Wernicke-Korsakoff.** High-output CHF, vascular leak.
B_2 (riboflavin)		Cheilosis, angular stomatitis, glossitis, weakness, corneal vascularization, anemia.
Niacin	Pellagra	**D**ermatitis, **D**iarrhea, **D**ementia (then **D**eath)—**the 3 (or 4) D's.**
B_6 (pyridoxine)		Peripheral neuropathy, **seizures,** anemia (may be **precipitated by INH**).
C (ascorbic acid)	Scurvy	Perifollicular hemorrhage, petechiae, bleeding gums, hemarthrosis, poor wound healing.
D		Osteomalacia in adults, rickets in children.
E (α-tocopherol)		Areflexia, ophthalmoplegia, decreased proprioception.

COMPLICATIONS

Cirrhosis and hepatocellular carcinoma; heart block; hypopituitarism, hypogonadism, hypoadrenalism; **diabetes**; arthropathy.

Vitamin Deficiencies

Table 9-37 outlines common vitamin deficiencies and their associated disorders.

CHAPTER 10

Hospital Medicine

Robert Trowbridge, MD

Pulmonary Embolism (PE)

Almost all PE patients have dyspnea, pleurisy, or tachypnea—and the absence of all three argues against the diagnosis.

Responsible for 50,000 deaths and up to 250,000 hospitalizations per year. The mortality rate for untreated venous thromboembolic disease exceeds 15%. Risk factors include **prior thromboembolic disease, malignancy, recent surgery, immobility, inherited thrombophilia, and certain medications** (OCPs, HRT). Tobacco use and obesity are also associated with venous thromboembolism.

Symptoms/Exam

- There are no specific signs or symptoms for PE.
- **Dyspnea and pleurisy** are each seen in > 50% of cases.
- Less common are hemoptysis, fever, and cough.
- **Tachypnea, rales,** and/or **tachycardia** may be seen.

Diagnosis

*A D-dimer test is more useful in **ruling out** PE when normal; an elevated D-dimer is not specific for PE.*

The results of the V/Q scan must be interpreted in conjunction with the pretest clinical probability.

- **D-dimer:** Elevated in most patients with PE, but variability in the assay.
- **ABGs:** Respiratory alkalosis with an increased A-a gradient is classically seen, although it may be normal.
- **ECG:**
  - Nonspecific anterior ST-T-wave abnormalities or sinus tachycardia is found in 40% of tracings.
  - A combination of an S wave in lead I and a Q wave with an inverted T wave in lead III (**S_1Q_3T3**) is uncommon but suggestive of the diagnosis.
- **CXR:** Often shows nonspecific pleural effusion or atelectasis. Two rare findings suggest PE:
  - **Hampton's hump:** A pleural-based density representing intraparenchymal hemorrhage.
  - **Westermark's sign:** The stump of a central pulmonary artery with focal oligemia (radiolucency).
- **Lower extremity venous Doppler ultrasound:** A thrombus is present in approximately 30% of PE patients.
- **Clinical gestalt** is a powerful predictor of the likelihood of PE (see Table 10-1).
- **Ventilation-perfusion (V/Q) scanning**—see Table 10-2.
- **CT angiogram**—see Table 10-3.
- **Pulmonary angiogram**—see Table 10-3.

TABLE 10-1. Performance of Clinical Gestalt in Determining the Likelihood of PE[a]

Clinical Likelihood of PE	Actual Incidence of PE
Low (< 20%)	9%
Moderate (20–80%)	30%
High (> 80%)	68%

[a]According to PIOPED.

TABLE 10-2. Probability of PE on the Basis of V/Q Results and Clinical Probability[a]

V/Q Scan Result	High Clinical Probability	Intermediate Clinical Probability	Low Clinical Probability
High	95[a]	86	56
Intermediate	66	28	15
Low	40	15	4
Normal perfusion	0	6	2

[a] That is, 95% of patients with a high-probability V/Q scan and a high clinical probability were found to have a PE on angiography.

Treatment

- **Anticoagulation:**
  - Start with **IV unfractionated heparin** or **low-molecular-weight heparin (LMWH).**
  - Once the patient is adequately anticoagulated with heparin, **warfarin** should be started.
  - The **duration of therapy** is somewhat controversial, but at least six months of therapy with an INR of 2–3 for a first episode is typical. Longer therapy is reserved for patients with recurrent events or with risk factors for thrombophilia.
- **IVC filters** are reserved for patients with contraindications to anticoagulation (see Table 10-4) or those with recurrent events despite adequate anticoagulation. IVC filters decrease the risk of PE in the short term (up to two weeks) but are associated with more recurrent lower extremity DVTs at two years.
- **Thrombolysis** is controversial:
  - Supported in massive PE (i.e., those with refractory hypotension due to PE).

TABLE 10-3. Pros and Cons of Diagnostic Tests in PE

	Pros	Cons	Comments
V/Q scan	Noninvasive; results are well characterized.	Often not available after normal business hours; frequently nondiagnostic.	Performs best when baseline CXR is normal.
CT angiography	Specific; may reveal alternative diagnosis; readily available in most hospitals.	Risk of contrast dye nephropathy; uncertain sensitivity, especially for smaller thrombi.	Role still evolving.
Pulmonary angiography	Gold standard.	Most invasive; requires local expertise.	Perform only if other tests fail to establish the diagnosis.

TABLE 10-4. Contraindications to Anticoagulation

Contraindications to Anticoagulation
Absolute:
■ Hemorrhagic stroke
■ Active internal bleeding
■ Suspected aortic dissection
Relative:
■ Recent internal bleeding (within six months)
■ Prior hemorrhagic stroke
■ Thrombocytopenia
■ CNS mass lesion (especially renal cell carcinoma, melanoma)

- Controversial whether to give in patients with PE and right heart strain who have normal hemodynamics.

- **Surgical or catheter thrombectomy:** Last-ditch options for patients with hemodynamic compromise who fail or are not candidates for thrombolysis.

Deep Venous Thrombosis (DVT)

Risk factors for DVT are the same as those for PE.

Symptoms/Exam

- **Pain, swelling** or **erythema** of the affected extremity is most common.
- **Palpable cord** and low-grade **fever** are less common.
- Most thrombi occur in the **lower extremities,** although upper extremity thrombosis is increasing in frequency coincident with the use of long-term central venous catheters.
- Rarely, **phlegmasia cerulea dolens** (complete venous obstruction resulting in a painful, swollen, and bluish extremity) may be seen.

Differential

- Musculoskeletal injury, including trauma.
- Cellulitis.
- **Ruptured Baker's cyst:** A bursal sac located behind the knee that, when ruptured, can cause pain, swelling, and erythema down into the calf region.
- **Reflex sympathetic dystrophy:** A neurally mediated syndrome of pain and swelling in an extremity, often occurring after minor trauma.

Diagnosis

Compression/duplex ultrasonography, impedance plethysmography, contrast venography (see Table 10-5).

Treatment

- **LMWH** (e.g., enoxaparin 1 mg/kg SQ q 12 h) or **IV unfractionated heparin** (using weight-based dosing adjusted to maintain PTT 1.5–2.0 times normal range) in all patients without contraindications. Outpatient therapy is appropriate in select patients (see Table 10-6).

TABLE 10-5. **Tests for DVT**

	PROS	CONS	COMMENTS
Compression/duplex ultrasonography	Noninvasive; sensitivity and specificity > 95%.	Poor for thrombosis in calf veins or above the inguinal ligament.	First-line test of choice. Consider repeat testing (in 3–5 days) if negative but high clinical suspicion.
Impedance plethysmography	Sensitive and specific.	Not widely available; cumbersome.	Rarely done.
Contrast venography	Gold standard.	Most invasive; requires contrast dye.	Perform only if other tests fail to establish the diagnosis.
D-dimer	Useful for ruling out the diagnosis when combined with low clinical suspicion.	Poor specificity; widespread assay variability.	Assay variability has limited widespread use.

- **Warfarin** can be started as soon as adequate anticoagulation with heparin has been achieved.
- **Duration of therapy** and indications for **IVC filter** are the same as those for PE.
- **Thrombolytic therapy** may result in fewer long-term complications (postphlebitic syndrome) at the expense of an increased risk of bleeding. Consider in patients (especially younger ones) with massive DVT, including phlegmasia cerulea dolens. IV therapy is equivalent to catheter-directed therapy.

Orthopedic patients or surgery patients with other major risk factors should be treated with LMWH or SCDs if anticoagulants are contraindicated.

PREVENTION

- Hospitalized medical and surgical patients are at risk for venous thromboembolic disease. Prophylaxis should thus be considered in all hospitalized patients.
- Although many regimens are effective, appropriate medications and doses vary by specific clinical scenario (see Table 10-7):
  - **SQ "minidose" heparin,** usually 5000 U SQ BID.
  - **SQ LMWH** at lower doses than those used for full anticoagulation.
    - Enoxaparin 30 mg BID or 40 mg QD; dalteparin 5000 U QD.
  - **Adjusted-dose warfarin.**
  - **Elastic stockings** (thromboembolic disease stockings, or TEDS) and **sequential compression devices (SCDs).**

Average-risk surgical patients (those without additional major risk factors) or medical patients should be treated with unfractionated heparin (5000 U SQ BID) or TEDS if anticoagulation is contraindicated.

TABLE 10-6. **Criteria for Outpatient Treatment of DVT**

- Clinical stability with normal vital signs
- Low risk of bleeding
- Normal or near-normal renal function
- Adequate outpatient follow-up to ensure compliance and to monitor for complications

TABLE 10-7. Selected Methods for the Prevention of Venous Thromboembolism

Risk Group	Recommendations for Prophylaxis
Surgical patients	
General surgery	
Low risk: Minor procedures, age < 40, and no clinical risk factors	Early ambulation.
Moderate risk: Minor procedures with additional thrombosis risk factors; age 40–60, and no other clinical risk factors; or major operations with age < 40 without additional clinical risk factors	Elastic stockings (ES), low-dose unfractionated heparin (LDUH),[a] or LMWH, or intermittent pneumatic compression (IPC) plus early ambulation if possible.
Higher risk: Major operation, age > 40 or with additional risk factors	LDUH, LMWH, or IPC.
Higher risk plus increased risk of bleeding	ES or IPC.
Very high risk: Multiple risk factors	LDUH or higher-dose LMWH plus ES or IPC.
Selected very high risk	Consider adjusted-dose perioperative warfarin (ADPW), INR 2.0–3.0, or postdischarge LMWH.
Orthopedic surgery	
Elective total hip replacement surgery	Subcutaneous LMWH, ADPW, or adjusted-dose heparin started preoperatively plus IPC or ES.
Elective total knee replacement surgery	LMWH, ADPW, or IPC.
Hip fracture surgery	LMWH or ADPW.
Neurosurgery	
Intracranial neurosurgery	IPC with or without ES; LDUH and postoperative LMWH are acceptable alternatives; IPC or ES plus LDUH or LMWH may be more effective than either modality alone in high-risk patients.
Acute spinal cord injury	LMWH; IPC and ES may have additional benefit when used with LMWH. In the rehabilitation phase, conversion to full-dose warfarin may provide ongoing protection.
Trauma	
With an identifiable risk factor for thromboembolism	LMWH; IPC or ES if there is a contraindication to LMWH; consider duplex ultrasound screening in very high risk patients; IVC filter insertion if proximal DVT is identified and anticoagulation is contraindicated.
Medical patients	
Acute MI	Subcutaneous LDUH or full-dose heparin; if heparin is contraindicated, IPC and ES may provide some protection.
Ischemic stroke with impaired mobility	LMWH, LDUH, or danaparoid; IPC or ES if anticoagulants are contraindicated.

TABLE 10-7. Selected Methods for the Prevention of Venous Thromboembolism (continued)

Risk Group	Recommendations for Prophylaxis
General medical patients with clinical risk factors, especially patients with cancer, CHF, or severe pulmonary disease	Low-dose LMWH or LDUH.
Cancer patients with indwelling central venous cathethers	Warfarin 1 mg/day or LMWH.

[a]LDUH 5000 U SQ q 8–12 h starting 1–2 hours before surgery.

Recommendations assembled from Geerts WH et al. Prevention of venous thromboembolism. *Chest* 2001;119(Suppl):132.

Reproduced, with permission, from Tierney LM et al. *Current Medical Diagnosis & Treatment 2005,* 44th ed. New York: McGraw-Hill, 2005:283.)

ACUTE PAIN MANAGEMENT

Several basic principles guide the management of acute pain in the hospitalized patient:

- The patient's description of symptoms is the most reliable indicator of pain. **Pain scales,** including the 10-point analog scale, should be used.
- Minor pain will respond to **nonopioid analgesics,** including acetaminophen and NSAIDs, or to low-potency opioids such as codeine.
- For moderate or severe pain, the **potent opioids (morphine, hydromorphone,** or **fentanyl)** should be used. An **appropriate loading dose** is necessary with repeat doses every 10–15 minutes until pain relief has been achieved (see Tables 10-8 and 10-9).
- Maintain pain relief with **patient-controlled anesthesia (PCA)** or **regularly scheduled** nurse-administered medication.
  - In chronically opioid-dependent patients, start continuous opioid infusions immediately.

The lack of an adequate loading dose may result in fruitless and frustrating efforts to "catch up" with the pain.

Regularly scheduled analgesics are the standard of care. "As needed" or "prn" dosing is inappropriate except as a backup for "breakthrough" pain.

TABLE 10-8. Initial Dosing of Opioids

	Parenteral Starting Dose	Oral Starting Dose
Hydromorphone	1.5 mg q 3–4 h	6 mg q 3–4 h
Hydrocodone	–	10 mg q 3–4 h
Oxycodone	–	10 mg q 3–4 h
Methadone	–	5 mg q 6–8 h
Morphine	5–10 mg q 3–4 h	30 mg q 3–4 h
Meperidine	50–100 mg q 3 h	–
Codeine	–	60 mg q 3–4 h

TABLE 10-9. Opioid Equivalency

MEDICATION	COMMON TRADE NAMES	EQUIVALENT PARENTERAL DOSE (mg)	EQUIVALENT PO DOSE (mg)	$T_{1/2}$ (hours)
Fentanyl	–	0.1	–	1–2
Hydromorphone	Dilaudid	1.5	7.5	2–3
Hydrocodone	Lortab, Vicodin	–	20	3–5
Oxycodone	Percocet, Percodan	–	20	3–5
Methadone	–	–	20	15–30
Morphine	Many	10	30	2–4
Meperidine	Demerol	75–100	–	2–4
Codeine	Many	–	200	2–3

- In opioid-naïve patients, start continuous infusion only after opioid requirement has been determined (12–18 hours)
- Pain control should be reassessed often and medications/doses adjusted frequently.
- Attempt a rapid transition to **long-acting preparations** once the amount of opioid required to relieve pain has been determined.
- **Adjunctive measures** should be considered in all patients. The use of **nonsteroidal agents** in conjunction with opioids may be especially effective for postoperative pain. TCAs and gabapentin may also be effective for neuropathic pain.

IV-equivalent doses can be remembered as differing (roughly) by a factor of 10 (i.e., fentanyl is 10 times as strong as hydromorphone, which is 10 times as strong as morphine, which is 10 times as strong as meperidine).

DELIRIUM

Occurs in up to 30% of hospitalized elderly patients. Patients often have multiple risk factors (see Table 10-10). Etiologies are as follows:

SYMPTOMS/EXAM

- **Underlying medical conditions,** especially **infection, fever, and metabolic derangements.** Although bacterial meningitis should always be considered, it is unlikely to develop de novo in a hospitalized patient
- **Alteration of the sleep-wake cycle** and disruption of normal life order, especially in the elderly.
- **Medications,** especially opioids, anticholinergics, and benzodiazepines.
- **Medical devices,** including indwelling urinary catheters.
- **Altered sensorium** is the most common clinical feature.
- The severity of impairment **waxes and wanes** over time.
- **Cognitive functioning** is usually significantly affected. Patients are easily distracted and often difficult to engage in conversation.
- **Paranoia** and **persecutory delusions** are common.

The 25/50/75 rule for the fentanyl patch: MS04 25 mg IV per day = fentanyl 50 μg/day patch = MS04 75 mg PO per day.

TABLE 10-10. Risk Factors for Delirium

- Advanced age
- Male gender
- Fever
- Ethanol use
- Prescription of multiple medications
- Preexisting dementia
- Depression

Diagnosis

- Detailed evaluation, including physical exam, review of the medication list, and appropriate laboratory studies (e.g., electrolytes, serum calcium, UA, and CXR if new pulmonary findings).
- **CT** of the head is rarely useful, but consider in patients who are anticoagulated or have a history of trauma.
- **LP** only in the rare patient in whom there is a clinical suspicion for meningitis.

Avoidance of unnecessary medications and medical devices is key to the prevention and treatment of delirium.

Treatment/Prevention

- **Recognition of risk** and **prevention** are key. Effective interventions include the following:
  - Frequent reorientation.
  - Maintenance of the sleep-wake cycle.
  - Hearing/visual aids.
  - Limitation of unnecessary medications and medical devices.
- **Treatment** of delirium should focus on:
  - Using the above measures in prevention.
  - Treating the underlying cause.
  - Removal of exacerbating factors (especially medications and medical devices).
  - **Haloperidol,** in low doses, can be effective as a second-line therapy.
  - **Risperidone** is associated with TIA and stroke in the elderly and should be avoided.

GI PROPHYLAXIS IN THE HOSPITALIZED PATIENT

GI bleeding secondary to stress-induced gastric mucosal disease **occurs in up to 5–6% of critically ill patients.** Hemodynamically significant bleeding is rare, but mortality is significantly increased. Risk factors include a history of trauma or burns, sepsis, and hepatic or renal dysfunction. **Coagulopathy** and **respiratory failure necessitating mechanical ventilation** are the most powerful risk factors for stress-related hemorrhage. Prophylactic measures include the following:

- **Sucralfate** and **H_2 receptor blockers** both result in at least a 50% reduction in the likelihood of bleeding (see Table 10-11).
- **Antacids** may be effective but are rarely used,
- **Enteral feeding** may decrease bleeding risk.
- PPIs are **relatively unproven for this indication** and are considered **second-line therapy.**

The absence of both coagulopathy and respiratory failure necessitating mechanical ventilation conveys less than a 0.1% chance of significant bleeding.

Perioperative β-blockers greatly decrease the risk of perioperative MI and mortality in patients with or at risk for CAD.

Patients who have cardiac disease or symptoms that require urgent or emergent evaluation and treatment, regardless of their pending surgery, should have their surgery delayed until their cardiac issues are addressed.

The indications for coronary revascularization in the preoperative patient are no different from those in patients not facing surgery. "Prophylactic" CABG and/or angioplasty/stenting should not be done unless it is likely to increase long-term survival.

TABLE 10-11. Prophylaxis for GI Bleeding

	Pros	Cons
Sucralfate	Effective.	Interferes with the absorption of multiple medications. Frequent dosing. Can only be given PO or through feeding tube.
H_2 receptor blockers	Effective; can be given IV or PO.	Possible increased risk of nosocomial pneumonia.

PERIOPERATIVE MANAGEMENT

Preoperative Cardiac Evaluation

Cardiac disease is a major cause of perioperative morbidity and mortality, with 50,000 patients developing perioperative MIs per year.

- **Preoperative cardiac risk assessment** is mandatory in all patients undergoing noncardiac surgery.
- Initial risk assessment may be completed using a validated **risk prediction score** (see Tables 10-12 and 10-13).
- Following this risk assessment, further evaluation and/or intervention may be appropriate in selected individuals with elevated risk (see Figure 10-1).

Preoperative Pulmonary Evaluation

The risk factors for perioperative pulmonary complications are outlined in Table 10-14. Preventive measures are as follows:

- **Smoking cessation** can significantly decrease complication risk, especially if completed at least two months preoperatively.
- **Incentive spirometry**, including deep breathing exercises, may decrease the risk of complications and should be taught to the patient preoperatively.
- **Optimization of chronic lung disease** is critical.
- **Pulmonary function testing** is not routinely useful in guiding treatment but can give an indication of the severity of underlying disease and may help evaluate unexplained pulmonary symptoms.

TABLE 10-12. Revised (Simplified) Cardiac Risk Index

One point each for:
■ Higher-risk surgery (thoracic, abdominal, or major vascular operation)
■ Ischemic heart disease
■ CHF
■ Diabetes requiring insulin
■ Cerebrovascular disease (history of stroke or TIA)
■ Renal insufficiency (Cr > 2)

TABLE 10-13. Risk of Major Perioperative Complications from Risk Index

Risk Points	Risk of Major Complications (%)
0	0.4
1	0.9
2	7
3 or more	11

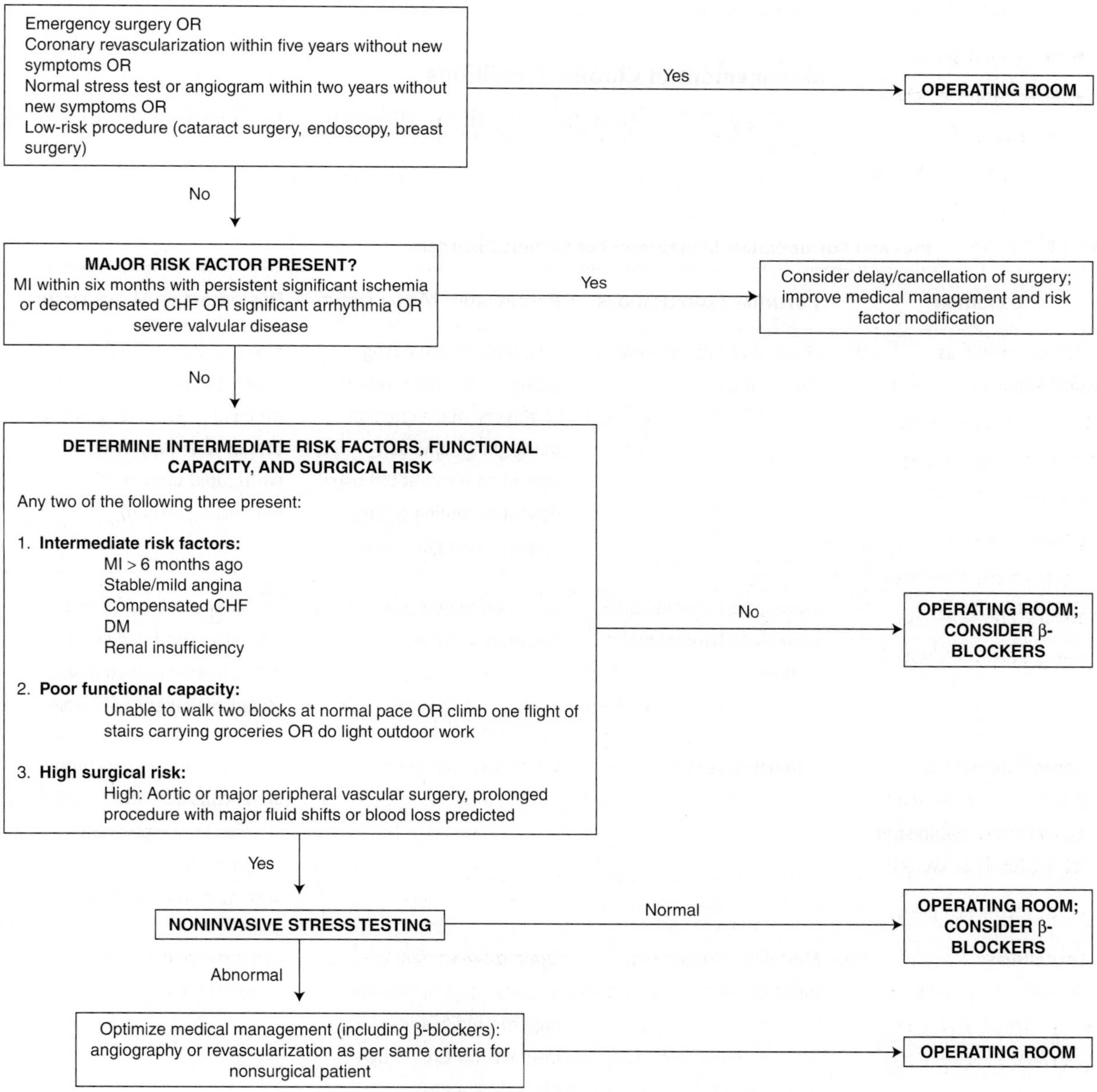

FIGURE 10-1. Algorithm for further cardiac evaluation and intervention.

PFTs and ABGs are not part of a routine preoperative pulmonary risk assessment. Obtain these only if you would do so even if the patient were not undergoing surgery.

TABLE 10-14. Risk Factors for Perioperative Pulmonary Complications

- Surgery on the chest or abdomen
- Chronic lung disease
- Current tobacco use
- Morbid obesity
- Age > 60
- Prior stroke
- Altered mental status
- Neck or intracranial surgery

- **ABG analysis** is not routinely necessary.
- **Antibiotics** should not be given routinely.

Management of Chronic Conditions

Table 10-15 lists guidelines for the perioperative management of chronic disorders.

TABLE 10-15. Pre- and Postoperative Management of Chronic Disorders

CONDITION	POTENTIAL COMPLICATIONS	PREOPERATIVE MANAGEMENT	POSTOPERATIVE MANAGEMENT
DM, on insulin as outpatient	Hypo- and hyperglycemia; DKA; infection.	Give 50% of usual long-acting insulin the morning of surgery (the exception being glargine, which should be given at the usual dose the evening before surgery) with glucose drip.	Strongly consider insulin drip titrating to normoglycemia; otherwise restart long-acting insulin with supplemental (with rapid titration of long-acting insulin).
DM, not on insulin	Hypo- and hyperglycemia; nonketotic hyperosmolar state.	Omit oral hypoglycemic the day prior to surgery.	Consider insulin drip; use regularly scheduled short-acting insulin if needed and restart oral agent once able.
Chronic steroid use (especially greater than equivalent of prednisone 20 mg for three weeks)	Adrenal crisis (rare).	Continue usual dose.	Can usually just give chronic dose; consider "stress-dose" steroids for longer/major surgeries: hydrocortisone 100 mg q 8 h × 2–3 days.
Liver disease	Mortality, hemorrhage, infection.	Optimize treatment of underlying complications; high morbidity and mortality for Child-Pugh Class C patients.	Optimize treatment of underlying complications.

NUTRITION IN THE HOSPITALIZED PATIENT

Nutritional guidelines for hospitalized patients are as follows (see also Table 10-16):

- **Oral supplements** are appropriate if the patient is able to tolerate oral intake.
- **Enteral tube feedings** are the mode of choice for patients with functional GI tracts who cannot be fed orally.
  - **NG or nasoduodenal tubes** (especially in patients at high risk for aspiration) are appropriate for patients needing temporary support.
  - **Tube enterostomies** are used when long-term nutritional support is anticipated. **Jejunostomy** may decrease the risk of aspiration but requires a surgical procedure, in contrast to the endoscopically placed **gastrostomy** tube.
- **Total parenteral nutrition (TPN),** delivered through dedicated central venous access, is another long-term option but is difficult to manage and is associated with multiple adverse events (see Table 10-17). It is appropriate for patients with significant GI tract disease or dysfunction.
- **Peripheral parenteral nutrition (PPN)** is another, albeit short-term, option.

Poor perioperative glycemic control is associated with a higher incidence of infection and delayed wound healing.

OVERDOSE/TOXIC INGESTION

General guidelines for overdose and toxic ingestion are as follows (see also Table 10-18):

- **Supportive care** is the mainstay of treatment.
  - **Airway protection,** including endotracheal intubation, if necessary.
  - **Volume/electrolyte repletion.**

TABLE 10-16. Indications for Enteral Feeding, TPN, and PPN

	Indications	Advantages	Disadvantages
Enteral feeding	Nutritional needs cannot be met through oral feeding and supplements.	Less invasive. Lower incidence of infectious complications. Preserved mucosal immunity and bowel integrity. More rapid transition to regular oral feeding.	Requires a functional GI tract. Requires tube placement. Associated with an increased incidence of aspiration, although risk may be lower with jejunal compared to gastric tubes.
TPN	Long-term need (> 1–2 weeks) for supplemental or replacement nutrition; unable to use GI tract.	Long-term therapy possible.	Need for maintenance of central venous access → catheter-related infectious complications (2–3%). Catheter-related thromboses. Metabolic complications (50%; see Table 10-17).
PPN	Short-term need (< 1–2 weeks) for supplemental or replacement nutrition; unable to use GI tract.	Does not require central venous access.	Effective only as a short-term option (1–2 weeks). Large-volume infusion.

Table 10-17. Metabolic Complications of TPN

Complication	Treatment
Abnormal LFTs	Decrease carbohydrate load; reconfigure balance between fats, carbohydrates, and amino acids.
Acalculous cholecystitis (4% with long-term TPN)	Surgery.
Elevated BUN	Assess volume status; if adequate, decrease infusion rate and/or amino acid load.
Hyperglycemia	Frequent glucose checks; addition of insulin to TPN.
Micronutrient deficiencies (zinc, selenium, vitamin B_{12}, copper)	Regular supplementation.
Refeeding syndrome (hypophosphatemia, hypokalemia, hypomagnesemia)	Consider decreasing infusion rate; electrolyte supplementation.

TABLE 10-18. Characteristics and Treatment of Common Ingestions

Substance	Manifestations	Laboratory Tests	Treatment	Comments
Acetaminophen	Initially nausea and vomiting; then an asymptomatic interval followed by recurrent nausea, abdominal pain, and jaundice.	Elevated acetaminophen level as a function of time of ingestion (> 150 μg/dL at four hours indicates a need for treatment). LFTs begin to rise within 12 hours, peaking at 4–6 days. AST and ALT may be markedly elevated (> 10,000 IU). PT is most indicative of prognosis (PT < 90 predicts an 80% survival rate). Hyperbilirubinemia. Renal failure in up to 50% of cases.	Activated charcoal if within four hours of ingestion or delayed absorption is suspected. *N*-acetylcysteine (140 mg/kg load followed by 70 mg/kg every four hours for 17 doses). IV preparation is available if the patient is unable to tolerate PO. Immediate transfer to liver transplant center for progressive coagulopathy. acidosis, or liver failure.	*N*-acetylcysteine is most effective within 10 hours but may be effective substantially later. Chronic alcoholics (not a single alcohol ingestion) may be subject to hepatotoxicity at lower doses of acetaminophen.

TABLE 10-18. Characteristics and Treatment of Common Ingestions (continued)

SUBSTANCE	MANIFESTATIONS	LABORATORY TESTS	TREATMENT	COMMENTS
Aspirin	Nausea and vomiting, tinnitus, GI bleeding and volume depletion, mental status changes.	Anion-gap metabolic acidosis with concomitant respiratory alkalosis. Elevated PT. Elevated serum salicylate level.	Activated charcoal and gastric lavage. Sodium bicarbonate with alkalinization of the serum and urine (goal pH 7.40–7.50) to decrease toxicity and promote renal elimination. Hemodialysis for severe acidosis, altered mental status, or levels > 80–100 mg/dL.	Threshold for hemodialysis lowered to 60 mg/dL for chronic ingestion.
Lithium	Altered mental status progressing to coma. Tremor, hyperreflexia, clonus. Vomiting, diarrhea.	Elevated serum lithium level (although toxicity may occur at low levels with chronic administration).	Volume repletion; consider alkalinization of urine. Dialysis for a lithium level > 4 mEq/L (2.5 mEq/L if significantly symptomatic) or with concomitant renal failure.	Levels may "rebound" after dialysis and require repeat dialysis. Not bound by activated charcoal.
SSRIs	Somnolence, agitation; nausea, vomiting, tachycardia.	None.	Supportive care.	Rarely fatal.
TCAs	Dilated pupils, dry mouth, tachycardia (almost always present), flushed skin, seizures, decreased mental status, ileus, urinary retention, hypotension, pulmonary edema.	Widened QRS (> 0.12). Pronounced R wave in aVR (> 3 mm). AV block and ventricular dysrhythmias.	Activated charcoal; consider gastric lavage (as anticholinergic effects may delay gastric emptying, consider up to 12 hours following ingestion). Alkalinization (with intermittent boluses of bicarbonate) may ameliorate cardiotoxicity.	Low threshold for admission (especially patients with anticholinergic symptoms/signs). Pronounced R waves in aVR may be most predictive of cardiac complications.

TABLE 10-18. Characteristics and Treatment of Common Ingestions (continued)

SUBSTANCE	MANIFESTATIONS	LABORATORY TESTS	TREATMENT	COMMENTS
TCAs *(continued)*			Lidocaine but **not** procainamide for ventricular dysrhythmia. Norepinephrine or epinephrine (not dopamine) for hypotension.	
Methanol	Altered mental status, seizures; nausea, vomiting; visual disturbances, blindness.	Anion-gap metabolic acidosis. Osmolar gap ($osm_{measured} - osm_{calculated}$). Elevated serum methanol level.	If within 1–2 hours of ingestion, gastric lavage. Charcoal is ineffective. **Immediate** hemodialysis for severe poisoning (level > 50 mg/dL or osmolar gap > 10, severe acidosis, mental status changes/seizures). IV fomepizole (ethanol titrated to a level of 100–200 mg/dL when fomepizole is not available) in less severe poisoning or as a temporizing measure. Sodium bicarbonate for acidosis.	Mortality > 80% with seizures or coma. Lethal dose 75–100 mL.
Ethylene glycol	Same as methanol. Oxalate crystals in the urine. Fluorescence of the urine with Wood's lamp. Acute renal failure.	Anion-gap metabolic acidosis. Osmolar gap ($osm_{measured} - osm_{calculated}$). Elevated serum ethylene glycol level.	Same as methanol, except hemodialysis with ethylene glycol level > 20 mg/dL.	Lethal dose 100 mL.

TABLE 10-18. Characteristics and Treatment of Common Ingestions (continued)

SUBSTANCE	MANIFESTATIONS	LABORATORY TESTS	TREATMENT	COMMENTS
Isopropyl alcohol	Altered mental status progressing to coma; ataxia; hypotension (secondary to myocardial depression).	Elevated osmolar gap ($osm_{measured} - osm_{calculated}$). Lack of metabolic acidosis. Ketonuria.	If within 1–2 hours of ingestion, gastric lavage. Hemodialysis for coma, plasma isopropanol level > 400 mg/dL; consider for hypotension and with concomitant hepatic or renal dysfunction.	Lethal dose 150 mL.
Carbon monoxide	Headache, altered mental status, seizures, coma. Also nausea, abdominal pain.	Elevated carboxyhemoglobin saturation (may normally be up to 15% in smokers). Pulse oximetry and Po_2 may be normal.	High-flow O_2 via endotracheal tube if severe. Hyperbaric oxygen if immediately available for severe poisoning and for pregnant patients (controversial).	Cherry-red lips infrequently seen. Po_2 and pulse oximetry falsely reassuring.

- **Activated charcoal** binds most medications and is given to most patients.
- **Gastric lavage** is associated with a high complication rate and should be considered only with recent (< 1–4 hours prior to presentation), serious ingestions or when delayed gastric emptying is suspected (e.g., anticholinergic agents). If mental status is an issue, intubate prior to lavage.
- **Emetic agents** (ipecac) are generally not used in adults because they increase the risk of aspiration and their efficacy is questionable when given > 1 hour after an ingestion.
- Screen all patients for **coingestions** for which there is a specific antidote or treatment (e.g., acetaminophen, aspirin).

*Agents **not** bound by activated charcoal include lithium, ethanol/methanol/ethylene glycol, hydrocarbons, and heavy metals.*

ACUTE COMPLICATIONS OF SUBSTANCE ABUSE

Table 10-19 delineates guidelines for treating acute complications associated with the ingestion of controlled substances.

Acetaminophen Toxicity—

The "140" rule:

An ingestion > **140 mg/kg** is usually toxic.

A four-hour level > **140–150 μg/dL** mandates treatment.

The loading dose of *N*-acetylcysteine is **140 mg/kg.**

WITHDRAWAL SYNDROMES

Ethanol Withdrawal

Most chronic alcoholics experience some withdrawal symptoms on cessation of drinking, although only a small minority will develop delirium tremens (DTs). Mortality is approximately 5%; risk factors include advanced age, temperature > 40°C, and preexisting hepatic or pulmonary disease.

TABLE 10-19. Manifestations and Treatment of the Acute Complications of Substance Abuse

Substance	Manifestations	Laboratory Tests	Treatment	Comments
Gamma hydroxybutyrate (GHB)	Somnolence and respiratory depression; bradycardia; muscle twitching and seizures.	None.	Consider activated charcoal if ingestion was very recent. Supportive care.	Most patients recover spontaneously within six hours.
Opioids	Somnolence followed by respiratory depression and coma. Constricted pupils, hypotension, bradycardia, apnea, hypothermia; pulmonary edema and aspiration possible. Meperidine and tramadol may cause seizures.	Positive urine tox screen (except methadone and tramadol).	Supportive care. Naloxone 0.4–1.0 mg as needed (the effect of naloxone lasts only two hours, and repeated doses may be necessary).	Fentanyl may require very high doses of naloxone. Patients should be observed for at least 24 hours; longer for methadone coingestion. Screen for coingestion (many opioids are compounded with acetaminophen, e.g., Tylox, Percocet).
Cocaine	Agitation, palpitations, chest pain. Tachycardia, hypertension. Myocardial ischemia/infarction. Stroke.	Tox screen. Always obtain ECG to assess for ischemic changes.	Benzodiazepines.	Avoid β-blockers with myocardial ischemia. If a β-blocker is used for hypertension, a vasodilating agent should be added.
Amphetamines (including MDMA)	Agitation, tachycardia, hypertension, hyperthermia, seizures, rhabdomyolysis.	Elevated CK with rhabdomyolysis.	Benzodiazepines. Specific treatment of complications (cooling for hyperthermia, hydration and alkalinization for rhabdomyolysis).	
Ethanol	Disinhibition, agitation, slurred speech. Somnolence progressing to stupor with respiratory depression and coma.	Elevated blood alcohol level.	Supportive care. Attention to nutritional deficiencies in chronic alcoholics. Screen for coingestions.	

HOSPITAL MEDICINE

Symptoms/Exam

- Symptoms usually begin 2–3 days (but occasionally up to seven days) after the last drink. Withdrawal seizures almost always happen within 36 hours of stopping drinking.
- **Tremulousness with anxiety** is most common and may progress to agitation and delirium with hallucinations.
- **DTs** usually occur several days after the last drink.
- **Hypertension, tachycardia,** and **hyperthermia** are common.

Treatment

- **Benzodiazepines** are the cornerstone of treatment.
  - **Symptom-triggered schedules** administer benzodiazepines as directed by the Clinical Institute Withdrawal Assessment for Alcohol Scale (CIWA) score. May result in the use of lower doses of medications than other schedules, but requires frequent reassessment.
  - **Fixed schedules** provide regular benzodiazepines regardless of symptoms; may result in oversedation.
- **β-blockers, clonidine, and carbamazepine** may be useful adjuncts, but their use should not supplant the role of benzodiazepines.
- Screen for nutritional deficiencies; all patients should receive **thiamine** supplementation.
- **Withdrawal seizures** are also treated with benzodiazepines (other antiseizure medications are generally not necessary). Consider prophylactic treatment with benzodiazepines at the time of admission in patients with a history of withdrawal seizures.

*Manifestations of tricyclic (anticholinergic) overdose: **"mad as a hatter, red as a beet, dry as a bone, blind as a bat, and hot as a hare"**–i.e., confused, flushed, dry mouth, visual changes.*

The combination of an elevated anion gap and an elevated osmolar gap suggests ingestion of ethanol, methanol, or ethylene glycol.

Opioid Withdrawal

Less likely to cause serious morbidity and mortality than ethanol withdrawal.

Symptoms/Exam

- Symptoms include **anxiety, nausea,** and **diarrhea** accompanied by **rhinorrhea, lacrimation,** and **diaphoresis.** More significant symptoms include **severe myalgias** and **tremulousness.**
- **Hypertension, tachycardia, tachypnea,** and **fever** may develop; pupils are enlarged.

Fluorescent urine and oxalate crystalluria indicate ethylene glycol ingestion.

Treatment

- **Methadone** is useful for moderate to severe symptoms.
  - Titrated to symptom relief at four- to six-hour intervals.
  - Symptom scale may be used to determine methadone dosage.
- **Clonidine** may also be useful as either adjunctive or primary therapy.

HYPERTENSIVE URGENCY AND EMERGENCY

A **hypertensive emergency** occurs when an elevated BP results in active end-organ damage that is likely to result in death or serious morbidity without immediate treatment.

- Includes **aortic dissection, hypertensive encephalopathy, myocardial ischemia/infarction, intracranial bleeding, CHF,** and **acute nephropathy.**
- BP must be lowered immediately in such situations, generally within one hour.

An inebriated patient with a focal-onset seizure or in status epilepticus should prompt a search for another cause of seizure, such as head trauma, infection, other overdose, or metabolic disturbance.

Hypertensive urgency occurs with severe hypertension (> 220/120) without end-organ complications.

Hypertensive emergencies may occur at BPs not considered "critically" high.

SYMPTOMS/EXAM

- Systolic BP (SBP) is usually > 220 mmHg, while diastolic BP (DBP) is usually > 120 mmHg. The BP level tolerated may be dependent on the chronic baseline BP.
- **Funduscopic exam** may reveal papilledema and flame hemorrhages.
- **Hypertensive encephalopathy** is marked by nausea/vomiting, headache, confusion, lethargy, and/or irritability.
- Focal neurologic deficits suggest **intracranial hemorrhage.**
- Severe chest pain radiating to the back and differential pulses in the upper extremities may occur with **aortic dissection.**
- **Ischemic chest pain** may be present as an individual process or as a complication of dissection.

Poorly controlled essential hypertension is by far the most common cause of hypertensive urgency/emergency.

DIFFERENTIAL

- Poorly controlled essential hypertension.
- Rebound hypertension after antihypertensive medication are abruptly stopped (e.g., oral clonidine or β-blockers).
- Pheochromocytoma.
- Hyperthyroidism.
- Volume overload (often with renal failure).

DIAGNOSIS

Evaluation is directed by the presence of suspected complications:

- **CT of the head** in patients with mental status changes or focal neurologic deficits to exclude intracranial hemorrhage.
- **MRI** in hypertensive encephalopathy may demonstrate **posterior leukoencephalopathy** (white matter edema in the parietal and occipital areas).
- **Emergent transesophageal echocardiography or thoracic CT** in suspected aortic dissection.
- **Electrocardiography** in patients with suspected myocardial ischemia.

The mean arterial pressure should be lowered by no more than 20–25% within the first hour. BP should subsequently be lowered to a level of approximately 160/100 over the ensuing 4–6 hours.

TREATMENT

- **Pharmacologic** treatment is dictated by the specific end-organ complications present (see Tables 10-20 and 10-21).
- **Nitroprusside** and **labetalol** are the most commonly used medications.
- In hypertensive emergency, **BP should be lowered within one hour,** and parenteral agents are almost always necessary.
- **The immediate goal is not normotension,** as a dramatic reduction in BP can overwhelm the cerebral autoregulatory mechanism, causing ischemic stroke.
- In hypertensive urgency, **oral medications are most useful** and BP may be controlled at a more leisurely rate. Outpatient treatment is appropriate in most instances.
- **Captopril** and **clonidine** are particularly effective in hypertensive urgency.

Rapid-acting oral or sublingual nifedipine should be avoided—it may lower BP too drastically and precipitate stroke.

TABLE 10-20. Medications for Hypertensive Emergency

MEDICATION	ADVANTAGES	DISADVANTAGES
Nitroprusside	Very effective; easily titrated. Predictable BP response. Short-acting.	May cause nausea and vomiting. Thiocyanate toxicity is possible, especially in patients with renal or hepatic insufficiency.
Fenoldopam	Useful in renal failure; predictable BP response.	May cause nausea, headache, and reflex tachycardia. Increases intraocular pressure (avoid with glaucoma).
Labetalol	Excellent for hyperadrenergic states.	May precipitate bronchospasm, heart block.
Enalapril	Easily transitioned to oral therapy.	Response may be extreme in high renin states. Use with care in renal insufficiency. Can cause hyperkalemia.
Nicardipine	Potent antihypertensive.	Avoid with dissection, myocardial ischemia.
Hydralazine	Useful in pregnancy.	May cause reflex tachycardia. Avoid with dissection, myocardial ischemia.

SYNCOPE

Defined as a transient loss of consciousness and postural tone; accounts for 3% of all ER visits and up to 6% of all hospital admissions.

The history and physical establish a diagnosis in nearly 50% of syncope cases.

SYMPTOMS/EXAM

The history and physical exam establish a diagnosis in almost 50% of patients with syncope. Specific findings, however, are dependent on the underlying etiology, and knowledge of the differential diagnosis is critical (see Table 10-22).

TABLE 10-21. Medications for Specific Complications of Hypertensive Emergency

INDICATION	DRUGS OF CHOICE	CONTRAINDICATED
Aortic dissection	Nitroprusside **and** labetalol	Nicardipine, hydralazine
Pulmonary edema	Nitroprusside, nitroglycerin	
Myocardial ischemia/infarction	Nitroglycerin, labetalol	Nicardipine, hydralazine
Hypertensive encephalopathy	Nitroprusside	
Eclampsia	Labetalol, hydralazine	Enalapril
Acute renal failure	Fenoldopam, labetalol	

TABLE 10-22. Differential Diagnosis of Syncope

Mechanism	Suggestive Features
Orthostatic hypotension	History of presyncope upon standing; advanced age; a drop in BP (SBP by 20 mmHg or DBP by 10 mmHg) upon standing.
Medication-related	Diuretics, antihypertensives, polypharmacy.
Autonomic insufficiency	Parkinson's (Shy-Drager).
Neurally mediated (vasovagal, vasomotor, neurocardiogenic)	Preceded by nausea, flushing, diaphoresis, and tachycardia; autonomic symptoms often persist upon awakening.
Vasovagal	Occurrence while under emotional stress, pain.
Situational	Occurrence in specific situations (while coughing, micturating, or defecating).
Carotid sinus hypersensitivity	Advanced age.
Cardiac arrhythmia (tachyarrhythmia, bradyarrhythmia)	No premonitory symptoms or residual symptoms upon awakening; history of cardiovascular disease.
Obstructive/low cardiac output	Signs and symptoms of cardiopulmonary disease.
Valvular heart disease (aortic stenosis, pulmonic stenosis)	Characteristic murmur on exam.
Myocardial ischemia/infarction	Associated chest pain; extracardiac sounds.
IHSS	Characteristic murmur on exam.
Aortic dissection	Chest pain radiating to the back; differential pulses in upper extremities.
PE	Pleurisy; dyspnea; history of venous thromboembolism.
Atrial myxoma	Tumor plop on auscultation.
Neurologic	
Migraine	Subsequent headache.
Vertebrobasilar insufficiency (VBI)	Tinnitus, dysarthria, diplopia; focal neurologic findings—very unusual to have VBI cause syncope without other brain stem symptoms.
Seizures (temporal lobe)	Postictal state.
Psychiatric	Signs and symptoms of psychiatric disease.

Patients < 45 years of age with a normal ECG and no history of structural heart disease are at low risk for an adverse outcome.

Diagnosis

Testing other than **history, physical exam, and ECG** is individualized to the patient. Extensive testing is often fruitless but should be considered in patients with risk factors for an adverse outcome (see Table 10-23).

- ECG identifies a definitive cause in only 5% of patients but may provide evidence of unsuspected cardiac disease and should be obtained in most patients.

TABLE 10-23. Risk Factors for Adverse Outcome in Syncope

- Age > 45
- History of CHF or ventricular arrhythmia
- Abnormal ECG

- **Ambulatory ECG (Holter) monitoring** detects arrhythmia as the cause of syncope in < 5% of patients but may note a normal rhythm during symptoms in 15%, effectively excluding an arrhythmic cause. The yield is somewhat higher with **loop recorders and event monitors,** especially in patients with infrequent symptoms.
- **Electrophysiologic testing** may be performed in those at high risk for arrhythmia.
- **Upright tilt-table testing** should be reserved for patients with recurrent events in whom an arrhythmic cause has been excluded and a neurally mediated cause suspected.
- **Carotid sinus massage** with cardiac monitoring should be completed in older patients without a readily identifiable cause of syncope or with symptoms suggestive of carotid sinus hypersensitivity. A three-second pause is diagnostic and may indicate the need for pacemaker insertion.
- **Echocardiography** if historical or physical findings suggest left ventricular dysfunction or valvular disease.
- Testing for CAD, including **stress electrocardiography and stress imaging studies,** is necessary when the history or ECG is suggestive of myocardial ischemia.
- **CT and MRI** of the head are rarely indicated unless there was concomitant head trauma. **EEG** is useful only when seizures are suspected.

Older patients—especially those with risk factors for or a history suggestive of cardiac disease or arrhythmia—should undergo more detailed testing, including echocardiography and noninvasive testing for CAD.

Testing for neurologic disease with CT and MRI in syncope is very low yield in the absence of specific neurologic signs and symptoms.

Treatment

- Treatment is directed at the underlying condition.
- Hospitalize if risk factors for cardiac syncope are present or syncope is suspected to be secondary to arrhythmic or obstructive/low cardiac output.

COMMUNITY-ACQUIRED PNEUMONIA

With > 3.5 million cases annually prompting > 1 million hospitalizations, community-acquired pneumonia is the sixth leading cause of death in the United States.

Symptoms/Exam

- **Fever, dyspnea,** or **cough** productive of **purulent sputum** are most common.
- **Pleuritic chest pain** and **chills/rigors** are also possible.
- Patients who are immunocompromised, reside in an institution, have recently been hospitalized, or are at risk for aspiration should be considered separately.

Diagnosis

- **CXR** shows an infiltrate, but radiographic findings cannot predict the microbiologic cause.
- **Sputum Gram stain and culture** are controversial and only marginally predictive of microbiology, but they are recommended for inpatients and can be considered in outpatients as well.
- **Blood cultures** provide reliable data and may allow for the tailoring of antimicrobial therapy. They are positive in approximately 10% of cases.
- Tests for specific etiologies, including serologies for Q fever and psittacosis as well as culture and antigen testing for *Legionella,* are obtained only when there is a high clinical suspicion (see Table 10-24).

Certain historical features may suggest a specific microbiologic etiology for community-acquired pneumonia, but none is adequately specific to establish a diagnosis.

TABLE 10-24. Causative Organisms and Historical Features of Community-Acquired Pneumonia

ORGANISM	CAUSE (%)	SUGGESTIVE HISTORICAL FEATURES
Streptococcus pneumoniae	20–60	Acute onset; often follows URI; underlying COPD.
Haemophilus influenzae	3–10	Often follows URI; COPD.
S. aureus	3–5	May follow influenza infection; cavitary disease.
Legionella spp.	2–8	Exposure to humidifier, hot tub, or air-conditioning cooling towers; pleuritic chest pain and pleural effusion are common; diarrhea; hyponatremia.
Klebsiella, other gram-negative rods	3–10	Ethanol abuse; DM; residence in nursing home.
Mycoplasma pneumoniae	1–6	Young adults in summer and fall; associated rash and bullous myringitis.
Chlamydia pneumoniae	4–10	Young adults; often follows prolonged sore throat.
Q fever (*Coxiella burnetii*)	Rare	Exposure to livestock (cattle, goats, sheep); elevated LFTs.
Chlamydia psittaci	Rare	Exposure to birds, including parrots, pigeons, and chickens; headache; temperature-pulse dissociation.

Blood cultures are the most definitive way to establish a diagnosis in community-acquired pneumonia.

TREATMENT

- **Outpatient therapy** is appropriate in many patients. The **Fine index (pneumonia severity index, or PSI)** can help guide decisions regarding the need for hospitalization (see Tables 10-25 and 10-26).
- **Antibiotic treatment** is largely empirical, covering typical and atypical agents. Appropriate choices include:
  - Extended-spectrum fluoroquinolones (e.g., moxifloxacin, levofloxacin).
  - A third-generation cephalosporin plus a macrolide.
  - A β-lactam/β-lactamase inhibitor combination plus a macrolide.
  - In **severe community-acquired pneumonia,** consider "double coverage" for *Pseudomonas* (i.e., two antibiotics with antipseudomonal activity).
- **Prompt initiation of antimicrobial therapy** (within eight hours of presentation) has a significant beneficial effect on mortality.
- **Early conversion from parenteral to oral therapy** should be considered in patients with decreasing leukocytosis, improvement in cough/dyspnea, and no fever for at least eight hours.
- Patients may be **discharged** without delay at the time of conversion to oral therapy as long as they meet discharge criteria (see Table 10-27).
- **Duration of treatment** is variable. Most clinicians prescribe 7–10 days of therapy, reserving longer courses (at least two weeks) for infections thought to be caused by *S. aureus, Legionella, Mycoplasma,* and *Chlamydia* spp.
- **Repeat CXR** is not indicated during hospitalization except when complications (e.g., pleural effusion) are suspected. A follow-up film to ensure clearing and to assess for underlying processes in 4–6 weeks is appropriate, especially in smokers and older patients.

There is no benefit to observing patients in the hospital after conversion to oral therapy once they have met the criteria for clinical stability.

Table 10-25. Scoring System for Risk Class Assignment of Community-Acquired Pneumonia (PORT Prediction Rule)

PATIENT CHARACTERISTIC	POINTS ASSIGNED[a]
Demographic factor	
Age: men	Number of years
Age: women	Number of years minus 10
Nursing home resident	10
Comorbid illnesses	
Neoplastic disease[b]	30
Liver disease[c]	20
CHF[d]	10
Cerebrovascular disease[e]	10
Renal disease[f]	10
Physical examination finding	
Altered mental status[g]	20
Respiratory rate ≥ 30 breaths/min	20
Systolic BP < 90 mmHg	
Temperature ≤ 35°C or ≥ 40°C	15
Pulse ≥ 125 bpm	10
Laboratory or radiographic finding	
Arterial pH < 7.35	30
BUN ≥ 30 mg/dL	20
Sodium < 130 meq/L	20
Glucose > 250 mg/dL	10
Hematocrit < 30%	10
Arterial Po_2 < 60 mmHg	10
Pleural effusion	10

Adapted, with permission, from Fine MJ et al. A prediction rule to identify low-risk patients with community-acquired pneumonia. *N Engl J Med* 1997;336:243.

[a] A total point score for a given patient is obtained by summing the patient's age in years (age minus 10 for women) and the points for each applicable characteristic.

[b] Any cancer except basal or squamous cell carcinoma of the skin that was active at the time of presentation or diagnosed within one year before presentation.

[c] Clinical or histologic diagnosis of cirrhosis or another form of chronic liver disease.

[d] Systolic or diastolic dysfunction documented by history, physical examination and CXR, echocardiogram, multigated angiogram (MUGA) scan, or left ventriculogram.

[e] Clinical diagnosis of stroke or TIA or stroke documented by MRI or CT scan.

[f] History of chronic renal disease or abnormal BUN and creatinine concentration documented in the medical record.

[g] Disorientation (to person, place, or time, not known to be chronic), stupor, or coma.

Table 10-26. Recommendations for Site of Care for Community-Acquired Pneumonia by PORT Risk Class

Number of Points	Risk Class	Mortality at 30 Days (%)	Recommended Site of Care
Absence of predictors	I	0.1–0.4	Outpatient
≤ 70	II	0.6–0.7	Outpatient
71–90	III	0.9–2.8	Outpatient or brief inpatient
91–130	IV	8.2–9.3	Inpatient
≥ 130	V	27.0–31.1	Inpatient

Data from Fine MU et al. A prediction rule to identify low-risk patients with community-acquired pneumonia. *N Engl J Med* 1997;336:243.

TABLE 10-27. Criteria for Discharge in Community-Acquired Pneumonia

- Clinical stability:
  - Improvement in cough/dyspnea
  - Adequate O_2 saturation (> 90%)
  - Afebrile (temperature < 37.8°C)
  - Resolution of tachycardia (< 100 bpm)
  - Resolution of tachypnea (RR < 24)
  - Resolution of hypotension (SBP > 90 mmHg)
- No evidence of complicated infection (e.g., extrapulmonary or pleural involvement)
- Ability to tolerate oral medications

ENVIRONMENTAL (ACCIDENTAL) HYPOTHERMIA

Residence in cold climate is not mandatory for hypothermia to develop.

Risk factors include **advanced age, alcohol or drug use, cognitive impairment, and psychiatric disease.** Additional features are as follows:

Symptoms/Exam

- **Cold water exposure is common.**
- **Temperature** is < 35°C.
  - **Mild hypothermia** occurs with temperatures 33–35°C.
  - **Moderate** and **severe hypothermia** occurs with temperatures < 33°C.
- **Lethargy, irritability,** and **confusion** are common.
- **Tachycardia, tachypnea, and shivering** occur with mild exposure.
- **Loss of shivering, bradycardia, hypotension, respiratory depression,** and **coma** are seen with more severe hypothermia.

Differential

The differential diagnosis of hypothermia is given in Table 10-28.

Diagnosis

- **Laboratory abnormalities** include metabolic acidosis, hypo- and hyperglycemia, DIC, hyperkalemia, and hyperamylasemia.

TABLE 10-28. Differential Diagnosis of Hypothermia

- Environmental (accidental) exposure
- Occult sepsis
- Myxedema
- Adrenal insufficiency
- Hypopituitarism
- DKA
- Hepatic failure

- ECG may show **Osborn or J waves (notching of the terminal aspect of the QRS complex, best seen in lead V_4), slow atrial fibrillation, and prolonged cardiac intervals** (see Figure 10-2).

Ventricular dysrhythmias occur during rewarming; ventricular fibrillation is treated with bretylium if available. Otherwise, the standard ACLS protocol is appropriate.

TREATMENT

The treatment of accidental hypothermia is as follows (see also Table 10-29):

- **Limit movement and manipulation of the patient;** unnecessary stimulation (including central line and NG tube placement) can result in ventricular dysrhythmias.
- **Empiric antibiotics** are unnecessary except in the immunocompromised and elderly.
- **Bradycardia** should generally not be treated, especially given the risk of ventricular fibrillation with placement of a pacing wire.
- If **cardiac arrest** occurs, resuscitation should not cease until the core temperature reaches at least 32°C—**"a patient with hypothermia is not dead until he/she is warm and dead."**

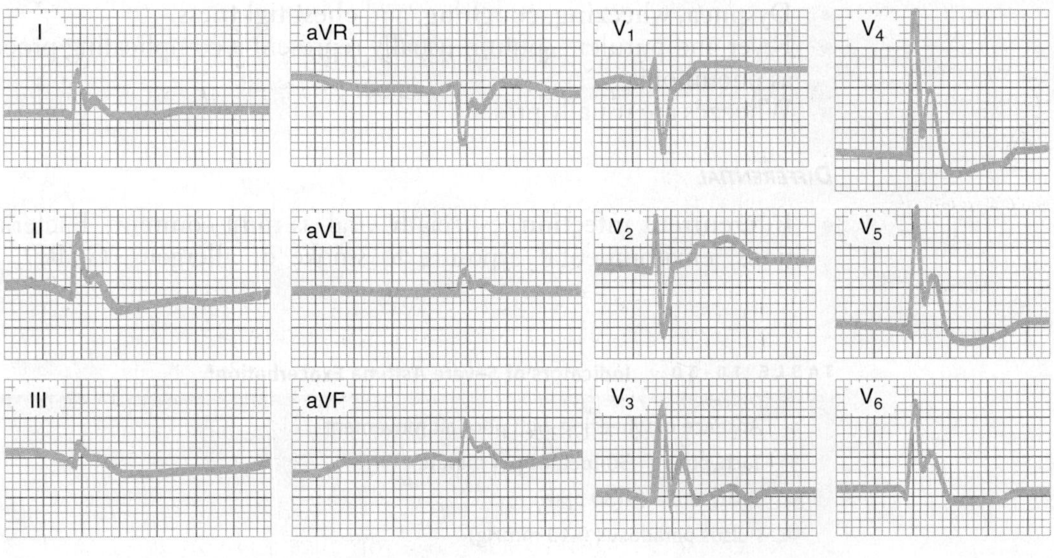

FIGURE 10-2. Osborn Wave in Hypothermia.

(Courtesy of R. Brindis. Reproduced, with permission, from Goldschlager N, Goldman MJ. *Principles of Clinical Electrocardiography*, 13th ed. New York: McGraw-Hill, 1989.)

TABLE 10-29. **Rewarming Techniques in Accidental Hypothermia**

METHOD	DESCRIPTION	INDICATIONS	COMMENTS
Passive external rewarming	Removal of wet clothes; coverage with blankets.	Mild hypothermia.	Limited efficacy.
Active external rewarming	Warmed blankets (including hot air blankets over torso only); warmed baths.	Mild hypothermia.	Limited efficacy; rewarming of the extremities can cause paradoxical worsening because of return of chilled blood from the extremities.
Active internal or core rewarming[a]	Warmed IV fluids; warmed humidified air.	Moderate and severe hypothermia.	Widely available; limited efficacy.
	Extracorporeal blood rewarming via cardiopulmonary, arteriovenous, or venovenous bypass.	Moderate and severe hypothermia; cardiac arrest.	Most effective technique; invasive; requires specialized knowledge and equipment.
	Peritoneal/pleural lavage with warmed fluids.	Moderate and severe hypothermia.	Useful when extracorporeal techniques are not available.

[a] The decision to proceed with invasive active internal rewarming is individualized to the patient and dependent on both temperature and clinical manifestations. Noninvasive measures may suffice for most patients with moderate hypothermia.

HOSPITAL MEDICINE

ACUTE EXACERBATIONS OF ASTHMA

Reactive airway disease is present in > 15 million Americans and results in almost 500,000 hospital admissions and 5000 deaths annually. Indicators and risk factors for death are outlined in Tables 10-30 and 10-31.

SYMPTOMS/EXAM

- **Dyspnea, wheezing, coughing,** and **chest tightness.**
- Fever and purulent sputum usually represent a complicating process such as pneumonia.
- **Wheezes** are usually present.

DIFFERENTIAL

- **Intercurrent infection,** especially viral, is most common. Bacterial infections, environmental exposure to smoke or allergens, GERD, medical

TABLE 10-30. **Indicators of Severe Asthma Exacerbation[a]**

- Absence of wheezing with poor air movement
- Tachypnea (> 30 breaths per minute)
- Tachycardia (>130 bpm)
- Pulsus paradoxus (>15 mmHg)
- Accessory respiratory muscle use
- Altered mental status

[a] Each indicator of severe asthma exacerbation presents individually in < 50% of cases.

TABLE 10-31. Risk Factors for Death in Asthma Exacerbations

- Previous severe exacerbations/ICU admissions/intubation
- > 2 hospitalizations or three ER visits in the past year
- Use of corticosteroids or > 2 canisters of β_2-agonist metered-dose inhalers (MDIs) per month
- Difficulty in perceiving presence or severity of airflow obstruction
- Low socioeconomic status
- Illicit drug use
- Serious comorbidities

noncompliance, and use of certain medications (NSAIDs, β-blockers) are also possible.

- **"All that wheezes is not asthma."** Consider CHF, PE, upper airway obstruction, and foreign body aspiration.

A PEF < 50% predicted indicates severe airflow obstruction.

DIAGNOSIS

- **Peak expiratory flow rate (PEF)** is most predictive of the severity of exacerbation and should guide therapy.
- **ABG analysis** is reserved for those with a severe decrease in PEF or suspected hypoventilation; usually shows a decreased P_{CO_2} unless the patient is developing ventilatory failure.
- **CXR** is usually normal and is necessary only when a secondary process is suspected.

A normal or increased P_{CO_2} indicates severe airway obstruction.

TREATMENT

Treatment should proceed as outlined below (see also Table 10-32):

- **Systemic corticosteroids** are the mainstay of treatment.
  - Decrease the need for hospitalization and subsequent relapse rate when begun immediately.
  - May require 6–8 hours to provide a significant effect.
  - Oral and IV preparations are equally effective.
- **Inhaled bronchodilator therapy:**
  - **Combination therapy** (β_2-agonists and ipratropium bromide) in all patients with moderate to severe exacerbations.
  - **Drug delivery is equivalent** with handheld MDIs and nebulizer therapy, although the latter may be more effective in patients who have difficulty using inhalers or are in respiratory distress.
- **Antibiotics** are generally unnecessary; reserve for patients with evidence of an underlying bacterial infection.
- O_2 therapy should be provided to keep O_2 saturations above 90%.

TABLE 10-32. Treatment of Acute Asthma Exacerbations

ALL PATIENTS	SELECTED PATIENTS	NOT USEFUL/HARMFUL
Corticosteroids	Antibiotics	Theophylline
Inhaled bronchodilators	O_2	Injected bronchodilators
	Mechanical ventilation	Chest physiotherapy
	? Noninvasive mechanical ventilation	Mucolytic agents
		Magnesium

TABLE 10-33. Indications for Mechanical Ventilation[a]

- Persistent hypercapnia
- Altered mental status
- Progressive and persistent acidemia (pH < 7.30)
- Respiratory fatigue

[a] If the patient does not respond to appropriate therapy. Most patients, even with hypercapnia, will respond to therapy and will not require intubation.

- **Endotracheal intubation and mechanical ventilation** (see Table 10-33) should be reserved for patients who do not respond to the above therapies and continue to experience severe airflow obstruction.
- **Noninvasive mechanical ventilation** is not well established.
- **Disposition:** The PEF should guide all decisions regarding disposition (see Figure 10-3).

ACUTE EXACERBATIONS OF CHRONIC OBSTRUCTIVE PULMONARY DISEASE

The fourth leading cause of death in the United States, COPD accounts for > 500,000 hospital admissions and > 100,000 deaths annually.

SYMPTOMS/EXAM

Three features are commonly present: worsening **dyspnea,** increased **cough,** and **change in sputum volume or purulence.**

- A **mild** exacerbation includes one of these symptoms, **moderate** two, and **severe** all three.

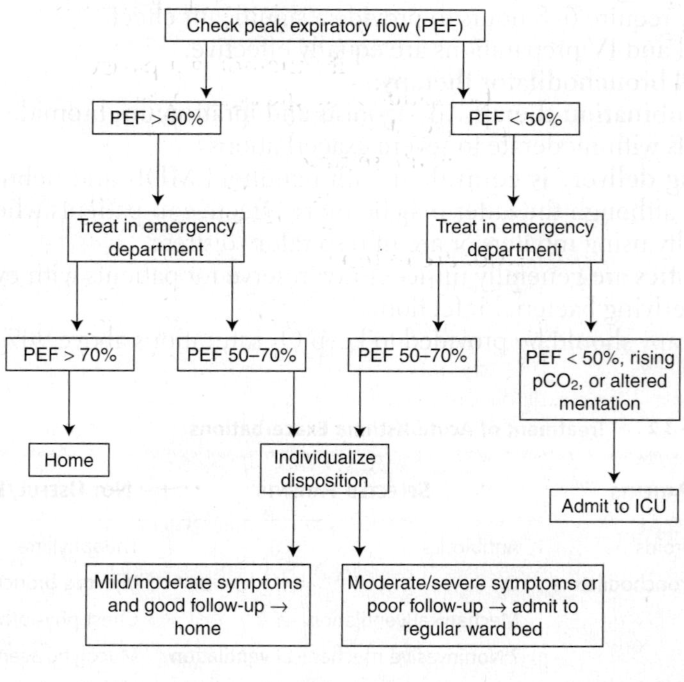

FIGURE 10-3. Determination of disposition on the basis of PEF.

TABLE 10-34. Causes of COPD Exacerbations

- Superimposed infection, most commonly viral
- PE
- Pneumothorax
- Myocardial ischemia/infarction
- CHF
- Environmental exposures (including cigarette smoke)

- Other symptoms are usually referable to a concomitant process (e.g., fever with pneumonia or pleurisy with PE).
- **Decreased air movement, prolonged expiratory time.** Wheezes and extra pulmonary sounds are not always present.
- **Use of accessory muscles of respiration, pursed-lip breathing, cyanosis.**

DIAGNOSIS

- The diagnosis is made clinically. A diligent search for exacerbating or concomitant processes should be completed in all patients (see Table 10-34).
- **Spirometry** is of low utility in guiding acute management and poorly predictive of disease severity when obtained in an acute setting.
- **PEF measurements** are far less reliable in COPD exacerbations than in asthma.
- A **CXR** should be obtained in all patients to assess the possibility of pneumonia and other exacerbating factors.
- **ABG analysis** is not mandatory but should be considered in those at risk for hypercarbia and those with altered mental status.

TREATMENT

- **Antibiotics** should be started in patients with exacerbations severe enough to warrant hospitalization (see Table 10-35). Antibiotics should cover *S. pneumoniae* and *H. influenzae.*
- **Bronchodilator therapy** in all patients, including a β_2-agonist (most commonly albuterol) and/or the anticholinergic agent ipratropium bromide.
  - Limited data exist to suggest the superiority of combination therapy over monotherapy in an acute setting.
  - Drug delivery is equivalent with handheld MDIs and nebulizer therapy, although the latter may be more effective in patients who have difficulty using inhalers or are in respiratory distress.
- **Corticosteroids** (oral and parenteral) result in an increased FEV_1.
  - A two-week course of therapy is as effective as an extended eight-week course.

TABLE 10-35. Factors Favoring Hospitalization for COPD

- Severe underlying disease
- Hypercarbia
- Hypoxemia
- Lack of response to ER treatment
- Lack of in-home support
- Poor baseline functional status

TABLE 10-36. Medicare Criteria for Long-Term O_2 Therapy

- $Pao_2 \le 55$ mmHg or O_2 saturation $\le 88\%$

OR

- Pao_2 56–59 mmHg or O_2 saturation $\le 89\%$ with
  - P pulmonale on ECG or
  - Lower extremity edema or
  - Hematocrit $\ge 55\%$

OR

- $Pao_2 \le 55$ mmHg or O_2 saturation $\le 88\%$ with exercise or sleep (for use with sleep or exercise)

> ***COPD treatment—***
>
> **ABC-ON**
>
> **A**ntibiotics
> **B**ronchodilators
> **C**orticosteroids
> **O**xygen
> **N**oninvasive mechanical ventilation

Oxygen should not be withheld when indicated because of fears of suppressing respiratory drive.

- Inhaled corticosteroids have no role in the treatment of hospitalized patients (with the possible exception of the continuation of chronic therapy).
- **O_2 therapy** should be considered in all patients and should not be withheld because of concerns about suppressing respiratory drive. O_2 should be titrated to provide an O_2 saturation of at least 88%.
- **Noninvasive mechanical ventilation** reduces the need for invasive mechanical ventilation and shortens the length of stay in the intensive care setting; it may also improve survival.
- **Smoking cessation counseling** and **nicotine replacement therapy** for all patients actively smoking.
- **Theophylline** and methylxanthines should not be initiated as therapy for an acute exacerbation but may be continued if taken as part of chronic maintenance therapy. Chest physiotherapy and mucolytic therapy are ineffective as acute interventions.
- **Long-term O_2 therapy (LTOT)** improves mortality in severe COPD, and all patients should be screened for eligibility (see Table 10-36).
- **Pulmonary rehabilitation,** including breathing exercises, support networks, and exercise education, can additionally improve quality of life.
- Differs from treatment of COPD exacerbations (see Table 10-37).

TABLE 10-37. Treatment of Acute Exacerbations of Asthma vs. COPD

TREATMENT	ASTHMA	COPD
PEF useful	Yes	No
Systemic corticosteroids	Yes	Yes
Antibiotics	No	Yes
O_2	Yes	Yes
Combination bronchodilator therapy[a]	Yes	Unclear
Noninvasive mechanical ventilation	Unclear	Yes

[a] β_2-agonist and ipratropium bromide.

CHAPTER 11

Infectious Diseases

José M. Eguía, MD

Flora

- Oropharynx 4S MNOPQ
  - Strep viridans
  - Staph
  - Strep. pyogenes
  - Strep pneumoniae
  - Moraxella Catarrhalis
  - Neiserria sp.
  - Obligate anaerobes (not B fragilis)
  - Parasites
  - Hemophilus sp.
  - Corynebacteria.
- Nasopharynx.
  - S
  - S
  - S
  - S
  - M
  - N
  - H
- Skin. Staph (including aureus)
  - coryne
  - propionibacteria
  - 3 Fungus - Candida
    - M. furfur
    - Dermatophytes
- Upper intestine:
  - Strep.
  - Lactobacilli
  - Candida
- Large intestine
  - Obligate anaerobe (including B. fragilis)
  - Aerobic gm Negative bacilli
  - Streptococci (including Enterococci.)
  - C. albicans
  - Protozoa.
- Conjunctiva
  - Staph
  - Corynebacteria
  - Hemophilus sp.
- lower GenitoUrinary
  - Staph
  - SLC
  - Anaerobes oblig
  - Bacilli Gm-ve
  - corynebac
  - Vaginalis
  - Neisseria sp.

ACTINOMYCES VS. NOCARDIA

Table 11-1 contrasts the clinical presentation, diagnosis, and treatment of *Actinomyces* infections with that of *Nocardia* infections.

Actinomycosis can spread without regard to tissue planes.

ASPLENIA-RELATED INFECTIONS

Postsplenectomy sepsis has a short viral-like prodrome followed by abrupt deterioration and shock. Encapsulated organisms involved include *Streptococcus pneumoniae* (> 50%), *Neisseria meningitidis,* and *Haemophilus influenzae.* Other organisms include *Capnocytophaga* (dog or cat contact), *Salmonella* (sickle cell anemia), *Babesia,* and malaria (more fulminant).

PREVENTION

- **Vaccinate** against *S. pneumoniae, H. influenzae* type b (unvaccinated older individuals), and *N. meningitidis.* Vaccinate ≥ 2 weeks before elective splenectomy or at hospital discharge.
- Give a supply of antibiotics to be taken as **self-administered therapy** for fevers (e.g., amoxicillin to be taken at the onset of fever, followed by immediate evaluation in urgent care). **Daily prophylaxis** for a defined period (e.g., penicillin for 3–5 years following splenectomy) is recommended for children but not adults.

BABESIOSIS

An *Ixodes* tick–borne illness caused by *Babesia microti,* an intracellular protozoan that infects RBCs. Found in coastal New England and Long Island and, to a lesser extent, in the upper Midwest and the West Coast. Infections peak in summer and early fall.

Think of babesiosis in a febrile elderly or asplenic patient who lives in the coastal Northeast and presents with hemolytic anemia and thrombocytopenia in the summer or early fall.

SYMPTOMS

Fever, chills, headache, myalgia, fatigue, anorexia, nausea, vomiting, abdominal pain, and **dark urine** may be seen, but most cases are asymptomatic. Healthy individuals may have mild illness with intermittent symptoms for weeks to months. Older, asplenic, or immunocompromised (including HIV-positive) patients present with more severe symptoms.

TABLE 11-1. Diagnosis and Treatment of *Actinomyces* and *Nocardia* Infections

	Actinomyces	*Nocardia*
Gram stain	Gram-positive, branching rod	Gram-positive, branching rod
Acid-fast stain	Negative	**Weakly AFB positive**
Pathology	Sulfur granules and draining sinuses	Abscess
Infected host	Poor dentition or IUD user	**Immunocompromised**
Sites of infection	Mandible, lung, abdomen/pelvis	Lung, CNS, skin
Treatment	Penicillin for 6–12 months	TMP-SMX for 3–6 months

EXAM

Fever, hepatosplenomegaly, and occasionally petechiae or ecchymoses.

DIAGNOSIS

- **Peripheral blood smears** show intracellular parasites in 1–10% of RBCs (or up to 85% if severe). The classic "Maltese cross" tetrads may be seen, but **more commonly *Babesia* parasites look like *Plasmodium falciparum* signet-ring forms with no other parasitic stages seen** (see Figure 11-1).
- Labs show **hemolytic anemia,** mild leukopenia, **thrombocytopenia,** elevated LFTs, and hemoglobinuria.
- Antibody tests are available.
- PCR may be more sensitive for detecting low levels of parasitemia.

TREATMENT

- Most infections are **self-limited.**
- For sicker, asplenic, or immunocompromised patients, use clindamycin + quinine or atovaquone + azithromycin (doxycycline and most antimalarial drugs are ineffective).
- **Exchange transfusion** has been used as adjunctive therapy in patients with a high degree of hemolysis or parasitemia (> 10%) or with the more severe European forms of the disease.

COMPLICATIONS

Patients may develop shock or ARDS. Deaths in the United States have occurred in patients both with and without spleens. **Coinfection with Lyme disease** should be suspected in any patient with babesiosis.

BARTONELLA

A pleomorphic gram-negative rod. *Bartonella henselae* is transmitted by kittens or feral cats, *Bartonella quintana* by body lice. The type of disease depends on the transmitted species and level of immune compromise. The spectrum of disease in *B. henselae* includes **cat-scratch disease,** bacillary

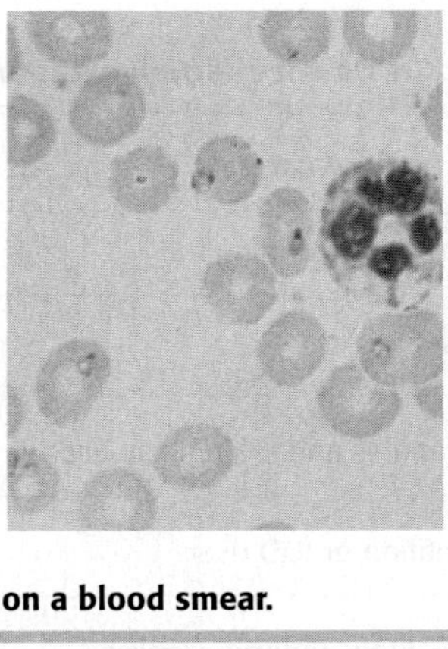

FIGURE 11-1. Babesiosis on a blood smear.

Note parasites within RBCs resembling malaria. Tetrads and classic "Maltese crosses" are rare but diagnostic of babesiosis. (Reproduced, with permission, from *Bench Aids for the Diagnosis of Malaria Infections*, 2nd ed. Geneva: World Health Organization, 2000.) (Also see Color Insert.)

angiomatosis, and peliosis hepatis; that of *B. quintana* includes **trench fever, bacteremia, endocarditis,** bacillary angiomatosis, and peliosis hepatis.

SYMPTOMS/EXAM

- **Cat-scratch disease (*B. henselae*; immune-competent patients):** Presents with fever, malaise, a papule or pustule at the site of the cat scratch or bite, and regional adenopathy (usually in the head, neck, or axillae).
- **Bacillary angiomatosis and peliosis hepatis (*B. henselae* and *B. quintana*; AIDS patients):** The skin nodules of bacillary angiomatosis are friable, red-to-purplish lesions that may ulcerate. Peliosis produces fever, weight loss, abdominal pain, and hepatosplenomegaly; imaging shows hypodense, cystic, blood-filled structures in the liver, spleen, or lymph nodes. May be a cause of fever of unknown origin (FUO) in AIDS patients.
- **Trench fever (*B. quintana*; immune-competent patients):** Relapsing febrile paroxysms last up to five days each and are sometimes accompanied by headache, myalgias, hepatosplenomegaly, and leukocytosis. Seen in the homeless and in those from war-torn regions.

DIFFERENTIAL

- **Cat-scratch disease:** TB, atypical mycobacterial infection, sporotrichosis, tularemia, plague, leishmaniasis, histoplasmosis, infectious mononucleosis.
- **Bacillary angiomatosis:** Kaposi's sarcoma, pyogenic granuloma.
- **Trench fever:** Endocarditis, TB, typhoid fever.

Consider bioterrorism-related disease when observing the sudden onset of multiple cases of severe illness (often with flulike prodromes) with a fulminant course and high mortality.

DIAGNOSIS

- Blood cultures (not sensitive), serologic tests.
- Lymph node aspirate in cat-scratch disease may show sterile pus.
- Lymph node biopsy shows stellate necrosis and bacilli on Warthin-Starry silver stain.

TREATMENT

- Erythromycin, azithromycin, doxycycline.
- Cat-scratch disease usually resolves in several months and may not require treatment other than needle aspiration for symptom relief.

BIOTERRORISM AGENTS

Table 11-2 outlines infectious agents that could potentially be used in bioterrorism.

Smallpox presents with deep, tense lesions that are at the same stage and may appear on the palms and soles. Varicella lesions are more superficial lesions, appear at different states of maturation, and are never found on the palms and soles.

CATHETER-RELATED INFECTIONS

Include catheter-related bloodstream infections (CRBSIs) as well as exit-site, tunnel, and pocket infections. The most commonly isolated etiologic agents are coagulase-negative staphylococci, *S. aureus*, enterococci, and *Candida albicans*.

SYMPTOMS/EXAM

Clinical findings are unreliable. Fever and chills are sensitive but not specific findings. Inflammation and purulence around the catheter and bloodstream infection are specific but not sensitive.

TABLE 11-2. **Potential Bioterrorism Agents**

AGENT/ DISEASE	CLINICAL FINDINGS	SYNDROME	DIFFERENTIAL	INITIAL DIAGNOSTIC TESTING	IMMEDIATE INFECTION CONTROL MEASURES	TREATMENT
Inhalational anthrax	Nonspecific flulike illness followed by abrupt onset of fever, chest pain, and dyspnea **without CXR findings of pneumonia;** progression to shock and death in 24–36 hours.	Acute respiratory distress with fever.	Pulmonary embolism, dissecting aortic aneurysm.	CXR with **widened mediastinum;** gram-positive rods in blood.	Standard precautions.	Ciprofloxacin, doxycycline, penicillin.
Pneumonic plague	Apparent severe community-acquired pneumonia, but with hemoptysis, cyanosis, GI symptoms, and progression to shock and death in 2–4 days.	Acute respiratory distress with fever.	Community-acquired pneumonia, hantavirus pulmonary syndrome, meningococcemia, rickettsial disease.	Gram-negative rods or coccobacilli with "safety pin" appearance in sputum, blood, or lymph nodes.	Standard and droplet precautions.	Ciprofloxacin, doxycycline, gentamicin, streptomycin.
Smallpox	Severe flulike prodrome followed by a generalized papular rash that **begins on the face and extremities** and uniformly progresses to vesicles and pustules, headache, vomiting, back pain, and delirium.	Acute rash with fever.	Varicella (chickenpox), disseminated herpes zoster, monkeypox.	Clinical diagnosis.	Standard, droplet, airborne and contact precautions.	Supportive care.
Viral hemorrhagic fever (e.g., Ebola)	Fever with **mucosal bleeding,** petechiae, thrombocytopenia, and hypotension.	Acute rash with fever.	Meningococcemia, malaria, typhus, leptospirosis, TTP, HUS.	Clinical diagnosis.	Standard and contact precautions.	Supportive care.

TABLE 11-2. Potential Bioterrorism Agents (continued)

Agent/ Disease	Clinical Findings	Syndrome	Differential	Initial Diagnostic Testing	Immediate Infection Control Measures	Treatment
Tularemia	Fever, rigors, headache, myalgia, coryza, and sore throat followed by substernal discomfort, dry cough, pleuritis, or pneumonitis.	Influenza-like illness.	Influenza, atypical pneumonia, SARS, anthrax, smallpox, plague, Q fever.	CXR with infiltrate, hilar adenopathy, or effusion; small gram-negative coccobacilli in sputum or blood.	Standard precautions.	Ciprofloxacin, doxycycline, gentamicin, streptomycin.
Cutaneous anthrax	Pruritic maculopapule that ulcerates by day 2, progressing to vesicles and a painless black eschar with extensive nonpitting edema.	Localized ulcer and extensive edema.	Staphylococcal lymphadenitis, ecthyma gangrenosum.	Gram-positive rods in vesicle fluid.	Standard precautions.	Ciprofloxacin, doxycycline, penicillin.

Adapted from the California State Department of Health and the Centers for Disease Control and Prevention.

Diagnosis

- **Blood cultures:** Obtain two sets of cultures, at least one of which is drawn percutaneously.
- **Catheter cultures:** Should be performed only if CRBSI is suspected. The **semiquantitative (roll plate) method,** in which the catheter tip is rolled across an agar plate, is most commonly used. A **colony count > 15** after overnight incubation suggests catheter-related infection.

Treatment

- **Catheter removal** in most cases of **nontunneled** CRBSI. For **tunneled catheters and implantable devices,** consider removal in the presence of severe illness or documented infection (especially *S. aureus*, gram-negative rods, or *Candida*) or if complications occur.
- **Initial antibiotic therapy:** Treatment is usually **empiric** with vancomycin (to cover methicillin-resistant *S. aureus*).
- **Duration of treatment:** Patients with **uncomplicated bacteremia** should be treated for **10–14 days;** those with **complicated infections** (e.g., persistently positive blood cultures after catheter removal, endocarditis, septic thrombophlebitis, osteomyelitis) should be treated for **4–8 weeks.**

Transesophageal echocardiography is a cost-effective means of ruling out endocarditis in S. aureus *CRBSI. Transthoracic echocardiography is less sensitive.*

Complications

Septic thrombophlebitis, infective endocarditis, septic pulmonary emboli, osteomyelitis, or other complications due to septic emboli.

CLOSTRIDIUM DIFFICILE COLITIS

Risk factors for *C. difficile* colitis include antibiotic use (particularly clindamycin, cephalosporins, and ampicillin), cancer chemotherapy, bowel surgery, and multiple-organ failure. Diarrhea usually occurs after **one week** of antibiotic therapy but may arise up to **six weeks** later.

SYMPTOMS/EXAM

Diarrhea (usually watery; **may be bloody**), abdominal pain and distention, fever, leukocytosis.

C. difficile is a common cause of otherwise unexplained leukocytosis in hospitalized patients.

DIFFERENTIAL

Antibiotic side effects without *C. difficile*, neutropenic enterocolitis/**typhlitis,** IBD, ischemic bowel.

DIAGNOSIS

- **Fecal WBCs and stool cultures are not useful.**
- **Toxin assays are necessary** because 5% of healthy patients and 25% of hospitalized patients have *C. difficile* in their stools, but only one-third have symptoms.
- **Radiographs** show colonic distention and thickening ("thumbprinting" may be seen on plain abdominal films).
- **Endoscopy** shows friable, edematous mucosa with raised yellow plaques (pseudomembranes); specific but not sensitive.

TREATMENT

Diarrhea that arises during antibiotic treatment may also be caused by adverse drug effects (amoxicillin, amoxicillin/clavulanic acid, erythromycin).

- **Stop antibiotics** if possible.
- Avoid antidiarrheal agents and opiates.
- Contact isolation.
- Give **PO** or IV **metronidazole** (PO is preferred) or PO vancomycin (oral vancomycin is as effective as metronidazole but is more costly and carries the risk of vancomycin-resistant enterococcus; IV vancomycin is ineffective).
- The **relapse** rate is 15%, with relapses usually occurring **within two weeks** of treatment cessation.
  - For first-time recurrences, treat again with the same regimen.
  - For refractory cases, consider tapering or pulse-dosing PO treatment, cholestyramine (binds toxin) or bacitracin, vancomycin + rifampin, or vancomycin enemas.

COMPLICATIONS

Ileus, toxic megacolon, perforation (all may be accompanied by a decrease in diarrhea), hemorrhage, sepsis.

EHRLICHIOSIS

A tick-borne illness caused by rickettsiae. Two main types:

- **Human monocytic ehrlichiosis (HME):** Caused by *Ehrlichia chaffeensis;* found in southern states such as Arkansas and Missouri (where Rocky Mountain spotted fever is also present).
- **Human granulocytic ehrlichiosis (HGE):** Caused primarily by *Anaplasma phagocytophila;* found in the Northeast and upper Midwest (where Lyme disease is also present).

SYMPTOMS/EXAM

Most cases are asymptomatic, but some may present with fever, malaise, myalgias, and headache (flulike symptoms occurring in the spring and summer months) as well as with nausea, arthralgias, anorexia, and chills. HME and HGE are clinically indistinguishable.

Ehrlichiosis has been called "spotless" Rocky Mountain spotted fever in that there is clinical and epidemiologic overlap.

DIFFERENTIAL

Rocky Mountain spotted fever, leptospirosis, influenza, infectious mononucleosis, aseptic meningitis, dengue fever, typhoid fever.

DIAGNOSIS

- **Leukopenia** and **thrombocytopenia;** often **elevated LFTs.**
- **Peripheral blood smear** may show **morulae** ("mulberries" in Latin), a cluster of organisms in the cytoplasm of WBCs. The test is insensitive, especially for HME.
- Acute and convalescent antibody titers are most sensitive (> 95% of patients develop antibodies within four weeks of symptom onset).
- PCR.

TREATMENT

Doxycycline (or chloramphenicol).

COMPLICATIONS

Pneumonitis, septic shock, hepatitis, renal failure, DIC. May be fatal, especially in older patients.

ENCEPHALITIS

HSV and arboviruses (e.g., **West Nile virus,** eastern and western equine virus, St. Louis virus) are the most common causes of encephalitis in the United States. Patients may report travel (e.g., Japanese B virus), tick bite (e.g., Rocky Mountain spotted fever, Lyme disease, ehrlichiosis), or animal bite (e.g., rabies). Postinfectious cases are seen 1–3 weeks after URI, measles infection, or smallpox vaccination.

In contrast with meningitis, encephalitis is an infection of the brain parenchyma and is characterized by cognitive deficits.

SYMPTOMS

Presents with **fever,** headache, neck stiffness, altered mental status (from mild lethargy to confusion, stupor, and coma), and alterations in speech and behavior.

EXAM

Focal neurologic signs, including motor weakness, accentuated DTRs, hemiparesis, cranial nerve palsies (especially CN III and CN VI), and seizures. A rash may be seen with Lyme disease, Rocky Mountain spotted fever, and VZV; weakness and flaccid paralysis may be seen with West Nile virus.

Encephalitis that develops in the summer or fall is often due to arboviruses. In late spring or early summer, think of tick-borne infections. In the winter or spring, think of measles, mumps, and VZV.

DIFFERENTIAL

Brain abscess, primary or secondary brain tumor, subdural hematoma, SLE, drugs/toxic encephalopathy.

DIAGNOSIS

The primary goal is to **distinguish HSV from other causes.**

- CSF findings are usually abnormal but nonspecific. May see **RBCs** in HSV encephalitis.
- EEG shows diffuse slowing of brain waves. **HSV encephalitis may localize to the temporal lobes** with highly characteristic slow-wave (2- to 3-Hz) complexes.
- MRI with gadolinium shows multifocal lesions (white matter demyelination may be seen in postinfectious cases). Temporal lobe involvement is seen with HSV.
- Acute and convalescent serologies.
- Special CSF testing for specific arboviral IgM antibodies. **PCR for HSV is sensitive and specific in most studies.**

TREATMENT

- Supportive care (antipyretics, antiseizure medications, lower ICP, mechanical ventilation). IV acyclovir for HSV and VZV.
- The effect of steroids or IVIG on postinfectious encephalitis is unclear.

COMPLICATIONS

Patients with HSV encephalitis have high mortality (70%) and serious sequelae, especially if treatment is delayed. Arboviral infections are largely subclinical except for eastern equine virus, which has > 50% mortality in infants and older adults but is the least common.

ENDOCARDITIS

Infection of the heart valves. Classified as **native-valve endocarditis (NVE)** or **prosthetic-valve endocarditis (PVE)**. IV drug users are a special population at risk, particularly for tricuspid valve endocarditis (see Table 11-3).

TABLE 11-3. Etiology of Endocarditis

TYPE	ETIOLOGY
NVE	Viridans streptococci, other streptococci, *S. aureus,* enterococci.
PVE	*S. epidermidis, S. aureus.*
IV drug use	*S. aureus.*
"Culture-negative" endocarditis	Recent antibiotic use. **HACEK** organisms (*Haemophilus, Actinobacillus, Cardiobacterium, Eikenella, Kingella*). *Candida* and *Aspergillus* (IV drug users, long-term indwelling catheters, immunosuppressed). Rare causes: *Chlamydia psittaci,* the "ellas" (*Bartonella, Legionella, Brucella, Coxiella*), and Whipple's disease.

Symptoms

- **Acute bacterial endocarditis:** High fever (80%), chills, and embolic phenomena; often no murmur.
- **Subacute endocarditis:** Indolent course; presents with low-grade fever and more immunologic manifestations.

Exam

Presents with fever, heart murmur, **Osler's nodes** ("OUCHler nodes"—painful nodules on the finger and toe pads), **splinter hemorrhages** (red-brown streaks in the proximal nail beds), **petechiae** (especially conjunctival and mucosal), **Janeway lesions** (nontender hemorrhagic macules on the palms and soles), and **Roth's spots** (retinal hemorrhages; see Figure 11-2). Patients with right-sided disease may develop right-sided heart failure or pulmonary findings, including pleuritic chest pain, cough, and radiographic abnormalities (multiple peripheral infiltrates with cavitation or effusions).

Differential

Atrial myxoma, marantic endocarditis (nonbacterial thrombotic endocarditis, seen in cancer and chronic wasting diseases), Libman-Sacks Endocarditis (seen in **SLE**; autoantibodies to heart valve), acute rheumatic fever, suppurative thrombophlebitis, catheter-related sepsis, renal cell carcinoma, carcinoid syndrome.

Diagnosis

- **Labs:** Leukocytosis with left shift, mild anemia, elevated ESR. UA may show proteinuria, **microscopic hematuria,** and RBC casts.
- **Blood cultures** are critical in establishing a diagnosis and are positive in 85–95% of cases. It is recommended that **three sets** of blood cultures be taken at least **one hour apart** (before antibiotics).
- **Echocardiography:** Transthoracic echo has 60–75% sensitivity, transesophageal echocardiography (TEE) 95% sensitivity. Both are 95% specific.

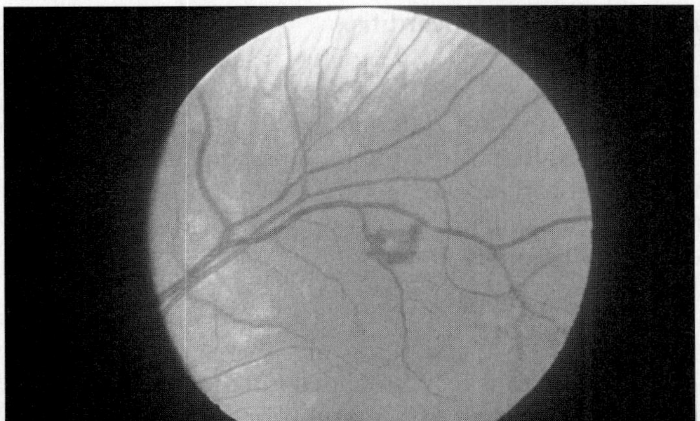

FIGURE 11-2. Roth's spot in endocarditis.

This retinal image shows a lesion with central clear areas surrounded by hemorrhage. (Courtesy of William E. Cappaert, MD. Reproduced, with permission, from Knoop KJ, Stack LB, Storrow AB. *Atlas of Emergency Medicine*, 2nd ed. New York: McGraw-Hill, 2002:80.) (Also see Color Insert.)

INFECTIOUS DISEASES

- Duke criteria:
  - **Major criteria: Positive blood cultures** (two or more sets drawn at separate sites and times) and either a **new murmur** or an **oscillating vegetation on echocardiogram.**
  - **Minor criteria: Predisposing conditions, fever, embolic disease** (pulmonary or intracranial infarcts, mycotic aneurysm, conjunctival hemorrhages, Janeway lesions), **immunologic phenomena** (glomerulonephritis, Osler's nodes, Roth's spots, RF), and a positive **blood culture** not meeting the major criteria.
  - Two major, one major + three minor, or five minor criteria support a diagnosis of **definite** endocarditis. Endocarditis is highly unlikely if none of these criteria are met.

Treatment

- **NVE (empiric):** Typically start with nafcillin + gentamicin or vancomycin + gentamicin. Gentamicin should be given q 8 h for synergistic killing (no once-daily dosing). Adjust antibiotics on the basis of culture results and treat for 4–6 weeks. Uncomplicated right-sided staphylococcal endocarditis (with no embolic disease) can be treated with nafcillin + gentamicin × 2 weeks.
- **PVE (empiric):** Vancomycin + rifampin + gentamicin. Adjust antibiotics on the basis of culture results and treat for six weeks.
- **Persistent fever** after **one week** suggests a septic embolic focus or inadequate antibiotic coverage.
- **Reappearance of fever** after initial defervescence suggests septic emboli, drug fever, interstitial nephritis, or, less commonly, the emergence of resistant organisms.
- **Indications for surgery during active infection:** Refractory CHF (50% mortality if surgery delayed), valvular obstruction, myocardial abscess, perivalvular extension (new conduction abnormalities), persistent bacteremia, fungal endocarditis, and most cases of PVE.

> Streptococcus bovis *and* Clostridium septicum *endocarditis/bacteremia are seen in patients with bowel pathology and should prompt upper and lower GI endoscopies.*

Complications

- **CHF:** Caused by valvular destruction or myocarditis. The **most common cause of death due to endocarditis.**
- **Embolic phenomena:** Mycotic aneurysms, infarcts, or abscesses in the CNS, kidney, coronary arteries, or spleen. Right-sided disease usually causes pulmonary emboli but may also cause systemic emboli with a **patent foramen ovale** (positive bubble study on echocardiogram).
- Arrhythmias and heart block.
- Myocardial or perivalvular abscess (especially with *S. aureus*); may extend to cause pericarditis and tamponade.

> *PR prolongation in a patient with endocarditis may suggest conduction abnormalities due to an aortic valve ring abscess.*

Prevention

- **Antibiotic prophylaxis** is recommended for known valvular disease (mitral valve prolapse only if there is a murmur or thickened leaflet), most congenital heart disease (except secundum ASDs or repaired VSDs/PDAs), hypertrophic cardiomyopathy, prosthetic valves, and prior endocarditis.
- **Procedures for which prophylaxis is recommended** (in which GI/GU mucosa may potentially be disrupted): Dental extractions, periodontal procedures, surgical/other procedures +/– biopsy (not flexible endoscopy), vaginal hysterectomy, vaginal delivery, C-section.

- **Procedures above the diaphragm:** PO amoxicillin, IV ampicillin, or IV/PO clindamycin 30–60 minutes before the procedure.
- **Procedures below the diaphragm:** IV ampicillin + gentamicin 30 minutes before the procedure followed by PO amoxicillin or IV ampicillin six hours after the procedure; or use IV vancomycin + gentamicin 30 minutes before.

FEBRILE NEUTROPENIA

Defined as a single oral temperature of ≥ 38.3°C (101°F) or ≥ 38°C (100.4°F) for ≥ 1 hour in a neutropenic patient (< 500 cells/mm^3 or < 1000 and expected to decrease to ≤ 500 cells/mm^3). Patients have usually received cancer chemotherapy in the **preceding 7–10 days.** Causes include infection, and, to a lesser extent, mucositis, drugs, and the malignancy itself.

SYMPTOMS

Patients may be asymptomatic with little or no inflammatory response.

EXAM

Subtle signs include pain at commonly infected sites—e.g., the periodontium, pharynx, lower esophagus, abdomen, lung, perineum/anus, eye (fundus), or skin (vascular catheter access sites, bone marrow aspiration sites, nails).

DIAGNOSIS

Physical examination (excluding rectal examination), CBC with differential, BUN, creatinine, transaminases, and blood cultures (peripheral and/or catheter); culture other inflamed or purulent sites for bacteria/fungi; CXR if there are respiratory signs/symptoms.

TREATMENT

- **If fever: Empiric antibiotics** after a prompt and thorough initial evaluation (cefepime, ceftazidime, imipenem, or meropenem +/– aminoglycoside +/– vancomycin).
- **If no fever:** Antibiotics if signs and symptoms are compatible with infection.
- Remove vascular access devices (e.g., Hickman-Broviac catheters, subcutaneous ports) in the presence of subcutaneous tunnel/periport infection, septic emboli, hypotension, or nonfunctioning catheters.
- **Low risk for developing severe infection:** Patients < 60 years of age; those with mild or no symptoms, no hypotension, no COPD, and no prior fungal infection; those with solid tumors; and those who are outpatients at the time of fever onset. If prompt access to medical care is available, can treat with a PO outpatient regimen. **Other patients are high risk** and should be hospitalized for IV antibiotics and further evaluation.
- **Indications for empiric vancomycin:** Hypotension, suspected serious catheter-related infections (e.g., cellulitis, bacteremia), known colonization with drug-resistant pneumococci or methicillin-resistant S. *aureus*, preliminary blood cultures with gram-positive bacteria.
- Granulocyte transfusions are not recommended for routine use.
- **Hematopoietic growth factors** (colony-stimulating factors) are recommended only if a long delay is expected in bone marrow recovery.

- Patients who remain febrile should be reassessed after **3–5 days.** Options are as follows:
  - Continue the **same regimen** if clinically stable.
  - **Change** or **add antibiotics** (e.g., vancomycin) if there is progressive disease.
  - Add an **antifungal agent** if the patient is expected to remain neutropenic for 5–7 more days.

FEVER OF UNKNOWN ORIGIN (FUO)

Defined as a temperature > 38.3°C (101°F) that lasts at least **three weeks** and remains undiagnosed despite evaluation over **three outpatient visits** or **three hospital days.** Etiologies include infection, cancer (each 25–40%), and, to a lesser extent, autoimmune diseases (15%). Infection is likely if the patient is older or from a developing country or in cases of nosocomial, neutropenic, or HIV-associated FUO.

FUO is most commonly due to unusual presentations of common diseases rather than to rare diseases.

Exam

Repeated physical exams may yield subtle findings in the fundi, conjunctivae, sinuses, temporal arteries, and lymph nodes. Heart murmurs, splenomegaly, and perirectal or prostatic fluctuance/tenderness should be assessed.

Differential

- **Infectious: TB, endocarditis,** and **occult abscesses** are the most common infectious causes of FUO in immune-competent patients. Consider primary HIV infection or opportunistic infections due to unrecognized HIV.
- **Neoplastic: Lymphoma** and **leukemia** are the most common cancers causing FUO. Other causes include hepatoma, renal cell carcinoma, and atrial myxoma.
- **Autoimmune:** Adult Still's disease, SLE, cryoglobulinemia, polyartertis nodosa, giant cell (temporal) arteritis/polymyalgia rheumatica (more common in the elderly).
- **Miscellaneous:** Other causes of FUO include drug fever, hyperthyroidism or thyroiditis, granulomatous hepatitis, sarcoidosis, Crohn's disease, Whipple's disease, familial Mediterranean fever, recurrent pulmonary embolism, retroperitoneal hematoma, and factitious fever.
- In roughly 10–15% of cases, the cause is not diagnosed. **Most of these cases resolve spontaneously.**

Diagnosis

- **History:** Ask about immune status, cardiac valve disorders, drug use, travel, exposure to animals and insects, occupational history, recent medications, sick contacts, and family history of fever.
- Obtain routine labs, blood cultures (off antibiotics; hold culture bottles for two weeks), CXR, and PPD. If indicated, obtain cultures of other body fluids (sputum, urine, stool, CSF) as well as a blood smear (malaria, babesiosis) and HIV test.
- Echocardiography for vegetations; CT/MRI if neoplasms or abscesses are suspected.
- Use more specific tests selectively (ANA, RF, viral cultures, antibody/antigen tests for viral and fungal infections).
- Invasive procedures are generally low yield except for temporal artery biopsy in the elderly, liver biopsy in patients with LFT abnormalities, and bone marrow biopsy for HIV.

Treatment

- If there are no other symptoms, treatment may be deferred until a definitive diagnosis is made.
- Broad-spectrum antibiotics if the patient is severely ill or neutropenic.

Incubation period is very helpful in determining the cause of food-related nausea, vomiting, abdominal pain, or diarrhea.

FOOD-BORNE ILLNESS

Table 11-4 outlines the causes and treatment of food-borne illness, grouped according to incubation period.

FUNGAL INFECTIONS

See Figure 11-3 for typical forms of fungi that might be seen in tissues examined by histopathology.

Patients are usually afebrile in toxin-mediated food-borne illness.

Candidiasis

The opportunistic yeast *Candida* is a commensal found on the skin and in the GI tract and female genital tract. **Superficial infection** is especially common among diabetics. Risk factors for **deep or disseminated infection** include immune compromise due to illness (HIV or malignancy) or treatment (neutropenia or steroids); multiple or prolonged antibiotic treatment; and invasive procedures.

Symptoms/Exam/Diagnosis

- **Candiduria:** Yeast in urine **usually represents colonization** and not infection. Seen in patients with Foley catheters or antibiotic use. Diagnose infection by detecting pyuria or yeast in urine casts; treat if the patient is symptomatic or neutropenic, has undergone renal transplant, or is awaiting urinary tract procedures.
- **Intertrigo ("diaper rash"):** Pruritic vesiculopustules rupture to form macerated or fissured beefy-red areas at skin folds. Satellite lesions may be present. Seen in both immune-competent and immunosuppressed patients.
- **Oral thrush:** Presents with burning sensations of the tongue or mucosa with white, curdlike patches that can be scraped away to reveal a raw surface. Seen in patients with AIDS or malignancy or in those who use inhaled steroids for asthma. Diagnosed by appearance or by scraping with KOH prep or Gram stain.
- **Candidal esophagitis:** Presents with dysphagia, odynophagia, and substernal chest pain. Seen in patients with AIDS, leukemia, and lymphoma. Diagnosed by the endoscopic appearance of white patches or from biopsy showing mucosal invasion. May occur concurrently with HSV or CMV esophagitis.
- **Candidemia and disseminated candidiasis:** Diagnose through cultures of blood, body fluids, or aspirates. Mortality is 40%. Candidemia may lead to endophthalmitis (eye pain, blurred vision), osteomyelitis, arthritis, or endocarditis.
- **Hepatosplenic candidiasis:** Presents with fever and abdominal pain that emerge as neutropenia resolves following bone marrow transplant. Associated with a high mortality rate. Diagnosed by ultrasound or CT imaging showing abscesses. Blood cultures are frequently negative.

TABLE 11-4. Causes of Food-Borne Illness

DISEASE/ASSOCIATIONS	AGENT	SYMPTOMS	TREATMENT
Incubation period < 2 hours: likely toxin/chemical agent			
Ciguatera (grouper, snapper)	**Neurotoxin** from algae that grow in **tropical** reefs.	**Perioral paresthesias** and **shooting pains in the legs** (may persist for months); bradycardia/hypotension if severe.	Emetics/lavage within three hours; IV fluids, atropine/pressors, mannitol.
Scombroid (tuna, mahi-mahi, mackerel)	Histamine-like substance in **spoiled fish.**	Burning mouth/metallic taste, **flushing,** dizziness, headache, GI symptoms; urticaria/bronchospasm if severe.	Antihistamines.
MSG poisoning ("Chinese restaurant syndrome")	Acetylcholine.	Burning sensation in the neck/chest/abdomen/extremities; sweating, bronchospasm, tachycardia.	No treatment.
Incubation period 2–14 hours: likely toxin			
S. aureus (dairy, eggs, mayonnaise, meat products)	Preformed heat-stable enterotoxin.	Vomiting, epigastric pain.	No treatment.
Bacillus cereus (cooked rice kept at room temperature)	Preformed toxin (like *S. aureus*) or sporulation and toxin production in vivo (like *C. perfringens*).	Vomiting, epigastric pain, diarrhea.	No treatment.
Clostridium perfringens (frequently from reheated meats, stews, gravies)	Toxin is released after heat-resistant clostridial spores germinate in the intestines.	Lower GI symptoms.	No treatment.
Incubation period > 14 hours: bacteria, viruses			
Campylobacter (most common)		Fever, diarrhea.	Cipro or azithromycin.
Salmonella		Fever, diarrhea.	Cipro or azithromycin.
Shigella	Shiga toxin.	Fever, diarrhea.	Cipro or azithromycin.

INFECTIOUS DISEASES

TABLE 11-4. Causes of Food-Borne Illness

Disease/Associations	Agent	Symptoms	Treatment
Enteroinvasive *E. coli* (EIEC)		Fever, diarrhea.	Cipro or azithromycin.
Yersinia		Fever, diarrhea.	TMP-SMX or cipro.
Vibrio parahaemolyticus (undercooked seafood)		Fever, diarrhea.	No treatment.
Enterohemorrhagic *E. coli* O157:H7 (EHEC) (undercooked ground beef, contaminated produce)	Shiga toxin.	Usually afebrile; bloody diarrhea, HUS in 5% of cases.	No antibiotics; may increase HUS risk.
Enterotoxigenic *E. coli* (ETEC) ("traveler's diarrhea")	Enterotoxins.	Usually afebrile; diarrhea.	Cipro.
Norwalk-like virus (cruise ship outbreaks)		Usually afebrile; vomiting, headaches, diarrhea.	No treatment.

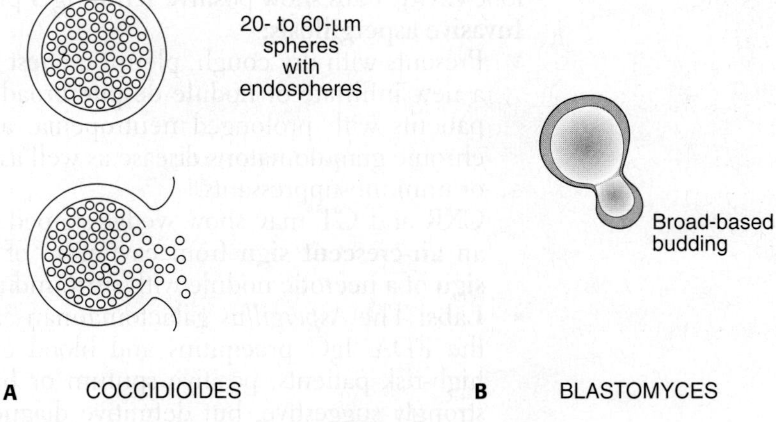

FIGURE 11-3. Characteristic tissue forms of fungi.

(Reproduced, with permission, from Bhushan V, Le T. *First Aid for the USMLE Step 1: 2004*. New York: McGraw-Hill, 2005:191.)

Treatment

- **Candiduria:** Most cases do not need treatment.
- **Intertrigo and oral thrush:** May be treated with topical antifungals (nystatin, clotrimazole or miconazole creams, or nystatin suspension swish and swallow).
- **Esophagitis and other deep or disseminated infections:** Options include fluconazole, amphotericin, voriconazole, and caspofungin.
- Replace vascular catheters at a new site (do not exchange over a wire!).
- *Candida albicans* is the most common cause and is usually susceptible to fluconazole. *C. albicans* can be distinguished from other etiologic agents within several hours by a positive germ tube test (i.e., the yeast grows a germ tube or pseudohyphae). Patients who have been on fluconazole prophylaxis may have resistant *C. albicans* or non-albicans species (e.g., *C. glabrata*, *C. krusei*).

Complications

Patients with persistent candidemia after catheter removal may have peripheral septic thrombophlebitis or septic thrombosis of the central veins.

Aspergillosis

Aspergillus fumigatus and other species are widespread in soil, water, compost, potted plants, ventilation ducts, and marijuana.

Symptoms/Exam

- **Harmless saprophytes:** Found in the ear canal and in burn wounds or eschars.
- **Allergic bronchopulmonary aspergillosis (ABPA):** Presents with episodic bronchospasm, fever, and brown-flecked sputum. Seen in patients with underlying asthma or CF. CXR shows patchy, fleeting infiltrates and lobar consolidation or atelectasis. Labs show eosinophilia, elevated serum IgE, and positive serum IgG precipitins.
- **Aspergilloma of the lungs or sinus:** May be asymptomatic or present with hemoptysis, chronic cough, weight loss, and fatigue. Seen in patients with previous TB, sarcoidosis, emphysema, or PCP. CXR and CT may show an **air-crescent sign** or a rim of air around a fungus ball in a preexisting upper lobe cavity. Labs show positive serum IgG precipitins.
- **Invasive aspergillosis:**
  - Presents with dry cough, pleuritic chest pain, and persistent fever with a new infiltrate or nodule despite broad-spectrum antibiotics. Seen in patients with prolonged neutropenia, advanced AIDS, diabetes, and chronic granulomatous disease as well as in those on high-dose steroids or immunosuppressants.
  - CXR and CT may show wedge-shaped lesions from tissue infarction, an **air-crescent sign** from cavitation of a necrotic nodule, or a **halo sign** of a necrotic nodule with surrounding hemorrhage.
  - **Labs:** The *Aspergillus* galactomannan assay was recently approved by the FDA. IgG precipitins and blood cultures are rarely positive. In high-risk patients, positive sputum or bronchial washing cultures are strongly suggestive, but definitive diagnosis requires a biopsy demonstrating tissue invasion.
  - **Patients are often severely ill, and empiric antifungal therapy may be reasonable in high-risk patients.**

DIFFERENTIAL

- **ABPA:** TB, CF, lung cancer, eosinophilic pneumonia, bronchiectasis.
- **Aspergilloma:** Invasive aspergillosis.
- **Invasive aspergillosis:** Aspergilloma, cavitating lung tumor, nosocomial *Legionella* infection.

TREATMENT

- **ABPA:** Systemic or inhaled corticosteroids for acute exacerbations. Itraconazole × 8 months improves lung function and decreases steroid requirements.
- **Aspergilloma:** Surgical excision for massive hemoptysis. Antifungals play a limited role.
- **Invasive aspergillosis:** Voriconazole, amphotericin, or caspofungin.

COMPLICATIONS

- **ABPA:** Bronchiectasis, pulmonary fibrosis.
- **Aspergilloma:** Massive hemoptysis; contiguous spread to the pleura or vertebrae.
- **Invasive aspergillosis:** High mortality, especially in bone marrow and liver transplant patients.

Cryptococcosis

Cryptococcus neoformans is an encapsulated budding yeast found worldwide in soil, bird (pigeon) droppings, and eucalyptus trees. Risk factors for the disease are HIV-related immune suppression, Hodgkin's disease, leukemia, and steroid use. *C. neoformans* is the most common fungal infection in AIDS patients (usually associated with a CD4 count < 100) and is the most common cause of fungal meningitis in all patients.

Cryptococcemia (a positive serum CrAg or blood culture) indicates disseminated disease even with a normal LP; immunosuppressed patients should be treated for life.

SYMPTOMS/EXAM

- **Meningitis:** Mental status changes, headache, nausea, cranial nerve palsies. HIV patients usually lack obvious meningeal signs.
- May also cause atypical pneumonia (pulmonary infection is usually asymptomatic) or skin lesions (umbilicated papules resembling molluscum contagiosum), or may involve the bone, eye, or GU tract.

DIFFERENTIAL

Meningitis due to TB, neurosyphilis, toxoplasmosis, coccidioidomycosis, histoplasmosis, HSV encephalitis, meningeal metastases.

Serum CrAg titers are not useful for monitoring treatment response of meningitis in immunosuppressed patients. CSF CrAg titers should decrease during successful treatment.

DIAGNOSIS

- **LP:** May show high opening pressure, low glucose, high protein, and lymphocytic pleocytosis. **Patients with more advanced immunosuppression may have a bland CSF profile even with meningitis.** India ink or Gram stain of CSF may show budding yeast with a thick capsule (both are < 50% sensitive).
- **Polysaccharide cryptococcal antigen (CrAg) in serum or CSF:** Serum CrAg is > 99% sensitive in AIDS patients with meningitis. CSF CrAg is only 90% sensitive. A serum CrAg titer of > 1:8 indicates active disease.
- **Fungal culture** of blood, CSF, urine, sputum, or bronchoalveolar lavage.
- CT or MRI may show hydrocephalus or occasionally nodules (cryptococcomas).

TREATMENT

- **HIV-negative patients:** For mild to moderate lung disease, treat with oral fluconazole × 6–12 months. For meningitis, cryptococcemia, or severe lung disease, treat with amphotericin + 5-flucytosine × 2 weeks followed by oral fluconazole 400 mg/day for at least 10 weeks.
- **HIV-positive patients:** For mild to moderate lung disease, treat with fluconazole 200–400 mg/day for life. For meningitis, severe lung disease, or disseminated disease, give **induction/consolidation therapy** with amphotericin + 5-flucytosine × 2 weeks or until symptoms improve, followed by oral fluconazole 400 mg/day × 10 weeks. Flucytosine has higher rates of myelosuppression in patients with HIV. In patients with less severe meningitis (normal mental status, CSF WBC > 20, CSF CrAg < 1:1024), fluconazole 400 mg/day may be used alone for 8–10 weeks as induction.
- Patients with HIV or ongoing immunosuppression need **long-term maintenance therapy** with oral fluconazole 200 mg/day. It may be reasonable to stop prophylaxis if the CD4 count increases to > 100 for > 3–6 months in response to antiretrovirals.
- **Repeat LP** until symptoms resolve in patients with coma or other signs of elevated ICP.

COMPLICATIONS

A poorer prognosis for meningitis is seen in patients with abnormal mental status, those > 60 years of age, and those with evidence of high organism load or lack of immune response (as indicated by cryptococcemia, high initial CrAg titer in CSF or serum, high CSF opening pressure, < 20 WBCs in CSF, low glucose, and positive India ink).

Coccidioidomycosis

Coccidioides immitis is found in the arid **southwestern United States,** central California, northern Mexico, and Central and South America. It is found in soil, and outbreaks occur after earthquakes or dust storms. Risk factors include exposure to soil and the outdoors (construction workers, archaeologists, farmers).

SYMPTOMS/EXAM

- **Primary infection ("valley fever," "desert rheumatism"):** Usually presents with self-limited flulike symptoms, fever, dry cough, pleuritic chest pain, and headache, often accompanied by **arthralgias, erythema nodosum, or erythema multiforme.** CXR may be normal or show unilateral infiltrates, nodules or thin-walled cavities. Some patients (5%) may develop chronic pneumonia, ARDS, or persistent lung nodules.
- **Disseminated disease (1%):** Chronic meningitis, skin lesions (papules, pustules, warty plaques), osteomyelitis, or arthritis.

DIFFERENTIAL

Atypical pneumonia, TB, sarcoidosis, histoplasmosis, blastomycosis.

DIAGNOSIS

- **Serologic tests** (complement fixation assays); titers ≥ 1:32 indicate more severe disease and a higher risk of dissemination.
- Pathology may show giant **spherules** in infected tissues.

- **Cultures** of respiratory secretions or aspirates of bone and skin lesions may grow the organism (alert the laboratory if the diagnosis is suspected; *Coccidioides* is highly infectious to lab workers).

TREATMENT

- Treatment may not be necessary for acute disease but may be reasonable in patients at risk for dissemination.
- Fluconazole, itraconazole, or amphotericin for disseminated disease.

COMPLICATIONS

Disseminated disease is more common in nonwhites, pregnant women, and patients with HIV, diabetes, or immunosuppression.

Histoplasmosis

Histoplasma capsulatum is found in the **Mississippi** and **Ohio River valleys.** The organism is found in moist soil and in bat and bird droppings. Risk factors include exploring caves and cleaning chicken coops or attics.

SYMPTOMS/EXAM

- **Primary infection:** Presents with fever, dry cough, and substernal chest discomfort. CXR may show patchy infiltrates that become nodular or exhibit multiple small nodules and hilar or mediastinal adenopathy. Some patients may develop chronic upper lobe cavitary pneumonia or mediastinal fibrosis (dysphagia, SVC syndrome, or airway obstruction).
- **Disseminated disease:** Presents with **hepatosplenomegaly,** adenopathy, **painless palatal ulcers,** meningitis, and pancytopenia from bone marrow infiltration. Patients with HIV may develop colonic disease (diarrhea, perforation or obstruction from mass lesions).

DIFFERENTIAL

Atypical pneumonia, influenza, coccidioidomycosis, blastomycosis, TB, sarcoidosis, lymphoma.

DIAGNOSIS

- **Urinary antigen test** is most useful, especially in disseminated disease.
- **Biopsy with silver stain** of bone marrow, lymph node, or liver.
- Cultures of blood or bone marrow are positive in immunosuppressed patients.
- Serologic tests (complement fixation and immunodiffusion assays) are less helpful acutely.

TREATMENT

- Treatment is not needed for acute pulmonary disease.
- Itraconazole or amphotericin for chronic cavitary pneumonia, mediastinal fibrosis, or disseminated histoplasmosis.

COMPLICATIONS

Disseminated disease is more common in elderly, immunosuppressed, and HIV patients.

Blastomycosis

Blastomyces dermatitidis is found in the **central United States** (as is *Histoplasma*) as well as in the upper Midwest and Great Lakes regions. Risk factors include exposure to woods and streams.

SYMPTOMS/EXAM

Acute pneumonia. May lead to warty, crusted, or ulcerated **skin lesions** or to osteomyelitis, epididymitis, or prostatitis.

DIAGNOSIS

Microscopy and culture of respiratory secretions; biopsy or aspirate material shows large yeast with **broad-based budding.**

TREATMENT

Itraconazole or amphotericin for all infected patients.

GUILLAIN-BARRÉ SYNDROME

Acute symmetric ascending weakness or paralysis with areflexia; paresthesias may also be present distally. Usually occurs within 30 days of a respiratory or GI infection, especially *Campylobacter* enteritis, CMV, EBV, or mycoplasma infection. Differential diagnosis includes the following:

- **Focal cord lesion:** Usually asymmetric; early sphincter involvement.
- **Rabies:** Follows wild animal exposure.
- **West Nile virus.**
- **Botulism:** Also presents with diplopia and ocular palsies.
- **Tick paralysis:** Look for an attached tick, frequently on the scalp.
- **Polio:** Usually asymmetric; fever is present.
- **Toxins:** Heavy metals, organophosphates.

HANTAVIRUS PULMONARY SYNDROME

First identified in the southwestern United Sates in 1993; cases have since been reported across the country. Infection follows inhalation of **aerosols of dried rodent urine, saliva, or feces.** The disease begins as a nonspecific **febrile syndrome** (sudden fever, myalgias) with **rapid progression** to respiratory failure/ARDS and shock. Patients have leukocytosis, hemoconcentration, and thrombocytopenia. Diagnose by serology or by immunohistochemical staining of sputum or lung tissue. **Ribavirin** has been used experimentally, but mortality remains 50%.

HUMAN IMMUNODEFICIENCY VIRUS (HIV)

HIV targets and destroys CD4+ T lymphocytes, leading to AIDS. Risk factors include unprotected sexual intercourse, IV drug use, maternal infection, needlesticks, and mucosal exposure to body fluids; also at risk are patients who received blood products before 1985. Prognostic factors are CD4 count and HIV RNA viral load. CD4 count measures the degree of immune compromise and predicts the risk of opportunistic infections; viral load measures HIV replication rate, gauges the efficacy of antiretrovirals, and predicts CD4 count decline.

Symptoms/Exam

- **Primary HIV infection:** Often asymptomatic. Otherwise, acute retroviral syndrome presents 2–6 weeks after initial infection with fever, sore throat, lymphadenopathy, and a truncal maculopapular rash or mucocutaneous ulcerations. Other signs and symptoms include myalgias or arthralgias, diarrhea, headache, nausea, vomiting, weight loss, and thrush.
- **Chronic HIV infection:** Fatigue, fevers, night sweats, diarrhea, persistent lymphadenopathy, and weight loss. Suspect in patients with thrush, oral hairy leukoplakia, herpes zoster, seborrheic dermatitis, oral aphthous ulcers, or recurrent vaginal candidiasis.

Differential

Acute retroviral syndrome resembles infectious mononucleosis, acute CMV infection, aseptic meningitis, and syphilis.

Diagnosis

- **ELISA/enzyme immunoassay (EIA):** Detects antiviral antibodies; used to diagnose HIV. Usually positive by **three months** after initial infection. Because false positive results may occur (especially in low-risk populations being screened), confirm by **Western blot.**
- **HIV RNA viral load:** Not approved by the FDA for **diagnosing** HIV. Has high sensitivity even in patients who have not yet developed antibodies. False positive results may occur, usually in the form of a low copy number (e.g., < 10,000 copies/mL); true positive results in antibody-negative patients with acute infection are usually > 100,000 copies/mL.
- **p24 core antigen:** Highly specific, but less sensitive (85–90%) and less readily available than HIV viral load. Approved by the FDA for diagnosing acute HIV.
- **Detuned ELISA:** Licensed for research only. ELISA antibody-positive serum samples are diluted and retested; if the ELISA test is negative after dilution, it indicates a lower concentration, less specific antibodies, and seroconversion within the last 4–6 months.

Treatment

- Current recommendations (International AIDS Society-USA, 2004; World Health Organization, 2002) are to start HIV treatment in all patients who are symptomatic. Treatment of asymptomatic patients should be started when the CD4 count is 200–350 cells/mm^3. Previous guidelines also recommended starting HIV treatment in patients with a viral load > 55,000 copies/mL.
- Consider initiating antiretrovirals in patients with acute retroviral syndrome.
- Use three drugs—usually two nucleoside analogs (AZT, 3TC, d4T, ddI, abacavir, tenofovir, emtricitabine) plus a non-nucleoside analog (nevirapine or efavirenz) **or** a protease inhibitor (amprenavir, fosamprenavir, indinavir, nelfinavir, saquinavir, atazanavir, or lopinavir/ritonavir) that may be ritonavir "boosted." Protease inhibitors can have significant drug interactions.
- During pregnancy, women should be offered standard therapy in the form of two nucleoside reverse transcriptase inhibitors (including AZT) + nevirapine or a protease inhibitor. Consider starting after 10–14 weeks of gestation to minimize risk of teratogenicity. **Efavirenz is contraindicated during pregnancy.**

COMPLICATIONS

Progressive immunosuppression from HIV leads to opportunistic infections and malignancies (see Figure 11-4). Prophylactic measures against some of these conditions are outlined in Table 11-5.

Vesicular rashes (chickenpox, zoster, smallpox) and SARS require both airborne and contact precautions.

INFECTION CONTROL PRECAUTIONS

Isolation and barriers are used to prevent transmission of microorganisms from patients to other patients, visitors, or health care workers (see Table 11-6).

INFECTIOUS MONONUCLEOSIS

Caused by the Epstein-Barr virus (EBV). Commonly seen in late adolescence and early adulthood (college or military populations). Clinical course is generally benign, with patients recovering in 2–3 weeks.

SYMPTOMS

Presents with the triad of **fever, sore throat** (may be severe), and **generalized lymphadenopathy,** often with an abrupt onset. Patients may have a viral-like prodrome as well as retro-orbital headache or abdominal fullness (from hepatosplenomegaly).

EXAM

Lymphadenopathy (especially of the posterior cervical nodes), pharyngitis, and splenomegaly. Rash occurs in 10% of cases (especially in patients given ampicillin), and palatal petechiae may be seen. RUQ tenderness is more common than hepatomegaly.

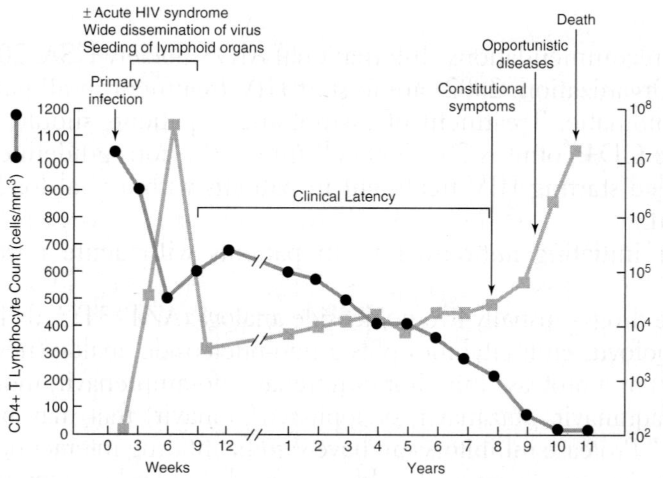

FIGURE 11-4. The course of HIV infection and disease in adults—clinical decision points.

(Adapted, with permission, from Fauci AS et al. Immunopathologic mechanisms of HIV infection. *Ann Intern Med* 1996;124:654.)

TABLE 11-5. Prophylaxis Against AIDS-Related Opportunistic Infections

Pathogen	Indication for Prophylaxis	Medication	Comments
Pneumocystis jiroveci cystic pneumonia (PCP)	CD4 count < 200/mm^3 or a history of oral thrush. Prophylaxis may be stopped if CD4 > 200 for ≥ 3 months on HAART.	TMP-SMX or dapsone +/− pyrimethamine or pentamidine nebulizers or atovaquone.	Single-strength tablets of TMP-SMX are effective and may be less toxic than double-strength tablets.
Mycobacterium avium complex (MAC)	CD4 count < 50/mm^3. Prophylaxis may be stopped if CD4 > 100 for ≥ 3 months on HAART.	Azithromycin or clarithromycin or rifabutin.	Azithromycin can be given once weekly; rifabutin can increase hepatic metabolism of other drugs.
Toxoplasma	CD4 count < 100/mm^3 and *Toxoplasma* IgG positive. Prophylaxis may be stopped if CD4 > 100–200 for ≥ 3 months on HAART.	TMP-SMX or dapsone +/− pyrimethamine or atovaquone.	Covered by all PCP regimens except pentamidine.
Mycobacterium tuberculosis	PPD > 5 mm; history of positive PPD that was inadequately treated; close contact to a person with active TB.	INH-sensitive: INH × 9 months (include pyridoxine).	For INH-resistant strains, use rifampin or rifabutin +/− pyrazinamide.
Candida	Frequent or severe recurrences.	Fluconazole or itraconazole.	
Herpes simplex virus (HSV)	Frequent or severe recurrences.	Acyclovir or famciclovir or valacyclovir.	
Pneumococcus	All patients.	Pneumococcal vaccine.	Some disease may be prevented with TMP-SMX, clarithromycin, and azithromycin. Repeat when CD4 > 200.
Influenza	All patients.	Influenza vaccine.	
HBV	All susceptible patients (i.e., hepatitis B core antibody negative)	Hepatitis B vaccine (three doses).	
HAV	All susceptible patients at increased risk for HAV infection or with chronic liver disease (e.g., chronic HBV or HCV).	Hepatitis A vaccine (two doses).	IV drug users, men who have sex with men, and hemophiliacs are at increased risk.

TABLE 11-6. Infection Control Measures

Precaution	Prevents Transmission of	Barriers to Be Used	Should Be Used for (Examples)
Standard	Transient flora from patients or surfaces.	Hand washing; gloves for contact with all body fluids and mucosa. Face shields and gowns if splashes of body fluids are possible.	Everybody!
Airborne	Droplet nuclei (≤ 5 μm) or dust particles that remain suspended for long distances.	Negative-pressure rooms and use of surgical masks when transporting patients. Health care workers use fitted N-95 masks. Consider face shields.	TB, measles, SARS, vesicular rashes (chickenpox, zoster, smallpox).
Droplet	Large droplets that travel < 3 feet and are generated by coughing, sneezing, talking, suctioning, or bronchoscopy.	Private rooms and use of surgical masks when patients are transported. Health care workers use surgical masks.	Meningococcal or *H. influenzae* meningitis, influenza, pertussis.
Contact	Direct and indirect contact.	Private rooms (patients may be grouped together); limit patient transport. Dedicated equipment (e.g., stethoscopes). Health care workers use gowns and gloves for all patients.	Some fecally transmitted infections (HAV, *C. difficile*), vesicular rashes (chickenpox, zoster, smallpox), SARS.

Differential

- **CMV:** Consider if there was a recent blood transfusion. Symptoms are usually systemic; sore throat and lymphadenopathy are uncommon. Diagnose with a positive CMV IgM.
- **Heterophil-negative EBV:** Usually affects children; has milder symptoms.
- **Acute toxoplasmosis:** Presents with nontender head and neck lymphadenopathy and mild lymphocytosis. Diagnose with *Toxoplasma* IgM and IgG seroconversion.
- **Primary HIV infection:** Fever, lymphadenopathy, pharyngitis, maculopapular rash, and, less commonly, aseptic meningitis.
- **HAV or HBV:** Characterized by markedly elevated AST and ALT.
- **Syphilis.**
- **Rubella:** A prominent rash begins on the face and progresses to the trunk and extremities. Has a shorter course (only several days).
- **Streptococcal pharyngitis:** Presents with fever, tender submandibular or anterior cervical lymphadenopathy, and pharyngotonsillar exudates with no cough. Splenomegaly is not seen. Diagnose with rapid streptococcal test and throat culture if antigen test is negative.

Diagnosis

- Neutropenia (mild left shift); **atypical lymphocytes** (see Figure 11-5) in 70% of cases (WBC 12,000–18,000 and occasionally 30,000–50,000); thrombocytopenia; mildly elevated LFTs.

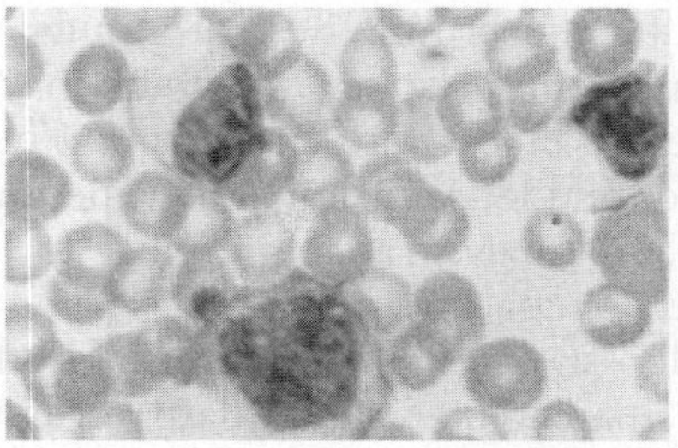

FIGURE 11-5. Atypical lymphocytosis seen in infectious mononucleosis and other infections.

These reactive T lymphocytes are large with eccentric nuclei and bluish-staining RNA in the cytoplasm. (Reproduced, with permission, from Braunwald E et al [eds]. *Harrison's Principles of Internal Medicine,* 15th ed. New York: McGraw-Hill, 2001.) (Also see Color Insert.)

- **Heterophil antibodies** (Monospot) are found in 90% of cases (may initially be negative and then turn positive in 2–3 weeks). Other EBV serologies are rarely needed.
- Anti-VCA IgM is positive at presentation; anti-EBNA and anti-S antibodies are positive in 3–4 weeks. Anti-VCA IgG antibodies are positive if patients were previously exposed. Cold agglutinins are found in 80% of cases after 2–3 weeks.

TREATMENT

None in the majority of cases. Steroids are used on rare occasions for tonsillar obstruction, severe thrombocytopenia, autoimmune hemolytic anemia, and CNS complications.

COMPLICATIONS

Autoimmune hemolytic anemia (< 3%). Splenic rupture is rare but may occur in weeks 2–3 (patients should avoid contact sports and heavy lifting). Meningoencephalitis is rare, and patients usually recover completely.

LYME DISEASE

A tick-borne illness caused by *Borrelia burgdorferi* (found in the Northeast, mid-Atlantic, and upper Midwest more than the West) and other *Borrelia* species (found in Europe and Asia). Prevalence is based on the distributions of the tick vectors *Ixodes scapularis* (found in the Northeast and upper Midwest) and *I. pacificus* (found in the West). Transmitted primarily by nymphal stages that are active in late spring and summer. Requires tick attachment > 24 hours.

The rash of early Lyme disease is often missed and resolves in 3–4 weeks without treatment.

SYMPTOMS/EXAM

- **Early localized infection:** Occurs one week (3–30 days) after tick bite. Presents with **erythema migrans** (60–80%), which appears as an expanding red lesion with "bull's eye" central clearing on the thigh, groin, or axilla (see Figure 11-6). Often accompanied by fever, myalgias, and lymphadenopathy.
- **Early disseminated infection:** Occurs weeks to months after tick bite. Skin lesions are like erythema migrans but are smaller, and they may ap-

pear several days after the primary lesion. Cranial neuritis (facial palsy), peripheral neuropathy, and aseptic meningitis may be seen. Cardiac abnormalities include AV block (rarely requiring a permanent pacemaker), myopericarditis, and mild left ventricular dysfunction. Migratory **myalgias, arthralgias, fatigue,** and malaise are common.

- **Late Lyme disease:** Occurs months to years later in untreated patients. Arthritis may develop in large joints (commonly the knee; shows PMN predominance) or small joints. Attacks last weeks to months **with complete remission between recurrences** and become less frequent over time. Chronic neurologic findings include subacute encephalopathy (memory, sleep, or mood disturbances) and peripheral sensory polyneuropathy (pain or paresthesias; abnormal EMG).

Lyme disease may present as asymmetric oligoarticular arthritis, frequently of the knee or other large joints.

Diagnosis

The testing strategy depends on the pretest probability of disease (per the American College of Physicians 1997 guidelines):

- **High likelihood (> 80%, e.g., erythema migrans in an endemic area):** Clinical diagnosis is sufficient. Serology is often negative in early disease and is not needed to confirm the diagnosis.
- **Low likelihood (< 20%, e.g., nonspecific complaints with no objective findings):** Serologic testing is not indicated, and patients should not be treated (positive results will likely be false positives).
- **Intermediate likelihood (20–80%, e.g., some typical findings and residence in an endemic area):** Combine ELISA with a confirmatory Western blot (as with HIV). In the first month of symptoms, test IgM and IgG antibodies in acute and convalescent sera; later, test only IgG antibodies.
- Patients with neuroborreliosis usually have a positive serum serology. CSF antibody testing is not necessary.
- PCR of plasma and tissue (but not CSF) is sensitive, but no guidelines exist.

Ixodes scapularis *bites can lead to coinfection with Lyme disease, human granulocytic ehrlichiosis, and/or babesiosis.*

FIGURE 11-6. Erythema chronicum migrans seen in Lyme disease.

The classic "bull's eye" lesion consists of an outer ring where the spirochetes are found, an inner ring of clearing, and central erythema due to an allergic response at the site of the tick bite. Note that some lesions may consist of just the outer annular erythema wth central clearing. (Reproduced, with permission, from Braunwald E et al [eds]. *Harrison's Principles of Internal Medicine,* 15th ed. New York: McGraw-Hill, 2001.) (Also see Color Insert.)

Treatment

- **Early Lyme disease:** Doxycycline or amoxicillin × 14–21 days (an alternative is cefuroxime). In the presence of meningitis, radiculopathy, or third-degree AV block, treat with ceftriaxone or cefotaxime × 14–28 days (or, alternatively, IV penicillin or doxycycline). Treatment response for early Lyme disease is excellent. Jarisch-Herxheimer reactions occur in 5–10% of patients during the first days of treatment.
- **Late infection (arthritis):** Doxycycline or amoxicillin × 28 days. For the first arthritis recurrence, repeat doxycycline or ceftriaxone × 14 days. For further recurrences, treat symptomatically and consider synovectomy. For late neurologic disease, treat with ceftriaxone × 14–28 days; response may be slow and incomplete.

Complications

- Some patients may have treatment-resistant (autoimmune) arthritis for months to years despite appropriate antibiotics. *B. burgdorferi* DNA is not found in the joint, and patients do not respond to antibiotics.
- Following appropriately treated Lyme disease, some patients may develop poorly defined, subjective complaints (myalgia, arthralgia, fatigue, memory impairment). **These patients do not benefit from repeated or prolonged antibiotic treatment.** The most common reason for apparent antibiotic failure in Lyme disease is misdiagnosis.

Patients with a tick attached for < 24 hours do not need treatment for Lyme disease.

Prevention

Patients in endemic areas with a tick that is partially engorged or attached **> 24 hours** may benefit from doxycycline 200 mg PO × 1 dose. Testing of ticks for infectious organisms is not recommended. Lyme disease vaccine is no longer available.

MENINGITIS

Symptoms/Exam

As for encephalitis. Atypical presentations are more likely in neonates, young children, and the elderly. Etiologies are as follows:

- **Acute meningitis:**
  - **Acute neutrophilic meningitis:** Caused by bacteria (see Table 11-7).
  - **Acute eosinophilic meningitis:** Caused by *Angiostrongylus cantonensis*, or rat lung worm; results from ingestion of undercooked mollusks or contaminated vegetables. Endemic in Southeast Asia and the Pacific Islands; associated with peripheral eosinophilia.
- **Chronic meningitis** (symptoms lasting from weeks to months with persistent CSF pleocytosis [usually lymphocytic]):
  - Etiologic agents include TB (40%), atypical mycobacteria, *Cryptococcus* (7%), *Coccidioides, Histoplasma, Blastomyces*, secondary syphilis, Lyme disease, and Whipple's disease. The etiology is frequently unknown (34%). Noninfectious causes include CNS or metastatic neoplasms (8%), leukemia, lymphoma, vasculitis, sarcoid, and subarachnoid or subdural bleeds.
  - **Chronic neutrophilic meningitis:** May be caused by *Nocardia, Actinomyces, Aspergillus, Candida*, SLE, or CMV in advanced AIDS.
  - **Chronic eosinophilic meningitis:** Associated with *Coccidioides*, parasites, lymphoma, and chemical agents.

TABLE 11-7. Initial Antimicrobial Therapy for Purulent Meningitis of Unknown Cause

Age Group	Common Microorganisms	Empiric Antibiotics—First Choice[a,b]	Severe Penicillin Allergy
Adults 18–50 years of age	*S. pneumoniae, N. meningitidis.*	Ceftriaxone/cefotaxime +/– vancomycin.[c]	Chloramphenicol + vancomycin.[c]
Adults > 50 years of age	*S. pneumoniae, Listeria monocytogenes,* gram-negative bacilli.	Ceftriaxone/cefotaxime + ampicillin +/– vancomycin.[c]	Chloramphenicol (*N. meningitidis*) + TMP-SMX (*Listeria*) + vancomycin.[c]
Impaired cellular immunity (or alcohol abuse)	*S. pneumoniae, L. monocytogenes,* gram-negative bacilli (*Pseudomonas*).	Ceftazidime + ampicillin +/– vancomycin.[c]	TMP-SMX + vancomycin.[c]
Postneurosurgery or post–head trauma	*S. pneumoniae, S. aureus,* gram-negative bacilli (including *Pseudomonas*).	Ceftazidime + vancomycin (for possible MRSA).	Aztreonam or ciprofloxacin + vancomycin.

[a] May add steroids (dexamethasone 10 mg q 6 h × 2–4 days) for patients who present with acute community-acquired meningitis that is likely to have been caused by *S. pneumoniae* (de Gans J et al. Dexamethasone in adults with bacterial menigitis. *N Engl J Med* 2002;347:1549.)

[b] Doses for meningitis are higher than those for other indications: ceftriaxone 2 g IV q 12 h, cefotaxime 2 g IV q 4 h, vancomycin 1 g IV q 12 h or 500–750 mg IV q 6 h, ampicillin 2 g IV q 4 h, or ceftazidime 2 g IV q 8 h.

[c] In areas where penicillin-resistant pneumococcus is prevalent, vancomycin should be included in the regimen.

Adapted, with permission, from Tierney LM et al (eds). *Current Medical Diagnosis and Treatment 2005.* New York: McGraw-Hill, 2005:1251.

   - **Chronic meningitis and cranial nerve palsies:** Caused by Lyme disease, syphilis, sarcoid (CN VII—Bell's palsy), and TB (CN VI—lateral rectus palsy).
- **Aseptic meningitis:**
   - Usually viral with a benign course. Treat with nonspecific supportive care.
   - Associated with enteroviruses and arboviruses in the late summer and early fall and with mumps in the spring.
   - Also associated with HSV-2 (recurrent—Mollaret's meningitis; unlike HSV-1 encephalitis, HSV-2 meningitis has a benign course, but treatment and/or suppression can be considered) as well as with HIV and drug reactions (TMP-SMX, IVIG, NSAIDs, carbamazepine).
   - Less common but treatable causes include secondary syphilis (penicillin), Lyme disease (ceftriaxone), and leptospirosis (doxycycline).

DIAGNOSIS/TREATMENT

- **Fulminant presentation (< 24 hours) or ill-appearing patient:** Give antibiotics **within 30 minutes;** give dexamethasone along with or prior to antibiotics. Then perform a history and physical and obtain CT/MRI (if indicated) and LP.
- **Subacute course and stable patient:** Perform a history and physical and obtain CT/MRI (if indicated), blood cultures, and LP; then give empiric treatment.

- Obtain head CT/MRI before LP if a mass lesion is suspected (e.g., with papilledema, coma, seizures, focal neurologic findings, or immunocompromised patients).
- CSF Gram stain sensitivity is 75% (60–90%); CSF culture sensitivity is 75% (70–85%) for bacterial meningitis (see Table 11-8). Sensitivity is unchanged if antibiotics are administered < 4 hours before culture.

PREVENTION

- ***N. meningitidis*** **chemoprophylaxis:** Given to household contacts, roommates, or cellmates; those with direct contact with the patient's oral secretions (kissing, sharing utensils, endotracheal intubation, suctioning, day care contacts if < 7 days); and special cases (immunocompromised, outbreaks). Also given to index patients if not treated with cephalosporin (penicillins and chloramphenicol do not reliably penetrate the nasal mucosa). Possible regimens include rifampin 600 mg PO BID × 4 doses, ciprofloxacin 500 mg PO × 1 dose, or ceftriaxone 250 mg IM × 1 dose.

TABLE 11-8. CSF Profiles in Various CNS Diseases

DIAGNOSIS	RBC (PER μL)	WBC (PER μL)	GLUCOSE (mg/dL)	PROTEIN (mg/dL)	OPENING PRESSURE (cm H_2O)	APPEARANCE
Normal[a]	< 10	< 5	~2/3 of serum	15–45	10–20	Clear
Bacterial meningitis	Normal	↑ (PMNs)	↓	↑	↑	Cloudy
Aseptic/viral meningitis, encephalitis	Normal	↑ (lymphs)[b]	Normal	Normal or ↑	Normal or ↑	Usually clear
Chronic meningtitis (TB, fungal)	Normal	↑ (lymphs)[b]	↓	↑	↑	Clear or cloudy
Spirochetal meningitis (syphilis, Lyme disease)	Normal	↑ (lymphs)[b]	Normal	↑	Normal or ↑	Clear or cloudy
Neighborhood reaction[c]	Normal	Variable	Normal	Normal or ↑	Normal or ↑	Usually clear
SAH, cerebral contusion	↑↑	↑	Normal	↑↑	Normal or ↑	Yellow or red

[a] With traumatic tap, usually have 1 WBC/800 RBCs and 1 mg protein/1000 RBCs.

[b] May have PMN predominance in early stages.

[c] May be seen with brain abscess, epidural abscess, vertebral osteomyelitis, sinusitis/mastoiditis, septic thrombus, and brain tumor.

Adapted, with permission, from Tierney LM et al (eds). *Current Medical Diagnosis and Treatment 2005.* New York: McGraw-Hill, 2005:1251.

- *N. meningitidis* vaccine (serotypes A, C, Y, and W-135, *not* B): Given for epidemics as well as to military recruits, pilgrims to Mecca, and travelers to the African Sahel (meningitis belt), Nepal, and northern India. May also be given to college freshman living in dormitories, asplenic patients, and those with terminal complement (C5–C9) and properdin deficiencies.
- *H. influenzae* type b chemoprophylaxis: Give rifampin to household contacts of unvaccinated children < 4 years of age; consider for day care contacts.
- *H. influenzae* type b vaccine: Routine childhood immunization; consider in adult patients with asplenia.

> ***To remember gram-positive cocci—***
>
> **The Grapes of Staph (like *"The Grapes of Wrath"*):** Staphylococci are frequently seen in grapelike clusters.
>
> ***Strep* = strip:** Streptococci are often seen in long strips or chains.

MICROBIOLOGY PRINCIPLES

Gram-Positive Cocci

- In clusters (sometimes chains or pairs): *Staphylococcus.*
  - Coagulase positive: *S. aureus.*
  - Coagulase negative: Examples—*S. epidermidis, S. saprophyticus.*
- In chains or pairs: *Streptococcus.*
  - Lancet-shaped pairs: *S. pneumoniae* (see Figure 11-7).
- In pairs: *Enterococcus.*

> ***To remember gram-positive rods—***
>
> **B**ad **C**h**OR**al **ACT**s **N**eed **CLOS**e and **PROP**er **LIST**ening
>
> ***B**acillus*
> ***COR**ynebacterium*
> ***ACT**inomyces*
> ***N**ocardia*
> ***CLOS**tridium*
> ***PROP**ionibacterium*
> ***LIST**eria*

Gram-Positive Rods

- Large, with spores: *Bacillus, Clostridium.*
- Small, pleomorphic (diphtheroids): *Corynebacterium, Propionibacterium.*
- Filamentous, branching, beaded:
  - Aerobic: *Nocardia.*
  - Anaerobic: *Actinomyces.*
- Other: *Listeria, Lactobacillus, Erysipelothrix.*

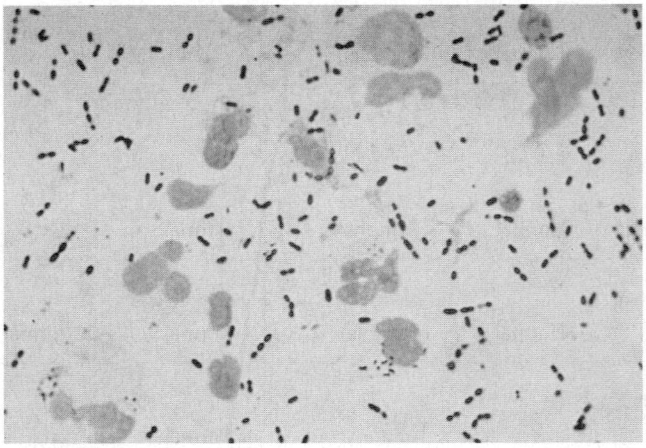

FIGURE 11-7. Pneumococcal pneumonia.

This Gram-stained sputum sample shows many neutrophils and lancet-shaped gram-positive cocci in pairs and chains, indicating infection with *S. pneumoniae.* (Courtesy of Roche Laboratories, Division of Hoffman-LaRoche Inc., Nutley, NJ.) (Also see Color Insert.)

Gram-Negative Cocci

- **In pairs (diplococci):** *Neisseria gonorrhoeae, N. meningitidis, Moraxella (Branhamella) catarrhalis.*
- **Other:** *Acinetobacter.*

Gram-Negative Rods

- **Enterobacteriaceae (lactose fermenters):** *E. coli, Serratia, Klebsiella, Enterobacter, Citrobacter.*
- **Nonfermenters:** *Proteus, Serratia, Edwardsiella, Salmonella, Shigella, Morganella, Yersinia, Acinetobacter, Stenotrophomonas, Pseudomonas.*
- **Anaerobes:** *Bacteroides, Fusobacterium.*
- **Fusiform (long, pointed):** *Fusobacterium, Capnocytophaga.*
- **Other:** *Haemophilus.*

Acid-Fast Bacteria

- Mycobacteria.
- *Nocardia* (weakly or partially acid-fast).

> ***To remember lactose fermenting gram-negative rods–***
>
> **SEEK** Carbs
>
> ***S**erratia*
> ***E**. coli*
> ***E**nterobacter*
> ***K**lebsiella*
> ***C**itrobacter*

OSTEOMYELITIS

Spread may be contiguous (80%) or hematogenous (20%).

- **Local spread:** Occurs in diabetics and in patients with vascular insufficiency, prosthetic joints, decubitus ulcers, trauma, and recent neurosurgery.
- **Hematogenous spread:** Affects IV drug users, those with sickle cell disease, and the elderly.

Common causes of osteomyelitis are as follows:

- Etiologic agents include *S. aureus* and, to a lesser extent, coagulase-negative staphylococci (prosthetic joints or postoperative infections), streptococci, anaerobes (bites, diabetic foot infections, decubitus ulcers), *Pasteurella* (animal bites), *Eikenella* (human bites), and *Pseudomonas* (nail punctures through sneakers).
- **Other causes:** *Salmonella* (sickle cell), *M. tuberculosis* (foreign immigrants, HIV), *Bartonella* (HIV), *Brucella* (unpasteurized dairy products).
- **By location:** *Pseudomonas* affects the sternoclavicular joint and symphysis pubis (in IV drug users); *Brucella* affects the sacroiliac joint, knee, and hip; and TB affects the lower thoracic vertebrae (Pott's disease).

SYMPTOMS/EXAM

- **Contiguous spread:** Local redness, warmth, and tenderness; patients are afebrile and are not systemically ill.
- **Hematogenous spread:** Sudden fever; pain, and tenderness over the affected bone. May present with pain only (no fever).
- **Vertebral osteomyelitis with epidural abscess:** Spinal pain followed by radicular pain and weakness.
- **Prosthetic hip and knee infections:** May present only as pain on weight bearing.

DIAGNOSIS

- **Probing to bone (diabetic patients):** Approximately 66% sensitive and 85% specific (PPV 89%).
- **Plain x-rays:** Reveal bony erosions or periosteal elevation ≥ 2 weeks after infection. Less helpful in trauma or diabetic/vascular patients with neuropathy (frequent stress fractures).
- CT scans.
- **MRI:** Approximately 90% sensitive and specific (abnormal marrow edema; surrounding soft tissue infection). Especially useful for diagnosing vertebral osteomyelitis.
- **Nuclear scans:** Three- or four-phase studies with technetium-99 are preferred. Most useful for distinguishing bone from soft tissue inflammation when the diagnosis is ambiguous.
- **Microbiology:** Obtain bone culture at debridement or by needle aspiration; sinus tract cultures are not reliable. With hematogenous osteomyelitis, positive blood cultures may obviate the need for bone biopsy.

TREATMENT

- After debridement of necrotic bone (with cultures taken), empiric antibiotics should be chosen to cover the likely pathogens (see above).
- IV antibiotics should be given for 4–6 weeks, although oral quinolones may be equally effective in some circumstances.
- The choice of agent is guided by microbiology. In patients who are not candidates for definitive therapy, long-term suppressive antibiotics may be used.
- Surgery is indicated for spinal cord decompression, bony stabilization, removal of necrotic bone in chronic osteomyelitis, and reestablishment of vascular supply.

COMPLICATIONS

Vertebral osteomyelitis with epidural abscess; chronic osteomyelitis.

PREVENTION

Diabetics with neuropathy (detected by the 10-g monofilament test) should be taught to examine their feet on a daily basis and should be examined by a clinician at least once every three months.

PYELONEPHRITIS

Caused by the same bacteria as those responsible for uncomplicated UTI. With the exception of *S. aureus*, most cases are caused by organisms ascending from the lower urinary tract; *S. aureus* is most frequently hematogenous and produces intrarenal or perinephric abscesses. Renal struvite stones (staghorn calculi) are frequently associated with recurrent UTI due to urease-producing bacteria (*Proteus*, *Pseudomonas*, and enterococci).

SYMPTOMS

Presents with flank pain and fever. Patients often have lower urinary tract symptoms (dysuria, urgency, and frequency) that sometimes occur 1–2 days before the upper tract symptoms, and they may also have nausea, vomiting, or diarrhea.

EXAM

Fever, CVA tenderness, mild abdominal tenderness.

DIFFERENTIAL

Renal stones, renal infarcts, cholecystitis, appendicitis, diverticulitis, acute prostatitis/epididymitis.

DIAGNOSIS

UA shows pyuria and bacteriuria and may also exhibit hematuria or WBC casts. CBC reveals leukocytosis with left shift. Urine culture is usually positive, and blood culture may be positive as well.

Fever and WBC casts on UA are seen in pyelonephritis but not in cystitis.

TREATMENT

- Fluoroquinolone × 7 days or ampicillin + gentamicin or ceftriaxone × 14 days.
- Radiologic evaluation for complications may be useful in patients who are severely ill or immunocompromised, who are not responding to treatment, or in whom complications are likely (e.g., pregnant patients, diabetics, and those with nephrolithiasis, reflux, transplant surgery, or other GU surgery).
  - X-rays can detect stones, calcification, masses, and abnormal gas collections.
  - Ultrasound is rapid and safe.
  - Contrast-enhanced CT is most sensitive but may affect renal function.

COMPLICATIONS

Perinephric abscess should be considered in patients who remain febrile 2–3 days after appropriate antibiotics; UA may be normal and cultures negative. Patients are treated by percutaneous or surgical drainage plus antibiotics. Intrarenal abscesses (e.g., infection of a renal cyst) < 5 cm in size usually respond to antibiotics alone. Diabetics may develop emphysematous pyelonephritis, which usually requires nephrectomy and is associated with a high mortality rate.

ROCKY MOUNTAIN SPOTTED FEVER

A tick-borne illness caused by *Rickettsia rickettsii*. The vector is the *Dermacentor* tick, which needs to feed for only 6–10 hours before injecting the organism (a much shorter attachment time than for Lyme disease). Most commonly occurs in the mid-Atlantic and South Central states (**not** the Rocky Mountain states). The highest rates are seen in late spring and summer and in children and men with occupational tick exposures.

Think of Rocky Mountain spotted fever and start treatment early in patients with a recent tick bite (especially in the mid-Atlantic or South Central states) along with fever, headache, and myalgias followed by a centripetal rash.

SYMPTOMS/EXAM

- **Initial symptoms (seven days after a tick bite)**: Fever, myalgias, and headaches.
- Maculopapular rash (in 90%) starts four days later and progresses to petechiae or purpura. The rash first appears on the wrists and ankles and then spreads centrally and to the palms and soles.
- Patients may develop severe headache, irritability, and even delirium or coma.

DIFFERENTIAL

Meningococcemia, measles, typhoid fever, ehrlichiosis (HME or HGE), viral hemorrhagic fevers (e.g., dengue), leptospirosis, vasculitis.

Diagnosis

Diagnosis is made clinically (symptoms and signs plus recent tick bite); treatment should be started as soon as Rocky Mountain spotted fever is suspected. Diagnosis can be made by biopsy of early skin lesions or confirmed retrospectively by serologic testing. Labs may show thrombocytopenia, elevated LFTs, and hyponatremia. The Weil-Felix test (for antibodies cross-reacting to *Proteus*) is no longer considered reliable.

Treatment

Doxycycline or chloramphenicol.

Complications

Pneumonitis, pulmonary edema, renal failure, and death after 8–15 days.

STRONGYLOIDIASIS

Infection with the helminth *Strongyloides stercoralis* is endemic in warm climates such as the southeastern United States, Appalachia, Africa, Asia, the Caribbean, and Central America. Unlike most other parasitic worms, *Strongyloides* can reproduce in the small intestine, leading to a high worm burden. Autoinfection and dissemination are seen in hosts with deficient cell-mediated immunity (e.g., AIDS, chronic steroids, organ transplants, leukemia, lymphoma).

Consider hyperinfection with Strongyloides stercoralis *in patients with vague abdominal complaints or fleeting pulmonary infiltrates plus eosinophilia, or in immunosuppressed patients who develop systemic gram-negative or enterococcal infection.*

Symptoms/Exam

- **Normal hosts:** May be asymptomatic or present with vague epigastric pain, nausea, bloating, diarrhea, or weight loss due to malabsorption. Serpiginous papules or urticaria ("larva currens") may be seen around the buttocks, thighs, and lower abdomen as larvae migrate from the rectum and externally autoinfect the host.
- **Immunocompromised hosts:** Hyperinfection or disseminated strongyloidiasis can develop. Worms leave the GI tract and travel to the lungs and elsewhere. Patients present with fever, severe abdominal pain, dyspnea, productive cough, hemoptysis, and local symptoms (e.g., CNS, pancreas, eyes).

Differential

Local enteric disease mimics PUD, sprue, or ulcerative colitis. Hyperinfection resembles overwhelming bacterial or fungal sepsis.

Diagnosis

Stool or duodenal aspirates can be tested for ova and parasites. In hyperinfection, larvae may be seen in sputum, bronchoalveolar lavage, CSF, and urine. Paradoxically, **eosinophilia is prominent in normal hosts with disease but is uncommon in patients with hyperinfection.** CXR shows transient (normal host) or diffuse, persistent pulmonary infiltrates (hyperinfection).

Treatment

Thiabendazole, albendazole, or ivermectin. Discontinue steroids and other immunosuppressive agents.

Complications

Ileus or small bowel obstruction can result from enteric worms. Hyperinfection and tracking of enteric bacteria (gram-negative rods, enterococci) can lead to bacteremia, meningitis, UTI, or pneumonia.

SOFT TISSUE INFECTIONS

Table 11-9 outlines the etiology, clinical presentation, and treatment of common soft tissue infections.

SYPHILIS

Caused by the spirochete *Treponema pallidum.*

SYMPTOMS/EXAM

- **Primary:** Usually presents with a chancre, a single painless papule that erodes to form a clean-based ulcer with raised/indurated edges (may be multiple or atypical if HIV-positive or minimal if previous syphilis). Also presents with **regional nontender lymphadenopathy.** Incubation period is three weeks (range of three days to three months). The chancre resolves in 3–6 weeks, but lymphadenopathy persists.
- **Secondary:** Presents with a **maculopapular rash** (may include the palms and soles), **condylomata lata** in intertriginous areas (painless, broad, gray-white to erythematous plaques that are highly infectious; see Figure 11-8), or a **mucous patch** (condylomata lata on the mucosa; see Figure 11-9). **Systemic symptoms** include low-grade fever, malaise, pharyngitis, laryngitis, lymphadenopathy (especially epitrochlear), anorexia, weight loss, arthralgias, headache, and meningismus (aseptic meningitis). Occurs 2–8 weeks after primary chancre, but may overlap.
- **Latent:** Positive serology but no current symptoms.
  - **Early latent** (< 1 year): Fourfold increase in antibody titer; known history of primary or secondary syphilis; infected partner.
  - **Late latent** (> 1 year or unknown duration): One-third progress to tertiary syphilis.
- **Tertiary syphilis:** May include **aortitis** (aneurysm rupture is the leading cause of death from syphilis) or destructive **gummas** (bone, skin, mucocutaneous areas). **Neurosyphilis** is usually asymptomatic (in CSF, WBC > 5, elevated protein, low glucose, positive CSF-VDRL). CNS symptoms include **tabes dorsalis** (demyelination of the posterior columns, leading to wide-based gait and foot slap), **Argyll Robertson pupil** (irregular, small pupil that accommodates but does not respond to light), and meningovascular syphilis (subacute encephalopathy with multifocal ischemic infarcts). Occurs 1–20 years after initial infection.

DIFFERENTIAL

The differential of genital ulcer disease follows. Table 11-10 outlines the differential diagnosis of lesions on the palms and soles.

- Primary syphilis, HSV.
- **Chancroid (*Haemophilus ducreyi*):** The papule progresses to a pustule that ulcerates (over 2–4 days) to form a nonindurated, **painful ulcer with yellow-gray exudates** and tender inguinal lymphadenopathy **(buboes).** A painful ulcer accompanied by tender inguinal lymphadenopathy strongly suggests chancroid. Diagnosis is clinical, as chancroid is difficult to culture. Drain buboes and treat with ceftriaxone 250 mg IM × 1 or azithromycin 1 g PO × 1. Associated with **high rates of HIV coinfection;** seen mainly in the tropics.
- **Lymphogranuloma venereum (*Chlamydia trachomatis* serovars L1–L3):** Presents with an evanescent genital ulcer (which has usually resolved by

TABLE 11-9. Common Soft Tissue Infections

Organism	Patient Characteristics	Source of Organism	Clinical Features	Treatment (Examples)
Group A streptococcus and occasionally groups B, C, and G	Normal.	Skin flora.	Cellulitis, erysipelas.	Dicloxacillin, cephalexin, clindamycin (penicillin if documented strep only).
S. aureus	Same as above.	Same as above.	Cellulitis, furunculosis.	Same as above.
Vibrio vulnificus, other *Vibrio* spp.	Cirrhosis.	Shellfish or seawater exposure.	Hemorrhagic bullae, septic shock.	Ceftazidime, doxycycline.
Mycobacterium marinum	Normal.	Fish tanks.	Nonhealing ulcer, nodular lymphangitis.	Rifampin + ethambutol, TMP-SMX.
Mycobacterium fortuitum	Normal.	Nail salon foot baths.	Furuncles.	Excision.
Pseudomonas, *Aeromonas*	Normal.	Hot tubs, freshwater exposure.	*Pseudomonas:* folliculitis; *Aeromonas:* spreading cellulitis.	Quinolones.
Pseudomonas	Neutropenia.	–	Ecthyma gangrenosum (hemorragic bullae that ulcerate; see Figure 11-10).	Quinolones.
Noninfectious agents	IBD, rheumatoid arthritis.	–	Pyoderma gangrenosum (pustule/nodule that ulcerates).	Steroids.
Erysipelothrix	Fishermen, meat handlers.	–	Hands, fingers.	Penicillin, ampicillin, quinolone.
Bacillus anthracis	Hide tanners and wool workers (postal workers).	Soil (bioterrorism agent).	Nonpainful ulcer/eschar, extensive edema.	Doxycycline, quinolones.
Francisella tularensis (tularemia)	Trappers and skinners of wild rodents.	Ticks, rabbits.	Regional lymphadenopathy, pneumonia.	Doxycycline, streptomycin.
Pasteurella, *Capnocytophaga*	Normal.	Animal bites or scratches.	*Pasteurella*, rapidly progressing cellulitis; *Capnocytophaga:* DIC, sepsis in asplenics and cirrhotics.	Amoxicillin/clavulanate.
Sporothrix schenckii	Gardeners, rose handlers.	Thorned plants.	Nodular lymphangitis.	Itraconazole.

TABLE 11-9. Common Soft Tissue Infections (continued)

Organism	Patient Characteristics	Source of Organism	Clinical Features	Treatment (Examples)
Pityriasis rosea	After a viral URI, patients develop a herald patch followed by a generalized eruption.	—	Round, pink, scaling patches; "Christmas tree" distribution on back.	UV light; topical steroids and antihistamines for itching.

the time patient seeks care) followed by painful lymphadenopathy (**buboes with groove sign** from the inguinal ligament separating the inguinal and femoral nodes) that may suppurate. Systemic symptoms are common. Complications include proctitis, fistulas, and strictures. Diagnose by serology (L1–L3 serovars). Drain buboes and treat with doxycycline × 3 weeks. Mainly seen in the tropics.

- **Granuloma inguinale, donovanosis (*Calymmatobacterium granulomatis*):** Nodules erode to painless, **beefy-red, friable lesions.** Lesions often have marked edema and **pseudobuboes** (subcutaneous granulomas that are not lymphadenopathy). Diagnose by scraping and biopsy (intracellular Donovan bodies are seen in mononuclear cells). Treat with doxycycline or TMP-SMX for at least three weeks until the lesions heal. Recurrences are common. This disease is rare in the United States.
- **Trauma, excoriation** (e.g., zippers, scabies).
- **Other:** Psoriasis, Behçet's, Reiter's, lichen planus.

Diagnosis

- Direct visualization of motile spirochetes by darkfield microscopy from condylomata lata or mucous patches.

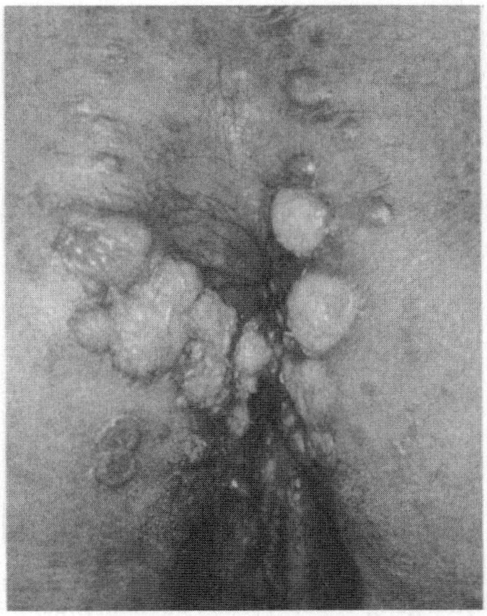

FIGURE 11-8. Condylomata lata in secondary syphilis.

(Reproduced, with permission, from Kasper DL et al [eds]. *Harrison's Principles of Internal Medicine,* 16th ed. New York: McGraw-Hill, 2005:979.) (Also see Color Insert.)

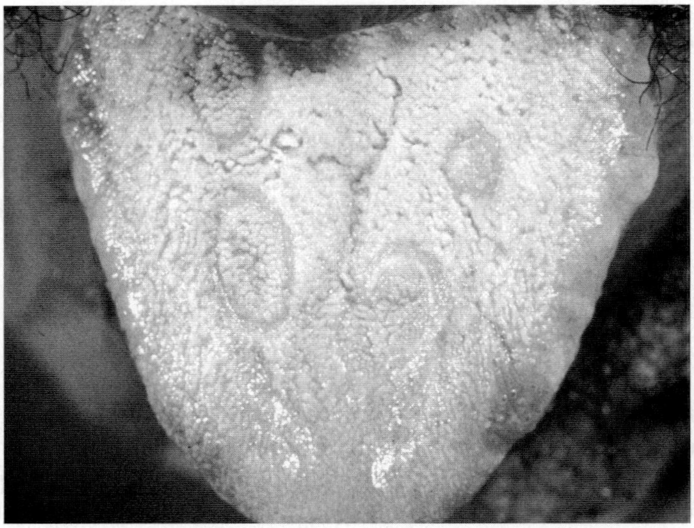

FIGURE 11-9. Mucous patches in secondary syphilis.

Note the multiple painless grayish-white erosions with a red periphery on the dorsal and lateral tongue. These highly infectious mucosal lesions contain large numbers of treponemes. (Courtesy of Ron Roddy. Reproduced, with permission, from Kasper DL et al [eds]. *Harrison's Principles of Internal Medicine*, 16th ed. New York: McGraw-Hill, 2005:980.) (Also see Color Insert.)

- **VDRL and RPR:** Nontreponemal, nonspecific antibody tests are useful for screening (detect antibodies that cross-react with beef cardiolipin). The **prozone effect** may be seen in secondary syphilis or pregnancy (high antibody titers produce negative tests that become positive as the sample is diluted). The sensitivity of VDRL/RPR is 70% in primary syphilis and 99% in secondary syphilis. False positives have a titer ≤ 1:8.
- **FTA-ABS and MHA-TP:** Specific treponemal antibody tests that are used to confirm VDRL and RPR. Remain positive for life (patients are "serofast").

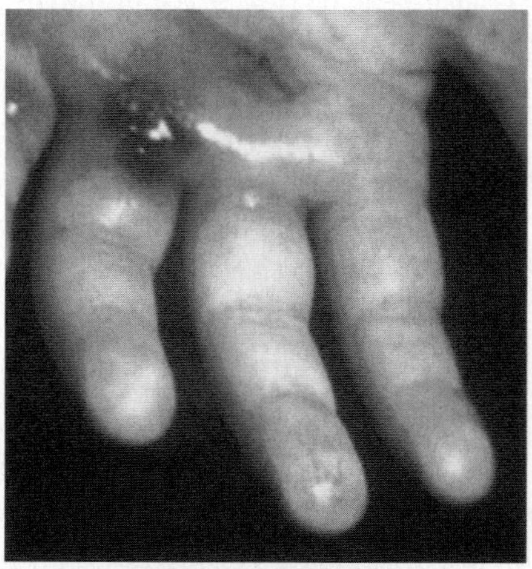

FIGURE 11-10. Ecthyma gangrenosum with *Pseudomonas* in a neutropenic patient.

Note the red papule with a necrotic center. (Reproduced, with permission, from Kasper DL et al [eds]. *Harrison's Principles of Internal Medicine*, 16th ed. New York: McGraw-Hill, 2005:890.) (Also see Color Insert.)

TABLE 11-10. Differential Diagnosis of Lesions on the Palms and Soles

	CAUSE	FEATURES OF LESIONS	DISTRIBUTION
Rocky Mountain spotted fever	*Rickettsia rickettsii.*	Macules, then petechiae (see Figure 11-11).	Wrists/ankles, then centrally, then palms and soles late in course.
Secondary syphilis	*Treponema pallidum.*	Red-brown, copper-colored papules: never vesicular (see Figure 11-12).	Condylomata lata or mucous patches on mucosa.
Erythema multiforme	Drug reaction, HSV, or *Mycoplasma* infection.	Target lesions (see Figure 11-13).	Symmetric over the elbows, knees, palms, and soles. May become diffuse and involve the mucosa.
Acute meningoccemia	*N. meningitidis.*	Blanching macules, then gun-metal gray petechiae and purpura (see Figure 11-14).	Distal extremities; then to trunk and "pressure spots" over hours.
Smallpox	Orthopoxvirus.	Deep, round, tense vesicles and pustules.	Start on the face and extremities; then move to the trunk (centrifugal).
Endocarditis	*Staphylococcus, Streptococcus,* etc.	Janeway lesions are painless, hemorrhagic macules (see Figure 11-15). Osler's nodes are subcutaneous, tender, pink or purplish nodules.	Janeway lesions appear on the palms and soles, Osler's nodes on the pads of digits.
Hand-foot-and-mouth disease	Coxsackie A16 virus.	Tender vesicles.	Peripheral and in mouth. Outbreaks occur within families.
Rat-bite fever	*Streptobacillus moniliformis.*	Maculopapules or purpura.	May be more severe at the joints of the arms and legs.
Atypical measles	Paramyxovirus (in patients who received killed virus vaccine from 1963 to 1967).	Maculopapules; may be hemorrhagic.	Most marked on the extremities. Typical measles has a central distribution (face/chest).

- Patients at high risk of developing neurosyphilis should undergo LP and have a **CSF-VDRL** test. CSF-VDRL is specific but not sensitive for neurosyphilis (sensitivity 30–70%).
- **Indications for LP:** Indicated for patients with neurologic symptoms, serum RPR ≥ 1:32, current aortitis or gummas, and previous treatment failure. LP for all HIV-positive patients has been recommended by some but is controversial.

TREATMENT

- Think of syphilis as **early** (primary, secondary, early latent), **late** (late latent or tertiary), or **neurosyphilis.**
- Patients with **early syphilis** get benzathine penicillin G 2.4 MU IM × 1 or doxycycline or ceftriaxone. Failures occur with azithromycin (especially if the patient is infected with HIV).

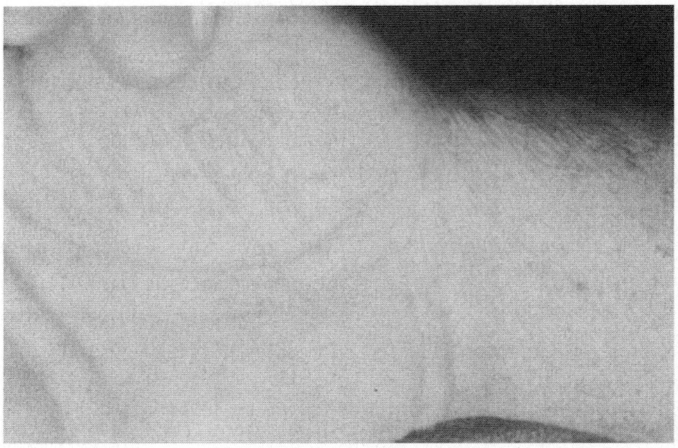

FIGURE 11-11. Rocky Mountain spotted fever.

(Reproduced, with permission, from Braunwald E et al [eds]. *Harrison's Principles of Internal Medicine,* 15th ed. New York: McGraw-Hill, 2001: Color Plate IID-45.) (Also see Color Insert.)

False positive VDRL tests–

VDRL FAIL

Viruses (hepatitis, HIV)
Drugs (IV drug users)
Rheumatic fever and **R**heumatoid arthritis
Lupus and **L**eprosy
Fever (relapsing or rat bite; both caused by other spirochetes)
Aging
Infectious mononucleosis
Lyme disease (caused by another spirochete)

- Those with **late syphilis** get benzathine penicillin G 2.4 MU IM q week × 3 or doxycycline.
- Patients with **neurosyphilis** require penicillin G 3 MU IV q 4 h × 10–14 days.
- **Pregnant women who are allergic to penicillin should be desensitized and treated with penicillin to prevent congenital syphilis.**
- Repeat RPR or VDRL at 3, 6, 12, and 24 months; titer should decrease **at least fourfold** 6–9 months after treatment of primary or secondary syphilis. If the test remains positive after that time period, it suggests treatment failure, reinfection, or HIV.
- Treat again if clinical signs persist or recur or if VDRL/RPR titer does not decrease **fourfold.**

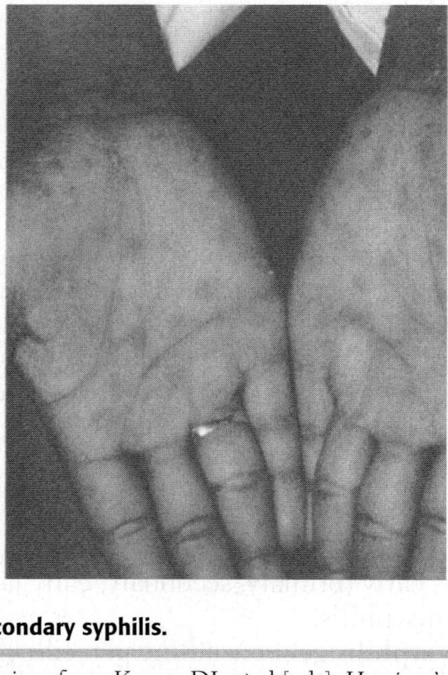

FIGURE 11-12. Secondary syphilis.

(Reproduced, with permission, from Kasper DL et al [eds]. *Harrison's Principles of Internal Medicine,* 16th ed. New York: McGraw-Hill, 2005:979.) (Also see Color Insert.)

INFECTIOUS DISEASES

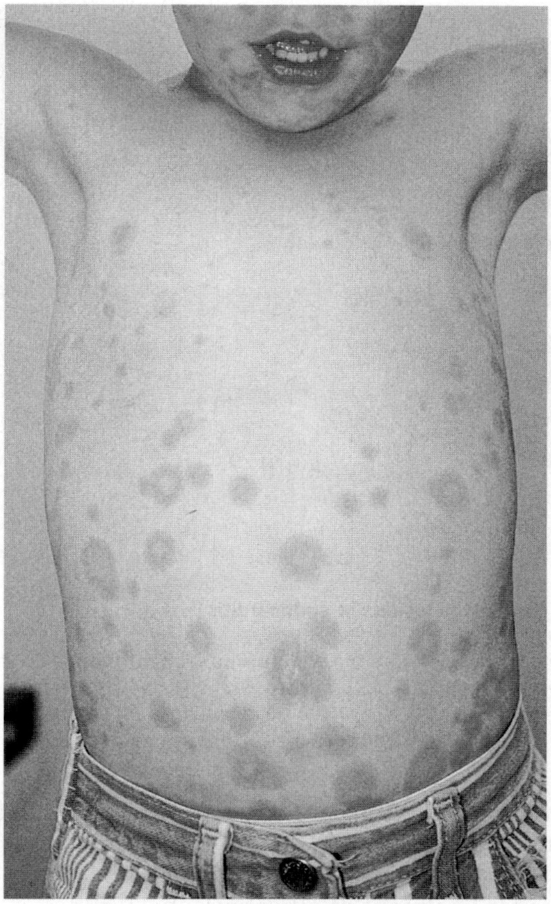

FIGURE 11-13. Erythema multiforme.

(Courtesy of Michael Redman, PA-C. Reproduced, with permission, from Knoop KJ, Stack LB, Storrow AB. *Atlas of Emergency Medicine*, 2nd ed. New York: McGraw-Hill, 2002:378.) (Also see Color Insert.)

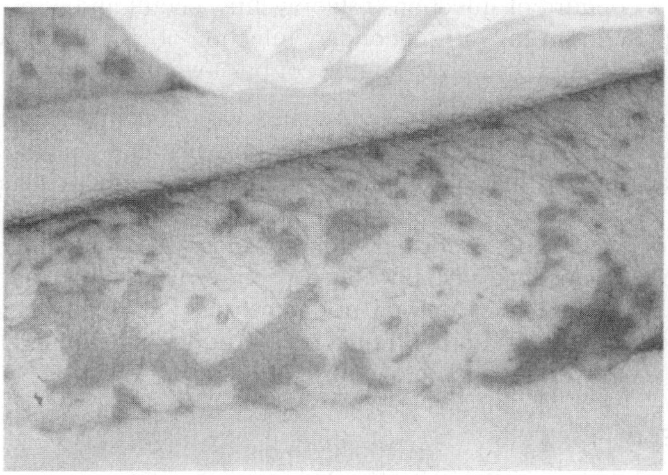

FIGURE 11-14. Acute meningococcemia.

(Courtesy of Stephen E. Gellis, MD. Reproduced, with permission, from Kasper DL et al [eds]. *Harrison's Principles of Internal Medicine*, 16th ed. New York: McGraw-Hill, 2005:284.) (Also see Color Insert.)

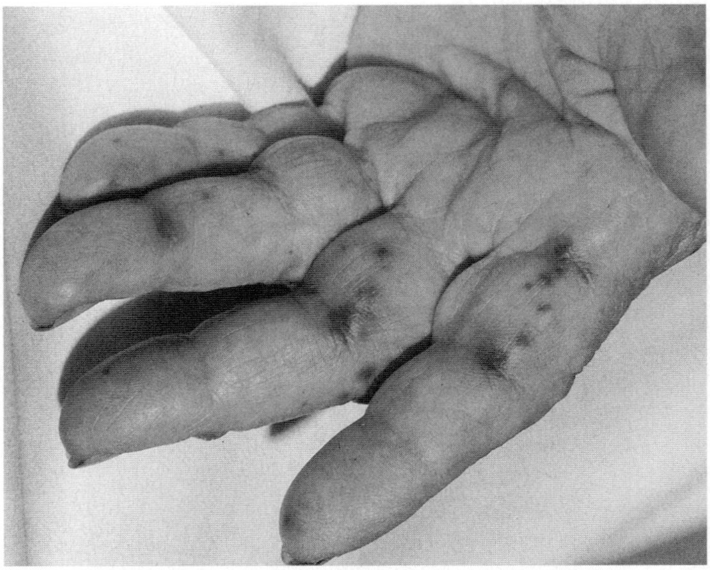

FIGURE 11-15. Janeway lesions in endocarditis.

(Reproduced, with permission, from Wolff K, Johnson RA, Suurmond D. *Fitzpatrick's Color Atlas and Synopsis of Clinical Dermatology*, 5th ed. New York: McGraw-Hill, 2005:636.) (Also see Color Insert.)

- **Jarisch-Herxheimer reactions** are commonly seen in the first 24 hours of treatment and are characterized by low-grade fever, headache, myalgias, malaise, and new skin lesions. Thought to be due to cytokine release, and may be seen after treatment of other spirochetal illnesses (e.g., Lyme disease, relapsing fever). Treat with antipyretics.

TOXIC SHOCK SYNDROME (TSS)

Usually affects healthy individuals; associated with **exotoxins** released by certain strains of *S. aureus* or group A streptococci (rarely groups B, C, or G). May cause a concurrent infection (osteomyelitis, occult abscesses, erysipelas, necrotizing fasciitis or myositis, secondary infection of chickenpox wounds) or simply colonize a mucosal, postoperative, or burn-wound surface.

- **Streptococcal TSS:** Commonly associated with concurrent invasive infections. Invasive group A streptococcal strains usually have type 1 M protein, a cell-surface protein that is antiphagocytic and may serve as a superantigen. Strains may also produce streptococcal pyrogenic exotoxins A, B, or C.
- **Staphylococcal TSS:** Associated with menses and with the use of hyperabsorbable tampons that have now been withdrawn from the market ("menstrual TSS"). Most cases are now nonmenstrual TSS due to vaginal or surgical wound colonization. Strains may produce superantigens TSST-1 (75%) or staphylococcal enterotoxins B and C.

Symptoms/Exam

- Staphylococcal or streptococcal isolation, evidence of end-organ damage (renal insufficiency, coagulopathy, abnormal LFTs), rash, ARDS, generalized edema or effusions, soft tissue necrosis.
- Staphylococcal TSS also requires fever and a diffuse macular rash that may subsequently desquamate (especially on the palms and soles). Other features include vomiting, diarrhea, severe myalgias, and confusion.

- Streptococcal TSS may be preceded by an influenza-like prodrome or increasing pain at a deep site of infection.
- TSS is rarely preceded by streptococcal pharyngitis.

DIFFERENTIAL

Gram-negative septic shock, Rocky Mountain spotted fever, leptospirosis, measles, DVT.

DIAGNOSIS

- Routine labs, including CK.
- Vaginal examination.
- Cultures of blood, wounds, and vaginal mucosa.
- Evaluate for invasive streptococcal infection or occult staphylococcal infection.

TREATMENT

Aggressive hydration and surgical debridement of deep-seated streptococcal infection and necrotic tissue are critical. Administer empiric broad-spectrum antibiotics. If the appropriate organism is isolated, narrow therapy to penicillin + clindamycin (for streptococci) or nafcillin/oxacillin (vancomycin for methicillin-resistant *S. aureus*) and perhaps clindamycin (for staphylococci). Clindamycin is added because it may decrease toxin production and is active against organisms in the stationary phase; the cell wall–acting penicillins are most effective against rapidly growing bacteria. Consider adding IVIG.

COMPLICATIONS

Death (in 30% of streptococcal or 3% of staphylococcal TSS), gangrene of the extremities, ARDS, chronic renal failure.

TRAVEL MEDICINE

General Guidelines

Most cases of fever in returned travelers are due to common illnesses such as influenza, viral URI, pneumonia, and UTI. The most common travel-related infections are malaria (see below), typhoid fever, hepatitis, dengue, and amebic liver abscess. Life-threatening infections that are treatable if diagnosed early include falciparum malaria, typhoid fever, and meningococcemia (consider these in all returned travelers with fever).

SYMPTOMS/EXAM

- **Careful travel history:** Determine the countries visited, urban vs. rural locales, accommodation type, immunizations, chemoprophylaxis, and sexual history.
- **Specific exposures:** Determine if there was freshwater contact (leptospirosis, schistosomiasis) or exposure to unpasteurized dairy (brucellosis), mosquitoes (malaria, dengue), ticks (rickettsial diseases, tularemia), or sick contacts (meningococcus, TB, viral hemorrhagic fevers).
- Examine for lymphadenopathy, maculopapular rash (dengue, leptospirosis, acute HIV, acute HBV), eschars at the site of a tick bite (rickettsial disease), and splenomegaly (malaria, typhoid, brucellosis).

DIFFERENTIAL

- Malaria (see below).
- **Typhoid fever:** Presents with fever, malaise, and abdominal discomfort, often without GI symptoms. Exam reveals splenomegaly, pulse-temperature dissociation, and evanescent rose spots. Diagnose by blood cultures growing *Salmonella;* treat with ciprofloxacin or levofloxacin. Vaccine is 70% effective.
- **Hepatitis:** HAV and HEV are transmitted by the fecal-oral route and may have nonspecific prodromes. HBV and HCV are transmitted by sexual contact, shared needles, or blood transfusions.
- **Dengue:** Endemic in equatorial and subtropical areas. Patients have abrupt onset of fever, retro-orbital headache, and myalgias. Exam shows a blanching rash. Treatment is supportive.
- **Leptospirosis:** Recent outbreaks have affected eco-travelers in Hawaii and Indonesia. May be biphasic, with fever, chills, and headache that resolve but are followed 1–3 days later by conjunctivitis, a maculopapular rash, hepatosplenomegaly, and aseptic meningitis. Severe cases (Weil's syndrome) have jaundice, renal failure, pulmonary hemorrhage, and hypotension. Treat with penicillin or doxycycline (patients may get **Jarisch-Herxheimer reactions**).
- **Rickettsial illnesses:** Include Mediterranean spotted fever and African tick typhus. Fever, headaches, myalgias, eschars, and maculopapular rashes spread from the trunk outward to the palms and soles (unlike rashes in Rocky Mountain spotted fever, which spread inward). Treat with doxycycline.
- **Amebiasis (*Entamoeba histolytica*):** May cause bloody dysentery or liver abscesses. Diagnose by stool microscopy showing cysts or trophozoites with ingested RBCs. Colonoscopy shows typical "flask-shaped" ulcers. Serologic tests are 95% sensitive for diagnosing liver abscess. Treat with metronidazole followed by paromomycin to eradicate stool cysts. **Amebic liver abscesses do not require drainage.**
- Acute schistosomiasis; acute HIV and other STDs.
- **Traveler's diarrhea:** Caused by ETEC (> 50%), *Campylobacter*, and, to a lesser extent, *Shigella, Salmonella* (< 15% each), and parasites (*Giardia, Entamoeba, Cryptosporidium*). Onset is usually within one week of arrival, with watery diarrhea lasting 2–4 days; patients are **usually afebrile.** Dysentery with bloody diarrhea and fever may be seen with *Shigella* or *Entamoeba.* Treat with hydration, antimotility agents (avoid in dysenteric cases), and antibiotics to shorten disease duration (ciprofloxacin × 1–3 days, azithromycin).

DIAGNOSIS

- Routine tests include CBC, liver and renal chemistries, UA, and CXR.
- Evaluate the differential for eosinophilia; obtain thick and thin blood smears for malaria (may need to repeat every 8–12 hours for two days). Blood cultures for typhoid fever and meningococcus; stool for culture and ova/parasites.

PREVENTION

- Avoid untreated water, ice cubes, undercooked foods ("boil it, cook it, peel it, or forget it"), stray or wild animals, swimming in fresh water, and insect bites (use insect repellents containing 30–35% DEET or permethrin to coat mosquito netting or clothes).
- Malaria prophylaxis (see below).

- Safe-sex counseling.
- **Regular adult immunizations:** Tetanus, diphtheria, measles/mumps/rubella (MMR), and polio vaccinations should be up to date. Influenza and pneumococcal vaccine for some adults; hepatitis B vaccine for sexually active adults and health care workers.
- **Vaccines for most travelers to developing countries:** Hepatitis A and typhoid (for rural areas). Consider immune globulin (for hepatitis A in travelers leaving < 2–3 weeks after vaccination), meningococcus (for Nepal, sub-Saharan Africa, and pilgrims to Mecca), Japanese encephalitis (for rural China and southern Asia), yellow fever (required by certain countries), and rabies.
  - **Live attenuated vaccines (avoid during pregnancy or if immunosuppressed):** MMR, **oral** polio, **oral** typhoid, yellow fever, and oral cholera (not recommended for use).
  - **Egg-based vaccines:** Influenza, yellow fever.

For fever after recent travel (< 21 days), consider malaria, typhoid fever, dengue, leptospirosis, rickettsial illnesses, and meningococcemia. For longer incubation periods (> 21 days), consider non-falciparum malaria, TB, hepatitis, amebic liver abscess, acute HIV, and brucellosis.

Malaria

A common cause of fever in the tropics and in returned travelers or immigrants. *Plasmodium falciparum* is the most dangerous species and has a high prevalence in sub-Saharan Africa. Other species include *P. vivax*, *P. malariae*, and *P. ovale*. Malaria is transmitted by Anopheles mosquitoes or is acquired congenitally, through blood transfusions, or from stowaway mosquitoes ("airport malaria"). Nonimmune individuals (e.g., young children, visitors, migrants returning to the tropics after living in nonendemic areas) and pregnant women are at risk for severe disease.

Symptoms/Exam

- Fever, chills, malaise, headache, myalgias, and GI symptoms occur primarily when parasitized RBCs burst open, eventually leading to cyclic symptoms every 48 or 72 hours.
- Signs include hemolytic anemia, splenomegaly, hypoglycemia, thrombocytopenia, transaminitis, indirect hyperbilirubinemia, and hemoglobinuria ("blackwater fever").
- Illness usually occurs 1–2 weeks after infection with *P. falciparum*, but incubation may be longer for other species.
- Nephrotic syndrome due to immune complexes is most common with *P. malariae*. Relapsing illness may be seen after months or years with *P. vivax* and *P. ovale* because these have dormant liver stages or hypnozoites.
- Mature *P. falciparum* parasites (schizonts) bind to vascular endothelium, leading to capillary obstruction and ischemia. If left untreated, this can in turn lead to hypoglycemia, cerebral malaria (seizures, coma), nephritis, renal failure, and pulmonary edema. Falciparum malaria also leads to high rates of parasitized RBCs, causing severe anemia.

A blood smear showing a banana-shaped gametocyte or RBCs infected with multiple signet-ring forms is diagnostic for Plasmodium falciparum *infection, the most severe form of malaria.*

Diagnosis

- **Order blood smears in all febrile travelers or returned immigrants.** Giemsa- or Wright-stained **thick and thin smears** are the best diagnostic tests.
- ***P. falciparum* must be distinguished from other species** (see Figure 11-16A) because it requires hospital admission and is the only species with significant drug resistance. *P. falciparum* is usually characterized by > 1% parasitized RBCs, > 1 parasite/RBC (see Figure 11-16B), banana-shaped gametocytes (see Figure 11-17), and lack of mature schizonts. It is also as-

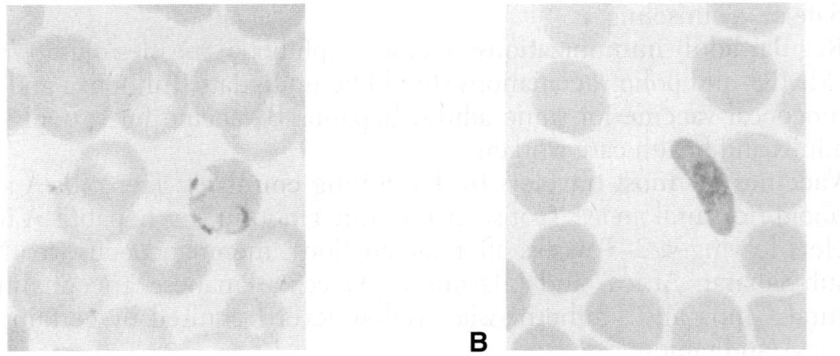

FIGURE 11-16. Falciparum malaria on a thin blood smear.

(**A**) Young signet-ring-shaped parasites are seen for all species of *Plasmodium*, but only *P. falciparum* shows multiple parasites within a single RBC. (**B**) Banana-shaped gametocytes are diagnostic for *P. falciparum*. (Reproduced, with permission, from *Bench Aids for the Diagnosis of Malaria Infections*, 2nd ed. Geneva: World Health Organization, 2000.) (Also see Color Insert.)

sociated with travel to Africa, severe disease, and symptoms that occur within two months of travel.

Treatment

- Treat *P. vivax*, *P. ovale*, and *P. malariae* with chloroquine. Treat *P. vivax* and *P. ovale* with primaquine as well to eradicate chronic liver stages (if patients have normal G6PD levels).
- **For *P. falciparum*, assume chloroquine resistance** (unless acquired in Central America, Haiti, or the Middle East) and treat with quinine + doxycycline, quinine + sulfadoxine/pyrimethamine (Fansidar), Fansidar alone, mefloquine, or atovaquone/proguanil (Malarone). Artesunate and artemisinin compounds are the fastest-acting malaricidal agents, but they are unavailable in the United States. **Repeat blood smears at 48 hours** to document > 75% decrease in parasitized RBCs. Exchange transfusion may be used for severe malaria or in the presence of > 15% parasitemia.
- In the United States, IV quinidine is often used because IV quinine may be unavailable. Primaquine may lead to severe hemolytic anemia, so screen for G6PD deficiency before using it. Adverse effects of mefloquine include irritability, bad dreams, GI upset, and, to a lesser extent, seizures and psychosis. Sulfadoxine/pyrimethamine is a sulfa drug and may lead to Stevens-Johnson syndrome. Atovaquone/proguanil has GI toxicities. Halofantrine (rarely used in the United States) may lead to QT prolongation. Doxycycline leads to photosensitivity and GI upset. During pregnancy, chloroquine is safe, and quinine, sulfadoxine/ pyrimethamine, and doxycycline may be used despite potential fetal risks because morbidity and mortality are so high.

P. ***V**ivax and P.* ***O**vale may lead to **V**ery **O**ld infections, presenting months or years after individuals leave an endemic area. Be sure to include primaquine at the end of treatment regimens to eradicate the chronic liver stages.*

Prevention

Avoid mosquito bites (use bed netting, window screens, insecticides, and insect repellents with 30–35% DEET). **Chloroquine is effective in Central America, Haiti, and parts of the Middle East.** For most other areas, the

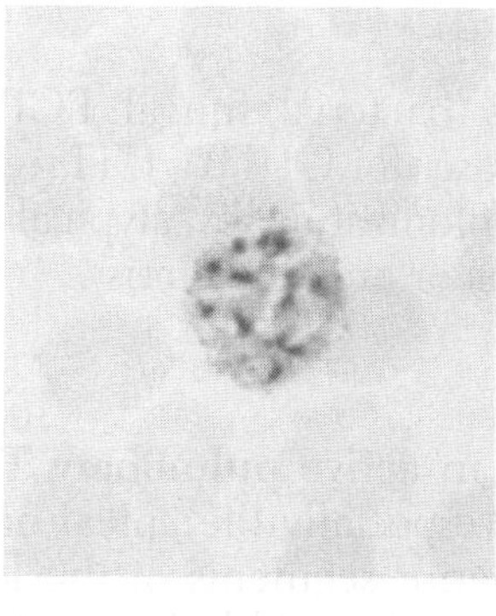

FIGURE 11-17. Vivax malaria on a thin blood smear.

Mature schizonts ready to burst and release many daughter parasites are seen in *P. vivax, P. ovale,* and *P. malariae* infections. They are not seen in the blood with *P. falciparum.* (Banana-shaped gametocytes are diagnostic for *P. falciparum.* (Reproduced, with permission, from *Bench Aids for the Diagnosis of Malaria Infections,* 2nd ed. Geneva: World Health Organization, 2000.) (Also see Color Insert.)

CDC recommends mefloquine or atovaquone/proguanil. For Southeast Asia (the Thai-Burmese and Thai-Cambodian border areas), use doxycycline because resistance to all other antimalarials is common.

TUBERCULOSIS (TB)

In the United States, *Mycobacterium tuberculosis* is most commonly found among the disadvantaged (homeless, malnourished, crowded living conditions) and in immigrants from developing countries.

SYMPTOMS/EXAM

- **Primary TB:** Usually asymptomatic with no radiographic signs, but 5% of patients (usually infants, elderly, and immunosuppressed) develop **progressive primary infection.**
- **Latent tuberculosis infection (LTBI):** Patients are infected (usually skin test–positive) but do not have symptoms of active disease. Bacilli are contained by granuloma-forming T cells and macrophages.
- **Active TB/reactivation disease:** Approximately 10% of LTBI patients develop active disease, **5% within the first two years of infection** and 5% over the rest of their lives. **Risk factors for reactivation** include recent infection (within two years), HIV, hematologic malignancy, immunosuppressive medications (e.g., steroids, especially > 15 mg prednisone daily), diabetes, illicit drug use, silicosis, and gastrectomy.
  - **Pulmonary TB:** Presents with subacute cough (initially dry and then productive, sometimes with blood-streaked sputum), malaise, fever, sweats, and weight loss. Exam is normal or reveals apical rales, rhonchi, or wheezing.
  - **Extrapulmonary TB:** Lymphatic (painless cervical lymph node swelling) and pleural disease are most common. Other sites of infection may be seen, especially in patients with advanced HIV. Fever may be seen with more extensive disease.

DIFFERENTIAL

Pneumonia or lung abscess (bacterial, fungal, PCP), malignancy (of the lung or elsewhere), Crohn's disease (for GI TB), UTI (renal TB may yield a "sterile pyuria"), HIV infection, colonization by atypical mycobacteria (in patients with underlying emphysema or bronchiectasis).

DIAGNOSIS

- **Radiographic findings in active pulmonary TB:** Infiltrates, nodules (including hilar), cavities (especially the apical or posterior segments of the upper lobes or the superior segments of the lower lobes), calcifications. **Advanced HIV patients and the elderly may have normal or atypical radiographs.**
- **Sputum smears** are most sensitive in patients with cavitary disease. Bacilli are visualized by acid-fast (Ziehl-Neelsen, Kinyoun) or fluorochrome (rhodamine-auramine) stain.
- **Cultures** of sputum, blood, or tissue are the **gold standard** but may take weeks to grow. Sensitivities help guide treatment.
- **Nucleic acid amplification and/or hybridization tests:** Adjuncts to smear and culture; approved by the FDA for rapid identification of TB in respiratory smears (not extrapulmonary sites). Not available in all laboratories.
- For extrapulmonary disease, **histopathology** shows granulomas with caseating necrosis; AFB stains may show bacilli. For pleural TB, biopsy of the pleura showing granulomas is more sensitive than pleural fluid culture.
- **Tuberculin skin testing** identifies patients with latent or active infection but is not 100% sensitive or specific; false negatives are seen in elderly, malnourished, and immunosuppressed patients as well as in those with overwhelming TB infection. A blood test that measures the release of γ-interferon from lymphocytes in response to PPD is also available for the diagnosis of LTBI.

TREATMENT

- Patients with suspected active TB should be placed in **respiratory isolation** if hospitalized. Cases should be reported to public health authorities.
- For most cases of TB, the CDC recommends starting **treatment with four drugs;** isoniazid, rifampin, pyrazinamide, and ethambutol are most commonly used. Modify once susceptibility results are available. Ethambutol may be omitted if the transmitted organism is known to be fully susceptible.
- In patients on protease inhibitors, non-nucleoside reverse transcriptase inhibitors, itraconazole, methadone, or other medications metabolized by the liver, **rifabutin** may be used instead of rifampin because it is associated with less cytochrome P-450 induction.
- Steroids may be helpful for meningitis and pericarditis.
- **Strongly consider using directly observed therapy** to maximize compliance. Treat most adults for six months. Patients with HIV/AIDS or miliary/meningeal disease are sometimes treated longer.

COMPLICATIONS

- Treatment failure is usually due to medication nonadherence (> 95%).
- While patients are on treatment, **monitor monthly for clinical symptoms.** Consider **monthly LFTs** for those with baseline liver disease. In the presence of severe hepatitis (e.g., AST and ALT five times greater than the up-

per limit of normal), discontinue all hepatotoxic drugs and reintroduce one at a time every 3–4 days while monitoring symptoms and liver tests.

- **Other baseline monitoring:** Visual acuity and color vision (patients on ethambutol), uric acid (pyrazinamide), and audiometry (streptomycin). Give **pyridoxine** (vitamin B_6) to HIV patients to decrease the risk of INH-related peripheral neuritis.

PREVENTION

- **Screening and treatment of latent TB infection:** Patients who are at risk for reactivation disease should be screened regardless of age ("a decision to screen is a decision to treat"). The Mantoux tuberculin skin test measures **induration** (not erythema) transversely on the forearm 2–3 days after intradermal injection of tuberculin; a visible wheal must be seen at the time of injection. Positive skin tests should be followed by a CXR to rule out active pulmonary disease. Table 11-11 outlines CDC guidelines governing tuberculin skin test positivity.
- The CDC recommends treatment of latent TB infection (formerly called "prophylaxis") in HIV-negative persons with INH QD or BIW × 9 months or with rifampin QD × 4 months. The use of combination rifampin/pyrazinamide for two months has been associated with severe and fatal hepatitis and should be avoided.
- New health care workers and others who will be tested repeatedly should have **two-step testing,** with a repeat skin test after 1–3 weeks if they are initially negative (≤ 10 mm). If the second test is positive, it is likely due to a boosting response, and the person is considered a "reactor" but not a "recent converter." A **skin-test conversion** indicating recent infection is defined as an increase of ≥ 10 mm of induration within a two-year period. **Anergy testing** is not recommended. **Previous BCG vaccination** should be disregarded, as persistent reactivity is unlikely after > 10 years.

VARICELLA-ZOSTER VIRUS (VZV)

Primary infection causes chickenpox. Reactivation of latent infection leads to herpes zoster, or "shingles." Immunosuppressed individuals can have more severe disease.

SYMPTOMS/EXAM

- **Chickenpox:** Incubation period is **10–20 days.** Presents with prominent fever, malaise, and a pruritic rash starting on the face, scalp, and trunk and spreading to the extremities. The rash starts as maculopapular and turns into vesicles ("dewdrops on a rose petal") and then into pustules that rupture, leading to crusts. **Multiple stages are present simultaneously.**
- **Herpes zoster:** Dermatomal tingling or pain followed by rash.

DIFFERENTIAL

- **Smallpox:** Lesions are deeper and painful; **all lesions occur at the same stage.**
- **Disseminated HSV:** Especially if skin disorder, diagnose by culture.
- **Meningococcemia:** Petechiae, purpura, sepsis.

TABLE 11-11. CDC Guidelines for Tuberculin Skin Test Positivity

≥ 5 mm OF INDURATION (FOR PATIENTS AT HIGHEST RISK OF REACTIVATION)	≥ 10 mm OF INDURATION	≥ 15 mm OF INDURATION (FOR PATIENTS AT LOWEST RISK OF REACTIVATION)
HIV. Immunosuppression due to organ transplants or other medications (prednisone ≥ 15 mg/day for one month or more). Close contacts of TB cases. CXR with fibrotic changes consistent with prior TB.	Recent immigrants (≤ 5 years) from developing countries. Residents or **established employees** of jails, long-term care facilities, or homeless shelters. IV drug users. Chronic illnesses such as silicosis, diabetes, chronic renal failure, leukemia, or lymphoma; head and neck or lung cancers; > 10% weight loss; gastrectomy.	Patients with no risk factors for TB. **New employees** of high-risk institutional settings (at work entry).

DIAGNOSIS

- Usually a clinical diagnosis.
- Confirm by scraping of lesions (culture or fluorescent staining for virus).
- Tzanck smear of vesicle base for multinucleate giant cells.
- PCR of CSF for CNS complications.

TREATMENT

Acyclovir, valacyclovir, and **famciclovir** reduce duration and severity and may prevent complications in adult chickenpox (if treated within **24 hours**) and shingles (if treated within **72 hours**). **VZIG** may prevent complications in immunocompromised or pregnant patients.

COMPLICATIONS

- Chickenpox:
  - **Interstitial pneumonia** may occur, especially in pregnant women.
  - **Bacterial infections** (group A strep).
  - **Encephalitis.**
  - **Transverse myelitis.**
  - Varicella may **disseminate** or be multidermatomal in immunosuppressed patients (HIV, steroids, malignancy).
  - **Reye's syndrome** (fatty liver, encephalopathy) may develop in children with chickenpox (or influenza) after taking **aspirin.**
- Herpes zoster:
  - **Postherpetic neuralgia** is most common in the elderly and may be prevented by starting antivirals **within 72 hours** of rash onset. The effect of steroids is less clear.
  - **Ophthalmic zoster** may lead to blindness; patients with lesions on the tip of the nose should have an ophthalmologic consult.

- **Ramsay Hunt syndrome:** Presents with vesicles on the ear, facial palsy, loss of taste on the anterior two-thirds of the tongue, and vertigo. Tinnitus/deafness may occur.

PREVENTION

- **Chickenpox:** Vaccine can be given up to three days after exposure to patients with active lesions. **This live attenuated vaccine should not be given to immunosuppressed patients.**
- **Herpes zoster:** None. The effect of vaccine on risk of shingles is unknown.

Smallpox rash starts on the face and extremities and moves to the trunk, where it is sparse. Generally, chickenpox rash also begins on the face and scalp and moves rapidly to the trunk, where it is denser, with relative sparing of the extremities.

NOTES

CHAPTER 12

Nephrology

Alan C. Pao, MD

Hyponatremia

Symptoms/Exam

- Symptoms and signs relate to the rate and severity of the decline in Na^+.
- May be asymptomatic or may present with symptoms ranging from nausea and vomiting to confusion and lethargy or seizures and coma.

The vast majority of clinically significant hyponatremias will have a P_{osm} < 280 mOsm/kg. The main reason to check plasma osmolality is to exclude the unusual isotonic and hypertonic causes.

Differential

The evaluation and differential diagnosis of hyponatremia are outlined in Figure 12-1.

Diagnosis

- Determine tonicity:

  Plasma osmolality (P_{osm}) = $(2 \times Na^+) + (BUN/2.8) + (glucose/18)$

- For hypotonic hyponatremias, determine volume status:
  - **Clinical exam:** Look for volume overload (elevated JVP, S3 gallop, ascites, edema) or volume depletion (dry mucous membranes, flat JVP).

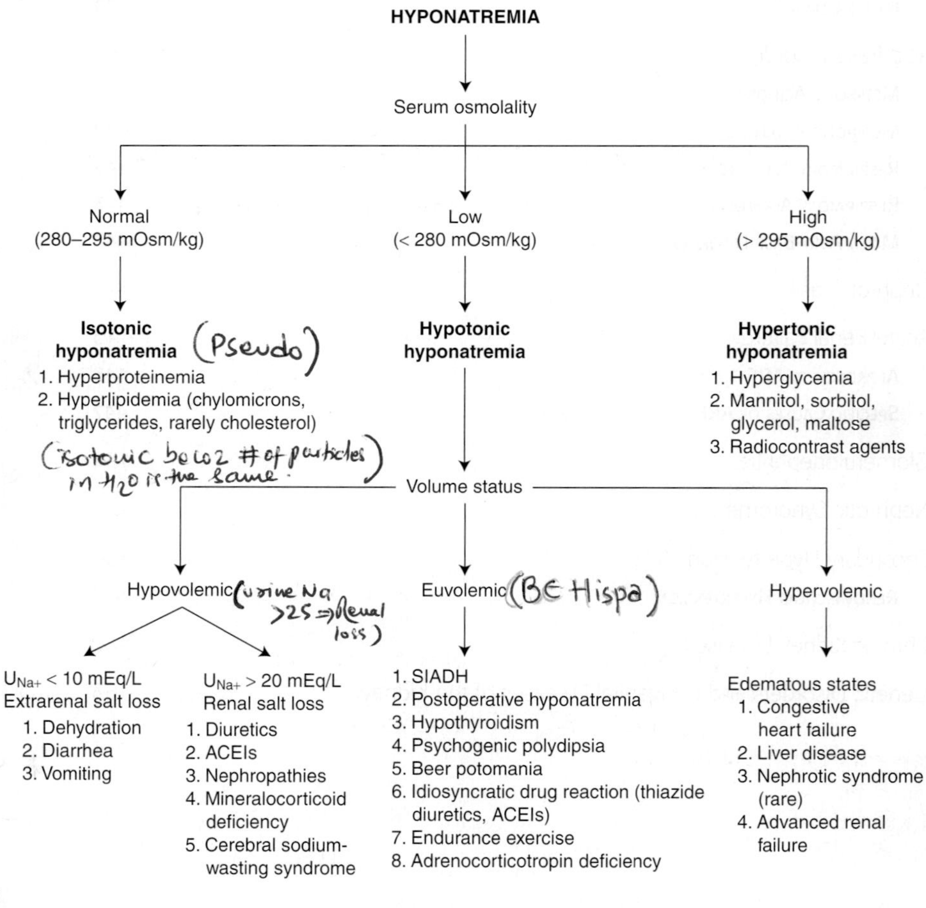

FIGURE 12-1. Evaluation of hyponatremia.

(Adapted, with permission, from Narins RG et al. Diagnostic strategies in disorders of fluid, electrolyte, and acid-base homeostasis. *Am J Med* 1982;72: 496.)

- A **urine $Na^+ < 10$** suggests hypovolemia.
- A **fractional excretion of Na^+ (Fe_{Na+}) < 1%** is a more accurate predictor of low volume status than urine Na (U_{Na}):

  Fe_{Na+} = excreted Na^+/filtered Na^+ = $(U_{Na+} \times P_{Cr}) / (P_{Na+} \times U_{Cr})$

  where P_{Cr} = plasma creatinine, P_{Na+} = plasma sodium, and U_{Cr} = urine creatinine.
- **$U_{osm} > P_{osm}$ or $U_{osm} > 1200$ mOsm/kg** suggests a high ADH state due to hypovolemia or SIADH.

Checking urine Na^+ or calculating Fe_{Na} is reliable only when the patient is oliguric and not taking diuretics.

TREATMENT

- Fluid management depends on the **volume status** of the patient.
  - **Hypervolemia:** Fluid restriction or diuretics.
  - **Euvolemia:** Fluid restriction.
  - **Hypovolemia:** Isotonic or hypertonic saline.
- The rate of correction of Na^+ depends on how quickly it dropped and how symptomatic the patient is.
  - **Acute symptomatic hyponatremia:** Na^+ should be raised until symptoms resolve (2 mEq/L per hour). Hypertonic (3%) saline is often required, usually with a loop diuretic.
  - **Symptomatic chronic hyponatremia:** Na^+ should be raised more slowly (1 mEq/L per hour). Hypertonic saline may be required.
  - **Asymptomatic chronic hyponatremia:** No immediate correction is required; fluid management as outlined above often suffices.
- Treat the underlying cause.

To prevent central pontine myelinolysis, do not increase Na^+ more than 12 mEq/L over a 24-hour period.

Syndrome of Inappropriate Antidiuretic Hormone Secretion (SIADH)

Although the classic etiology tested on the boards is **small cell lung cancer,** remember the **"big three"** causes: any CNS disorder, any pulmonary disorder, and medications (especially psych meds).

SYMPTOMS/EXAM

Symptoms are those due to hyponatremia and to the underlying cause of SIADH.

DIFFERENTIAL

- **CNS disorders:**
  - **Head trauma:** SAH, subdural hematoma.
  - **Infection:** Meningitis, encephalitis, brain abscess.
  - **Other:** Tumors, CVA, MS.
- **Pulmonary disorders:** Small cell lung cancer, pneumonia, lung abscess, TB, pneumothorax.
- **Drugs:** Chlorpropamide, TCAs, haloperidol.
- **Malignant neoplasia.**

DIAGNOSIS

- Low P_{osm}.
- Hyponatremia with normal volume status.
- $U_{osm} > P_{osm}$.
- Rule out other causes of hyponatremia. **SIADH is a diagnosis of exclusion.**

Treatment

- **Water restriction.**
- **Second-line agents:** Hypertonic saline and loop diuretic.
- **Chronic SIADH:** Demeclocycline.

Hypernatremia

Symptoms/Exam

Hypernatremia is almost always due to free water deficits (and only rarely to an increase in body sodium).

- Hypernatremia leads to hyperosmolality, which pulls water from cells, leading to cellular dehydration and to **CNS symptoms** (lethargy, weakness, irritability, altered mentation, seizures, coma).
- **Volume depletion:** Dry mucous membranes, hypotension, low urine output.

Differential

*If U_{osm} is **low** in a hypernatremic patient, consider DI.*

- **Increased water loss (U_{osm} > 600 mOsm/kg):**
  - **Insensible loss:** Increased sweating, burns.
  - **GI loss:** Diarrhea.
- **Renal loss (polyuria):**
  - Postobstructive or post-ATN diuresis.
  - Diabetes mellitus (DM).
  - **Diabetes insipidus (DI) (U_{osm} < 600 mOsm/kg)**—suspect in a hypernatremic patient with copious amounts of dilute urine (see Chapter 6 for a full discussion).
- **Excess Na^+ retention:** Rare; due to hypertonic saline infusion.

Diagnosis

- Diagnosis is usually apparent from the clinical presentation.
- Measure U_{osm}; it should be high in the hypovolemic patient (the kidney is trying to hold on to water, so the urine becomes concentrated).

Treatment

- **Calculate free-water deficit:**

$$\text{Normal body water (NBW)} - \text{current body water (CBW)} = 0.5 \times \text{body weight in kg } [(\text{plasma } Na^+ - 140)/140]$$

- Replace the calculated free-water deficit. Na^+ should be lowered 1 mEq/L per hour, not to exceed 12 mEq/L in a 24-hour period.
- If the patient is hypotensive and volume depleted, isotonic saline should be used initially; hypotonic saline can be used once tissue perfusion is adequate.

POTASSIUM DISORDERS

Hyperkalemia

Symptoms/Exam

May be asymptomatic or may present with symptoms ranging from muscle weakness to ventricular fibrillation (VF).

Differential

- **High K⁺ dietary intake.**
- **Extracellular K⁺ shift:** Metabolic acidosis, insulin deficiency, β-adrenergic blockade, rhabdomyolysis, tumor lysis syndrome, digitalis overdose, succinylcholine, periodic paralysis–hyperkalemic form.
- **Low urine K⁺ excretion:** Renal failure, decreased effective circulating volume, hypoaldosteronism.
  - **Decreased renin-angiotensin system activity:** Hyporeninemic hypoaldosteronism, ACEIs, NSAIDs, cyclosporine.
  - **Decreased adrenal synthesis:** Addison's disease.
  - **Aldosterone resistance:** High-dose trimethoprim, pentamidine, K⁺-sparing diuretics.

Diagnosis

- The cause is often apparent after a careful history, a review of meds, and basic labs (chemistry panel with BUN, creatinine, and CK).
- Check ECG as an indicator of severity:
  - **Mild:** Normal or peaked T waves.
  - **Moderate:** QRS prolongation or flattened P waves.
  - **Severe:** VF.
- Additional labs for special situations include the following:
  - **Tumor lysis syndrome:** High LDH, uric acid, and phosphorus; low calcium.
  - **Hypoaldosteronemic states:** Check **transtubular K⁺ gradient (TTKG):**

$$TTKG = (U_{K+}/P_{K+}) / (U_{osm}/P_{osm})$$

where U_{K+} = urine potassium and P_{K+} = plasma potassium.

A TTKG < 5 in a hyperkalemic patient is highly suggestive of hypoaldosteronism.

Treatment

- **Reduce cardiac excitability:** IV calcium.
- **Shift K⁺ entry into cells:** Glucose and insulin, β_2-adrenergic agonists (e.g., inhaled albuterol), $NaHCO_3$.
- **Remove excess K⁺:** Diuretics, cation-exchange resin (Kayexalate), dialysis.

Hypokalemia

Symptoms/Exam

- **Symptoms usually occur when P_{K+} < 2.5–3.0 mEq/L.**
- Presents with weakness, rhabdomyolysis, and cardiac arrhythmias.

Differential

- **Low K⁺ dietary intake.**
- **Intracellular K⁺ shift:** Alkalemia, increased insulin availability, increased β-adrenergic activity, periodic paralysis (classically associated with thyrotoxicosis).
- **GI K⁺ loss:** Diarrhea.
- **Renal K⁺ loss:**
  - Diuretics.
  - Vomiting
  - **Mineralocorticoid excess:** Primary hyperaldosteronism, Cushing's disease, European licorice ingestion and syndrome of apparent mineralocorticoid excess, hyperreninemia.
  - Hypomagnesemia.
  - Bartter's and Gitelman's syndromes.

Diagnosis

- 24-hour urine collection for K^+:
  - **< 25 mEq/day:** Extrarenal loss.
  - **> 25 mEq/day:** Renal K^+ wasting.
- Spot urine collection for K^+ (less accurate but easier to obtain):
  - **< 15 mEq/L:** Extrarenal loss.
  - **> 15 mEq/L:** Urine K^+ wasting. Check plasma renin activity and serum/urine aldosterone levels (see Chapter 6).
- **Additional labs for special situations:** Periodic paralysis may be associated with thyroid disease; check TSH.

Treatment

- **Replete KCl.** The average total body K^+ deficit is 200–400 mEq when P_{K+} = 3.0 mEq/L.
- The IV K^+ correction rate should **not** exceed 10 mEq/L per hour for a peripheral line or 20 mEq/L per hour for a central line.

ACID-BASE DISORDERS

Metabolic Acidosis

- There are **two main categories** of metabolic acidosis: **anion-gap and non-anion-gap.**
- Calculate anion gap (AG):

$$AG = (Na^+) - [(Cl^-) + (HCO_3^-)]$$

- A normal AG is approximately 12.
- An elevated AG **always** implies an AG metabolic acidosis even if the plasma HCO_3 is normal.

> ***Differential diagnosis of anion-gap metabolic acidosis–***
>
> **MUDPILES**
>
> **M**ethanol ingestion–can cause blindness, optic disk hyperemia
> **U**remia
> **D**iabetic ketoacidosis
> **P**araldehyde ingestion
> **I**soniazid overdose
> **L**actic acidosis–commonly due to tissue hypoxia from circulatory shock
> **E**thylene glycol ingestion–look for calcium oxalate crystals in urine
> **S**alicylate ingestion–classically presents with concomitant respiratory alkalosis

Anion-Gap Metabolic Acidosis (AG > 12)

Accumulation of unmeasured anions.

Differential

The differential is summarized in the mnemonic **MUDPILES.**

Diagnosis

- Check renal function.
- Check lactate.
- Check serum or urine ketones.
- Calculate the osmolal gap to rule out ingestion of an alcohol:

$$\text{Osm gap} = \text{measured osm} - \text{calculated osm}$$

$$\text{Calculated osm} = (2 \times Na^+) + (BUN/2.8) + (glucose/18)$$

- An osm gap > 20 indicates the ingestion of an alcohol:
  - Ethanol, methanol, ethylene glycol.
  - Isopropyl alcohol should be suspected in the setting of normal electrolytes and ketones in urine (isopropyl alcohol is metabolized to acetone).
- Check salicylate level.

NON-ANION-GAP (HYPERCHLOREMIC) ACIDOSIS

Loss of bicarbonate balanced by accumulation of chloride.

DIFFERENTIAL

- **GI loss of HCO_3:** Diarrhea.
- **Renal loss of HCO_3:** Renal tubular acidosis (RTA). The causes of RTA are further discussed in Table 12-1.

DIAGNOSIS

- **Urine anion gap (UAG)** estimates the amount of urine NH_4^+.

UAG = urine cations – urine anions = (urine Na^+) + (urine K^+) – (urine Cl^-)

  - A **positive UAG** usually indicates low urine NH_4^+, which is associated with **RTA.** The characteristics of the different types of RTA are summarized in Table 12-1.

In patient with non-anion-gap metabolic acidosis, a history of diarrhea points to GI bicarbonate loss; if no diarrhea, consider RTA. The urine anion gap can confirm clinical suspicion.

TABLE 12-1. Characteristics of Different Types of Renal Tubular Acidosis[a]

	TYPE 1 (DISTAL)	TYPE 2 (PROXIMAL)	TYPE 4
Basic defect	Decreased distal acidification.	Diminished proximal HCO_3^- reabsorption.	Aldosterone deficiency or resistance.
Urine pH during acidemia	> 5.3.	Variable: > 5.3 if above reabsorptive threshold; < 5.3 if below.	Usually < 5.3.
Plasma [HCO_3^-], untreated	May be < 10 mEq/L.	Usually 14–20 mEq/L.	Usually > 15 mEq/L.
Fractional excretion of HCO_3^- at normal plasma [HCO_3^-]	< 3% in adults; may reach 5–10% in young children.	> 15–20%.	< 3%.
Diagnosis	Response to $NaHCO_3$ or NH_4Cl.	Response to $NaHCO_3$.	Measure plasma aldosterone concentration.
Plasma [K^+]	Usually reduced or normal; elevated with voltage defect.	Normal or reduced.	Elevated.
Dose of HCO_3^- to normalize plasma [HCO_3^-], mEq/kg per day	1–2 in adults; 4–14 in children.	10–15.	1–3; may require no alkali if hyperkalemia is corrected.
Nonelectrolytic complications	Nephrocalcinosis and renal stones.	Rickets or osteomalacia.	None.

[a] What had been called type 3 RTA is actually a variant of type 1 RTA.

Reproduced, with permission, from Rose BD, Post TW. *Clinical Physiology of Acid-Base and Electrolyte Disorders,* 5th ed. New York: McGraw-Hill, 2001:613.

- A **negative UAG** indicates intact ammonium production, which is associated with **diarrhea.**
- Diagnosis of specific RTA.
  - First examine the **serum K^+**.
    - **If high:** Type 4 RTA.
    - **If normal or low:** Go to the next step.
  - Look at the **urine pH.**
    - **If urine pH > 5.5:** Distal RTA.
    - **If urine pH < 5.0:** Proximal RTA.
  - To confirm proximal RTA, look for **other signs of generalized proximal tubular dysfunction**—e.g., glycosuria, low-grade proteinuria, hypophosphatemia.

TREATMENT

See Table 12-1.

Metabolic Alkalosis

Due to one of four main causes: Volume depletion, chloride depletion, potassium depletion, or hyperaldosteronism. **Urine chloride** concentration is the key test to distinguish various causes.

DIAGNOSIS/TREATMENT

- **Urine Cl^- < 10 mEq/L implies hypovolemia** (the kidney is trying to retain Na^+ and Cl^-, so urine Cl^- is low).
  - **GI loss:** Vomiting, NG suction, or chloride-losing diarrhea.
  - Diuretics.
  - **Gain of HCO_3:** Administration of $NaHCO_3$ or antacids.
  - **Treatment:** NaCl infusion.
- **Urine Cl^- > 10 mEq/L** = chloride-resistant metabolic alkalosis. **Broken down according to BP.**
  - **Hypertension:** Implies excess mineralocorticoid action (retain Na; lose H^+ and K^+):
    - Primary hyperaldosteronism or hyperreninemia.
    - Liddle's syndrome.
    - European black licorice ingestion or syndrome of apparent mineralocorticoid excess.
    - 11- or 17-hydroxylase deficiency.
  - **Normal BP:** Profound hypokalemia (leads to increased ammonium production), Bartter's syndrome, refeeding alkalosis.
  - Treat the underlying cause.

Respiratory Acidosis

SYMPTOMS/EXAM

- **CNS symptoms:** Headache, blurred vision, restlessness, anxiety.
- **CO_2 narcosis:** Tremors, asterixis, delirium, somnolence.

DIFFERENTIAL

- **Depressed medullary respiratory center:**
  - **Drugs:** Opiates, anesthetics, sedatives.
  - Central sleep apnea.
- **Obstructed upper airway:** Obstructive sleep apnea, aspiration.
- **Impaired respiratory muscle or chest wall function:** Guillain-Barré syndrome, myasthenia gravis, severe hypokalemia, severe hypophosphatemia, spinal cord injury, poliomyelitis, MS, myxedema, kyphoscoliosis.

- **Impaired alveolar gas exchange:** Exacerbation of underlying chronic lung disease, cardiogenic pulmonary edema, ARDS, pneumothorax, COPD.

DIAGNOSIS

- The diagnosis is usually apparent from the clinical picture.
- An arterial $pH < 7.40$ and an arterial $pCO_2 > 40$ mmHg confirm respiratory acidosis.
- Calculate the alveolar-arterial (A-a) O_2 gradient to differentiate intrinsic pulmonary from extrapulmonary disease where:
  - Alveolar pO_2 (pAO_2) = FiO_2 (atmospheric pressure − water vapor pressure) − (pCO_2/0.8).
    - For patients at sea level breathing room air, pAO_2 can be estimated by **$pAO_2 = 150 - (pCO_2/0.8)$.**
  - Arterial pO_2 (paO_2) as measured by ABG:
  - The normal ($pAO_2 - paO_2$) gradient is 10–20 mmHg.
    - An A-a gradient > 20 implies intrinsic pulmonary disease causing impaired gas exchange.
- Compensation for acute vs. chronic respiratory acidosis:
  - **Acute:** For every 10-mmHg increase in pCO_2, plasma HCO_3 increases 1 mEq/L.
  - **Chronic** (after 3–5 days): For every 10-mmHg increase in pCO_2, plasma HCO_3 increases 3 mEq/L.

TREATMENT

- Correct the underlying disorder.
- Mechanical ventilation if necessary.

Respiratory Alkalosis

SYMPTOMS/EXAM

- **Tachypnea.**
- **CNS symptoms:** Lightheadedness, altered mental status.
- **Hypocalcemia symptoms:** Paresthesias, circumoral numbness, carpopedal spasms.

DIFFERENTIAL

The differential diagnosis of respiratory alkalosis is outlined in Table 12-2.

DIAGNOSIS

- $pH > 7.40$ and $pCO_2 < 40$ constitute respiratory alkalosis.
- Compensation for acute vs. chronic respiratory alkalosis:
  - **Acute:** For every 10-mmHg decrease in pCO_2, plasma HCO_3 decreases 2 mEq/L.
  - **Chronic** (after 3–5 days): For every 10-mmHg decrease in pCO_2, plasma HCO_3 decreases 4 mEq/L.

TREATMENT

Correct the underlying disorder.

Mixed Acid-Base Disorders

MIXED METABOLIC ACIDOSIS AND ALKALOSIS

- Calculate the delta anion gap (ΔAG):

$$\Delta AG = \text{calculated AG} - 12$$

TABLE 12-2. Differential Diagnosis of Respiratory Alkalosis

■ **Hypoxia:**
Decreased inspired oxygen tension
High altitude
Ventilation/perfusion inequality
Hypotension
Severe anemia
■ **CNS-mediated disorders:**
Voluntary hyperventilation
Anxiety-hyperventilation syndrome
Neurologic disease
CVA (infarction, hemorrhage)
Infection
Trauma
Tumor
Pharmacologic and hormonal stimulation
Salicylates
Nicotine
Xanthines
Pregnancy (progesterone)
Hepatic failure
Gram-negative septicemia
Recovery from metabolic acidosis
Heat exposure
■ **Pulmonary disease:**
Interstitial lung disease
Pneumonia
Pulmonary embolism
Pulmonary edema
■ **Mechanical overventilation**

Adapted, with permission, from Gennari FJ. Respiratory acidosis and alkalosis. In Narins RG (ed). *Maxwell and Kleeman's Clinical Disorders of Fluid and Electrolyte Metabolism,* 5th ed. New York: McGraw-Hill, 1994.

- Using the ΔAG, calculate the corrected plasma HCO_3:

$$\text{Corrected plasma } HCO_3 = \text{actual plasma } HCO_3 + \Delta AG$$

- The patient's expected bicarbonate concentration should be reduced to the same extent that his anion gap is increased.
  - If corrected plasma $HCO_3 > 26$ mEq/L, concomitant metabolic alkalosis exists.
  - If corrected plasma $HCO_3 < 22$ mEq/L, concomitant non-anion-gap acidosis exists.

Mixed Respiratory and Metabolic Disorders

- Calculate the expected arterial pCO_2:
  - **Winter's formula: Expected $pCO_2 = 1.5 \times HCO_3 + 8$.**
  - Can be used only to calculate pCO_2 in the setting of metabolic acidosis.

- **Faster method: Expected $pCO_2 = HCO_3 + 15$.**
  - If measured pCO_2 > expected pCO_2, concomitant respiratory acidosis exists.
  - If measured pCO_2 < expected pCO_2, concomitant respiratory alkalosis exists.

*Respiratory acidosis and respiratory alkalosis can **never** be present simultaneously–you can't hypoventilate and hyperventilate at the same time!*

TRIPLE ACID-BASE DISORDERS—THE "TRIPLE RIPPLE"

- Defined as metabolic acidosis + metabolic alkalosis + respiratory acidosis or alkalosis.
- Classic causes:
  - **Diabetic or alcoholic ketoacidosis:** Non-anion-gap and anion-gap metabolic acidosis (ketoacidosis), metabolic alkalosis (vomiting and hypovolemia), and compensatory respiratory alkalosis.
  - **Salicylate toxicity:** Anion-gap metabolic acidosis (from salicylic acid), metabolic alkalosis (vomiting), and primary respiratory alkalosis (salicylates directly stimulate the respiratory center).

NEPHROLITHIASIS

Calcium stones account for the vast majority of cases. Four times more common in men; peak incidence is between the ages of 20 and 40.

SYMPTOMS/EXAM

- Flank pain +/– radiation to the groin.
- Urinary frequency, urgency, and dysuria.
- Microscopic or gross hematuria.

A 24-hour urine collection is warranted for recurrent nephrolithiasis (volume, pH, Na, Ca, oxalate, phosphorus, citrate, uric acid, cystine, creatinine).

DIAGNOSIS

- Collect and analyze the stone!
- Labs:
  - UA (look for blood, assess urine pH, rule out UTI).
  - Plasma Ca^{++}, phosphorus, uric acid, electrolytes (assess renal function, acidosis, hypokalemia).
  - PTH level.

TREATMENT

- **General treatment for all stones is a high volume of daily fluid intake.**
- Specific treatment guidelines are outlined in Table 12-3. Clues from the history are as follows:
  - **Recurrent UTIs**: Struvite stones.
  - **Prior malignancies:** Uric acid stones (tumor lysis).
  - **IBD**: Oxalate stones.
  - Medications, family history.

ACUTE RENAL FAILURE (ARF)

Approach to ARF

Some accepted definitions of ARF include serum creatinine > 0.5 mg/dL, doubling of serum creatinine, and a 25–50% increase in serum creatinine. ATN and volume depletion account for the majority of hospital cases.

TABLE 12-3. Types, Mechanisms, and Treatment of Kidney Stones

Type	Mechanisms and Disease Associations	Treatment[a]	Notes
Calcium oxalate	Hypercalciuria: **hyperparathyroidism, malignancy, granulomatous diseases.** Hyperoxaluria: short gut syndrome, **IBD.** Hypocitraturia: metabolic acidosis from RTA, chronic kidney disease, chronic diarrhea.	Ca^{++} restriction is **not** helpful. (may lead to hyperoxaluria) Thiazides, potassium citrate, moderate protein intake.	Citrate is the primary stone formation inhibitor.
Uric acid	Acidic urine (pH < 5.5): high animal protein diet. Hyperuricosuria: **gout, tumor lysis syndrome.**	Allopurinol, potassium citrate, moderate protein intake.	
Cystine	Hypercystinuria: **cystinuria.**	Tiopronin (Thiola).	
Struvite ($Mg\text{-}NH_4$ + phosphate)	Alkaline urine (pH > 6.5): UTI with urease-splitting organisms (***Proteus mirabilis***).	Treat the underlying infection.	Recurrent UTIs may be due to a residual nidus of infection from the stone.
Medication-related	Triamterene, acyclovir, indinavir.		

[a] In addition to large-volume water intake.

The differential diagnosis of ARF with a low Fe_{Na} (< 1%) includes:

- *Prerenal azotemia*
- *Glomerulonephritis*
- *Contrast nephropathy*
- *Rhabdomyolysis*
- *Early obstructive nephropathy*

DIFFERENTIAL

Table 12-4 outlines the differential diagnosis of ARF.

DIAGNOSIS

Guidelines for the diagnosis of ARF are as follows (see also Table 12-5):

- Review medications for nephrotoxic drugs.
- Assess volume status.
- Urine electrolytes to calculate Fe_{Na} (if oliguric).
- Assess urine sediment.
- Renal ultrasound to rule out obstruction.

In the setting of oliguric renal failure, the clinician must distinguish prerenal azotemia from ATN. Table 12-6 outlines the differences between these two states.

TREATMENT

- Treat the underlying cause or remove the offending agent.
- Support renal function through dialysis if necessary (see the mnemonic AEIOU).
- There is **no role for "renal dose" dopamine!**

TABLE 12-4. Causes of ARF

PRERENAL	INTRINSIC RENAL	POSTRENAL
Volume depletion Circulatory shock Severe CHF Severe cirrhosis (hepatorenal syndrome)	Acute tubular necrosis (ATN): ■ Ischemia ■ Contrast dye ■ Myeloma ■ Heme pigment (rhabdomyolysis and hemolysis) ■ Aminoglycosides Acute interstitial nephritis (AIN): ■ Allergic and drug reactions (especially NSAIDs) Glomerulonephritis Cholesterol emboli syndrome	Urinary tract obstruction

Specific Causes of ARF

ACUTE TUBULAR NECROSIS (ATN)

SYMPTOMS/EXAM

Urine sediment shows a muddy brown cast (see Figure 12-2).

DIFFERENTIAL

- **Ischemic:** Prolonged prerenal azotemia; **sepsis;** massive hemorrhage; NSAIDs, ACEIs, ARBs; contrast dye.
- **Toxic:**
  - Endogenous toxins:
    - Myoglobin → rhabdomyolysis (see Table 12-7).
    - Hemoglobin.
    - **Light chain deposition.**
    - Urate.
  - Exogenous toxins:
    - **Radiocontrast** (see Table 12-7).
    - Oxalate (ethylene glycol ingestion).
    - **Meds:** Antimicrobials (**aminoglycosides,** pentamidine, **amphotericin B**), antivirals (ritonavir), chemotherapy (cisplatin, ifosfamide, 5-FU), lithium.

> ***Indications for dialysis—***
> **AEIOU**
> **A**cidosis
> **E**lectrolytes: hyperkalemia
> **I**ngestions: severe acidemia
> **O**verload: pulmonary edema
> **U**remia

ACUTE INTERSTITIAL NEPHRITIS (AIN)

SYMPTOMS/EXAM

- Fever, rash, eosinophilia, arthralgias.
- Sudden-onset renal failure.

DIFFERENTIAL

- **Drugs** (bolded items are most common):
  - **Antimicrobials:** β-lactams (penicillin, ampicillin, methicillin), fluoroquinolones, rifampin, sulfonamides.
  - **NSAIDs** and **COX-2 inhibitors.**
  - **Other:** Phenytoin, allopurinol, cimetidine, furosemide, indinavir.

TABLE 12-5. Clinical Features, Urinary Findings, and Confirmatory Tests in the Differential Diagnosis of ARF

Cause of Acute Renal Failure	Suggestive Clinical Features	Typical UA	Some Confirmatory Tests
I. **Prerenal ARF**	Evidence of true volume depletion (thirst, postural or absolute hypotension and tachycardia, low JVP, dry mucous membranes/axillae, weight loss, fluid output > input) or decreased "effective" circulatory volume (e.g., heart failure, liver failure), treatment with NSAIDs or ACEIs.	Hyaline casts. $Fe_{Na} < 1\%$. $U_{Na} < 10$ mmol/L. Specific gravity SG > 1.018.	Occasionally requires invasive hemodynamic monitoring; rapid resolution of ARF upon restoration of renal perfusion.
II. **Intrinsic renal ARF**			
A. Diseases involving large renal vessels			
1. Renal artery thrombosis	History of atrial fibrillation or recent MI; flank or abdominal pain.	Mild proteinuria. Occasionally red cells.	Elevated LDH with normal transaminases, renal arteriogram.
2. Atheroembolism	Age usually > 50 years, recent manipulation of aorta, retinal plaques, subcutaneous nodules, palpable purpura, livedo reticularis, vasculopathy, hypertension, anticoagulation.	Often normal, eosinophiluria, rarely casts.	Eosinophilia, hypocomplementemia, skin biopsy, renal biopsy.
3. Renal vein thrombosis	Evidence of nephrotic syndrome or pulmonary embolism, flank pain.	Proteinuria, hematuria.	Inferior vena cavagram and selective renal venogram.
B. Diseases of small vessels and glomeruli			
1. Glomerulonephritis/vasculitis	Compatible clinical history (e.g., recent infection), sinusitis, lung hemorrhage, skin rash or ulcers, arthralgias, new cardiac murmur, history of HBV or HCV infection.	Red cell or granular casts, red cells, white cells, mild proteinuria.	Low C3, C4, ANCA, anti-GBM Ab, ANA, ASO, anti-DNase, cryoglobulins, blood cultures, renal biopsy.
2. HUS/TTP	Compatible clinical history (e.g., recent GI infection, cyclosporine, anovulants), fever, pallor, ecchymoses, neurologic abnormalities.	May be normal, red cells, mild proteinuria, rarely red cell/granular casts.	Anemia, thrombocytopenia, schistocytes on blood smear, increased LDH, renal biopsy.

TABLE 12-5. Clinical Features, Urinary Findings, and Confirmatory Tests in the Differential Diagnosis of ARF (continued)

Cause of Acute Renal Failure	Suggestive Clinical Features	Typical UA	Some Confirmatory Tests
3. Malignant hypertension	Severe hypertension with headaches, cardiac failure, retinopathy, neurologic dysfunction, papilledema.	Red cells, red cell casts, proteinuria.	LVH by echocardiography/ECG, resolution of ARF with control of BP.
C. ARF mediated by ischemia or toxins (ATN)			
1. Ischemia	Recent hemorrhage, hypotension (e.g., cardiac arrest), surgery.	Muddy brown granular or tubular epithelial cell casts. $Fe_{Na} > 1\%$. $U_{Na} > 20$ mmol/L. SG < 1.015.	Clinical assessment and UA usually sufficient for diagnosis.
2. Exogenous toxins	Recent radiocontrast study, nephrotoxic antibiotics or anticancer agents often coexistent with volume depletion, sepsis, or chronic renal insufficiency.	Muddy brown granular or tubular epithelial cell casts. $Fe_{Na} > 1\%$. $U_{Na} > 20$ mmol/L. SG < 1.015.	Clinical assessment and UA usually sufficient for diagnosis.
3. Endogenous toxins	History suggestive of rhabdomyolysis (seizures, coma, ethanol abuse, trauma).	Urine supernatant positive for heme.	Hyperkalemia, hyperphosphatemia, hypocalcemia, increased circulating myoglobin, CPK (MM), and uric acid.
	History suggestive of massive hemolysis (blood transfusion).	Urine supernatant pink and positive for heme.	Hyperkalemia, hyperphosphatemia, hypocalcemia, hyperuricemia, pink plasma positive for hemoglobin.

TABLE 12-5. Clinical Features, Urinary Findings, and Confirmatory Tests in the Differential Diagnosis of ARF (continued)

Cause of Acute Renal Failure	Suggestive Clinical Features	Typical UA	Some Confirmatory Tests
3. Endogenous toxins (continued)	History suggestive of tumor lysis (recent chemotherapy), myeloma (bone pain), or ethylene glycol ingestion.	Urate crystals, dipstick-negative proteinuria, oxalate crystals, respectively.	Hyperuricemia, hyperkalemia, hyperphosphatemia (for tumor lysis); circulating or urinary monoclonal spike (for myeloma); toxicology screen, acidosis, osmolal gap (for ethylene glycol).
D. Acute diseases of the tubulointerstitium			
1. Allergic interstitial nephritis	Recent ingestion of drug and fever, rash, or arthralgias.	White cell casts, white cells (frequently eosinophiluria), red cells, rarely red cell casts, proteinuria (occasionally nephrotic).	Systemic eosinophilia, skin biopsy of rash (leukocytoclastic vasculitis), renal biopsy.
2. Acute bilateral pyelonephritis	Flank pain and tenderness, toxic, febrile.	Leukocytes, proteinuria, red cells, bacteria.	Urine and blood cultures.
III. **Postrenal ARF**	Abdominal or flank pain, palpable bladder.	Frequently normal, hematuria if stones, hemorrhage, malignancy, or prostatic hypertrophy.	Plain film, renal ultrasound, IVP, retrograde or anterograde pyelography, CT scan.

Adapted, with permission, from Brady HR, Brenner BM. Acute renal failure. In Kasper DL et al (eds). *Harrison's Principles of Internal Medicine,* 16th ed. New York: McGraw-Hill, 2005.

- **Infections:** Many bacteria, viruses, and parasites.
- **Systemic disease:** Sarcoidosis, Sjögren's syndrome, SLE.
- **Idiopathic.**

DIAGNOSIS

- Urine microscopy reveals **WBC casts.**
- Hansel stain on urine WBCs yields > 1% eosinophils (low sensitivity).

TABLE 12-6. Distinguishing Prerenal Azotemia from Acute Tubular Necrosis

	PRERENAL AZOTEMIA	ATN
Fe_{Na}	< 1%	> 1%
BUN/Cr	> 20:1	10–15:1
U_{osm}	High.	Similar to serum osm.
Urine sediment	Bland.	Muddy brown casts.
Response to fluids	Rapidly improves.	Poor; may take 2–3 weeks for recovery. Often requires dialysis in the interim.

- Peripheral blood eosinophilia (low sensitivity).
- Renal biopsy typically shows interstitial inflammation with mononuclear cells, with normal glomeruli.

TREATMENT

- Withdraw or eradicate the offending agent.
- Corticosteroids.

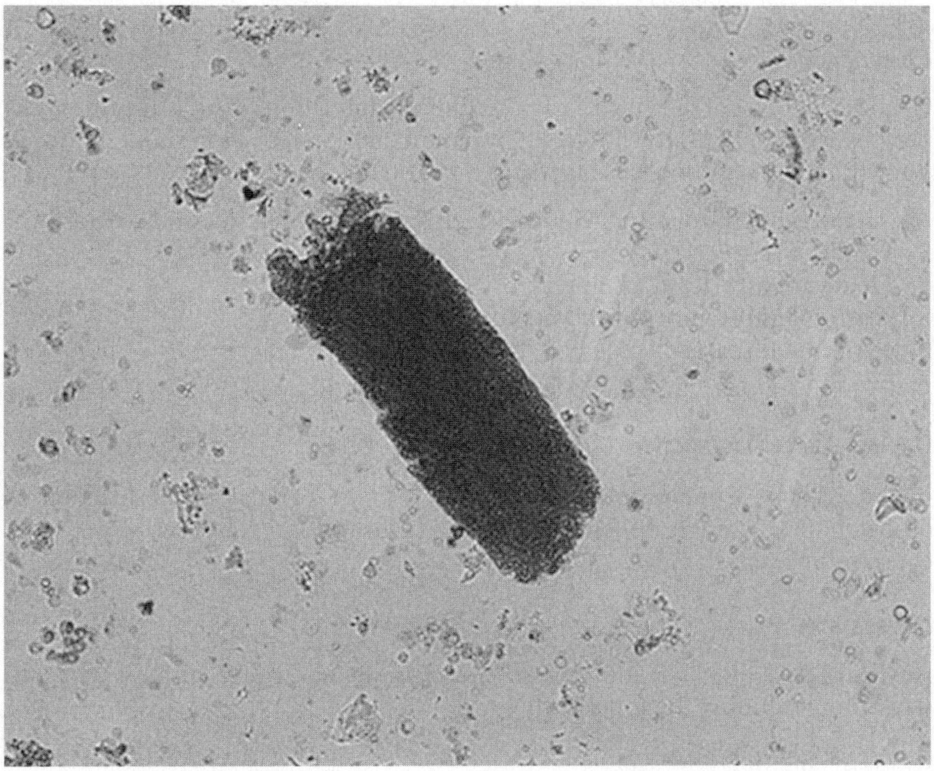

FIGURE 12-2. Muddy brown cast.

(Courtesy of R. Rodriguez.)

TABLE 12-7. Features of Contrast Dye Nephropathy and Rhabdomyolysis

	Contrast Nephropathy	Rhabdomyolysis
Risk factors	Underlying kidney disease. Diabetes. Concomitant use of ACEIs, ARBs, or NSAIDs. Volume depletion or sepsis.	Muscle trauma, ischemia, or inflammation. Toxins: alcohol, cocaine, statins, reverse transcriptase inhibitors. Metabolic: hypokalemia, hypophosphate. Genetic: McArdle's disease.
Other clinical features	Creatinine peaks 24–72 hours after dye load and then typically improves.	**Elevated serum CK.** Urine dipstick positive for blood, but no RBCs on microscopy. Other lab changes: hyperkalemia, hyperphosphatemia, hyperuricemia, and hypocalemia.
Treatment	Fluids: Isotonic $NaHCO_3$ 3 mL/kg bolus over 1 hr followed by 1 mL/kg/hr for 6 hrs. *N*-acetylcysteine (600 mg BID the day before and the day of contrast). Dialysis is rarely needed.	Early, aggressive volume repletion. Urine alkalization with $NaHCO_3$ may help. Dialysis may be needed.
Notes	Unlike other ATNs, **Fe_{Na+} is low** (due to intrarenal vasoconstriction).	Positive urine dipstick for blood due to myoglobin pigments in urine.

NSAID-induced nephropathy may include the following:

- *ARF from afferent arteriolar vasoconstriction in the setting of prerenal azotemia.*
- *AIN and minimal change disease.*
- *Analgesic nephropathy (papillary necrosis–chronic interstitial nephritis).*

Complications

Chronic interstitial nephritis is a potential complication of AIN. It presents as progressive renal failure with mild proteinuria and inactive sediment. Chronic interstitial nephritis may also be caused by the following:

- **Analgesic nephropathy** (papillary necrosis and chronic interstitial nephritis).
- **Chronic reflux.**
- **Heavy metals** (**lead**, arsenic).
- ***Aristolochia*** (Chinese herb nephropathy).
- **Systemic diseases:** Sickle cell, SLE, Sjögren's.

Urinary Tract Obstruction

In order for obstruction to cause ARF, there must be bilateral obstruction or obstruction of a single functioning kidney. Obstruction > 2 weeks is likely to cause permanent damage.

Differential

Anything that blocks urine flow to the outside may cause urinary tract obstruction, including the following:

- **Neurogenic bladder.**
- **Malignancies:** Prostatic hypertrophy or malignancy, cervical cancer, bladder cancer, lymphoma, pelvic lymphadenopathy.
- **Kidney stones.**
- **Retroperitoneal fibrosis.**

DIAGNOSIS

- Oliguria or anuria.
- **Labs:** Type 4 RTA, elevated creatinine.
- **Fe_{Na}:** Low (< 1%) early after obstruction, higher later in course.
- Foley catheter placement reveals large postvoid residual.
- **Ultrasonography** reveals **hydronephrosis.**

TREATMENT

- Relieve the obstruction.
- Volume repletion during postobstructive diuresis.

HEPATORENAL SYNDROME (HRS)

Renal failure in severe liver disease is not always HRS! HRS is a diagnosis of exclusion.

Seen in severe liver disease with portal hypertension. Pathophysiology is characterized by intense renal salt and water retention leading to oliguric renal failure.

DIAGNOSIS

- **Major criteria:**
  - Low GFR.
  - No preexisting renal disease.
  - Absence of shock, sepsis, fluid loss, or nephrotoxic drugs.
  - No improvement of renal function with 1.5 L of plasma expander.
- **Supporting criteria:**
  - Urine volume < 500 cc/day.
  - U_{Na+} < 10 mEq/L.
  - $U_{osm} > P_{osm}$.
  - Serum Na^+ < 130 mEq/L.
  - Low Fe_{Na+} (< 1%).

HRS is a marker of severe liver disease that can be reversed only by liver transplantation.

TREATMENT

- Albumin infusion.
- **Splanchnic vasoconstrictors:** Vasopressin analogues (terlipressin, ornipressin), midodrine, octreotide.
- Transjugular intrahepatic portosystemic shunt (TIPS).
- Renal replacement therapy, as a bridge to liver transplantation.
- **Liver transplantation** is definitive therapy.

CHOLESTEROL EMBOLI SYNDROME

SYMPTOMS/EXAM

- Acute is more common than chronic.
- Usually follows recent arterial manipulation (e.g., angiogram) or initiation of anticoagulation.
- Sites of embolization:
  - **Skin:** Livedo reticularis.
  - **Viscera:** Splenic infarct, ischemic bowel.
  - **Eye:** Retinal embolization (Hollenhorst plaques).
  - **Kidney:** Renal failure.

Diagnosis

- **Labs:** High ESR, low complement levels, high liver and muscle enzymes, **peripheral eosinophilia.**
- **Renal biopsy:** Elongated cholesterol crystals within the lumina of small vessels.

Treatment

Supportive.

GLOMERULONEPHRITIS (GN)

Symptoms/Exam

Hypertension, edema, and oliguria +/– hematuria.

Differential

The differential diagnosis of GN can be broken down on the basis of **serum complement levels** (see Figure 12-3).

Diagnosis

- Urine microscopy reveals **RBC casts** (see Figure 12-4).
- **Renal biopsy** is definitive.

Treatment

See Tables 12-8 through 12-10.

NEPHROTIC SYNDROME

Diabetes mellitus is the most common systemic disease that results in nephrotic syndrome in U.S. adults. The most common pathologic subtype of "idiopathic" nephrotic syndrome in adults is **membranous nephropathy.**

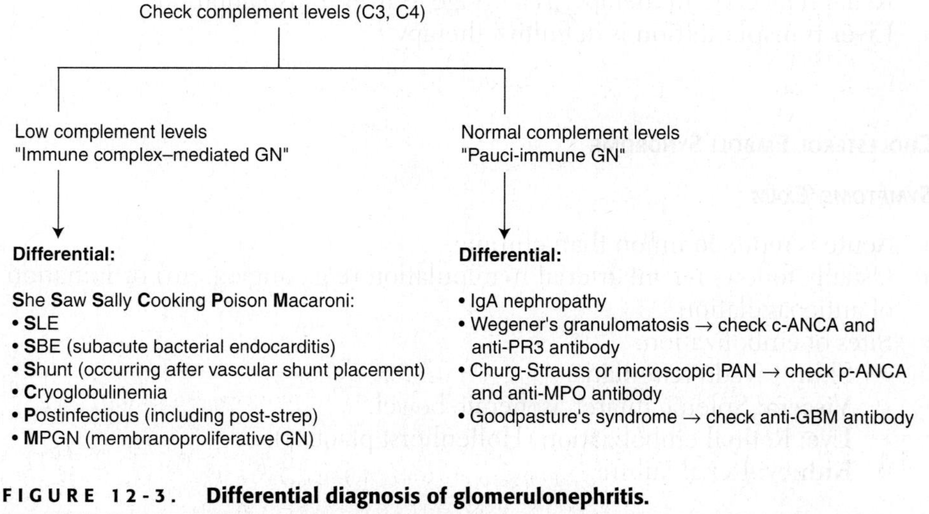

FIGURE 12-3. Differential diagnosis of glomerulonephritis.

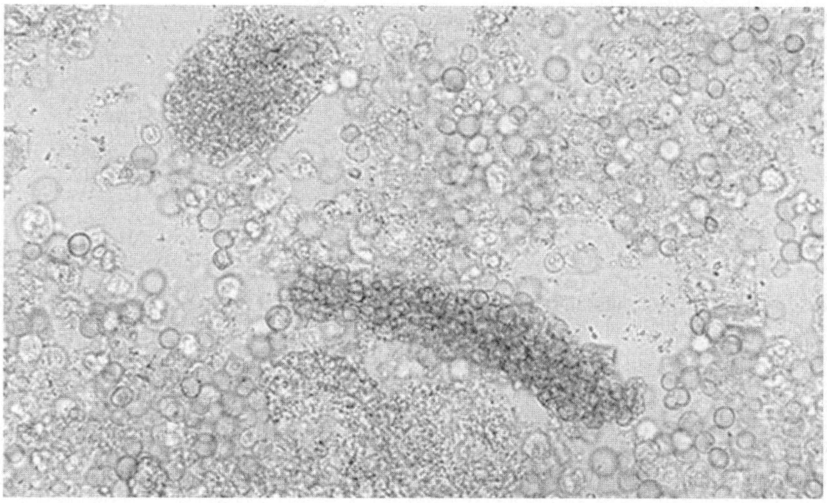

FIGURE 12-4. Red blood cell cast.

(Courtesy of R. Rodriguez.)

TABLE 12-8. Low-Complement Glomerulonephritis

DISEASE	PRESENTATION	DIAGNOSIS	PATHOLOGY	TREATMENT
SLE	Any of the 11 criteria for SLE (see Chapter 17). Lupus nephritis can be the presenting feature.	Anti-dsDNA, anti-Smith antibodies.	See Table 12-9.	See Table 12-9. End-stage renal disease (ESRD) occurs in 8–15% of SLE patients.
Postinfectious	**2–3 weeks after pharyngitis or skin infection.** Classically seen with streptococcal infections, but other infections may trigger GN as well.	**Elevated ASO** and anti-DNase B antibodies (for poststreptococcal GN).	Diffuse proliferative GN. Electron microscopy (EM) shows **subepithelial "humps."**	Renal failure typically resolves in six weeks. Only 5% require dialysis acutely.
Membranoproliferative glomerulonephritis (MPGN)	Cryoglobulin-related MPGN: arthralgias, palpable purpura, history of HCV infection. Microscopic hematuria with mild to heavy proteinuria. May be chronic or rapidly progressive.	Positive cryoglobulins, rheumatoid factor. Check **HBV, HCV,** and HIV serologies.	Hypercellular glomerulus. EM reveals **subendothelial deposits.**	HCV-related disease and cryoglobulinemia → α-interferon and ribavirin.
Endocarditis	Fevers, new heart murmur in patient with predisposition (e.g., abnormal heart valves, recent dental procedure, injection drug abuse, etc.).	Blood cultures, echocardiography.	May have renal impairment due to crescentic GN, cryoglobulinemia, ATN, or AIN.	Antibiotics. General rule: If endocarditis is cured, renal impairment will be cured.

TABLE 12-9. Pathology of Lupus Nephritis

WHO Classification	Pathology	Treatment	Notes
Class I	Normal.	Observe.	< 5% of all biopsies.
Class II	Mesangial.	Observe.	Microscopic hematuria.
Class III	Focal proliferative.	Observe (mild). Pulse steroids and IV cyclophosphamide (severe).	Similar to class IV but milder.
Class IV	Diffuse proliferative.	Pulse steroids and IV cyclophosphamide.	**Most common** at the time of biopsy; most aggressive course if untreated.
Class V	Membranous.	Observe.	Nephrotic syndrome.

Symptoms/Exam

- **Four features comprise nephrotic syndrome:**
  - Anasarca/peripheral edema
  - Hypoalbuminemia (serum albumin < 3 g/dL)
  - Hyperlipidemia
  - Proteinuria > 3.5 g/day
- Additional features include hypercoagulability.

Multiple myeloma may affect the kidney in many ways:

- *Cast nephropathy (most common): due to light chains*
- *Amyloidosis → nephrotic syndrome*
- *Proximal tubule involvement → Fanconi syndrome*
- *Hypercalcemia*
- *Hyperuricemia*
- *Hypovolemia*

Differential

- **Idiopathic or primary nephrotic syndrome:** Four main pathologic subtypes (see Table 12-11).
- **Secondary to systemic disease:** Long list includes malignancy (classically lymphoma or myeloma), infections (HIV, HBV or HCV, syphilis, leprosy, malaria), amyloidosis, and a variety of others. See Table 12-12 for the most common causes.

Diagnosis

As in the Symptoms/Exam section above, plus:

- **UA:** In addition to proteinuria, oval fat bodies or "**Maltese crosses**" may be visualized under polarized light.
- A 24-hour urine protein is the best way to quantify the extent of proteinuria. The spot urine protein-creatinine ratio can approximate 24-hour protein excretion in grams.
- Renal biopsy is definitive.
- Additional labs to search for secondary causes include hemoglobin A_{1c}, SPEP/UPEP, and serologies for HBV, HCV, HIV, and syphilis.

TABLE 12-10. Normal-Complement Glomerulonephritis

Disease	Presentation	Diagnosis	Pathology	Treatment	Clinical Course
IgA nephropathy	More common in Asians and Hispanics. Episodic hematuria with or without proteinuria (usually within 24 hours of URI).	Renal biopsy.	Normal or mesangial expansion. Immunofixation shows diffuse mesangial IgA immune deposits.	All patients: ACEIs. If proteinuria < 3 g/day: **fish oil.** If proteinuria > 3 g/day: steroids.	20% have progressive renal failure in 20 years. 10–20% progress to ESRD in 10 years. Worse prognosis with hypertension, elevated creatinine, or proteinuria.
Wegener's granulomatosis	Upper respiratory tract disease and nodular cutaneous lesions are more common. Rapidly progressive glomerulonephritis (RPGN).	c-ANCA and antiproteinase 3 (PR3) antibody positive. Renal biopsy.	Segmental fibrinoid necrosis. Crescentic formation. Immunofluorescence (IF) negative.	Steroids with PO cyclophosphamide. Plasmapheresis.	Variable course depending on localized indolent vs. systemic fulminant presentation.
Microscopic polyarteritis nodosa (PAN)	Upper respiratory tract disease is less common. RPGN.	p-ANCA and antimyeloperoxidase (MPO) antibody positive. Renal biopsy.	As above.	Steroids with PO cyclophosphamide.	As above.
Churg-Strauss syndrome	Asthma and eosinophilia. Peripheral neuropathy is more common.	p-ANCA and anti-MPO antibody positive. Renal biopsy.	As above.	Steroids with PO cyclophosphamide.	Renal involvement usually mild.
Goodpasture's syndrome	Pulmonary hemorrhage. RPGN.	Anti-GBM antibody positive. Renal biopsy.	Diffuse proliferative GN. Variable necrosis and crescent formation. IF linear deposition IgG along GBM.	Steroids with PO cyclophosphamide. Plasmapheresis.	RPGN is associated with poor renal survival.

TREATMENT

- **General measures:**
  - Control peripheral edema with loop diuretics.
  - Maintain good nutrition.
  - ACEIs to slow proteinuria.
  - Lipid lowering—generally target LDL < 100.
- **Treat the underlying disease.**

The five causes of large kidneys on ultrasound:

- *Diabetes*
- *HIV-associated nephropathy*
- *Amyloidosis*
- *Lymphoma*
- *Polycystic kidney disease*

SECONDARY HYPERTENSION

Comprises 5% of cases of hypertension.

SYMPTOMS/EXAM

Suspect secondary hypertension if:

- Age at onset of hypertension is < 30.
- Age at onset of hypertension is > 50.
- Rapid onset of severe hypertension in < 3–5 years.
- Hypertension is refractory to multiple medications.
- Hypokalemia.

DIFFERENTIAL

- **Renal:** Renovascular disease, renal parenchymal disease, polycystic kidney disease, Liddle's syndrome, syndrome of apparent mineralocorticoid excess, hypercalcemia.
- **Endocrine:** Hyper- or hypothyroidism, primary hyperaldosteronism, Cushing's syndrome, pheochromocytoma, congenital adrenal hyperplasia (see also Chapter 6).
- **Drugs:**
  - **Prescription:** Estrogen, cyclosporin A, steroids.
  - **OTC:** Pseudoephedrine, NSAIDs.
  - **Illicit:** Smoking, ethanol, cocaine.
- **Neurogenic:** Increased ICP, spinal cord section.
- **Miscellaneous:** Aortic coarctation, obstructive sleep apnea, polycythemia vera.

DIAGNOSIS

- **History, physical exam.**
- Medication review.
- Electrolytes and renal labs (see Table 12-13).

TREATMENT

- **Hypertensive emergency:** See Chapter 3.
- If possible, correct the underlying disorder:
  - **Renal:** See below.
  - **Endocrine:** See Chapter 6.
  - **Drugs:** Stop ingestion.
- **Antihypertensive medications:** See Chapter 2.

Renovascular Hypertension

Diminished renal blood flow causes elevated renin and aldosterone levels, which eventually results in hypertension (see Table 12-14).

TABLE 12-11. Primary Causes of Nephrotic Syndrome

DISEASE	PRESENTATION	PATHOLOGY	TREATMENT	CLINICAL COURSE
Minimal change disease	Sudden onset with heavy proteinuria. More common in **children.**	Normal light microscopy. EM shows epithelial foot process fusion.	Steroids.	Responds to steroids but often relapses. **Renal failure is uncommon.**
Focal segmental glomerulosclerosis	Increased frequency in **African-Americans.**	Focal segmental glomerulosclerosis.	Steroids, cyclosporin A; cyclophosphamide.	Higher frequency of ESRD compared to minimal change disease.
Membranous nephropathy	Increased frequency in **Caucasians.** Proteinuria with microhematuria. **Predilection to clotting:** renal vein thrombosis.	Thickened capillary loops with **subepithelial "spikes."** EM shows subepithelial deposits.	Observation if slow progression. Steroids alternating with either cyclophosphamide or chlorambucil.	25% spontaneously remit. Slow progression to renal failure.
MPGN	Can present with either nephritic or nephrotic features.	Hypercellular glomerulus with lobular architecture. EM shows **subendothelial deposits.**	Non-nephrotic: observe. Nephrotic or worsening renal function: steroids.	50% die or progress to ESRD within five years of renal biopsy.

SYMPTOMS/EXAM

- Age at onset of hypertension is < 30 or > 50 years.
- Rapid onset of hypertension in < 3–5 years.
- Severe hypertension despite an appropriate three-drug regimen.
- Flash pulmonary edema.
- Hypokalemia.
- **Serum creatinine increases after initiation of ACEI treatment.**

DIAGNOSIS

Imaging (duplex ultrasonography, MRA, CT angiography, angiography) reveals > 75% stenosis. Sensitivity and specificity are operator dependent.

TREATMENT

- **Medical therapy:** If BP control is adequate, it is **not** necessary to proceed with a revascularization procedure.
- Percutaneous transluminal angioplasty (PTA): Effective for fibromuscular dysplasia.

TABLE 12-12. Secondary Causes of Nephrotic Syndrome

DISEASE	PRESENTATION	PATHOLOGY	TREATMENT	CLINICAL COURSE	NOTES
HIV-associated nephropathy	High viral load. Low CD4 count. Nephrotic-range proteinuria. No peripheral edema.	Focal segmental glomerulosclerosis. Large dilated microcysts. Interstitial inflammatory infiltrate.	Initiation of HAART. Steroids if there is evidence of interstitial nephritis.	If untreated, may progress to ESRD within a few months. ESRD patients have been known to come off dialysis with the initiation of HAART.	Most common in African-Americans and Hispanics. **Kidneys are large and echogenic on renal ultrasound.**
Diabetic nephropathy	Onset 5–10 years after diagnosis in type 1 DM; more variable in type 2.	Mesangial expansion. Kimmelstiel-Wilson nodule. Tubulointerstitial fibrosis.	Glycemic control. Target LDL < 100. Target BP < 130/80.	Progresses from hyperfiltration to microalbuminuria to nephrotic to ESRD.	**Leading cause of ESRD in the United States.** **ACEIs** are first-line agents for type 1 DM. **ACEIs or ARBs** are first-line agents for type 2 DM.
Multiple myeloma (light chain deposition disease)	More severe renal failure with cast nephropathy.	$\kappa > \lambda$ light chain involvement. Glomerular or tubulointerstitial **Congo-red stain** (–) deposits.	Melphalan and prednisone. Plasma exchange if light chains in serum.	Mean survival is 44 months if no cast nephropathy.	**Monoclonal gammopathy on on SPEP/UPEP.** **Light chains will not be detected by urine dipstick for protein.**
AL amyloidosis	25% with overt multiple myeloma. More severe proteinuria. Less ARF.	$\lambda > \kappa$ light chain involvement. Glomerular or tubulointerstitial deposition **Congo-red stain** (+) deposits.	Melphalan and prednisone.	Mean survival 4–13 months.	

- **PTA/stent:** May be effective for atherosclerotic patients.
- **Surgical intervention:** Benefit is unclear.

CHRONIC KIDNEY DISEASE (CKD)

CKD is defined as permanent loss of renal function of > 3 months' duration. **ESRD** is defined as permanent loss of renal function that requires renal replacement therapy; GFR < 10 cc/min.

TABLE 12-13. Laboratory Tests for Evaluation of Hypertension

Basic tests for initial evaluation:

1. Always included:
   a. Urine for protein, blood, and glucose
   b. Microscopic UA
   c. Hematocrit
   d. Serum potassium
   e. Serum creatinine and/or BUN
   f. Fasting glucose
   g. Total cholesterol
2. Usually included, depending on cost and other factors:
   a. TSH
   b. WBC count
   c. HDL and LDL cholesterol and triglycerides
   d. Serum calcium and phosphate
   e. CXR; limited echocardiogram

Special studies to screen for secondary hypertension:

1. Renovascular disease: ACEI radionuclide scan, renal duplex Doppler flow studies, and MRI angiography.
2. Pheochromocytoma: 24-hour urine assay for creatinine, metanephrines, and catecholamines.
3. Cushing's syndrome: overnight dexamethasone suppression test or 24-hour urine cortisol and creatinine.
4. Primary aldosteronism: plasma aldosterone:renin activity ratio.

Adapted, with permission, from Fisher ND, Williams GL. Hypertensive vascular disease. In Kasper DL et al (eds). *Harrison's Principles of Internal Medicine,* 16th ed. New York: McGraw-Hill, 2005:1469.).

TREATMENT

The treatment of risk factors associated with the progression of renal disease is as follows:

- Proteinuria:
  - The most important predictor of progression of renal disease.
  - **ACEIs/ARBs are beneficial for diabetic** and nondiabetic nephropathies.

TABLE 12-14. Causes of Renovascular Hypertension

	ATHEROSCLEROSIS (MORE COMMON)	FIBROMUSCULAR DYSPLASIA
Affected gender	Men and women	Women
Age	> 50	15–40
Total occlusion	Common	Rare
Ischemic atrophy	Common	Rare
Angioplasty	Less amenable	Very amenable
Cure rate	Poor	Good

- **Hypertension:**
  - Target BP < 130/80.
  - **First-line agents: ACEIs.**
  - **Second-line agents: Diuretics** are effective in BP control owing to increased Na^+ retention in CKD patients.
- **Lipids:** Target LDL < 100.
- Smoking cessation.
- **Nutrition:** Protein restriction is controversial.

COMPLICATIONS

Complications from CKD/ESRD should be managed as follows:

- **Anemia:**
  - Erythropoietin (EPO) injections if hematocrit < 33%.
  - Replete iron stores if ferritin < 100 ng/mL or transferrin saturation (T_{sat}) < 20% (can use IV iron in hemodialysis patients).
- **Renal osteodystrophy** (see Figure 12-5):
  - Control phosphate with calcium-based phosphate binder ($CaCO_3$ or calcium acetate) when:
    - GFR < 60 mL/min and serum phosphorus > 4.6 mg/dL, or
    - ESRD and serum phosphorus > 5.5 mg/dL.
  - Control PTH with 1,25-OH vitamin D (calcitriol) when:
    - GFR < 60 mL/min and serum PTH > 70 pmol/L, or
    - ESRD and serum PTH > 300 pmol/L.
- **Hyperkalemia:** Dietary restriction, diuretics.
- **Acidosis:**
  - $NaHCO_3$ supplementation to prevent negative bone balance.
  - Titrate therapy by measuring 24-hour urine for citrate.
- **Pericarditis:** Initiate dialysis or increase dialysis dose.
- **Dialysis-related problems:**
  - **Vascular catheter–related infections:**
    - *S. aureus* is the most likely cause, followed by coagulase-negative staphylococcus.
    - Empiric treatment with first-generation cephalosporin (IV); add vancomycin if there is a high local prevalence of methicillin-resistant *S. aureus* (MRSA).
    - The definitive treatment should be tailored to the results of blood cultures drawn through a catheter and from a peripheral site.
    - Remove the catheter in the presence of a fungal infection, sepsis, endocarditis, or persistent bacteremia.
  - **Peritoneal catheter–associated peritonitis:**
    - *S. aureus*, *S. epidermidis*, and enteric gram-negative rods are the dominant organisms.
    - The first clues are a cloudy appearance to peritoneal fluid, fever, or abdominal pain.
    - Diagnose with Gram stain and culture of peritoneal fluid.
    - Can often be treated with infusion of antibiotics into the peritoneum. For severe cases, add IV antibiotics and possibly catheter removal.
    - If peritoneal fluid WBC count > 100 WBC/mm^3 or there is persistent infection after 96 hours of proper treatment, consider catheter removal.
    - If peritoneal culture grows fungus, anaerobes, or multiple organisms, suspect secondary peritonitis due to a perforated abdominal viscus.
  - **AV fistula (AVF) thrombosis:**

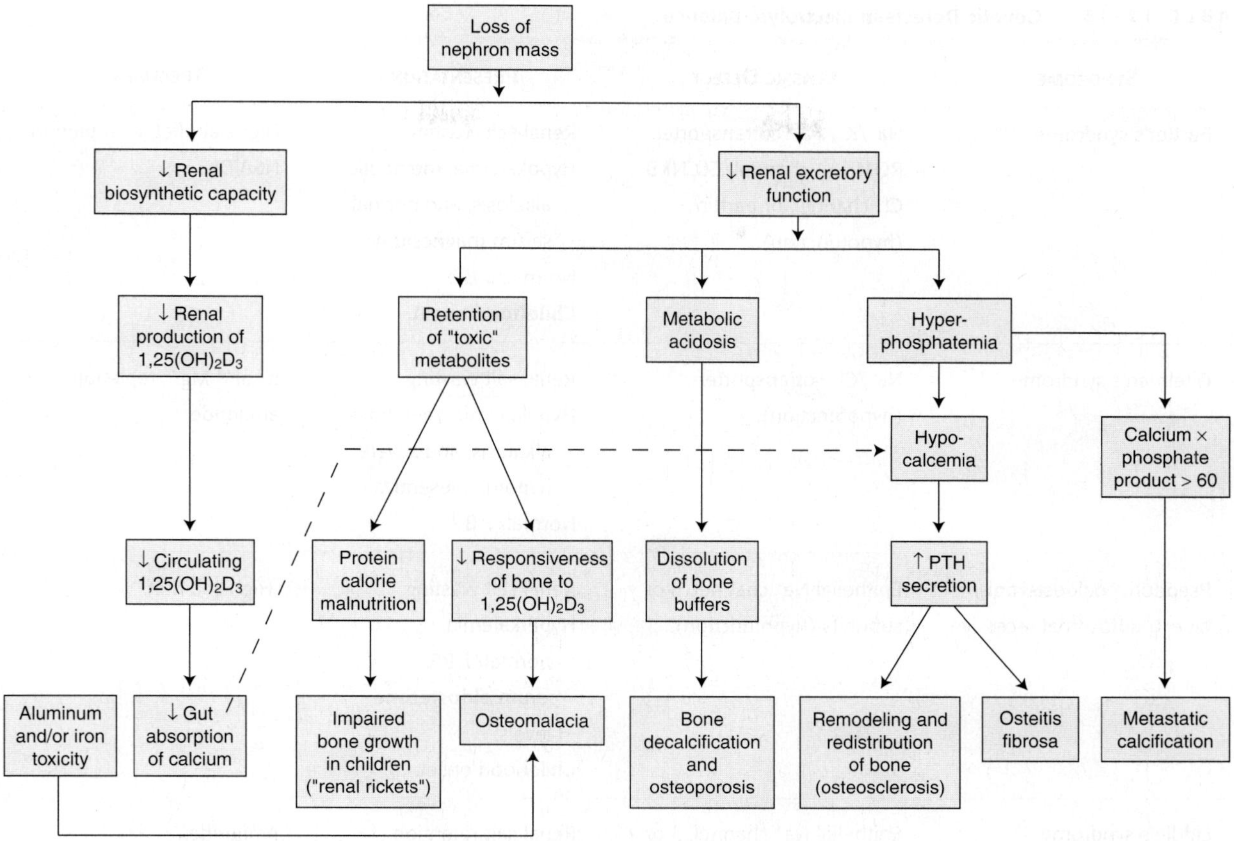

FIGURE 12-5. Pathogenesis of bone disease in chronic kidney disease.

(Reproduced, with permission, from Brenner BM, Lazarus JM. Chronic renal failure. In Wilson JD et al [eds]. *Harrison's Principles of Internal Medicine,* 12th ed. New York: McGraw-Hill, 1991.)

- Suspect if there is no palpable thrill or loss of audible bruit over the AVF site.
- Suspect if high venous access pressures are seen on dialysis or if the dialysis dose is inadequate owing to high recirculation.
- Diagnose with ultrasound or fistulogram.
- Treatment options are intravascular clot removal or thrombolytics.

GENETIC DISORDERS AND CONGENITAL DISEASES OF THE KIDNEY

Table 12-15 outlines genetic defects related to electrolyte balance. Table 12-16 presents the relationship of various genetic disorders to congenital diseases.

TABLE 12-15. Genetic Defects in Electrolyte Balance

Syndrome	Classic Defect	Presentation	Treatment
Bartter's syndrome	$Na^+/K^+/2Cl^-$ cotransporter, ROMK K^+ channel, CLCNKB Cl^- channel, or barttin (hypofunction).	Renal salt wasting. Hypokalemia, metabolic alkalosis, and normal serum magnesium. Normal/↓ BP. **Childhood onset.**	High-salt diet, K^+ repletion, NSAIDs.
Gitelman's syndrome	Na^+/Cl^- cotransporter (hypofunction).	Renal salt wasting. Hypokalemia, metabolic alkalosis, and severe hypomagnesemia. Normal/↓ BP.	K^+ and Mg^{2+} repletion, amiloride.
Pseudohypoaldosteronism, type 1, autosomal recessive	Epithelial Na^+ channel, β or γ subunits (hypofunction).	Renal salt wasting. Hyperkalemia, normal/↓ BP. ↑ serum **aldosterone** levels. Childhood onset.	High-salt diet.
Liddle's syndrome	Epithelial Na^+ channel, β or γ subunits (hyperfunction).	Renal salt retention. Hypokalemia, metabolic alkalosis, **hypertension.** ↓ serum aldosterone levels.	Amiloride.
Syndrome of apparent mineralocorticoid excess	11β-hydroxysteroid dehydrogenase 2 (failure to inactivate cortisol).	Renal salt retention. Hypokalemia, metabolic alkalosis, **hypertension.** ↓ serum aldosterone levels.	Spironolactone, K^+-sparing diuretics, dexamethasone.

TABLE 12-16. Genetic Disorders and Congenital Diseases of the Kidney

DISEASE	DEFECT	PRESENTATION	DIAGNOSIS	NOTES
Alport's syndrome	Type IV collagen of the GBM, cochlea, and lens.	**Hematuria:** affects males and female carriers of X-linked Alport's syndrome; can worsen after URI. **ESRD:** affects all males with X-linked Alport's syndrome; female carriers of X-linked Alport's syndrome do not have significant renal disease. **Sensorineural deafness.** **Ocular defects.**	Renal biopsy showing thickened GBM with splitting and splintering of the lamina densa on EM.	Renal transplantation. Reports of de novo Goodpasture's syndrome after renal transplantation due to exposure of type IV collagen from the allograft to the Alport's syndrome recipient.
Autosomal dominant polycystic kidney disease (ADPKD)	*PKD1* or polycystin-1; *PKD2* or polycystin-2.	Kidney enlargement due to multiple cyst formation. Hypertension. Mitral valve prolapse. Polycystic liver disease. Intracranial aneurysms (familial clustering).	Family history of ADPKD. Renal ultrasound showing: ▪ Two cysts with age < 30 years. ▪ Two cysts in each kidney with age > 30–59 years. ▪ Four cysts in each kidney with age > 60 years.	ACEIs or ARBs blockers for hypertension. Renal transplantation for ESRD.
Medullary sponge kidney	Developmental abnormality characterized by dilated medullary and papillary collecting ducts, leading to a "spongy-looking" medulla.	Patients can be asymptomatic. Hematuria. Calcium oxalate or phosphate nephrolithiasis.	Intravenous pyelogram. Retention of contrast media in the collecting ducts of the medulla, leading to "bouquet of flowers" appearance.	Benign clinical course.
Thin basement membrane disease	Unclear.	Microhematuria. Proteinuria is rare.	Thin GBM on renal biopsy.	Benign clinical course, but there is a small risk for progression to chronic kidney disease.

TABLE 12-16. Genetic Disorders and Congenital Diseases of the Kidney (continued)

Disease	Defect	Presentation	Diagnosis	Notes
Cystinuria: the classic aminoaciduria	rBAT/$b^{0,+}$AT transporter, leading to incomplete reabsorption of dibasic amino acids (**C**ystine, **O**rnithine, **L**ysine, and **A**rginine—**"COLA"**) in the proximal tubule of the nephron.	Cystine nephrolithiasis (cystine calculi are radiopaque on plain films).	24-hour urine collection for cystine and dibasic amino acids.	Decrease urine cystine concentration < 300 mg/L. Increase fluid intake. Tiopronin (forms a more soluble form of cystine through a mixed disulfide thiol-cystine complex).
Fabry's disease	α-galactosidase A (αGalA gene) leads to intracellular accumulation of neutral glycosphingolipids with terminal-linked galactosyl moieties.	**Abnormal glycosphingolipid accumulation.** ■ **Renal:** moderate proteinuria by age 30, occasional microhematuria, gradual progression to ESRD. ■ **Cardiovascular:** CAD, CHF, arrhythmias. ■ **Autonomic dysfunction:** hypohidrosis, acral paresthesias, altered intestinal mobility. ■ **Dermatologic:** angiokeratomas.	Reduced αGalA levels in serum or urine. Renal biopsy: glomeruli packed with clear vacuoles filled with glycosphingolipid deposits (myelin figures and zebra bodies).	Agalsidase β (Fabrazyme), renal transplantation.

CHAPTER 13

Neurology

Joey English, MD, PhD
Michael Rafii, MD, PhD

NEUROLOGIC HISTORY AND EXAM

Basic Exam

The most important part of the workup of any neurologic disorder—and a critical part of any attempt to localize a lesion—is the history and physical exam. The history should focus on the following factors:

- Symptom onset:
  - Acute onset (seconds to minutes): Most likely caused by a **vascular event** (e.g., stroke), a **seizure,** or a complicated **migraine.**
  - Subacute onset (hours to days): More likely caused by **infectious processes, inflammatory diseases,** or **autoimmune disorders** (e.g., MS).
  - Insidious onset (months to years): More likely caused by slowly growing **structural lesions** (e.g., tumors) or **neurodegenerative disorders.**
- Age/gender: In young patients, especially women, consider **autoimmune processes** high on the differential.
- **Location of symptoms:** Classic symptoms of common neurologic disease processes by location are as follows:
  - **Myopathies (muscle): Symmetric proximal weakness** of all extremities.
  - **Neuromuscular junction: Rapidly fluctuating weakness** (eyes, proximal extremities).
  - Polyneuropathy: **Symmetric distal sensory loss** and **weakness of all extremities.**
  - Myelopathy (spinal cord): **Symmetric weakness** of **both legs** and of **bowel and bladder.**
  - **Brain stem: Cranial nerve deficits, double vision.**

Coma Exam

Coma refers to a condition in which patients are unresponsive, show no purposeful movement, and do not open their eyes to painful stimuli. It requires the impairment of either **both cerebral hemispheres** or the reticular activating system of the **brain stem.**

- Generally caused by one of three processes:
  - A **structural** problem affecting the **brain stem** (e.g., mass effect, herniation).
  - An **electrical** problem (ongoing seizure activity not clinically apparent—e.g., nonconvulsive status epilepticus).
  - A **metabolic** process (e.g., anoxic brain injury, hepatic encephalopathy, infection).
- Exam:
  - Evaluate brain stem function by reviewing cranial nerve reflexes—i.e., pupillary response to light; oculovestibular responses of the eyes to either turning the head side to side or placing cold water in one ear (should not be done if the status of cervical spine stability is unknown); corneal reflexes; gag reflex; cough reflex.
  - Motor response to central and peripheral pain is also critical, as asymmetric responses suggest a focal intracranial lesion.
  - Patients with coma caused by a structural problem generally have **abnormal brain stem reflexes,** as their coma is caused by direct compression of the brain stem.
  - Patients with metabolic or electrical coma typically have intact brain stem reflexes.

- **Diagnosis/Treatment:**
  - Focus on correctable problems, including easily detectable metabolic disorders (e.g., hypoglycemia, drug overdose, electrolyte abnormalities, uremia, liver failure) and structural problems (e.g., subdural hematoma). Patients need urgent imaging of the brain as well as basic laboratory workup.
  - Patients with unexplained coma should also have an EEG to rule out nonconvulsive status epilepticus as well as CSF studies to rule out infectious causes of encephalopathy.

NEURODIAGNOSTIC TESTING

Lumbar Puncture (LP)

Used for the measurement of CSF pressure, for CSF analysis, and occasionally for therapeutic removal of CSF.

- Most often performed in the L3 and L4 interspaces (at the level of the superior iliac crests). The needle is advanced to the subarachnoid space.
- Opening pressure should be measured but is valid only when obtained with the patient in the lateral decubitus position (i.e., spinal needle located at the same level as the heart).
- Patients with papilledema or focal neurologic signs should have imaging prior to LP to evaluate for mass effect and risk of herniation. Imaging of the spine should precede LP for patients with spinal cord signs or symptoms.

Electroencephalography (EEG)

A tool for the investigation of seizure disorders, unexplained coma, metabolic encephalopathies, viral encephalitis, prion diseases, anoxic brain injury, and sleep disorders. Conditions with notable EEG findings include the following:

- **Metabolic encephalopathy:** Hepatic encephalopathy is the classic metabolic coma. EEG typically shows generalized periodic triphasic waves.
- **Viral encephalitis:**
  - **HSV encephalitis:** The classic EEG finding consists of periodic lateralizing epileptiform discharges (PLEDs) originating over one or both temporal lobes.
  - **Subacute sclerosing panencephalitis (SSPE):** EEG typically shows a flat background punctuated by periodic generalized large-amplitude slow-wave discharges.
- **Prion disease:** EEGs in patients with Creutzfeldt-Jakob disease show generalized sharp waves occurring at a frequency of 1 Hz.

Computed Tomography (CT)

CT imaging of the brain is inferior to MRI for most studies but is the imaging study of choice for investigating **acute hemorrhage** (e.g., SAH, epidural hematoma) and **bone pathology** (e.g., skull or vertebral fractures).

Magnetic Resonance Imaging (MRI)

The best imaging modality for most diseases of the brain and spinal cord, including neoplastic, vascular (except acute hemorrhage), demyelinating, infectious, and structural diseases (e.g., spondylosis of the spine).

Cerebral Angiography

The gold standard for investigating vascular abnormalities of the CNS, including stenosis, aneurysms, AVMs, and cerebral vasculitis. Also useful for preoperative evaluation of vascular supply to intracranial tumors (e.g., meningiomas). Cerebral **venography** is the gold standard for diagnosing venous sinus thrombosis.

Electromyography/Nerve Conduction Studies (EMG/NCS)

EMGs examine spontaneous and voluntary muscle activity by using a needle electrode placed directly into the muscle. They are useful for studying radiculopathies (spinal root injuries), motor neuron disease, neuropathies, neuromuscular junction diseases, and myopathies. NCSs are obtained by stimulating peripheral nerves and recording either sensory or motor responses along the course of the nerve.

Evoked Potentials (EPs)

Obtained by measuring the time course of a specific CNS response to a given stimulus.

- **Visual EPs** are generated by recording cortical response (using EEG electrodes) elicited by a monocular visual stimulus. A delay in response suggests that the conduction velocity along the visual pathway is low, a sign of demyelination (e.g., in **MS**).
- **Brain stem and sensory EPs** are useful for evaluating potential demyelinating lesions of the brain stem and dorsal columns of the spinal cord. Often used to obtain supportive evidence of CNS demyelination.
- **Sensory and motor EPs** are used for intraoperative monitoring during neurosurgical procedures involving the spinal cord or brain stem.

EPs are often used in patients with contraindications to MRI such as pacemakers and implanted defibrillators.

HEADACHE

All patients presenting with headache merit a detailed history and neurologic evaluation, including funduscopic evaluation for papilledema. The following findings in patients with headache should prompt further investigation (e.g., imaging, basic labs, LP):

- **Symptoms:** Abrupt-onset severe headache; progressive persistent headache; visual complaints; fever; jaw claudication; exacerbation of headache by maneuvers that increase ICP (e.g., Valsalva, cough); onset of headaches after age 40–50; awakening from sleep with headache.
- **Exam:** Focal neurologic deficits, papilledema, meningeal signs, scalp tenderness.
- Diseases to remember when evaluating a patient with headache include SAH, temporal arteritis, venous sinus thrombosis, pseudotumor cerebri (intracranial hypertension), intracranial hypotension, meningitis/encephalitis, and brain tumor.

Migraine Headache

Roughly 10–20% of the U.S. population have experienced migraine headaches, with 80% beginning before age 30. Most patients are **young**

women (the female-to-male ratio is 3:1). Ninety percent of patients have a strong family history.

Symptoms

- **Benign, recurrent headaches** that classically produce **unilateral pulsating pain** associated with symptoms such as **photophobia,** phonophobia, anorexia, **nausea,** and vomiting.
- Episodes typically last 4–72 hours, and patients often report improvement with resting in a **dark, quiet room.**
- Subtypes are as follows:
  - **Classic migraine (migraine with aura)**: Occurs in 20% of patients. The most common auras are **visual sensations,** including "fortification spectra" and scotoma (blind spots).
  - **Common migraine:** Most migraine patients do not have preceding auras.
  - **Migraine variants:** Named for associated focal neurologic deficits and/or vascular territories; include hemiplegic migraine, basilar migraine (brain stem symptoms such as ataxia, vertigo, and slurred speech), and ophthalmoplegic migraine (unilateral CN III palsy and pupillary abnormality).

Exam

- Patients with classic and common migraines have **normal neurologic exams.**
- In patients with headache and focal neurologic deficits, a migraine variant remains a diagnosis of exclusion. These patients require workup for other causes of headache and focal deficits (e.g., vascular event, infection, intracranial mass).

Tension headache is usually a nonthrobbing, bilateral occipital head pain that is not usually associated with nausea, vomiting, or prodromal visual disturbances.

Differential

Other headache syndromes, including tension and cluster headache.

Diagnosis

Based on history, with a focus on the exact character of the headaches as well as the presence of a strong family history.

Treatment

Management is divided into two categories: **abortive therapy** for the migraine itself (taken only at the time of migraine) and **prophylactic therapy** for preventing future attacks (taken daily). Prophylactic therapy is given only to patients with frequent severe migraines and includes **TCAs** (e.g., amitriptyline), β-blockers (e.g., propranolol), calcium channel blockers (e.g., verapamil), and **antiseizure medications** (e.g., valproic acid, topiramate). **Abortive therapy** includes the following:

- **Vasoconstrictors:**
  - **Triptans:** 5-HT_1 serotonin receptor agonists (e.g., sumatriptan, frovatriptan, eletriptan, naratriptan, almotriptan, rizatriptan, zolmitriptan) produce vasoconstriction. **Do not** use in patients with vascular disease (e.g., CAD, peripheral vascular disease) or in pregnant women.
  - **Ergotamines:** Also to be avoided in patients with vascular disease and in pregnant women.

- Others:
  - **Acetaminophen/butalbital/caffeine** (Fioricet). Butalbital is a barbiturate and has addictive properties.
  - **Isometheptene/dichloralphenazone/acetaminophen** (Midrin). Avoid in patients taking MAOIs.
  - **Antiemetics:** Prochlorperazine, promethazine.

Cluster Headache

Classically occur in **young men** 20–40 years of age (the male-to-female ratio is 5:1). A family history of similar headaches is uncommon.

Symptoms

- The cardinal feature is **periodicity.** Headaches occur **2–3 times daily** at **distinct times** over several weeks; onset with **sleep** is especially characteristic.
- Clusters spontaneously remit for months to years before recurring, typically at the same time of year as previous attacks. **Alcohol** is a classic trigger.
- Cluster headaches do not have auras (vs. migraines). A typical attack is characterized by abrupt-onset, severe **unilateral "icepick-like" periorbital pain** with associated **ipsilateral autonomic symptoms** (tearing of the eye and nares; rarely Horner's). Typically last 30–120 minutes.

Exam

- Patients are restless and agitated, often pacing the room (vs. migraine patients).
- Look for tearing, nasal discharge, and/or ptosis (e.g., **Horner's**) ipsilateral to the location of eye pain.

Differential

Other headache syndromes, including migraine (see Table 13-1) and **paroxysmal hemicrania** (similar symptoms, but with multiple (20–40) daily attacks lasting 5–10 minutes each and no periodicity; exquisitely sensitive to **indomethacin**).

TABLE 13-1. Cluster Headache vs. Migraine

	MIGRAINE	CLUSTER HEADACHE
Typical patient	Young woman	Young man
Triggered by alcohol	No	Yes
Periodicity	No	Yes
Aura	Yes (with classic form)	No
Autonomic symptoms	No	Yes
Response to O_2	No	Yes

TREATMENT

As with migraines, treatment includes abortive and prophylactic therapies. **Prophylactic** medications are started once cluster headaches begin but are not used during remissions given that months to years may pass between clusters. They include **verapamil** (first-line prophylactic treatment for cluster headache), **prednisone** (a taper of oral steroids is often used at the beginning of a cluster), lithium, valproate, and methysergide. **Abortive therapy** includes the following:

- **O_2 inhalation:** The **most effective abortive treatment** (5–10 L/min for 10–15 minutes).
- **Intranasal lidocaine ointment:** Produces a block of the sphenopalatine ganglion and aborts the headache.
- **Triptans:** Also useful for acute attacks.

Trigeminal Neuralgia (Tic Douloureux)

A **unilateral** facial pain syndrome affecting middle-aged and elderly patients. Most commonly occurs in the sixth decade. Onset in young patients should raise suspicion for an underlying disorder (e.g., MS, brain stem neoplasm).

SYMPTOMS

Characterized by abrupt-onset, short-duration (seconds) episodes of severe **unilateral lancinating electrical pain,** typically **radiating along the jaw** in the distribution of the second and third divisions of CN V_2 and V_3 (trigeminal nerve). Attacks are often **triggered by sensory stimuli** to the face (e.g., touch, wind, shaving, chewing).

EXAM

Neurologic exam is **normal.** Any abnormalities on exam, including sensory loss of the face in the distribution of the pain, suggests an alternative diagnosis and mandates further evaluation (e.g., imaging, LP).

DIFFERENTIAL

Cluster headache, paroxysmal hemicrania, dental abscess, internal jugular thrombophlebitis. Distinguishable by history and physical.

TREATMENT

Carbamazepine is first-line therapy. Alternatives include valproate, phenytoin, baclofen, gabapentin, and benzodiazepines.

Benign Intracranial Hypertension (Pseudotumor Cerebri)

A headache syndrome related to chronically elevated ICP. Classically seen in **young, obese women.** Associations have been noted with medications such as tetracycline derivatives and vitamin A as well as with diseases such as SLE, Behçet's disease, and uremia.

SYMPTOMS

- Patients usually note a progressive **global headache** that worsens when they lie flat, often worsening at night and **upon awakening.**
- Exacerbated by maneuvers that elevate ICP (e.g., Valsalva, cough, sneeze).

- Elevated ICP can produce **transient visual obscurations** (blurring or blackout of vision in either or both eyes for seconds); double vision from CN VI palsies; and/or progressive loss of peripheral vision. Total blindness can result.

EXAM

Papilledema is the key finding. Patients may also have decreased visual acuity and/or **loss of peripheral vision.** CN VI palsies may result from elevated ICP.

DIFFERENTIAL

Intracranial mass, venous sinus thrombosis, migraine variant (see Table 13-2).

DIAGNOSIS

- Patients with headache and papilledema should first undergo **brain imaging,** preferably with MRI. In patients with pseudotumor, MRI is normal, including ventricular size.
- **MR venography** to examine for venous sinus thrombosis.
- **LP** should be performed with the patient in the lateral decubitus position, with pressure measured after the patient's legs are extended and relaxed. LP reveals an **opening pressure > 250 mm H_2O,** normal protein and glucose, and no cells.

TREATMENT

Based on lowering ICP. **Acetazolamide,** a carbonic anhydrase inhibitor that reduces CSF production and ICP, is first-line therapy. Lasix can also be used. Serial LPs and permanent shunting of CSF are used for refractory cases. **Weight loss** is an important component of management in most patients. Serial **ophthalmology** evaluation is mandatory for these patients, as visual loss can be severe and permanent.

Medication Rebound Headache

Overuse of analgesic medications for headache syndromes (e.g., narcotics, triptans, ergotamines, barbiturates) can paradoxically produce refractory chronic daily headaches. Prophylactic medications are ineffective until pa-

TABLE 13-2. Classic Case Presentations of the Various Headache Syndromes

- **Migraine:** A 25-year-old woman resting uncomfortably in a dark, quiet room complains of unilateral head pain associated with nausea and photophobia; the headache was preceded by an aura of flashing colored lights.
- **Cluster headache:** A 32-year-old man pacing the ER has severe unilateral periorbital pain associated with tearing of the ipsilateral eye and nose. He has had three attacks per day over the past week, occurring at the exact same time every day and lasting 20–40 minutes each. The headache began after he drank alcohol at a party.
- **Trigeminal neuralgia:** A 58-year-old woman presents with attacks of brief, unilateral, severe electrical sensations radiating along the jaw.
- **Pseudotumor cerebri:** A 22-year-old obese woman presents with a two-month history of progressive headaches that were initially associated with intermittent blurry vision but are now accompanied by a progressive decrease in visual acuity.

tients have been weaned off the offending analgesic medications; often requires a slow taper of the analgesic to prevent withdrawal symptoms.

CEREBROVASCULAR DISEASE

Approximately 75% of strokes are ischemic (due to occlusion of arterial flow), with the remaining 25% caused by hemorrhage either in or around the brain (due to rupture of cerebral arteries or veins).

- A **stroke** is characterized by acute-onset focal neurologic deficits due to disruption of blood flow (either by occlusion or rupture) to a given area of the brain. By traditional definition, the neurologic deficits last > 24 hours. The residual deficit is related to underlying infarction of the brain.
- A **transient ischemic attack (TIA)** is fundamentally similar to stroke, but by traditional definition the deficits resolve within 24 hours. (In the overwhelming majority of TIAs, the deficits actually resolve in < 1 hour.) In TIAs, a region of brain is briefly ischemic, but flow is restored before permanent infarction occurs.

The nature of the focal neurologic deficits caused by strokes depends on the vascular territory involved and the region of brain supplied. Such deficits can first be divided into either anterior circulation or posterior circulation symptoms.

- **Anterior circulation:** Arise from the **internal carotid artery (ICA)** and include the **ophthalmic artery**, the **anterior cerebral artery (ACA)**, and the **middle cerebral artery (MCA)** (see Table 13-3).
- **Posterior circulation** (see Table 13-4):
  - Arise from **both vertebral arteries** as they travel up along the upper cervical spinal cord and fuse to form the **basilar artery.** The basilar artery travels along the brain stem, ultimately dividing into the **two posterior cerebral arteries (PCAs)** that supply the occipital lobes.
  - Three large pairs of arteries come off the vertebrobasilar system to supply the cerebellum: the **anterior inferior cerebellar arteries (AICA), posterior inferior cerebellar arteries (PICA),** and **superior cerebellar arteries (SCA).** Small perforating arterioles coming directly off the basilar artery provide vital supply to the brain stem.

Ischemic Stroke

Caused by occlusion of arterial blood flow to the brain, which in turn is caused by either **extracranial embolism** of clot to the large intracranial vessels or **progressive thrombosis** of small intracranial arterioles. Fairly easy to differentiate using imaging techniques such as MRI.

TABLE 13-3. Strokes Affecting the Anterior Circulation

AREA AFFECTED	SIGNS/SYMPTOMS
Ophthalmic artery	Ipsilateral monocular vision loss (amaurosis fugax).
ACA	Contralateral leg weakness.
MCA	Dominant hemisphere: aphasia, contralateral face/arm weakness. Nondominant hemisphere: contralateral face/arm weakness.

TABLE 13-4. Strokes Affecting the Posterior Circulation

AREA AFFECTED	SIGNS/SYMPTOMS
PCA	Contralateral visual field deficits (homonymous hemianopsia).
Cerebellum	Vertigo, nystagmus, nausea, vomiting, ipsilateral incoordination.
Brain stem	Double vision, vertigo, nausea, vomiting.

EMBOLIC STROKE

Occurs when an extracranial thrombus dislodges and embolizes to and occludes one of the large intracranial vessels (ophthalmic, ACA, MCA, PCA, vertebral, basilar, AICA, PICA, or SCA). Emboli most commonly arise from atherosclerotic plaques of the extracranial **ICA** (artery-to-artery emboli) or from the **heart.** Common sources include the following:

- **Atrial fibrillation (AF),** with clot arising in the left atrial appendage.
- **Valvular disease** (e.g., endocarditis, prosthetic valves) is also associated with cardiogenic emboli.
- Patients with severe left ventricular dysfunction and regional wall motion abnormalities following MI can form **ventricular thrombi** that embolize.
- Severe atheromatous disease of the proximal **aortic arch** can also generate cerebrovascular emboli.
- **Paradoxical emboli** can arise from right-to-left shunting of venous thrombi and emboli across an atrial defect.

EXAM

Patients with embolic stroke need aggressive investigation of the potential embolic source to determine if specific intervention is warranted. Key points to direct workup are as follows:

- An embolic stroke involving the posterior circulation (cerebellum, brain stem, occipital lobes) is most likely cardiogenic in nature, as this region is not supplied by the ICA.
- **Amaurosis fugax** (acute transient monocular vision loss) is most commonly caused by cholesterol emboli from an atherosclerotic plaque of the **ipsilateral ICA.**
- Embolic strokes involving the anterior circulation (ACA or MCA) can be secondary to either internal carotid emboli or cardiogenic emboli.

Amaurosis fugax = retinal angina.

DIAGNOSIS

- **Imaging studies** are as follows:
  - **Brain:** A head CT is the initial study of choice for acute stroke, primarily to evaluate for intracranial hemorrhage. MRI is best for characterizing the location and size of ischemic strokes.
  - **Internal carotid:** Use Doppler ultrasound or MRA of the extracranial carotid arteries to evaluate for significant stenosis (> 70%).
  - **Heart:** Transesophageal echocardiography (TEE) is superior to transthoracic echocardiography (TTE) for evaluating potential cardiac sources of emboli.
- Other important studies include the following:
  - **ECG:** Initial screening test for cardiac arrhythmias, especially AF or flutter.

- **Cardiac telemetry:** Monitoring patients on continuous cardiac telemetry for 24–48 hours can help detect paroxysmal AF.
- Patients < 50 years of age with unexplained embolic stroke should be evaluated for underlying hypercoagulable states (e.g., antiphospholipid syndrome, antithrombin III, protein S and C deficiency, factor V Leiden mutation).

TREATMENT

Specific treatments to decrease the risk of recurrent embolic strokes are as follows:

- **Symptomatic internal carotid stenosis:** Patients with embolic stroke involving the anterior circulation who are found to have > 70% **stenosis** of the ipsilateral ICA benefit from **carotid endarterectomy.**
- **Atrial fibrillation:** Warfarin therapy with a goal INR of 2–3 is the optimal treatment for patients with paroxysmal or chronic AF.
- **Cardiogenic emboli:** In practice, identifiable cardiac sources (e.g., aortic arch thrombi) are typically treated with warfarin for 4–6 months.
- **Cryptogenic embolic stroke:** In embolic stroke patients for whom no clear source is identified, aspirin appears to be equivalent to warfarin in preventing recurrent strokes.

THROMBOTIC STROKE

Occurs when a small cerebral artery gradually occludes secondary to progressive local thrombosis. The classic vessels involved are the small penetrating terminal arterioles that supply the **brain stem** and the **deep structures of the cerebral hemispheres,** including the basal ganglia, thalami, and internal capsule.

Think brain stem lesion if there are crossed symptoms.

- The internal capsule is of particular importance in that it contains the **descending motor fibers** from the motor cortex as they travel toward the brain stem and spinal cord. Occlusion of these small arterioles produces a discrete **"lacunar" infarct** of the small area of brain supplied by the terminal arteriole.
- Lacunar infarcts typically occur in vital structures (e.g., brain stem, internal capsule) and, despite their small size, can have devastating effects. The four classic "lacunar" strokes are as follows:
  - **Pure motor hemiparesis:** Presents with isolated weakness of the face, arm, and leg on one side of the body. Sensation is normal, and no "cortical signs" (e.g., aphasia, visual field deficits) are present.
  - **Dysarthria–clumsy hand syndrome:** Essentially a variant of pure motor hemiparesis, with isolated slurred speech and unilateral hand weakness and incoordination.
  - **Ataxia hemiparesis:** Patients have mild weakness of the face, arm, and leg on one side associated with marked ataxia of the same side of the body.
  - **Pure sensory loss:** Patients have complete loss of sensation on one side of the body.
  - **Other lacunar strokes.** The "named" brain stem strokes (e.g., Wallenberg's; see Table 13-5) are typically caused by a small-vessel lacunar stroke from thrombosis.

DIAGNOSIS

Imaging studies, particularly with MRI, are key in demonstrating strokes caused by small-vessel thrombosis. This can limit the necessary workup (e.g.,

TABLE 13-5. Specific Brain Stem Strokes

NAME	LOCATION	SYMPTOMS
Wallenberg's syndrome	Lateral medulla	Ipsilateral loss of pain and temperature on the face. Contralateral loss of pain and temperature on the body. Ipsilateral Horner's, vertigo, slurred speech.
"Locked-in" syndrome	Pons	Intact mental status; quadriparesis; able to do no more than move eyes up and blink.
Weber syndrome	Midbrain	Ipsilateral CN III palsy; contralateral hemiparesis.

do not need to pursue aggressive diagnostic tests for an embolic source) and focus treatment (e.g., warfarin therapy is not appropriate treatment for small-vessel thrombotic strokes).

TREATMENT

- The **primary risk factors** for small-vessel thrombotic strokes are **hypertension, diabetes, hyperlipidemia,** and **smoking.** Prevention of small-vessel thrombotic ischemic strokes rests primarily on aggressive control of these risk factors.
- Antiplatelet therapy reduces the risk of recurrent strokes in this patient population; choices include aspirin, clopidogrel, and ASA/dipyridamole.
- **Acute management of ischemic stroke** is as follows:
  - Only patients with acute ischemic stroke symptoms of < 3 hours' duration can receive IV thrombolysis with **tPA.** Other exclusions for tPA include coagulopathy (INR > 1.7), thrombocytopenia (platelets < 100,000), uncontrolled hypertension (SBP > 185), and prior intracranial hemorrhage. The primary risk of tPA treatment is intracranial hemorrhage.
  - Use of IV heparin in patients with ischemic stroke who do not qualify for tPA remains controversial. Available data suggest that antiplatelet therapy is the most appropriate treatment for this patient population. Heparin is more commonly used in arterial dissection and symptomatic posterior circulation stenosis.

Hemorrhagic Stroke

Caused by rupture of blood vessels within the brain parenchyma. As with ischemic stroke, focal symptoms depend on the location of the hemorrhage. In contrast to ischemic stroke, intraparenchymal hemorrhages are usually associated with **headache** and rapid **deterioration in level of consciousness.**

- The leading cause of hemorrhagic strokes is **hypertension. Hypertensive hemorrhages classically occur in four subcortical structures: the basal ganglia, thalamus, cerebellum, and pons (part of the brain stem).**
- Intraparenchymal hemorrhages occurring within the cortical white matter (so-called **lobar hemorrhages**) can be caused by hypertension but raise suspicion for other etiologies, such as metastatic lesions, vascular abnormalities (e.g., AVMs), hemorrhagic conversion of an ischemic stroke, infections (especially septic emboli), and cerebral amyloid angiopathy.

- **Treatment** is largely supportive. **Cerebellar hemorrhages** should be considered a neurosurgical emergency, as swelling and herniation onto the brain stem can be lethal.

Extraparenchymal Bleeds

The three types of extraparenchymal intracranial hemorrhages are **epidural, subdural,** and **subarachnoid.** The most common cause of all extraparenchymal intracranial hemorrhages is **head trauma.**

Epidural Hematomas

- Typically caused by trauma to the side of the head, usually near the ear, resulting in injury to the **middle meningeal artery** (MMA). The MMA runs between the skull and the dura, and injury thus produces bleeding into the epidural space. Such hematomas can expand rapidly, as they are produced by **arterial bleeding.**
- **Symptoms/Exam:** Although seen in < 25% of patients, the classic presentation is of head trauma with brief (seconds to minutes) loss of consciousness followed by a "lucid period" in which mental status and level of alertness are normal for minutes to hours. Followed by a rapid decline in mental status.
- **Diagnosis:** Since the dura is tacked down to the skull at the suture lines, epidural bleeds will tamponade in a confined space and will not cross the sutures, leading to the characteristic "lens-shaped" hematoma on CT scan.
- **Treatment:** Symptomatic epidural hematomas must be treated with neurosurgical decompression.

Subdural Hematomas

- Typically caused by head trauma that leads to a rapid deceleration of the skull (e.g., car accident) and subsequent shearing of the cerebral bridging veins as they travel through the subdural space into the draining venous sinuses. Most often seen in **elderly** who have **falls.** Spontaneous subdural hematomas may also occur, particularly in patients with underlying coagulopathy or thrombocytopenia.
- **Symptoms/Exam:** Can produce mass effect, which typically manifests as a progressive decline in mental status.
- **Diagnosis:** Head CT reveals hematoma layering along the outer surface of the cerebral cortex. Must be in the differential of any elderly patient with dementia.
- **Treatment:** As with epidural hematomas, symptomatic subdural hematomas require neurosurgical decompression.

Subarachnoid Hemorrhage (SAH)

- The most common cause of nontraumatic SAH is a **ruptured intracranial aneurysm.**
- **Symptoms/Exam:** Patients experience abrupt-onset severe headache ("**worst headache of my life**" or "thunderclap" headache) associated with nausea and vomiting. There may also be decreased level of consciousness and focal neurologic deficits.

- **Diagnosis:**
  - **Head CT** is the initial imaging study of choice. If CT is negative, do an **LP** to look for **xanthochromia.**
  - Patients with a confirmed SAH should then have conventional **cerebral angiography** to determine the presence, location, and anatomy of the aneurysm.
- **Treatment:** The first priority is to secure the aneurysm as soon as possible, as the risk of rebleeding is significant in the first 48 hours. Currently, aneurysms are treated with either **neurosurgical clipping** or **endovascular coiling.**
- **Complications:**
  - The major complications following SAH are related to **vasospasm** of the cerebral vessels. **Nimodipine** reduces complications from vasospasm and is given to all patients with SAH. Vasospasm is also treated with **"triple H therapy"** (hypertension, hypervolemia, and hemodilution) in an effort to augment blood flow in areas of vasospasm
  - Other complications include obstructive hydrocephalus and hyponatremia from **cerebral salt wasting.**

SEIZURES

A **seizure** is a paroxysmal neurologic event caused by abnormal, synchronous discharges from populations of cortical neurons. Symptoms can vary widely and can include overt convulsions, subtle alterations of consciousness (e.g., staring spells), or simple sensations (e.g., odd smells or sounds). **Epilepsy** is a condition in which patients have **unprovoked recurrent seizures.** The key step in diagnosis and treatment is to determine whether the initial seizure activity is **generalized** or **focal** in onset.

Primary Generalized Seizures

Originate with abrupt-onset, simultaneous synchronized discharges of neurons throughout both cerebral hemispheres. Given this origin, **no warning or aura** is noted. Selected subtypes are as follows:

- **Tonic-clonic (grand mal):**
  - The most common generalized seizure type; typically seen in genetic epilepsy syndromes and in seizures arising from metabolic abnormalities (e.g., hyponatremia, alcohol withdrawal, medications, CNS infections).
  - Begin with stiffening of the extremities (**tonic** phase), often associated with a guttural cry from contraction of the expiratory muscles, followed by rhythmic **clonic** jerking of the extremities.
  - There typically is associated urinary incontinence, tongue biting, and postictal confusion.
- **Myoclonic:**
  - A **myoclonic jerk** is an abrupt, brief, single contraction of a muscle group that produces a quick contraction and movement. **Myoclonic seizures** are characterized by frequent but asynchronous, nonrhythmic multifocal myoclonic jerks. Most commonly seen with metabolic derangements (especially **uremia** and **anoxic brain injury**).
  - An important genetic cause of myoclonic seizures is **juvenile myoclonic epilepsy**; patients often have "staring spells" during childhood (brief alterations in consciousness often associated with eye blinking or chewing movements) and subsequently develop both myoclonic and

tonic-clonic seizures in adolescence. They also experience myoclonic jerks when entering into or emerging from sleep.

- **Atonic:** Characterized by the abrupt loss of all muscle tone associated with a brief loss of consciousness. Primarily seen with inherited forms of childhood epilepsy.

Symptoms/Exam

Although symptoms can vary, most generalized seizures are associated with a period of postictal confusion and lethargy.

Diagnosis

- **Labs:** Routine evaluation of patients with new seizures includes metabolic labs, including electrolytes such as sodium and calcium as well as screening for renal or liver dysfunction. LP should be considered when infection or inflammatory disease is a concern.
- **Imaging:** Brain MRI should be done to investigate for structural abnormalities, with particular attention paid to the temporal lobes.
- **EEG:** EEG obtained prior to and during a seizure shows symmetric and synchronous generalized epileptiform discharges at the onset.

Treatment

- "Broad-spectrum" anticonvulsants such as **valproic acid,** topiramate, and lamotrigine are considered first-line treatment for primary generalized seizures.
- Although phenytoin and carbamazepine may be helpful in patients with primary generalized tonic-clonic seizures, these medications can actually exacerbate seizures and should thus be avoided.
- Two unique types of generalized epilepsy are **juvenile myoclonic epilepsy,** which is best treated with **valproic acid,** and **absence epilepsy,** which is classically treated with **ethosuximide.**

Complications

Table 13-6 outlines the side effects associated with common anticonvulsants used for seizure treatment. Other medication-related complications are as follows:

- **Anticonvulsants and OCPs:** Drugs that induce the liver cytochrome P-450 system (e.g., phenytoin and carbamazepine but not valproic acid) can lead to decreased effective levels of other medications, including OCPs. All female patients taking such anticonvulsants should be counseled to consider other means of birth control.

TABLE 13-6. Classic Anticonvulsant Side Effects

Drug	Side Effects
Phenytoin	**Gum hyperplasia,** ataxia, **peripheral neuropathy,** lymphoproliferative disorder, Stevens-Johnson syndrome.
Carbamazepine	**Hyponatremia, lymphopenia,** Stevens-Johnson syndrome. **Induces its own metabolism;** the initial dose can then become ineffective.
Valproate	**Tremor,** drowsiness, **weight gain,** hirsutism, thrombocytopenia, liver failure.

- **Anticonvulsants and birth defects:** Use of anticonvulsants during pregnancy is associated with an increased risk of birth defects, particularly **neural tube defects.** All women of childbearing age who use anticonvulsants should be advised to take 0.4 mg/day of folate. Pregnant women with epilepsy should be treated with a single anticonvulsant at the lowest therapeutic dose.

Focal (Partial) Seizures

Originate from a small, discrete focal lesion within the brain that gives rise to abnormal synchronized neuronal discharges. This activity may then spread to involve other areas of the brain. Subtypes are as follows:

- **Simple partial seizures:**
  - Focal seizures in which **no alteration of consciousness** is noted.
  - Initial symptoms depend on the location of the seizure focus and commonly include twitching/jerking of one side of the body (focal motor seizures) or sensations of strange smells or sounds.
- **Complex partial seizures:**
  - Evolve from simple partial seizures as the initial focal seizure activity spreads to involve some but not all of both cerebral hemispheres. In fact, the **stereotypical warning or aura** that many patients report is simply the manifestation of the initial simple partial seizure.
  - As seizure activity spreads, patients develop an **impairment of consciousness** and **behavioral arrest** during which they display stereotypical behaviors known as **automatisms** (e.g., lip smacking, chewing, pulling at clothes).
  - In contrast to simple partial seizures, complex partial seizures are associated with postictal confusion and lethargy.
- **Complex partial seizures with secondary generalization:**
  - In many patients with prolonged complex partial seizures, seizure activity can ultimately spread to involve the entire cerebral cortex. The manifestation of the "secondary generalization" of the initial focal seizure activity is usually generalized tonic-clonic activity.
  - Generalized seizures can thus be either **primary** (generalized seizure activity at onset) or **secondary** (initial focal activity that spreads to involve the entire cortex).
- **Todd's paralysis:**
  - Patients with focal-onset seizures often have transient (minutes to hours) focal weakness or paralysis following seizure termination. This weakness usually involves the area of the body first affected by the seizure, providing an important clue to the locus of seizure onset.
  - A patient with a generalized tonic-clonic seizure who is subsequently noted to have a postictal left hemiparesis likely had a focal-onset seizure that began in the right hemisphere and secondarily generalized.
- **Temporal lobe epilepsy:** The most common cause of simple and complex partial seizures is **temporal lobe pathology,** most commonly secondary to abnormalities of the **hippocampus.** Hippocampal sclerosis/calcification is seen on imaging. The classic auras of odd smells, sounds, or tastes are associated with temporal lobe epilepsy.

Prolonged simple partial seizures are called epilepsia partialis continua and are difficult to control.

DIAGNOSIS

Given that focal (partial) seizures arise from focal lesions, brain imaging studies are typically abnormal; EEG often shows localized (i.e., asymmetric) epileptiform activity. HSV encephalitis must be ruled out via CSF studies in patients with new-onset temporal lobe seizures.

Treatment

- **Medications:** Focal-onset seizures are best treated with anticonvulsants such as **phenytoin, carbamazepine,** phenobarbital, and valproic acid. Newer medications such as gabapentin, levetiracetam, lamotrigine, and topiramate are also useful.
- **Vagal nerve stimulators:** Although their mechanism of action remains unclear, vagal nerve stimulators can decrease the frequency of focal-onset seizures by 25% in patients with medically refractory seizures. A pacemaker-like device is implanted in the chest with leads attached to one of the vagal nerves.
- **Surgery:** Patients with focal-onset seizures often have an identifiable brain lesion on imaging studies. This is particularly true of temporal lobe epilepsy secondary to hippocampal lesions. In such patients with medically refractory seizures, **surgical resection** of the causative lesion (e.g., temporal lobectomy) can produce striking results, with up to 50–75% of patients becoming seizure free.

Complications

See Table 13-6 and the accompanying discussion.

Status Epilepticus

Traditionally defined as (1) continuous seizure activity lasting > 30 minutes, or (2) recurrent seizures without return of normal consciousness between seizures. Practically speaking, seizure activity lasting > 5 minutes is unlikely to remit spontaneously and carries the risk of permanent neuronal injury. Generally, ongoing or recurrent seizure activity lasting > 5 minutes is thus considered a medical emergency and treated as status epilepticus. Guidelines for treatment are given in Table 13-7.

TABLE 13-7. Basic Guidelines for the Treatment of Status Epilepticus

- ABCs.
- Draw labs for metabolic abnormalities (e.g., glucose, sodium, calcium).
- Administer **thiamine and glucose.**
- **Benzodiazepines are first-line anticonvulsants for status epilepticus.**
  - **Lorazepam: 0.1 mg/kg IV, given at** < 2 mg/min.
  - **Phenytoin or fosphenytoin** should then be started immediately even if seizures terminate with lorazepam.
    - **Phenytoin: 20 mg/kg IV at** < 50 mg/min; watch for hemodynamic instability.
    - **Fosphenytoin: 20 mg/kg "phenytoin equivalents" IV at** < 150 mg/min.
  - **If seizures persist,** the next step is to give a **second load** of phenytoin or fosphenytoin using an additional **5–10 mg/kg** IV load.
  - **If seizures continue,** the next step is to administer pentobarbital, midazolam, or propofol. Use of any of these medications typically requires continuous EEG recordings, mechanical ventilation, and cardiac pressors.

MOVEMENT DISORDERS

Hypokinetic Disorders

PARKINSON'S DISEASE

An idiopathic progressive neurodegenerative disorder affecting the dopaminergic neurons of the substantia nigra (see Figure 13-1). Incidence is 10–20 in 100,000, and prevalence is 100–150 in 100,000. Average age of onset is 60, and the male-to-female ratio is 1.5:1.

> ***Parkinson's features—***
>
> ***TRAP***
>
> **T**remor
> **R**igidity
> **A**kinesia
> **P**ostural instability

SYMPTOMS/EXAM

The **cardinal features** are **resting tremor ("pill rolling"), bradykinesia, "cogwheel" rigidity, postural instability,** and **response to levodopa.** Symptoms typically begin **asymmetrically,** usually in one extremity. Cognition is preserved in idiopathic Parkinson's.

DIFFERENTIAL

Parkinson-plus syndromes present with parkinsonian features as well as with additional symptoms (see below). Other causes of parkinsonism include cerebrovascular disease; recurrent head trauma (e.g., boxing); toxin exposure (including illicit drugs such as MPTP and heavy metals such as manganese); and antidopaminergic medications (e.g., traditional antipsychotics).

DIAGNOSIS

The diagnosis of idiopathic Parkinson's disease relies on the history and physical combined with response to levodopa. Young patients as well as those with atypical features should undergo further workup (e.g., imaging studies, toxin screens).

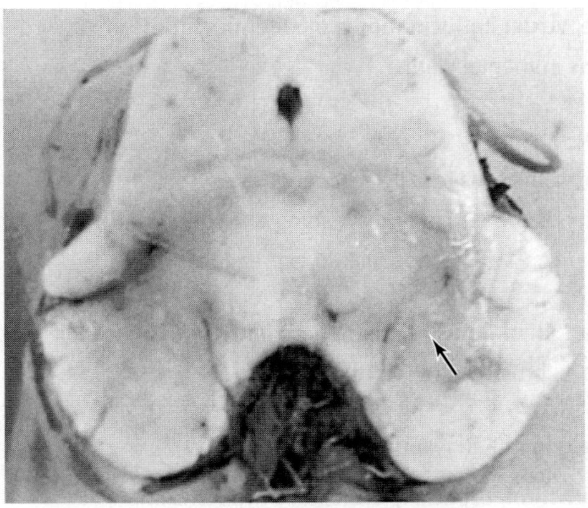

FIGURE 13-1. Midbrain of a 45-year-old woman with Parkinson's disease, showing depigmentation of the substantia nigra (arrow).

(Reproduced, with permission, from Waxman S. *Clinical Neuroanatomy*, 25th ed. New York: McGraw-Hill, 2003: Figure 13-9.) (Also see Color Insert.)

Treatment

Medical treatment includes the following:

- **Levodopa/carbidopa:** The gold standard for symptomatic treatment. Levodopa, a precursor of dopamine, is administered with carbidopa, a decarboxylase inhibitor that inhibits peripheral conversion of levodopa to dopamine. Should be taken on an empty stomach to maximize absorption.
- **Dopamine agonists:** Direct agonists of D2 dopamine receptors.
- **Catechol-O-methyltransferase (COMT) inhibitors:** One pathway of dopamine degradation is via COMT; inhibition of this enzyme raises endogenous dopamine levels.
- **MAOIs:** Another pathway of dopamine degradation is via MAO; inhibition of this enzyme likewise raises endogenous dopamine levels.

Parkinson-Plus Syndromes

A number of neurodegenerative diseases produce parkinsonian features along with a variety of other symptoms, including cognitive decline and cerebellar abnormalities (see Table 13-8). In general, Parkinson-plus syndromes respond poorly if at all to levodopa. A Parkinson-plus syndrome should thus be considered in **any patient who presents with parkinsonism associated with cerebellar or cognitive symptoms,** especially when the parkinsonian features do not respond to levodopa therapy.

Hyperkinetic Disorders

Huntington's Disease

An **autosomal-dominant** disorder characterized by progressive **chorea, dementia,** and **psychiatric** symptoms. Huntington's is a neurodegenerative dis-

TABLE 13-8. Clinical Features of Parkinson-Plus Syndromes

Syndrome	Key Features
Dementia with Lewy bodies	Cognitive decline, **visual hallucinations, misidentifications** of family/friends, marked **daily fluctuations** in mental status.
Progressive supranuclear palsy	Cognitive decline. Extraocular abnormalities, especially **vertical gaze.** Prominent **rigidity of the entire body,** leading to frequent **falls** and a **characteristic facial appearance** ("wide-eyed," scared expression).
Corticobasal degeneration	Cognitive decline; **"alien limb"** phenomenon; **limb apraxia;** inability to perform learned motor tasks (e.g., brush teeth, salute).
Multiple-system atrophy (MSA)	Encompasses a group of Parkinson-plus syndromes.
Shy-Drager syndrome	**Autonomic dysfunction,** especially orthostatic hypotension.
Olivopontocerebellar atrophy	**Ataxia;** incoordination with mild parkinsonism.
Striatonigral degeneration	**Isolated parkinsonism;** no tremor; **no response to levodopa.**

order of the **caudate nucleus** of the basal ganglia and is caused by a **polyglutamine (CAG) trinucleotide repeat expansion** in the Huntington gene on **chromosome 4.** This repeat can expand with successive generations, leading to the phenomenon of **anticipation**—earlier age of onset and more severe symptoms in successive generations.

Diagnosis

The clinical presentation combined with a strong family history suggests the disease. CT/MRI show marked **atrophy of the caudate nucleus** and exclude other structural abnormalities. Genetic testing now provides definitive evidence of the trinucleotide repeat expansion.

Treatment

No treatment is currently available for the underlying disease process. Chorea can be treated symptomatically with neuroleptics (e.g., haloperidol), dopamine-depleting agents (e.g., reserpine), or GABAergic agents (e.g., clonazepam). Genetic counseling is indicated for patients' children.

Wilson's Disease

An **autosomal-recessive** disorder characterized by progressive neuropsychiatric symptoms and liver dysfunction. Caused by mutations of a copper ATPase transporter gene on chromosome 13. Copper deposition occurs most prominently in the liver and basal ganglia (specifically the lentiform nuclei) of the brain; asymptomatic deposition is also seen in Descemet's membrane of the cornea. Liver dysfunction is typically seen prior to neuropsychiatric illness (onset of liver disease occurs at 10–15 years of age); most patients present as adolescents and young adults.

Symptoms

Patients have prominent extrapyramidal symptoms (tremor, dystonia, rigidity, bradykinesia) and cerebellar symptoms (ataxia, incoordination, slurred speech); common psychiatric symptoms include depression, psychosis, and personality changes.

Exam

As a rule, all Wilson's disease patients with neuropsychiatric symptoms will have **Kayser-Fleischer rings** (greenish-brown rings along the limbus of the cornea from copper deposition); a **slit-lamp** evaluation is often necessary to detect them. The tremor of Wilson's disease is a coarse proximal upper-extremity tremor classically described as a **"wing-beating" tremor.**

Diagnosis

Consider in any young patient presenting with progressive neurologic (especially extrapyramidal) or psychiatric symptoms, even in the absence of liver disease. Diagnosis is supported by laboratory evidence of low serum copper and ceruloplasmin (a protein into which copper is normally incorporated in the hepatocyte) and high urinary copper. Liver biopsy reveals copper deposition.

Treatment

Penicillamine, a copper chelating agent, has classically been used to treat Wilson's disease, although side effects are common; in particular, a **myasthe-**

nia gravis syndrome with positive titers of anti-ACh receptor antibodies can be induced by penicillamine therapy.

ESSENTIAL TREMOR

An idiopathic **postural** or **kinetic tremor** that typically affects the **hands** and **head.** It is seen equally in men and women, although hand tremor is most prominent in men and head tremor most prominent in women. Tremor onset occurs between 35 and 45 years of age. Family history is often strongly positive.

SYMPTOMS

In contrast to Parkinson's, essential tremor is not seen at rest but rather comes out with activity. The tremor is slightly faster than that of Parkinson's disease (8–10 Hz vs. 4–5 Hz). Most patients report a temporary but **striking improvement** in tremor **with alcohol** ingestion; conversely, physical and emotional stress exacerbate the tremor, as do medications such as caffeine and steroids.

EXAM

Postural tremor of the hands is tested by having patients maintain their arms extended fully from their bodies. Hand tremor can also come out with activity, although this should not be confused with a cerebellar tremor, in which tremor is worse as the hands approach a target. Tremor of the jaw is frequently seen. In patients with essential tremor, strength is normal. In contrast to Parkinson's disease, no abnormalities in muscle tone are present.

DIFFERENTIAL

In a young patient, Wilson's disease should be considered. Other causes of tremor include endocrine disorders (especially thyroid dysfunction), electrolyte abnormalities (including calcium and sodium), medications (especially lithium, antidepressants, and neuroleptics), and **Parkinson's disease.**

TREATMENT

The classic treatments are **β-blockers (e.g., propranolol)** and **primidone** (which is metabolized to phenobarbital). Benzodiazepines and gabapentin have also been used when first-line treatments fail.

TOURETTE'S SYNDROME

A disorder characterized by **brief involuntary actions (motor and vocal tics)** and **psychiatric disturbances.** Onset typically occurs in adolescents < 18 years of age, with a male-to-female ratio of 5:1. Two-thirds of patients have some amelioration of symptoms in adulthood, but complete remission is rare.

SYMPTOMS/EXAM

Motor tics can be simple (e.g., eye twitching, blinking, shoulder shrugging) or complex (e.g., mimicking another's actions—**echopraxia**). **Vocal tics** can be simple sounds (e.g., barking) or single words; classic vocal tics include **speaking obscenities (coprolalia)** and **mimicking another's speech (echolalia).** Tics are often exacerbated by physical or emotional stress. Neuropsychiatric problems include **obsessive-compulsive disorder,** learning disabilities, and attention-deficit disorder.

Differential

The differential for motor tics includes dystonia (see below) and ballismus. Primary psychiatric illness must also be considered in patients with vocal tics.

Treatment

Neuroleptics (e.g., haloperidol, risperidone) and **benzodiazepines** (e.g., clonazepam, diazepam) often help reduce the frequency of tics.

Dystonia

A syndrome characterized by repetitive, sustained contractions of agonist/antagonist muscles groups that typically produce painful **twisting/writhing movements** and/or **abnormal tonic postures** of the head or extremities. Can be focal or generalized.

- Etiologies include inherited/genetic, neurodegenerative (e.g., Huntington's, Wilson's, Parkinson's), rheumatologic (e.g., SLE, antiphospholipid syndrome), metabolic (e.g., thyroid disease), and toxin/medication related (e.g., **neuroleptics,** OCPs).
- Treat **focal** dystonia with **selective injection of botulinum toxin.** For **generalized** dystonia, stop the offending medication and treat with **anticholinergics** such as benztropine or diphenhydramine.

Neuroleptics such as prochlorperazine and promethazine can cause an acute dystonic reaction. Treat with anticholinergics.

Restless Leg Syndrome (RLS)

Characterized by intense, uncomfortable paresthesias of the legs (often described as a "crawling" or "creeping" sensation) that are relieved by leg movement. Generally idiopathic, but also seen in patients with a wide variety of chronic illnesses (e.g., Parkinson's, anemia, diabetes, COPD, thyroid disease, connective tissue diseases) and as a side effect of drugs (e.g., caffeine, lithium, calcium channel blockers).

Symptoms/Exam

Paresthesias are most severe when the legs are **at rest** (e.g., while sitting or lying), especially at night as patients try to sleep, and are **relieved by continued movement** of the legs. In addition, patients typically have periodic limb movements in sleep (PLMS)—frequent stereotypical movements of the leg. Neurologic exam is normal unless RLS is related to an underlying neurologic disorder.

Treatment

Dopaminergic medications (e.g., levodopa/carbidopa, pramipexole) are the **standard treatment** for RLS. Other useful agents include **benzodiazepines, narcotics,** and **gabapentin.**

MULTIPLE SCLEROSIS (MS)

An autoimmune inflammatory disease affecting the myelin of the CNS. Characterized by focal demyelinating plaques that occur at different times and locations within the CNS. Typically affects the optic nerves, corpus callosum, periventricular white matter, brain stem, and spinal cord. Generally seen in **younger women.** Incidence increases with latitude of birth and is twice as high in patients of Northern European descent as in patients of African descent.

SYMPTOMS

In addition to focal abnormalities, patients often suffer from chronic **fatigue.** Symptoms are **exacerbated by heat and exercise** (the Uhthoff phenomenon); old deficits are also worsened by underlying illness, especially infections such as UTIs or URIs.

EXAM

Classic lesions and exam findings include the following:

- **Optic nerve: Optic neuritis** presents as unilateral subacute vision loss associated with pain on eye movement. Exam shows pallor of the optic nerve, decreased visual acuity, difficulty with color discrimination, and a **relative afferent pupillary defect** (RAPD, or Marcus Gunn pupil) (see Figure 13-2).
- **Brain stem:** A demyelinating lesion of the medial longitudinal fasciculus (MLF) that yields an **internuclear ophthalmoplegia** (INO). Patients complain of double vision when looking to one side; exam reveals inability to adduct the eye ipsilateral to the lesion when looking to the contralateral

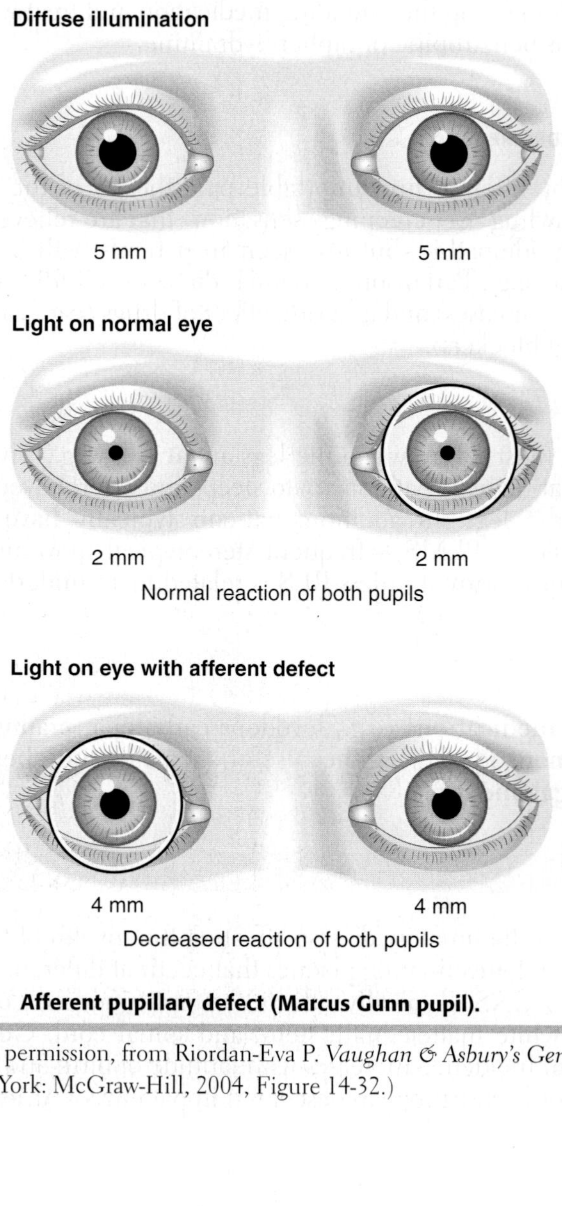

FIGURE 13-2. Afferent pupillary defect (Marcus Gunn pupil).

(Reproduced, with permission, from Riordan-Eva P. *Vaughan & Asbury's General Ophthalmology*, 16th ed. New York: McGraw-Hill, 2004, Figure 14-32.)

side. Adduction of the eye can be brought out by testing convergence, which remains normal (see Figure 13-3).

- **Spinal cord:** Transverse myelitis symptoms (**paresthesias,** sensory level, bowel/bladder dysfunction, **UMN signs**) are common. Involvement of the dorsal column tracts in the spinal cord is common, leading to **impaired vibration and joint position sense** in the lower extremities. **Lhermitte's sign** (electrical radiation down the spine elicited by neck flexion) is a classic finding and is likely related to dorsal column involvement.
- **Paroxysmal symptoms:** Patients often experience brief tonic **muscle spasms** of an isolated limb. Trigeminal neuralgia (brief lancinating electrical shocks along the angle of the jaw) is also seen and, when observed in a young person, should raise the possibility of MS.

Diagnosis

- **Clinical criteria:** No laboratory or imaging test is diagnostic for MS, and thus the diagnosis must be based on clinical criteria. Definitive diagnosis requires evidence from the history and exam of at least two distinct attacks involving two separate CNS regions. Imaging and laboratory data support the diagnosis.
- **MRI:** MRI abnormalities are seen in > 90% of patients. Most have multiple punctate/ovoid lesions involving the periventricular white matter ("Dawson's finger" lesions extending from the ventricles at right angles), **corpus callosum,** brain stem, and spinal cord. These are best seen on T2-weighted images. "Active" lesions enhance with gadolinium contrast (see Figure 13-4).
- **CSF:** Typical findings include normal opening pressure, mild lymphocytic pleocytosis (5–40 WBCs/mm^3), normal glucose, and normal to mildly increased protein. Eighty percent of patients have > 2 **oligoclonal bands** and an elevated CSF **IgG index,** but neither is specific for MS.
- **EPs:** Occasionally used to obtain supportive evidence of demyelination if MRI and CSF results are inconclusive. For evaluation of MS, visual EPs are often used.

Treatment

- **Disease-modifying therapies** include the following:
  - **β-interferon—"ABC drugs" (Avonex, Betaseron, Copaxone):** These drugs have been shown to decrease the frequency and severity of relapses in patients with relapsing-remitting MS. Table 13-9 outlines the administration of these drugs and delineates their potential side effects.
  - **Glucocorticoids:** High-dose IV glucocorticoids (Solu-Medrol 1 g IV QD × 3–5 days), which are typically used to treat acute attacks and the

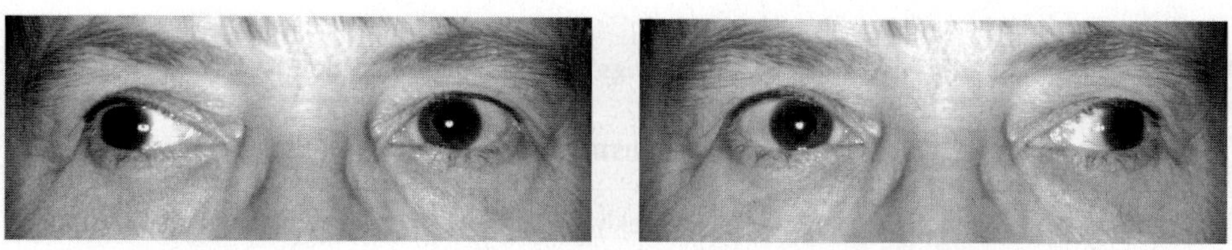

FIGURE 13-3. Bilateral internuclear ophthalmoplegia due to multiple sclerosis.

(Reproduced, with permission, from Riordan-Eva P. *Vaughan & Asbury's General Ophthalmology*, 16th ed. New York: McGraw-Hill, 2004: Figure 14-12.) (Also see Color Insert.)

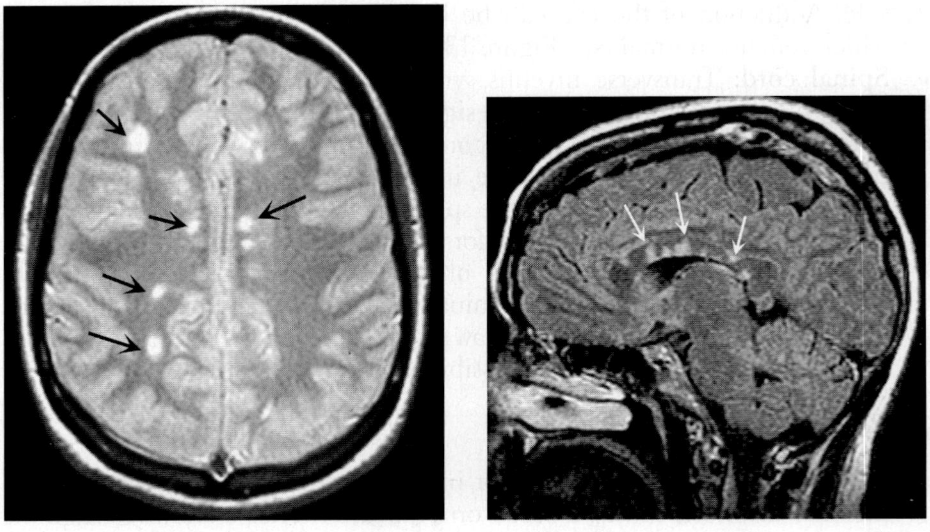

FIGURE 13-4. MRI findings in MS.

(A) Axial image from T2-weighted sequence demonstrates multiple bright signal abnormalities in white matter, typical for MS. (B) Sagittal T2-weighted FLAIR (fluid-attenuated inversion recovery) image in which the high signal of CSF has been suppressed. CSF appears dark, while areas of brain edema or demyelination appear high in signal, as shown here in the corpus callosum (*arrows*). Lesions in the anterior corpus callosum are frequent in MS and rare in vascular disease. (Reproduced, with permission, from Kasper DL et al [eds]. *Harrison's Principles of Internal Medicine*, 16th ed. New York: McGraw-Hill, 2005:2464.)

Consider MS in a young patient presenting with any of the following: optic neuritis, RAPD, INO, Lhermitte's sign, Uhthoff's phenomenon, and subacute spinal cord symptoms.

presence of new enhancing lesions on MRI, appear to be superior to oral steroids (especially for treating optic neuritis). Administration of glucocorticoids, however, has no impact on overall disease progression or long-term disability.

- **Specific symptoms** are targeted with appropriate medication:
  - **Hyperreflexic bladder:** Oxybutynin.
  - **Fatigue:** Amantadine.
  - **Paroxysmal symptoms** (e.g., tonic spasms): Carbamazepine.
  - **Spasticity:** Baclofen, diazepam.

TABLE 13-9. Administration of "ABC Drugs" and Associated Side Effects

DRUG	ADMINISTRATION	SIDE EFFECTS
Interferon-β_{1a} (Avonex)	Weekly IM	Flulike symptoms, depression
Interferon-β_{1b} (Betaseron)	QOD SQ	Flulike symptoms
Glatiramer acetate (Copaxone)	Daily SQ	Flushing, chest tightness

NEUROMUSCULAR JUNCTION DISORDERS

Myasthenia Gravis (MG)

An **autoimmune** disease caused by autoantibodies to the nicotinic ACh receptor (nAChR), resulting in impaired transmission at the neuromuscular junction. Occurs in **young women** (ages 20–30) and **older men** (ages 50–70). Associated with other autoimmune diseases, particularly **thyroid** disorders.

Symptoms

The hallmark is **fluctuating, fatigable weakness** classically affecting the **eye muscles.** There are two forms: (1) **ocular,** which is isolated to the extraocular and eyelid muscles, giving double vision and ptosis; and (2) **generalized,** which typically involves ocular, facial, and proximal limb muscles, giving rise to ocular symptoms as well as to facial weakness, trouble swallowing and speaking, and limb weakness. Patients with ocular MG typically progress to generalized MG.

Exam

- **Ptosis,** often asymmetric, can be brought out by testing prolonged upgaze; an ice pack briefly placed on the eye will improve ptosis.
- **Extraocular muscle palsies** are typically seen on lateral gaze.
- **Easy fatigability** of proximal muscles with repeated strength testing.
- **Preserved DTRs** and sensation.

Differential

- Lambert-Eaton myasthenic syndrome.
- Drug-induced MG. **Penicillamine** can cause a reversible antibody-positive MG syndrome.
- Botulism typically presents with cranial nerve palsies, including the extraocular muscles. Patients have fever and CSF pleocytosis.

Diagnosis

- **Anti-nAChR antibodies:** Present in > 80% of generalized MG and 50% of ocular MG cases.
- **Anti-MuSK antibodies:** Present in 20% of "seronegative" MG patients.
- **Tensilon test:** Tensilon (edrophonium), a short-acting AChE inhibitor, can give instantaneous improvement to an objectively weak muscle.
- **EMG/NCS:** Direct testing of the muscle with EMG/NCS remains the **best test for MG.** Repetitive nerve stimulation reveals a **decremental** motor response, the correlate of clinical fatigability.

Treatment

- **AChE inhibitors** (e.g., pyridostigmine).
- **Immunomodulators** include glucocorticoids, cytotoxic drugs, plasma exchange, and IVIG.
- **Thymectomy:** Patients require **imaging of the chest** to evaluate for thymic abnormalities, as 70% have hyperplasia and 10% have thymomas. Thymectomy is recommended for most patients < 60 years of age with generalized MG.
- **Myasthenic crisis:** Elective intubation if **FVC** falls < 15 cc/kg.

> ***The 5 W's of MG:***
>
> **W**axing and
> **W**aning (fluctuating)
> **W**eakness with
> **W**ork (fatigability),
> mostly in
> **W**omen

COMPLICATIONS

Often exacerbated by stress, fever, infections, and certain medications, including antibiotics (especially **aminoglycosides**), as well as by antiarrhythmics such as procainamide and β-blockers.

Lambert-Eaton Myasthenic Syndrome (LEMS)

An **autoimmune paraneoplastic** syndrome caused by autoantibodies to presynaptic voltage-gated calcium channels, leading to impaired transmission at the neuromuscular junction. Typically seen in men and women > 40 years of age. More than half have an underlying malignancy, with the majority being **small cell lung cancer.**

SYMPTOMS

- Proximal muscle weakness, especially in the legs, which **briefly improves with exertion** before eventually fatiguing.
- Muscle aches.
- **Autonomic symptoms** (dry mouth, impotence, constipation, postural hypotension).
- In contrast to MG, LEMS patients do **not** experience double vision or ptosis (see Table 13-10).

EXAM

Normal cranial nerve exam; proximal weakness of the legs and arms that **initially improves** with repeated testing; **hyporeflexia.**

DIFFERENTIAL

MG, **myopathy** (e.g., polymyositis/dermatomyositis).

DIAGNOSIS

- EMG/NCS: Direct testing of the muscle with EMG remains the **best test for LEMS.** In contrast to MG, high-frequency repetitive nerve stimulation

TABLE 13-10. MG vs. LEMS

CHARACTERISTIC	MG	LEMS
Antibody target channel	nAChR	Voltage-gated calcium
Associated cancer	Thymoma	Small cell lung cancer
Eye muscle involvement	Yes	No
Autonomic symptoms	No	Yes
Reflexes	Normal	Hypoactive
Repetitive strength testing	Rapid fatigue	Initial improvement
Repetitive nerve stimulation	Decremental response	Initial enhancement

in LEMS reveals an **initial enhancement** of motor responses, the correlate of clinical improvement upon initial exertion.

- **Neoplastic workup.** Diagnosis of LEMS often precedes the diagnosis of cancer by one year. Initial evaluation should be directed at possible small cell lung cancer.

TREATMENT

- Primary treatment is directed at treating the underlying malignancy.
- 3,4-diaminopyridine (DAP) may facilitate neuromuscular transmission.
- IVIG and plasma exchange may improve symptoms.

AMYOTROPHIC LATERAL SCLEROSIS (ALS)

A progressive degenerative disease of the UMNs (arising in the motor cortex) and LMNs (arising in the brain stem and anterior horn of the spinal cord). Affects males and females equally, with onset between 50 and 70 years of age. Life expectancy is 3–5 years, with death usually occurring secondary to aspiration pneumonia or respiratory failure. 5–10% of cases are familial. One genetic cause is autosomal-dominant transmission of a mutation in the copper-zinc superoxide dismutase (SOD1) gene on chromosome 21.

SYMPTOMS

Difficulty swallowing, nasal speech, "head drop" from neck weakness, shortness of breath, "muscle twitches," muscle cramps, progressive generalized weakness. Eye muscles are typically spared; bowel and bladder function is typically preserved.

EXAM

Exam findings include both UMN and LMN signs.

- **Signs of UMN injury:** Spasticity (increased muscle tone), hyperreflexia, Babinski sign.
- **Signs of LMN injury:** Atrophy (especially of the tongue and muscles of the hands); fasciculations (muscle twitches) in at least three limbs.

DIFFERENTIAL

Cervical spondylosis resulting in cervical cord injury, hexosaminidase A deficiency (Tay-Sachs), West Nile viral LMN syndrome, syringomyelia, thyrotoxicosis, hyperparathyroidism, paraneoplastic syndromes.

DIAGNOSIS

- **EMG/NCS:** Reveal evidence of widespread LMN injury (e.g., fibrillations, **fasciculations**) and UMN injury (large motor units) that does not fall in a nerve root distribution. Sensory nerve studies are normal.
- **Spinal fluid** analysis is normal.
- **Cervical spine imaging** to evaluate for the possibility of cervical spondylosis, a surgically treatable disease.

TREATMENT

- **Riluzole,** a presumed glutamate antagonist, is the only FDA-approved medication for ALS. Improves survival by approximately six months.

- **Noninvasive positive-pressure ventilation** improves survival and should be offered if **FVC** falls to < 50% predicted.
- **Percutaneous endoscopic gastrostomy (PEG) tube placement** allows for increased nutrition in the face of dysphagia and leads to increased muscle mass and longer survival.

NEUROPATHIES

General Characteristics

A large group of heterogeneous diseases of the peripheral nerves. Overall prevalence is approximately 3% but increases to 8% in older patient populations. The character, distribution, and progressive course of symptoms are vital for directing workup and treatment.

CHARACTER

Peripheral nerves carry distinct fiber types: sensory, motor, and autonomic. Many diseases selectively attack specific fiber types, while others indiscriminately affect all types. The nature of symptoms depends on which fiber types are injured.

- **Sensory nerves:** Paresthesias (burning, numbness, tingling) are common initial symptoms, with overt sensory loss occurring with progression of disease.
- **Motor nerves:** Weakness, atrophy, twitching (fasciculations).
- **Autonomic nerves:** Postural hypotension, impotence, nausea, diarrhea, dry mouth.

DISTRIBUTION

- **Polyneuropathies:** Result from diseases that affect multiple peripheral nerves in a diffuse and synchronous fashion. Many polyneuropathies are "length dependent," affecting the longest nerves first. Produces the classic "stocking-glove distribution" of symmetric involvement of all four distal extremities.
- **Mononeuropathies:** Diseases of an individual peripheral nerve (e.g., radial nerve palsy), with symptoms restricted to its specific innervation.
- **Mononeuritis multiplex:** A unique syndrome in which multiple individual peripheral nerves are progressively injured in an asymmetric and asynchronous fashion.

PATHOLOGY

The location of injury in peripheral neuropathies involves either the **axon** or its insulating **myelin** covering. Identifying its location helps focus the differential and direct treatment.

- **Axonal** neuropathies are more likely **metabolic** in nature. As they involve direct injury to the nerve, recovery is often more limited and slow. NCS shows **low amplitude.**
- **Demyelinating** neuropathies are often **inflammatory** and thus treatable; as the neuron itself is not directly injured, recovery is often possible as remyelination occurs. NCS shows **slow conduction velocity.**

Acute Polyneuropathies

Acute-onset, rapidly progressive polyneuropathies, particularly those with motor or autonomic involvement, can produce life-threatening complications over days to weeks. These require aggressive workup and treatment. Many are inflammatory or toxic in nature.

GUILLAIN-BARRÉ SYNDROME (GBS)

A postinfectious autoimmune **acute demyelinating polyneuropathy.** Given the decline of polio, it is now the most common cause of acute flaccid paralysis. GBS classically follows an acute GI illness caused by ***Campylobacter jejuni,*** as antibodies directed toward its bacterial lipopolysaccharide cross-react with peripheral nerve myelin; other infections (e.g., HIV, *Mycoplasma*) have also been associated with GBS.

SYMPTOMS

- Symptoms such as back pain or lower extremity paresthesias typically begin 1–2 weeks after the infection, followed by **symmetric weakness that begins in the feet** and gradually ascends over hours to days. Weakness severity can range from mild to complete quadriplegia with respiratory failure. Autonomic symptoms are prominent, and cardiac instability can be life-threatening.
- A unique variant, Miller-Fisher syndrome, produces symptoms of ophthalmoplegia, ataxia, and areflexia, with little weakness of the extremities.
- Overall, GBS is a **monophasic** disease, with maximal symptoms seen by four weeks.

EXAM

Cardinal features on exam are **areflexia** and **symmetric progressive weakness.**

DIAGNOSIS

- CSF shows "albuminocytologic dissociation"—**isolated elevated protein** with normal WBC counts.
- Miller-Fisher syndrome is associated with anti-GQ1B antibodies.
- NCS reveals demyelination changes of the proximal peripheral nerves.
- Serial PFTs with **maximum inspiratory force** and **FVC** are important for following diaphragmatic function.

TREATMENT

Standard treatment is either **IVIG** or **plasmapheresis;** steroids are not beneficial. Mechanical ventilation should be considered when FVC falls to 15 mL/kg. Do not wait for P_{CO_2} to rise. Keep patients with autonomic symptoms on **cardiac telemetry.**

VASCULITIC NEUROPATHIES

Acute axonal neuropathies are seen in a wide variety of systemic vasculitides and connective tissue diseases. Vasculitic infarction of individual peripheral nerves occurs in an asynchronous and asymmetric fashion, producing a multifocal neuropathy involving both sensory and motor fibers; this random involvement of multiple individual peripheral nerves is called **mononeuritis multiplex.**

- **Symptoms/Exam:** Include severe **pain, paresthesias,** and **weakness.** Progression occurs over days to weeks.
- **Diagnosis:** NCS reveals axon injury to multiple unrelated peripheral

nerves; nerve biopsy typically shows axonal injury and inflammatory cell involvement of the nerve's vascular supply. Check c-ANCA and p-ANCA to evaluate for vasculitis.

- **Treatment:** Requires aggressive treatment with both steroids and an immunomodulator such as cyclophosphamide or methotrexate.

OTHER ETIOLOGIES

Additional etiologies of acute-onset, rapidly progressive polyneuropathies include brachial neuritis, acute intermittent porphyria, toxin exposure (arsenic, lead), and infections (diphtheria, Lyme disease).

Chronic Polyneuropathies

Most polyneuropathies are indolent in onset and progression, with symptoms noted gradually and advancing over months to years.

CHARCOT-MARIE-TOOTH (CMT) DISEASE

The classic inherited polyneuropathy. Prevalence is 1 in 2500, making it the most common inherited neurologic disorder. Family history is strongly positive, with most forms being autosomal dominant.

- **Symptoms/Exam:** Begin in the first and second decades, usually with distal weakness in the legs. Patients have high-arched feet (pes cavus) and hammer toes; progressive atrophy and weakness of the hands and feet; distal sensory loss; and reduced or absent reflexes. Life expectancy is typically normal, but significant morbidity results from progressive weakness.
- **Treatment:** No treatment currently exists.

CHRONIC INFLAMMATORY DEMYELINATING POLYNEUROPATHY (CIDP)

A symmetric, insidious-onset demyelinating disease of the peripheral nerves. Often considered to be related to but distinct from **GBS,** as both share similar clinical and pathologic findings (including areflexia, weakness, elevated CSF protein, demyelination, and response to IVIG or plasmapheresis). CIDP, however, has **no associated antecedent illness** and evolves over **weeks to months,** often with a **relapsing and remitting** course.

DIABETIC NEUROPATHY

Diabetes is the most common cause of peripheral neuropathy in the United States, typically presenting as a slow-onset, distal, symmetric axonal polyneuropathy. Approximately 8–10% of all patients with diabetes develop neuropathy, usually associated with onset of diabetic retinopathy and nephropathy.

- **Symptoms/Exam:** This "length-dependent" neuropathy affects the longest nerves first, initially producing paresthesias and pain in the feet; progression leads to a "stocking-glove" distribution of sensory and motor deficits. Sensory, motor, and autonomic nerves can be affected, with sensory symptoms predominating.
- **Treatment:** Prevention of onset or progression depends on tight glycemic control. Neuropathic pain symptoms (burning, pain) can be treated with

TCAs such as amitriptyline and with anticonvulsants such as gabapentin or carbamazepine.

METABOLIC/INFECTIOUS NEUROPATHIES

Many insidious and chronic polyneuropathies are **metabolic** in nature, with common causes being nutritional deficiencies (e.g., vitamin B_{12}), toxin exposure (e.g., alcohol), and drug exposure (e.g., vincristine, INH, dapsone). In addition, many **infections** cause indolent polyneuropathies, including HIV and HSV; leprosy (Hansen's disease, caused by *Mycobacterium leprae*) remains one of the most common causes of polyneuropathy worldwide.

Mononeuropathies

CARPAL TUNNEL SYNDROME

The most common mononeuropathy; caused by compression of the **median nerve** at the carpal ligament of the wrist. Risk factors include repetitive hand-finger activities such as typing.

- **Symptoms:** Classic symptoms include progressive wrist pain; awakening at night with hand numbness; and paresthesias and weakness of the thumb and index finger.
- **Exam:**
  - Findings include **atrophy of the thenar eminence** (the palmar muscle bulk at the base of the thumb), weakness of thumb opposition, and sensory abnormalities of the thumb and index finger.
  - Two classic bedside tests for carpal tunnel are **Phalen's sign** (hyperflexion of the wrists leading to increased paresthesias) and **Tinel's sign** (tapping over the median nerve at the level of the wrist eliciting electrical radiating sensations along the thumb and index finger).
- **Diagnosis:** NCS provides the best objective test for median nerve abnormalities at the wrist.
- **Treatment:** Options include immobilization with wrist splints, NSAIDs, local steroid injections, and surgical release of the carpal ligament.

Patients with carpal tunnel syndrome often find relief "wringing" their hands.

RADIAL NERVE PALSY

Typically results from acute injury to the nerve in the spiral groove of the humerus, most commonly by **fracture of the humerus** or direct compression of the nerve ("**Saturday night palsy**").

- **Symptoms/Exam:** The most prominent symptom is "**wrist drop**" due to paralysis of the wrist extensor muscles; weakness of elbow extension (triceps) is also common.
- **Diagnosis:** NCS helps identify the exact location and extent of the injury.

ULNAR NEUROPATHY

This is an overuse injury, commonly caused by repetitive elbow flexion during the course of the day leading to trauma or compression at the elbow, particularly near the medial epicondyle. Common in thin women.

- **Symptoms/Exam:** Presents with paresthesias involving the fourth and fifth fingers, with weakness of the muscles that spread the fingers apart (the interossei), leading to the appearance of a **"claw hand."**

- **Treatment: Splinting the elbows** at night is first-line treatment and is most helpful in conjunction with NSAIDs if there is pain. Surgical release of the nerve near the elbow is often tried but not always beneficial.

PERONEAL NERVE COMPRESSION

- **Symptoms/Exam:** Compression of the **peroneal nerve** near the fibular head produces a **"foot drop"** secondary to weakness of foot dorsiflexors, as well as paresthesias along the lateral aspect of the lower leg. Compression can be secondary to frequent leg crossing, trauma, or local masses (e.g., cysts).
- **Treatment:** Involves identifying the risk factors for compression, initiating physical therapy, and using an ankle-foot orthosis; surgery is occasionally needed when a local mass is identified as the etiology of compression.

BELL'S PALSY

An acute-onset, unilateral paralysis of CN VII (the **facial nerve**).

- **Symptoms/Exam:**
  - The upper and lower halves of one-half of the face are affected, resulting in inability to fully close the eye or move the mouth on that side. Facial weakness from a central cause (e.g., a stroke) typically spares the upper half of the face, producing unilateral lower facial weakness.
  - In most cases, the etiology remains unclear, although an infectious or postinfectious cause is considered likely. Ramsay Hunt syndrome, in which unilateral facial paralysis is associated with herpetic blisters in the external auditory canal, supports this hypothesis.
- **Treatment:** Treatment of idiopathic Bell's palsy with steroids and antivirals such as acyclovir remains controversial but is common. Eye protection (artificial tears; use of eye patch at night) is crucial for preventing corneal abrasions.

MYOPATHIES

Diseases of skeletal muscle associated with slowly **progressive, symmetric weakness,** fatigue, and/or pain, classically involving the **proximal extremities.** Patients typically complain of difficulty reaching above their heads, combing their hair, rising from a chair, or walking up and down stairs. Other than pain, **no sensory symptoms** are noted. Major types include inherited, mitochondrial, inflammatory, metabolic, and toxic. Key diagnostic tests are serum CPK, EMG/NCS, and muscle biopsy.

- Patients with **elevated CPK levels** and symptoms suggestive of a myopathy should undergo **EMG/NCS testing,** which can more definitively identify the injury's location (e.g., peripheral nerve vs. neuromuscular junction vs. muscle) and distribution (e.g., proximal vs. distal), thus focusing the differential.
- **Muscle biopsy** is generally reserved for patients in whom EMG identifies a myopathy but not its cause. The target should be a symptomatic muscle (e.g., a proximal muscle such as the deltoid or quadriceps). Like EMG/NCS, muscle biopsy helps determine the location of injury (e.g., peripheral nerve vs. muscle) and its underlying cause.

NEUROLOGY

Inflammatory Myopathies

Presumed autoimmune diseases of skeletal muscles. Major types are **polymyositis, dermatomyositis,** and **inclusion body myositis,** each of which has distinctive patterns of muscle weakness, associated symptoms, and muscle pathology. Both polymyositis and dermatomyositis are most commonly seen in patients 40–60 years of age, occurring twice as frequently in women; inclusion body myositis is most commonly seen in patients > 50 years of age and occurs three times more frequently in men than in women.

POLYMYOSITIS

- Most commonly seen in patients 40–60 years of age, occurring twice as frequently in women than in men.
- **Symptoms/Exam:** Typically presents as slowly progressive, symmetric weakness in the **proximal extremities** and the **neck flexors.** Many patients develop slurred speech as well as muscle pain and tenderness.
- **Diagnosis:**
  - Serum CPK and ESR are usually elevated.
  - EMG shows nonspecific myopathic changes.
  - Muscle biopsy reveals a characteristic pattern and distribution of inflammation that can help distinguish polymyositis from dermatomyositis and inclusion body myositis.
- **Treatment: Initial** treatment is with high-dose prednisone. Patients who fail to respond require more aggressive treatment with immunomodulators such as azathioprine or methotrexate. Overall response to treatment is good, but long-term management may be required.

DERMATOMYOSITIS

- Like polymyositis, most commonly seen in patients 40–60 years of age, occurring twice as frequently in women.
- **Symptoms/Exam:** An inflammatory myopathy characterized by progressive proximal weakness associated with multiple distinct skin changes. These include the following:
  - Periorbital edema and a purplish discoloration **(heliotrope rash)** of the upper eyelids, nose, and cheeks.
  - **Gottron's papules,** the classic purplish papules that develop on the dorsal surface of the MCP and interphalangeal joints.
- **Diagnosis:**
  - As with polymyositis, CPK and ESR are elevated and EMG shows nonspecific myopathic changes. Muscle biopsy shows a distinct pattern of inflammation characteristic of dermatomyositis, helping distinguish it from polymyositis and inclusion body myositis.
  - In children, it is often associated with systemic vasculitis; in adults, it is occasionally the result of a paraneoplastic process from an underlying malignancy. Thus, adults usually have a screening evaluation for underlying malignancy.
- **Treatment:** The treatment of idiopathic dermatomyositis is the same as that of polymyositis.

INCLUSION BODY MYOSITIS

- A unique inflammatory myopathy that primarily affects older men.
- **Symptoms:**

    - Preferentially affects the finger and forearm flexors of the upper extremities and the quadriceps of the lower extremities.
    - Onset is insidious, with most patients complaining of difficulty with finger dexterity and grip strength.
- **Exam:** Presents with prominent wasting of the finger and forearm flexors and quadriceps.
- **Diagnosis:**
    - CPK is often normal; EMG shows nonspecific myopathic changes.
    - Muscle biopsy reveals inflammatory changes as well as the presence of rimmed vacuoles (inclusion bodies) within abnormal muscle fibers.
- **Treatment:** Despite its apparent inflammatory nature, inclusion body myositis does not respond well to either steroids or immunomodulators, and most patients lose the ability to ambulate within 10 years of diagnosis.

Metabolic Myopathies

Multiple endocrine abnormalities are associated with myopathies; CPK is often normal, and EMG shows nonspecific myopathic changes. Hyperthyroidism can lead to severe proximal muscle weakness and atrophy; hypothyroidism usually produces more muscle cramps with delayed relaxation of DTRs, although weakness is actually uncommon. These abnormalities are usually reversible with correction of the thyroid abnormality. Glucocorticoid excess, whether endogenous (e.g., Cushing's) or exogenous (e.g., steroid treatment), produces a myopathy with a typical proximal muscle pattern. Muscle biopsy reveals selective atrophy of type II muscle fibers.

Toxic Myopathies

Many medications are associated with toxic myopathies, and the condition is usually reversible upon withdrawal of the offending toxin. As with other myopathies, the usual pattern is of progressive, symmetric proximal muscle weakness. Common offending medications include statins, cimetidine, penicillamine, chloroquine, niacin, and zidovudine (AZT). Other toxins associated with myopathy include alcohol and heroin.

PARANEOPLASTIC SYNDROMES

Most result either from substances produced by tumor cells or from autoimmune complications of the response of the innate immune system to the cancer. Neurologic paraneoplastic syndromes appear to be caused by antibodies that cross-react with specific neuronal populations (see Table 13-11). Symptom onset is gradual, occurring over weeks to months; constitutional symptoms of the underlying tumor often lag by many months. Neurologic symptoms often become prominent even when the underlying tumor is difficult to detect. Thus, early identification of a neurologic paraneoplastic syndrome provides an opportunity to search for and aggressively treat the underlying tumor.

Lambert-Eaton Myasthenic Syndrome

The classic neurologic paraneoplastic syndrome; described above.

TABLE 13-11. Etiologies and Associated Antibodies of Paraneoplastic Syndromes

SYNDROME	UNDERLYING CANCER	ASSOCIATED ANTIBODY
Lambert-Eaton myasthenic syndrome	Small cell lung cancer	Anti-calcium channel
Subacute cerebellar degeneration	Ovarian cancer	Anti-Yo (Purkinje cells)
Limbic encephalitis	Small cell lung cancer	Anti-Hu
Sensory neuronopathy	Small cell lung cancer	Anti-Hu
Opsoclonus-myoclonus	Breast cancer	Anti-Ri

Subacute Cerebellar Degeneration

Associated with **ovarian cancer** and **anti-Yo antibodies** (which cross-react specifically with cerebellar Purkinje cells). Most patients are middle-aged women who experience subacute-onset, progressive slurred speech as well as ataxia and limb incoordination.

Limbic Encephalitis

Associated with **small cell lung cancer** and **anti-Hu antibodies.** Patients present with subacute behavioral problems, memory difficulties, and focal-onset seizures. The clinical picture is similar to that of HSV encephalitis (both primarily affect the limbic system), but the latter is acute onset and often fulminant, whereas paraneoplastic limbic encephalitis is more subacute and slowly progressive.

Sensory Neuronopathy

Also associated with **small cell lung cancer** and **anti-Hu antibodies.** Patients present with slowly progressive sensory loss that first affects the lower extremities. Neurologic exam reveals preserved motor strength, sensory loss, incoordination related to loss of proprioception, and areflexia.

Opsoclonus-Myoclonus

In adults, associated with **breast cancer** and occasionally small cell lung cancer; in **children,** classically associated with a **neuroblastoma** tumor. The associated antibody is anti-Ri. Patients experience opsoclonus (involuntary, erratic, rapid jerking of the eyes in either the horizontal or vertical direction) and myoclonus (brief, quick, jerklike contractions).

NOTES

CHAPTER 14

Oncology

Jonathan Rosenberg, MD

Chemotherapeutic Drugs

Principles of Chemotherapy

- Chemotherapeutic agents interfere with the mechanisms of cell division. There are two categories:
  - **Cell-cycle-specific drugs:** Methotrexate, vincristine, paclitaxel.
  - **Cell-cycle-nonspecific drugs:** Cyclophosphamide.
- Targets include DNA synthesis, microtubules, and direct DNA damage.

Classes of Drugs

- **Alkylating agents:** Form covalent bonds with DNA, RNA, and proteins (cyclophosphamide, ifosfamide, chlorambucil, cisplatin, carboplatin).
- **Antimetabolites:** Interfere with DNA and RNA synthesis (5-FU, methotrexate, fludarabine, cytarabine, mercaptopurine, thioguanine, cladribine, pentostatin, capecitabine, gemcitabine, hydroxyurea).
- **Natural products:** Bleomycin, daunorubicin, doxorubicin, epirubicin, mitoxantrone, mitomycin, etoposide, vincristine, vinorelbine, vinblastine, paclitaxel, docetaxel, irinotecan, topotecan.
- Table 14-1 outlines the phase dependence of different classes of chemotherapeutic agents.

Patterns of Toxicities

- **Cardiotoxicity:** Cardiomyopathy—dose dependent; evaluate EF prior to therapy.
  - **Anthracyclines:** Doxorubicin, daunorubicin, epirubicin, idarubicin.
  - **Mitoxantrone** (less likely).
- **Pulmonary toxicity:** Pulmonary fibrosis (e.g., bleomycin).
- **Cell-mediated immune defect:** Fludarabine, cladribine, pentostatin.
- **Hemorrhagic cystitis:** Alkylating agents, particularly cyclophosphamide and ifosfamide (mesna is a bladder-protective agent).

TABLE 14-1. Mitotic Phase Dependence of Chemotherapeutic Agents

S-Phase Dependent (Antimetabolites)	M-Phase Dependent	G2-Phase Dependent	G1-Phase Dependent
Capecitabine	Vinblastine	Bleomycin	Asparaginase
Cytarabine	Vincristine	Irinotecan	
Decitabine	Vinorelbine	Topotecan	
Doxorubicin	Etoposide		
Fludarabine	Docetaxel		
Floxuridine	Paclitaxel		
Gemcitabine			
Hydroxyurea			
Mercaptopurine			
Methotrexate			
Procarbazine			

- **Neuropathy:** Paclitaxel, docetaxel, cisplatin, vincristine, vinorelbine, vinblastine.
- **Hand-foot syndrome:** Liposomal doxorubicin, capecitabine, 5-FU.

Imatinib has markedly improved the treatment of CML, GI stromal tumor, and hypereosinophilic syndrome, among others.

TARGETED THERAPIES

Defined as novel agents or standard treatments that have a specific molecular target. May include hormonal therapy (leuprolide, tamoxifen, aromatase inhibitors, bicalutamide), small molecules that target enzymes (gefitinib, imatinib), or monoclonal antibodies (rituximab, trastuzumab, gemtuzumab). Often have fewer and less severe side effects than conventional chemotherapy.

Principles of Oncology

COMBINATION REGIMENS

- **Rationale:**
  - Maximum cell kill within the limits of toxicity.
  - Non-cross-resistance (different drugs lead to different mechanisms of resistance).
  - Synergistic effects between drugs.
- **Dose-dense therapy:** An active research area.
  - Does not let tumor cells recover before the next dose of chemotherapy; prevents "kinetic failures."
  - Minimizes chances for resistance to develop.
  - Still experimental.

RESPONSE TO THERAPY

- **Complete response:** Disappearance of all evidence of disease for at least four weeks.
- **Partial response:** Reduction by at least 50% of the sum of the diameter of all measurable lesions with no new disease appearing, maintained for at least four weeks.
- **Progressive disease:** Any growth of existing disease or new lesions during treatment.

CHEMOTHERAPY RESISTANCE

- **MDR1:** Multidrug resistance gene; encodes a pump that remove toxins from cancer cells.
- **Drug-specific resistance mechanisms:** Upregulation of downstream enzymes, antiapoptotic proteins, etc.

Radiation Therapy

MECHANISM

- Radiation induces ionization in biological tissues.
- Mediated by damage to DNA (cancer cells are less able to repair than normal cells).

ADMINISTRATION

- **External beam radiation therapy:** The most common modality. Toxicities can be minimized by the following:
  - **Conformal radiation therapy:** Shaping the radiation beam to fit the tumor outline precisely.
  - **Intensity-modulated radiation therapy (IMRT):** Shaping the intensity of the radiation beam.
- **Brachytherapy (implants):** The radiation source is implanted within the tumor.
- **Stereotactic radiosurgery:** A three-dimensional technique that delivers the radiation dose in one session, with a high dose of radiation to a very small volume. Used primarily for treating brain tumors.

Surgical Oncology

- Surgical intervention is employed as a therapeutic measure, a diagnostic maneuver, or both.
- **Therapeutic surgical intervention:** May have either curative or palliative intent.
  - Resection is predicated on the ability to achieve negative margins, usually with at least 1 cm of normal tissue if possible, or more in special circumstances.
  - Direct manipulation of tumor is avoided where possible to prevent local recurrence.
- **Diagnostic:** Lymph node biopsy; biopsy of a soft tissue mass.

ONCOLOGIC EMERGENCIES

Superior Vena Cava (SVC) Syndrome

Compression of the SVC by tumor or thrombosis of the SVC.

Lung cancer, especially small cell, is the most common cancer cause of SVC syndrome.

SYMPTOMS

Facial edema or erythema, shortness of breath, orthopnea, hoarseness, arm or neck swelling.

EXAM

Edema of the face, neck, and arms; dilation of upper body veins; plethora of the face.

DIAGNOSIS

CT of the chest and neck, Doppler ultrasound, CXR.

TREATMENT

- Corticosteroids and diuretics provide symptomatic relief of edema and dyspnea.
- Initiate radiotherapy or chemotherapy depending on the malignancy.
- Thrombolytic therapy, stent, or anticoagulation if due to thrombosis.

COMPLICATIONS

Laryngeal and cerebral edema are life-threatening complications.

Spinal Cord Compression

Affects 1–5% of patients with metastatic cancer. Diagnostic and treatment delays are associated with paralysis and loss of bladder and bowel control. Extradural metastases from vertebral involvement press on the spinal cord; more rarely, there is epidural involvement only.

Once patients with spinal cord compression lose their ability to ambulate, they usually do not recover it.

SYMPTOMS

- **Early:** Pain localized to the spine or radicular pain due to nerve root compression. Pain is exacerbated with movement, coughing, lying down, sneezing, or Valsalva/straining. Pain generally precedes functional loss by weeks to months.
- **Late:** Muscle weakness, sensory loss/sensory level, urinary retention, constipation, sphincter dysfunction, paralysis, autonomic dysfunction.

> ***Tumors that commonly metastasize to bone–***
>
> **BLT *with* Mayo, Mustard, and Kosher Pickle**
>
> **B**reast
> **L**ung
> **T**hyroid
> **M**ultiple **M**yeloma
> **K**idney (renal cell) and
> **P**rostate

EXAM

- Tenderness to palpation or percussion over the affected area of the spine.
- Focal neurologic findings, UMN signs, abnormal plantar responses, sensory loss.

DIAGNOSIS

- Conduct a history and neurologic examination.
- **Plain films are not helpful in ruling out cord compression.**
- **MRI** is the gold standard for diagnosis. Gadolinium enhances the ability to visualize epidural metastases without bony involvement.
- If MRI is unavailable, CT scan or CT myelogram can make the diagnosis.

TREATMENT

- Outcome depends on rapid assessment and diagnosis.
- If patients can walk at diagnosis, they will likely preserve their function after appropriate treatment.
- Early steroid administration reduces swelling and pressure on the cord. Administer high-dose bolus dexamethasone 100 mg IV followed by 10–24 mg IV q 6 h.
- Definitive treatment options include immediate surgical decompression, radiation therapy (for radiation-sensitive malignancies), or, rarely, chemotherapy.

Tumor Lysis Syndrome

Rapid release of intracellular contents due to rapid lysis of cancer cells with life-threatening metabolic consequences. Most commonly found in acute leukemias and lymphomas (particularly Burkitt's lymphoma); also seen in bulky metastatic testicular cancer. Almost never seen in other solid tumors.

SYMPTOMS/EXAM

- Hyperuricemia, hyperkalemia, hypocalcemia, hyperphosphatemia.
- Markedly elevated LDH indicates risk of tumor lysis.
- May lead to oliguric renal failure.

DIAGNOSIS

Closely monitor of serum laboratory values, including potassium, uric acid, calcium, phosphorus, and creatinine (q 3–4 h initially; then as clinically indicated).

TREATMENT

- Identify patients at risk before starting chemotherapy.
- Alkalinize urine; give IV hydration.
- Allopurinol should be started before chemotherapy to reduce the level of hyperuricemia (monitor for changes in renal clearance and adjust dose if necessary).
- Treatment is directed at managing electrolyte abnormalities, maintaining adequate hydration, and instituting dialysis if necessary.

Neutropenic Fever

Defined as a fever generally > 38.3°C with an absolute neutrophil count (ANC) of 500/μL or less. An ANC < 100/μL carries the highest risk. Associated with a high susceptibility to rapidly fatal infections. Etiologies are as follows:

- **Bacteria** (gram-negative bacilli, gram-positive cocci): The primary pathogens (increasing in incidence owing to increased use of indwelling catheters).
- **Fungal infections:** More common in patients on broad-spectrum antibacterial therapy, in those on steroids, or after allogeneic bone marrow transplant. The most common fungal pathogens are *Candida* and *Aspergillus.*
- **Viruses:** Viral infections occurring during neutropenia include the herpesviruses (CMV, HSV, VZV, EBV) and respiratory viruses (RSV, influenza A and B, parainfluenza, rhinovirus, adenovirus).

EXAM

Physical examination is directed at uncovering potential sources of infection.

DIAGNOSIS

- Obtain two sets of blood cultures, urine culture, culture of any catheter or catheter drainage, and CXR.
- Additional evaluation is dictated by signs and symptoms.

TREATMENT

- **Initial empiric antibiotic therapy**: Administer broad-spectrum antibiotics covering gram-negative bacilli (including *Pseudomonas*), taking into account local drug resistance patterns.
- **Monotherapy**: Ceftazidime, cefepime, imipenem-cilastatin, meropenem.
- **Combination therapy**: Aminoglycoside + antipseudomonal penicillin +/– β-lactamase inhibitors.
- Vancomycin is generally not used as part of first-line empiric therapy unless:
  - Evidence exists to support gram-positive infection.
  - Patients were receiving quinolones as prophylaxis prior to the onset of neutropenic fever.
  - Blood culture shows gram-positive cocci prior to identification and susceptibility testing.

- **Duration of treatment:**
  - If fever resolves and the organism is identified, coverage can be tailored, but broad-spectrum therapy must continue for at least seven days.
  - If fever resolves and no organism is identified, IV broad-spectrum antibiotics should continue for at least seven days; then consider switching to oral medications.
  - If fever is unresponsive after four days, consider adding vancomycin and/or amphotericin B.

BREAST CANCER

Risk increases with age. The lifetime risk for women is roughly 1 in 10. Risk factors are as follows:

Genetic syndromes markedly increase the risk for breast cancer, though they account for a minority of cases of breast cancer.

- **Genetic syndromes:** Those with a genetic predisposition should be screened beginning at least 10 years before the earliest-onset cancer in the family history.
  - **BRCA1:** Associated with a dramatic risk of breast cancer (56–85% over lifetime), ovarian cancer (15–45% over lifetime), and prostate cancer (less frequent). Autosomal-dominant inheritance.
  - **BRCA2:** Associated with breast and ovarian cancer. Also associated with pancreatic cancer and melanoma.
  - BRCA1 and 2 account for 50% of all inherited breast cancers.
  - **Cowden's syndrome:** PTEN gene mutation. Rare; risk of breast cancer is 25–50% over lifetime.
  - ATM mutation.
  - **Li-Fraumeni syndrome:** Breast cancer along with sarcomas, brain tumors, leukemia, lymphoma, and adrenal cancer.
  - For most patients, no identified genetic predisposition exists.
- **Other risk factors:** Family history of early-age breast cancer diagnosis in family members, early menarche, late menopause, obesity, nulliparity or late age at first pregnancy, estrogen replacement therapy (controversial).
- Tamoxifen can reduce the risk of breast cancer for women at high risk but is associated with an increased risk of blood clots and endometrial cancer.

DIFFERENTIAL

Fibrocystic disease, fibroadenoma, abscess, adenosis, scars, mastitis.

DIAGNOSIS

- Breast cysts can be evaluated with ultrasound and then aspirated.
- Breast masses require either FNA or core needle biopsy, possibly followed by excisional biopsy.
- Any mass that is felt on exam **must** be further evaluated with biopsy even if no abnormality is seen on mammogram.
- **Algorithm:** Mass → bilateral mammogram → tissue sampling → possible further workup depending on tissue findings.

TREATMENT

- **Treatment of early-stage breast cancer is as follows:**
  - **Ductal carcinoma in situ (DCIS):** A premalignant condition that is at high risk of turning into a cancer. Treatment involves excision with negative margins (lumpectomy) and radiation therapy to the breast.
  - **Lobular carcinoma in situ (LCIS):** A condition associated with an increased risk of breast cancer arising elsewhere in the breast. Treatment

with tamoxifen may be considered, but close follow-up and observation are usually indicated.
- **Invasive ductal or lobular carcinoma:**
  - Lumpectomy followed by radiation therapy is equivalent to mastectomy.
  - **Sentinel lymph node:** Injecting dye or tracer in the tumor and identifying which lymph node takes it up. The node or nodes are excised and assessed for metastasis. Axillary node dissection may then be warranted only in sentinel-node or clinically node-positive tumors.
  - Mastectomy for large tumors or for patient preference.
- **Determining who needs adjuvant therapy:**
  - In general, any patient with an **infiltrating** ductal or lobular cancer > 1 cm or with **positive lymph nodes** should receive adjuvant therapy.
  - Hormone therapy with **tamoxifen** (for **five years**) is effective **only** in patients with **estrogen- or progesterone-receptor-positive** (ER- or PR-positive) breast cancers.
  - Tamoxifen reduces the risk of recurrence by about 40%.
  - Polychemotherapy reduces the risk of recurrence by 25%.

- **Treatment of advanced (metastatic) breast cancer is as follows:**
  - **First-line treatment** for ER/PR-positive postmenopausal women is an aromatase inhibitor. Aromatase inhibitors prevent conversion of adrenal androgens into estrogens by aromatase enzymes in muscle and fat.
  - **Second-line hormonal therapy** includes megestrol acetate or tamoxifen.
  - If patients progress or are **hormone receptor negative,** treat with chemotherapy.
    - Initial chemotherapy can be multiagent, but once patients progress after first-line treatment, single-agent treatment is commonly used.
    - Active drugs include paclitaxel, docetaxel, doxorubicin, methotrexate, vinorelbine, capecitabine, and 5-FU.
  - Trastuzumab (Herceptin) is a humanized monoclonal antibody against the HER2 receptor found on breast cancer cells.
  - Overexpression of HER2 is associated with a poorer prognosis in breast cancer. Patients with HER2 overexpression (3+ by immunohistochemistry or gene amplification by fluorescence in situ hybridization) show responses to trastuzumab alone or in combination with chemotherapy.

PREVENTION

Screening recommendations are as follows:

- **Breast self-exam:** Data on efficacy conflict, but it is generally recommended that monthly exams start at age 20.
- **Clinical breast exam:** Annual after age 40; every three years between 20 and 40 years of age.
- **Mammography:** Every 1–2 years starting at 40; annually after age 50.

LUNG CANCER

The best way to prevent lung cancer (and recurrent lung cancer) is smoking cessation. Eighty-seven percent of all cases of lung cancer are related to smoking (risk is very high in patients who have been exposed to asbestos and who also smoke).

- Presents with weight loss, cough, hemoptysis, fatigue, recurrent bronchitis, and chest pain.
- Divided into two categories based on pathology and natural history (see below).

Non–Small Cell Lung Cancer (NSCLC)

The most common lung cancer; has multiple histologies (bronchoalveolar, adeno, and squamous), all with the same treatment and natural history. Squamous cell cancers cavitate and cause hypercalcemia due to parathyroid hormone–related protein (PTHrP) secretion. **Accurate staging is key to determining proper therapy.**

DIAGNOSIS

CXR, CT of the chest and abdomen, blood work (including liver panel), possibly PET scan.

TREATMENT

- Treat according to stage.
  - **Stage I or II:** Consider surgical resection.
  - **Stage IIIA (spread to ipsilateral mediastinal lymph nodes):** May warrant resection. Adjuvant chemotherapy may be administered after surgery.
  - **Stage IIIB (spread to contralateral mediastinal lymph nodes):** Consider chemotherapy and radiation.
  - **Stage IV (metastatic disease):** Chemotherapy has been shown to improve quality of life and modestly prolong survival compared with the best supportive care.
- Other commonly used drugs for NSCLC include cisplatin, carboplatin, paclitaxel, docetaxel, gemcitabine, and vinorelbine.

Majority of paraneoplastic syndromes are seen with small cell lung cancer. The exception is hypercalcemia due to PTHrP secretion which is due to squamous cell cancer.

Small Cell Lung Cancer (SCLC)

Characterized by early metastasis; surgical resection is not part of therapy. Often associated with neuroendocrine and paraneoplastic features.

DIAGNOSIS

Has two stages:

- **Limited:** All the visible cancer can be encompassed by a single radiation port in the chest.
- **Extensive:** Anything that is not limited.

TREATMENT

- Chemotherapy and radiation given together improve outcomes in limited-stage disease, but prognosis is still poor.
- Chemotherapy alone is the treatment of choice for patients with extensive-stage disease, yielding high response rates, but virtually all patients relapse.
- Since SCLC has high rates of brain metastasis (up to 35%), prophylactic cranial irradiation should be considered in all patients with a complete response to chemotherapy or chemoradiotherapy.
- Drugs of choice include etoposide, cisplatin, irinotecan, and topotecan.

MESOTHELIOMA

A neoplasm arising from the mesothelial surfaces of the peritoneum and pleural cavities, pericardium, and tunica vaginalis. Asbestos exposure increases risk. Smoking and asbestos exposure are synergistic.

Symptoms/Exam

Presents with dyspnea and nonpleuritic chest pain.

Diagnosis

- Thoracocentesis or pleural biopsy. Occasionally video-assisted thoracoscopic (VATS) biopsy is needed.
- Approximately 60% have right-sided disease on x-ray; 5% are bilateral. Most commonly presents with large unilateral pleural effusion.

Treatment

- Surgical resection if possible.
- Debulking of tumor, thoracocentesis, pleurodesis, supportive measures to decrease the impact of pleural-based disease.
- Chemotherapy is only modestly effective.

THYMOMA

An anterior mediastinal tumor that is often detected during workup of myasthenia gravis. Most are benign, but some progress to thymic carcinoma. Other paraneoplastic syndromes associated with thymoma include pure red cell aplasia.

Thirty percent of patients with myasthenia gravis will have thymoma.

Differential

Germ cell tumor, lymphoma, thyroid mass.

Treatment

Resection is the most effective treatment. If spread occurs outside the mediastinum, chemotherapy and radiation therapy may be used as well, but with limited efficacy.

SQUAMOUS CELL CARCINOMA OF THE HEAD AND NECK

Many of these cancers are curable. Major risk factors include tobacco (cigarettes, chewing tobacco, cigars), alcohol use, and HPV. Lesions progress as follows: leukoplakia → erythroplakia → dysplasia → carcinoma in situ → carcinoma.

Symptoms

Hoarse voice, globus sensation, otalgia, a sore in the mouth or throat, a lump in the throat, numbness in the face or throat, odynophagia, dysphagia, lymphadenopathy, tinnitus.

Exam

Evaluate the scalp, cranial nerves, lymph nodes, and oral cavity.

Diagnosis

- Pan-upper endoscopy to evaluate the entire aerodigestive tract.
- FNA is standard for neck nodes.
- Core needle biopsy is not done on newly diagnosed lesions owing to concerns over tumor recurrence in the needle tract.
- MRI or CT of the head and neck; CXR.

Treatment

Treatment depends on the anatomical site (e.g., oral cavity, base of tongue, oropharynx, pharynx, hypopharynx, larynx).

- **Early-stage tumors in the oral cavity, base of tongue, or lips:** May be treated with radiation or surgery alone.
- **Early-stage tumors of the oropharynx:** Radiation is the preferred modality.
- In the presence of cervical lymph node involvement, treat with surgery, radiation, or chemoradiation.
- For some patients with laryngeal cancer, voice-sparing treatments (partial laryngectomy, chemoradiotherapy) should be considered, as many (25%) can avoid laryngectomy.
- Commonly used chemotherapeutic agents include cisplatin and 5-FU.

NASOPHARYNGEAL CARCINOMA

Associated with EBV infection, not tobacco or alcohol. Endemic to China and parts of Africa.

Symptoms/Exam

Presents with a change in hearing, a sensation of ear stuffiness, tinnitus, nasal obstruction, and a mass in the neck.

Diagnosis

Same as that for squamous cell carcinoma of the head and neck.

Treatment

Not a surgical disease; requires chemotherapy (cisplatin) with concurrent radiation. Two-thirds of patients are cured.

THYROID CANCER

Thyroid nodules are more common in women than in men. A solitary thyroid nodule is found in 10–20% of cases. Risk is related to radiation exposure. There are four subtypes:

Medullary cancer can produce elevated levels of calcitonin and is often associated with MEN 2A or 2B.

- **Papillary:** Carries the best prognosis.
- **Follicular:** Has the second-best prognosis.
- **Medullary: From C cells of the thyroid** associated with MEN 2A and MEN 2B-RET proto-oncogenes.
- **Anaplastic:** Has a poor prognosis.
- Follicular and papillary are the most common diagnoses (> 90%).

Symptoms/Exam

Most thyroid cancers present as asymptomatic thyroid nodules; rarely, they may present with change in voice or lymphadenopathy.

DIAGNOSIS

- FNA of the nodule.
- A thyroid isotope scan can differentiate "hot" from "cold" nodules. Most cancers occur in cold nodules, but only 10% of cold nodules are malignant.
- Obtain calcitonin level to rule out medullary carcinoma.

TREATMENT

- **Local disease:** Thyroidectomy; possible lymph node sampling.
- Radioactive iodine is used to treat patients with high-risk tumors after surgery or metastatic disease, as these tumors take up iodine.

ESOPHAGEAL CANCER

Risk factors include cigarette smoking, alcohol use, obesity, and Barrett's esophagus.

SYMPTOMS/EXAM

Dysphagia, odynophagia, weight loss, cough, hoarseness.

DIAGNOSIS

- **Staging evaluation:** Endoscopy and biopsy, chest CT, endoscopic ultrasound, bronchoscopy (to rule out tracheal invasion).
- **Pathology:** Squamous cell and adenocarcinoma (increasing in incidence; associated with obesity)

TREATMENT

- **Localized esophageal cancer:** Treat with chemoradiation (5-FU + cisplatin and external beam radiotherapy) or surgery. Postoperative chemoradiation should be considered for locally advanced cancers.
- **Metastatic disease:** Few good options are available; drugs include cisplatin, paclitaxel, 5-FU, and gemcitabine.

GASTRIC CANCER

The most common cancer in China; associated with a diet of smoked and pickled foods that is high in nitrates and low in vegetables. Working in coal mining and in nickel, rubber, and timber processing are also risk factors.

SYMPTOMS/EXAM

Pain, anorexia, weight loss, vomiting, GI bleeding.

DIAGNOSIS

- Endoscopy and biopsy.
- Staging evaluation includes CT of the chest, abdomen, and pelvis as well as endoscopic ultrasound.
- Adenocarcinoma is the predominant histology.

TREATMENT

- Surgery is the preferred therapy for resectable gastric cancer.
- Adjuvant chemoradiotherapy for patients with locally advanced gastric cancer is indicated after surgery.

- Treat metastatic gastric cancer with chemotherapeutic agents such as ECF (epirubicin, cisplatin, 5-FU).

Gastrointestinal Stromal Tumors (GISTs)

Sarcoma of the stomach wall. Associated with an activating mutation in the c-kit oncogene.

Treatment

- Standard treatment is surgery.
- Conventional chemotherapy is ineffective.
- For patients with metastatic GIST, targeted therapy with imatinib (Gleevec); inhibits c-kit, leading to dramatic and prolonged responses in patients with previously untreatable and incurable disease.

PANCREATIC CANCER

A highly lethal cancer. Has a median survival of 9–12 months and a five-year survival of 3%. At diagnosis, > 50% are metastatic or unresectable. Risk factors include tobacco exposure and DM.

Symptoms/Exam

- Presents with pain, jaundice, glucose intolerance, palpable gallbladder (Courvoisier's sign).
- Painless jaundice is a sign of intrapancreatic bile duct obstruction and may allow early detection of resectable disease.
- **Serum marker:** CA 19-9.

Diagnosis

- CT of the abdomen with fine cuts through the pancreas.
- Endoscopic ultrasound.
- Endoscopic retrograde cholangiopancreatography (ERCP).

Treatment

- The only curative therapy is pancreaticoduodenectomy (Whipple procedure).
- **What is resectable:** Disease that does not involve the major vessels or celiac axis, with no distant metastases.
- **Adjuvant therapy after the Whipple procedure:** Chemoradiation with 5-FU.
- Treatment for unresectable patients includes the following:
  - Palliation of symptoms with chemotherapy (gemcitabine), radiation, biliary stent, or choledochojejunostomy to decrease jaundice.
  - Nerve block to the celiac plexus may relieve pain.
- **Advanced pancreatic cancer:** Gemcitabine gives symptom relief but is associated with a low response rate.

CARCINOID TUMORS

The majority of carcinoid tumors are hormonally inert, but some can secrete excessive serotonin, prostaglandins, kinins, and the like. The most common are carcinoids of the small bowel.

Symptoms/Exam

Flushing, diarrhea, abdominal cramps, bronchospasm, valvular heart disease.

Diagnosis

- Assess 24-hour urine for 5-HIAA.
- Indium-labeled octreotide scan can detect occult lesions.

Treatment

Primarily surgical removal, although somatostatin analogs (e.g., octreotide) have activity in controlling symptoms.

HEPATOCELLULAR CARCINOMA

Risk factors include HBV (especially vertical transmission), HCV, alcohol abuse (especially in combination with HCV), hemochromatosis, α_1-antitrypsin deficiency, and androgen and estrogen therapy.

Diagnosis

- High-risk patients should be screened with α-fetoprotein (AFP) and hepatic ultrasound, although the appropriate interval has not been established.
- Markedly elevated AFP in concert with imaging findings and risk factors may be diagnostic.
- The fibrolamellar variant is associated with the best prognosis.

Treatment

- Resection is the treatment of choice if liver function is adequate and anatomy permits.
- Patients with cirrhosis may be offered transplant for single tumors < 5 cm or three tumors < 3 cm each.
- Chemoembolization, intratumoral ethanol injection, cryotherapy, and radiofrequency ablation are all options for unresectable patients.
- There is no standard chemotherapy with proven efficacy.

COLORECTAL CANCER

Genetic syndromes include the following:

- **Hereditary nonpolyposis colorectal cancer (HNPCC):** Characterized by few polyps (nonpolyposis); associated with endometrial, gastric, renal, ovarian, and skin cancer and with mismatch repair genes MLH1/2 and MSH1/2.
- **Familial adenomatous polyposis (FAP):** Characterized by thousands of polyps; the treatment of choice is colectomy. Associated with a mutation in the APC gene.
- **Li-Fraumeni syndrome:** Associated with the p53 mutation.

Remember, HNPCC has few polyps, but FAP has thousands of polyps and thus treatment for FAP is colectomy.

Symptoms/Exam

Presentation is highly variable. May be asymptomatic or present with symptoms ranging from abdominal pain to colon obstruction to lower GI bleeding.

Lymph node involvement by colon cancer implies at least stage III disease and merits adjuvant chemotherapy.

TREATMENT

- **Treat according to stage.**
  - **Stage I:** Partial colectomy; no further therapy.
  - **Stage II:** Partial colectomy; no standard therapy. Consider adjuvant chemotherapy for certain high-risk features (obstruction, perforation, very large tumors).
  - **Stage III:** Partial colectomy. These lymph node–involved cancers all merit adjuvant chemotherapy. The standard is 5-FU or 5-FU/leucovorin/oxaliplatin.
  - **Stage IV:** Palliative colectomy or colon diversion to prevent obstruction. Chemotherapy for metastatic disease is generally palliative. The exception is stage IV due to a solitary hepatic metastasis, which may be cured with surgery +/– chemotherapy.
- **Chemotherapy:** Two medications are the backbone of chemotherapy for colon cancer:
  - **5-FU:** Converted to F-dUMP; inhibits thymidine production and interferes with DNA synthesis.
  - **Leucovorin (folinic acid):** Stabilizes the bond between F-dUMP and thymidylate synthetase, enhancing the efficacy of 5-FU.
  - Other drugs include irinotecan, oxaliplatin, cetuximab (an anti-EGFR antibody), and bevacizumab (an anti-VEGF antibody).
- **Rectal cancer:** Owing to the anatomy of the rectum, surgical approaches have less room for adequate margins. Therefore, radiation therapy is often given after surgery in addition to or in combination with chemotherapy.

PREVENTION

Annual fecal occult blood test (FOBT); sigmoidoscopy every three to five years or colonoscopy every ten years starting at age 50.

PROSTATE CANCER

The most common cancer diagnosed in men. A positive family history and African-American ethnicity are both risk factors.

SYMPTOMS/EXAM

- Often associated with urinary obstruction and concurrent prostatitis.
- **Screening measures** are as follows:
  - All patients with nodules warrant biopsy.
  - Those with a PSA > 4 merit biopsy.
  - A PSA that is < 4 but rapidly rising should be considered for biopsy.
  - **Percent free PSA:** A lower percent free PSA is associated with a higher risk of prostate cancer being present. May help in patients with a PSA < 4 in determining whether to biopsy.

DIAGNOSIS

- DRE, transrectal ultrasound biopsy.
- **Gleason score:** Evaluation of grade under the microscope; graded from 2 to 10, with 2 being almost benign and 10 being highly aggressive. Has a prognostic impact on outcomes in almost every stage of prostate cancer.

Treatment

- Three major options are available for the treatment of **localized prostate cancer:**
  - **Watchful waiting:** For patients with significant comorbidities, elderly patients, or those with indolent disease.
  - **External beam radiation therapy:** For patients with a risk of extraprostatic spread or contraindications to surgery.
  - **Brachytherapy:** Implantation of radioactive seeds in the prostate gland.
  - **Radical prostatectomy:** For patients with long life expectancies a high likelihood that cancer is confined to the prostate.

Most men die with their prostate cancer, not from it.

- **Advanced prostate cancer** (recurrence after local therapies or metastatic disease) is treated in the following manner:
  - The most effective medical therapy is **androgen deprivation.** Methods are as follows:
    - Bilateral orchiectomy.
    - LHRH agonists (suppress testosterone secretion by inhibiting FSH/LH release from the pituitary).
    - LHRH agonists + oral antiandrogen = combined androgen blockade.
    - High-dose oral antiandrogens are least proven but have fewer side effects.
    - Medical complications of androgen deprivation include hot flashes, anemia, weight gain, osteopenia, and osteoporosis.
- **Hormone-refractory prostate cancer** warrants the following approach:
  - Treat with chemotherapy using mitoxantrone or docetaxel.
  - Adjunctive therapy with zoledronic acid (bisphosphonate) to strengthen bones and prevent skeletal complications.

Decision to screen for prostate cancer should include a thorough discussion with patient about risks (false positives, bleeding, uncertain efficacy in reducing death from prostate cancer) and benefits (earlier diagnosis and treatment may improve survival).

Prevention

Annual DRE and PSA starting at age 50 (controversial) or age 40 for African-Americans and those with a positive family history.

KIDNEY CANCER

Risk factors include obesity, smoking, and von Hippel–Lindau syndrome (associated with retinal angiomas, CNS hemangioblastomas, and kidney cancer).

Exam/Diagnosis

- Must be ruled out in the workup of hematuria.
- Involves IVP or CT with contrast.
- Rarely, patients may present with polycythemia due to excess erythropoietin production.

Treatment

- For localized disease, treatment is nephrectomy.
- No adjuvant therapy has been proven beneficial.
- Cytokine-based therapy (IL-2, interferon) can cause regression of tumors in metastatic disease (10–20%).
- Nephrectomy may be indicated in the setting of metastatic disease if the kidney tumor itself represents the bulk of the cancer.

TESTICULAR CANCER

The most common cancer in younger men aged 15–35; a secondary peak occurs in men > 60 years of age. Undescended testicle is a major risk factor. Other risk factors include prior testicular cancer, Klinefelter's syndrome, and a positive family history. The five-year survival rate for all patients with germ cell tumors is about 95%.

SYMPTOMS/EXAM

- Scrotal mass; low back pain (from retroperitoneal lymphadenopathy).
- Testicular pain does **not** indicate a benign etiology.

DIAGNOSIS

- Approximately 10% present as extragonadal germ cell tumors with no testis primary.
- Evaluate with testicular ultrasound to identify a mass.
- Never biopsy the testis; an inguinal orchiectomy is needed to make the diagnosis.
- Serum markers elevated in 80% of germ cell patients are AFP and β-hCG.
- There are two major pathologic classifications:
  - **Seminoma:** Never has an elevated AFP; may have elevated β-hCG.
  - **Nonseminoma:** Includes embryonal carcinoma, yolk sac carcinoma, choriocarcinoma, teratoma, and seminoma when it is combined with these other histologies. May have elevated AFP and β-hCG.

TREATMENT

The treatment of germ cell cancers is determined by prognostic features and stage.

- **Early-stage seminoma:**
  - If disease is limited to the testis, treat with inguinal orchiectomy alone.
  - Observation, chemotherapy, and radiation therapy are all appropriate if the patient is felt to be at high risk for retroperitoneal lymph node metastasis.
  - If there is evidence of retroperitoneal metastasis on imaging, treat with radiotherapy.
- **Advanced seminoma:** Chemotherapy is standard and results in high cure rates (> 85%).
- **Early-stage nonseminoma:** Inguinal orchiectomy +/– retroperitoneal lymph node dissection and +/– adjuvant chemotherapy.
- **Advanced nonseminoma:** Treat with chemotherapy; results are almost as good as those with seminoma.
- Adverse prognostic factors include high tumor markers, presence of visceral metastasis outside the lungs (e.g., liver, soft tissue, brain), and a mediastinal primary site.
- **Chemotherapy regimens for germ cell tumors** include bleomycin, etoposide, and cisplatin (BEP) or etoposide and cisplatin (EP).
- Intensive follow-up is essential, as even relapsed patients have high rates of cure. Follow-up regimens include CT scans, markers, and physical examination at frequent intervals.

COMPLICATIONS

- Fertility problems persist in 50% of germ cell tumor patients and are thought to be related to underlying pathology as much as to treatment.

- Other long-term complications include increased cardiovascular disease, hypertension, and secondary malignancies (new testicular primary or secondary acute leukemia are the most likely).

BLADDER CANCER

Risk factors include cigarette smoking, analgesic abuse (phenacetin), chronic urinary tract inflammation, and Balkan nephropathy (a rare inherited disorder).

SYMPTOMS/EXAM

Hematuria, difficulty voiding, renal failure, bladder irritation/pain.

DIAGNOSIS

- Cystoscopy and biopsy, cytology, CT of the abdomen and pelvis, CXR, and bone scan if alkaline phosphatase is elevated.
- The most common pathology in the United States is transitional cell carcinoma, although squamous cell carcinoma is also found, most frequently in parts of the world where schistosomiasis is common.

TREATMENT

- **Superficial bladder cancer** (not penetrating into the detrusor muscle): Treat with local therapies such as excision, intravesical BCG, or intravesical chemotherapy.
- **Muscle invasive bladder cancer:** Radical cystectomy.
- Neoadjuvant combination chemotherapy may reduce the risk of recurrence and improve survival.
- Adjuvant chemotherapy is not yet proven but is often administered.
- For metastatic disease, the standard of care is gemcitabine and cisplatin as first-line chemotherapy.

CERVICAL CANCER

Almost half of women with cervical cancer are diagnosed before age 35. Risk factors include sexual activity at an early age, HPV infection (subtypes 16, 18, 31, 33, and 35), multiple partners, cigarette smoking, and concurrent HIV infection.

SYMPTOMS

The most common presenting symptom is vaginal bleeding between menses.

DIAGNOSIS

- Colposcopy and biopsy.
- The majority are squamous cell, although adenocarcinoma accounts for 20% of all cervical cancers.

TREATMENT

- Options for early-stage disease include radiation therapy, cone excisional biopsy, and simple hysterectomy.
- For more advanced disease, combined chemotherapy and radiation therapy is standard; radical hysterectomy/pelvic exenteration is also used.

PREVENTION

- Although the Pap smear has dramatically reduced the incidence of invasive cervical cancer in the United States, the disease remains a major cause of morbidity and mortality in underdeveloped nations.
- It is recommended that all women ≥ 18 years of age receive annual Pap smears.

ENDOMETRIAL CANCER

The most common genital tract malignancy in women; occurs primarily in postmenopausal women. Risks include unopposed estrogen (either endogenous or exogenous), obesity (due to increased aromatization of androgens to estrogens), and high levels of animal fat in diet. Childbearing reduces the risk; tamoxifen carries an increased risk after five years of use.

SYMPTOMS/EXAM

Postmenopausal uterine bleeding always requires evaluation.

DIAGNOSIS

- Transvaginal ultrasound, endometrial sampling, or dilation and curettage.
- Adenocarcinoma (endometrioid) is the most common.

TREATMENT

- Radical hysterectomy, bilateral salpingo-oophorectomy, and lymph node sampling are the treatment of choice, with adjuvant radiation therapy for selected patients.
- Progestins and doxorubicin/cisplatin play a role in treating metastatic disease.

OVARIAN CANCER

Epithelial ovarian cancer arises from cells that coat the ovary, which are similar to peritoneal epithelial cells. Risk is reduced by multiparity, OCP use, breastfeeding, and tubal ligation. BRCA1, BRCA2, and HNPCC are genetic risk factors; a positive family history is a risk factor even in the absence of a genetic syndrome.

SYMPTOMS/EXAM

- There are very few symptoms in early-stage disease.
- Increased abdominal girth, early satiety, rectal pressure, and urinary frequency are found in advanced disease.

DIAGNOSIS

- Close surveillance is warranted for patients with a genetic predisposition.
- Although an optimal regimen has not been identified, annual examination, transvaginal ultrasound, and CA-125 are often performed and prophylactic oophorectomy considered.
- Different pathologies are associated with different prognoses:
  - Mucinous and clear cell cancers have a poorer prognosis.
  - Borderline tumors have a good prognosis.

TREATMENT

- TAH-BSO.
- Early-stage tumors can be treated with adjuvant chemotherapy (often paclitaxel/carboplatin) for high-risk features.
- Advanced tumors require surgical debulking of peritoneal metastasis followed by chemotherapy.
- The treatment of ovarian germ cell tumors is similar to that of testicular cancer.

SARCOMA

Sarcomas are a heterogeneous group of cancers of mesenchymal tissue. Genetic risk factors include familial retinoblastoma associated with osteosarcoma. Other risk factors include prior radiation therapy and chronic lymphedema. Subtypes are as follows:

- **Bone sarcomas:**
  - **Osteosarcoma:** Affects long bones in children and adolescents; associated with Paget's disease in the elderly.
  - **Chondrosarcomas:** Affects older adults.
  - **Malignant fibrous histiocytoma:** Affects older adults.
  - **Ewing's sarcoma:** Affects children and adolescents, classically arising in the diaphysis.
- **Soft tissue sarcomas:** Sites involved include the extremities, trunk, retroperitoneum, and visceral organs (e.g., leiomyosarcomas, GI stromal tumors).

SYMPTOMS/EXAM

Symptoms depend on the site but often include swelling and pain of the extremities.

DIAGNOSIS

- FNA or open biopsy.
- Needle tract from biopsy must be excised at surgery to prevent seeding of tumor.
- MRI is often more effective at imaging sarcomas.
- Sarcomas rarely metastasize to the lymph nodes; the most common metastatic site is the lung.

TREATMENT

- Most bone sarcomas receive neoadjuvant chemotherapy followed by wide excision and then postoperative chemotherapy.
- Pre- and postoperative chemotherapy for other sarcomas is controversial but is often administered.
- Radiotherapy is often given after surgery to achieve local tumor control.
- Limb salvage procedures should be attempted when possible.
- Patients with surgically resectable metastases should undergo surgery, which may cure selected patients.
- Ewing's sarcoma is highly sensitive to combination chemotherapy; five-year survival rates are high.
- Give combination chemotherapy for metastatic disease; MAID (mesna, Adriamycin, ifosfamide, and DTIC) is the current regimen of choice.

ANAL CANCER

The most common histologies are squamous cell and cloacogenic (transitional cell), which behave similarly. The least common type is large bowel cancer, which is associated with high cure rates. The major risk factor is anal intercourse leading to HPV infection; potentiated by HIV infection, genital warts are a risk factor.

HIV and genital warts due to HPV are independent and additive risk factors for anal cancer.

SYMPTOMS/EXAM

- Patients often present with anal bleeding, pain, or the sensation of a mass in the anal canal.
- Lymph node drainage is to the inguinal lymph nodes, which are the first site of metastasis.
- Spreads stepwise from the anus to the inguinal lymph nodes and then hematogenously to the liver.

TREATMENT

- Very small tumors can be surgically removed.
- Larger tumors or those with spread to the lymph nodes require chemoradiotherapy.

PREVENTION

Screen with anal Pap smear in high-risk patients.

PRIMARY BRAIN TUMORS

Characterized by a bimodal age distribution; affect pediatric patients and those > 20 years of age (peak between 75 and 85 years). Subtypes are as follows:

- **Gliomas:** Most common; range from low grade to high grade (glioblastoma multiforme). Genetic syndromes that may predispose include tuberous sclerosis, NF1, Turcot's syndrome, and Li-Fraumeni syndrome, but these are rare causes.
- **Meningiomas:** Benign tumors that cause morbidity by mass effect.

> ***Tumors that metastasize to brain—***
>
> ***"Lots of Bad Stuff Kills Glia"***
>
> **L**ung
> **B**reast
> **S**kin (melanoma)
> **K**idney (renal cell CA)
> **G**I

SYMPTOMS/EXAM

- Presents with symptoms referable to ICP (headache, nausea, vomiting).
- Neurologic deficits, seizures, and strokelike phenomena are also seen.

DIAGNOSIS

Diagnosis is best made on MRI followed by biopsy or surgical resection.

TREATMENT

- Surgery is the definitive therapy for brain tumors.
- Radiation may be considered for recurrent disease.
- Stereotactic or gamma-knife radiotherapy may be used for small tumors,
- Chemotherapy has limited utility in malignant gliomas, although oligodendrogliomas are highly chemosensitive (associated with chromosome 1p and 19q loss).
- Chemotherapeutic agents for primary brain tumors include temozolomide and combination PCV (procarbazine, CCNU, vincristine).

BRAIN METASTASES

Occur in 15% of patients with solid tumors; most common in lung and breast cancer. In general, metastases point to a poor prognosis.

Metastasis reaches the brain via hematogenous spread, often passing through the lung first, so check a CXR in any patient with brain metastasis.

TREATMENT

- Patients with a solitary metastasis and no other evidence of cancer may be candidates for surgical resection followed by whole brain radiotherapy to prevent new metastases.
- For patients with multiple brain metastases, whole brain radiotherapy is the treatment of choice.
- Stereotactic radiosurgery or gamma-knife radiotherapy may be considered for those with solitary or few metastases.
- Brain metastases usually respond poorly to systemic chemotherapy.

CARCINOMA OF AN UNKNOWN PRIMARY SITE

Comprise 5% of all cancer diagnoses. Subsets of patients can benefit from treatment.

DIAGNOSIS

- Pathologic evaluation is the key component of workup.
- Immunohistochemical stains or electron microscopy may reveal the likely tissue of origin.
- Evaluation focuses on age- and gender-specific risk factors:
  - CT of the chest, abdomen, and pelvis.
  - Mammography and breast examination in women.
  - Testicular examination, DRE, and PSA testing in men.
  - Colonoscopy in all.

TREATMENT

Some special scenarios are as follows:

- **Women with axillary lymph nodes containing adenocarcinoma:** Should be treated like breast cancer—with mastectomy and axillary lymph node dissection; consider adjuvant therapy.
- **Patients with cervical lymph nodes and squamous cell carcinoma:** Should be treated like squamous cell cancer of the head and neck after thorough ENT evaluation.
- **Patients with inguinal lymph nodes and squamous cell carcinoma:** Careful evaluation of the anal canal, the penis in men, and the vagina, uterus, cervix, and vulva in women.
- **Young men with poorly differentiated carcinoma and mediastinal or retroperitoneal mass:** Treat as germ cell tumor patients; evaluate for occult testicular cancer.
- **Men with bone metastasis:** Evaluate with PSA testing for prostate cancer.
- **Women with peritoneal carcinomatosis:** Treat as if they have ovarian cancer.
- **Chemotherapy regimen for patients not falling into the above categories:** Etoposide and a platinum (cisplatin or carboplatin). Addition of paclitaxel may improve response and survival.

ACUTE LEUKEMIAS

Genetic disorders associated with acute leukemia include Down's syndrome, Bloom's syndrome, Fanconi's anemia, and ataxia-telangiectasia. Risk factors include chemical exposure (benzene, petroleum products), hair dyes, smoking, and prior chemotherapy or radiation.

SYMPTOMS/EXAM

Suppression of normal hematopoiesis (anemia, leukopenia, thrombocytopenia), bone pain, leukostasis (with very high WBC counts).

DIAGNOSIS

Evaluation of peripheral blood smear, bone marrow aspirate and biopsy, immunohistochemistry, cytogenetic evaluation, flow cytometry.

Acute Lymphoblastic Leukemia (ALL)

May have either B- (75%) or T-cell lineage. The Philadelphia chromosome t(9;22) is common and points to a poor prognosis. Adult ALL is more aggressive and less curable than childhood ALL. Patients with T-cell ALL should be tested for HTLV-1 (endemic to southern Japan, the Caribbean, the South Pacific, and sub-Saharan Africa).

DIFFERENTIAL

ALL is distinguished from lymphoblastic lymphoma by more extensive bone marrow involvement (> 25%).

TREATMENT

- **Combination chemotherapy:** Vincristine, prednisone, methotrexate, daunorubicin, and asparaginase.
- **Treatment regimen:**
  - Induction chemotherapy.
  - Several cycles of high-dose consolidation chemotherapy.
  - Prolonged maintenance low-dose chemotherapy.
- CNS prophylaxis with intrathecal chemotherapy is mandatory for **all** patients (systemic chemotherapy does not penetrate the blood-brain barrier well enough).

Acute Myeloid Leukemia (AML)

DIAGNOSIS

- Bone marrow biopsy with > 20% marrow blasts and associated cytopenias.
- **FAB classification** is as follows:
  - **M0:** Undifferentiated
  - **M1:** Myeloid
  - **M2:** Myeloid with differentiation
  - **M3:** Promyelocytic leukemia (APL)
  - **M4:** Myelomonocytic leukemia
  - **M5:** Monocytic
  - **M6:** Erythroid
  - **M7:** Megakaryocytic

Treatment

- Induction chemotherapy with Ara-C and anthracycline.
- Consolidation therapy using high-dose Ara-C may lead to durable remission or cure.
- Bone marrow transplant may be considered in patients who relapse

Acute Promyelocytic Leukemia (AML-M3, APL)

Characterized by heavily granulated promyelocytic blasts; associated with t(15;17) involving the retinoic acid receptor. DIC is present in the majority of patients at diagnosis.

AML-M3 is unique among AMLs for its propensity to cause DIC and for its high curability when treated with ATRA.

Treatment

- Treatment involves the differentiating agent *all*-trans retinoic acid (ATRA), given during induction chemotherapy and as maintenance chemotherapy.
- **Retinoic acid syndrome:** Characterized by pulmonary infiltrates, respiratory failure, fever, capillary leak syndrome, and cardiovascular collapse. Treated early with high-dose corticosteroids and temporary cessation of ATRA.
- APL is highly curable owing to ATRA therapy.

CHRONIC LEUKEMIAS

Chronic Myelogenous Leukemia (CML)

A myeloproliferative disorder resulting from malignant transformation of hematopoietic stem cells. Characterized by translocation of the BCR gene adjacent to ABL kinase, leading to a fusion protein (BCR-ABL), the Philadelphia chromosome t(9;22).

Symptoms/Exam

- **Chronic phase:** Usually asymptomatic, but some patients present with fatigue, early satiety, LUQ pain, or weight loss. Hepatosplenomegaly is common. The WBC count is elevated but stable (predominantly myeloid series).
- **Accelerated phase:** Presence of increased blasts and early forms in the peripheral blood; transition phase to more aggressive disease.
- **Blast phase:** Presentation is similar to that of acute leukemia. Highly refractory to conventional therapy; most often symptomatic (night sweats, weight loss, bone pain, fevers, cytopenias).

Diagnosis

Physical exam, review of peripheral blood smear, bone marrow biopsy with cytogenetics.

Treatment

- The old standard of care was allogeneic bone marrow transplant within two years of diagnosis or α-interferon and Ara-C for patients who could not undergo allogeneic transplant.
- Busulfan and hydroxyurea play a role in reducing blood counts but are palliative and not curative.

- **Imatinib (STI571):**
  - A specific tyrosine kinase inhibitor targeting fusion protein BCR-ABL.
  - More than 90% of patients in the chronic phase will have complete normalization of blood counts and 65% normal cytogenetics after one year of imatinib therapy.
  - Only 10% of patients in blast phase have complete hematologic remission; 15% have major cytogenetic response.
  - Side effects are mild (nausea, rash).
  - The optimal way to use imatinib in CML has yet to be determined, and long-term outcomes are not yet clear.

Chronic Lymphocytic Leukemia (CLL)

The most common leukemia in adults. Median survival is 10–15 years.

Exam/Diagnosis

- More patients are identified in the early stage owing to elevated lymphocyte count.
- Most patients are asymptomatic.
- Evaluation includes a detailed physical exam for lymphadenopathy/organomegaly, flow cytometry of peripheral blood, and optional bone marrow biopsy.
- **Evans' syndrome:** Common in CLL; presents with autoimmune hemolytic anemia and thrombocytopenia.
- **Rai staging** is as follows:
  - 0: Lymphocytosis alone
  - 1: Lymphocytosis and lymphadenopathy
  - 2: Lymphocytosis and enlarged spleen or liver
  - 3: Lymphocytosis and anemia
  - 4: Lymphocytosis and thrombocytopenia

Treatment

- Treatment should be directed toward relieving disease-related symptoms, rapidly progressive disease, and autoimmune hemolytic anemia or thrombocytopenia.
- Many different treatment approaches are available, including alkylating agents (chlorambucil, cyclophosphamide), nucleoside analogs (fludarabine, cladribine, pentostatin), and monoclonal antibodies (alemtuzumab).
- Highly effective in palliation, but not curative.
- For young patients, allogeneic BMT should be considered.
- **Richter's transformation:** CLL may transform into a large cell lymphoma in 3–10% of patients; associated with a very poor prognosis.

HODGKIN'S LYMPHOMA

The malignant cell is the Reed-Sternberg cell ("owl-eye" cell). Has a bimodal age distribution.

Symptoms/Exam

- Some 40% of patients present with systemic symptoms (B symptoms), which consist of weight loss, fever, and night sweats.
- Symptoms are also related to the site of involvement.

Diagnosis

- Excisional biopsy for architecture.
- Staging includes physical examination of lymph nodes, examination of Waldeyer's ring, detection of hepatosplenomegaly, CT of the chest/abdomen/pelvis, CXR, and measurement of laboratory values, including CBC, LDH, ESR, and alkaline phosphatase.
- Routine staging laparotomy (splenectomy) has fallen out of favor.

Treatment

- **Early-stage disease (localized lymphadenopathy):**
  - Subtotal nodal irradiation or mantle irradiation.
  - Chemotherapy with ABVD (Adriamycin, bleomycin, vincristine, and dacarbazine) or Stanford V followed by radiation of the involved field.
  - Combination chemotherapy with ABVD.
- **Advanced disease:** Combination chemotherapy with ABVD is standard.
- Patients with refractory disease should be considered for high-dose chemotherapy.

Complications

Long-term complications include myelodysplasia and acute leukemia, secondary cancers (breast cancer in women treated with nodal irradiation), cardiomyopathy (secondary to doxorubicin), pulmonary toxicity (secondary to bleomycin), infertility, hypothyroidism, and neuropathy.

NON-HODGKIN'S LYMPHOMA (NHL)

A heterogeneous group of cancers of B and T cells. Incidence is increasing for unknown reasons.

Symptoms/Exam

Include B symptoms (weight loss, fever, night sweats) and symptoms referable to lymph node masses or extranodal masses.

Diagnosis/Treatment

- Diagnosis is based on histology, immunohistochemistry, and flow cytometry.
- Both FNA and excisional biopsy are now acceptable.
- **Classification schemes:** Rappaport classification, Working Formulation, Revised European-American Lymphoma (REAL) classification, WHO classification.
- Can be roughly divided into three subtypes based on natural history:
  - **Low grade:** Indolent; high response rates to chemotherapy, but generally not curable. Treatment is based on reducing symptoms. Median survival is 6–10 years.
  - **Intermediate grade:** Curable. The standard chemotherapy, CHOP (cyclophosphamide, doxorubicin, vincristine, and prednisone), cures approximately half of patients and is given in 6–8 cycles of therapy. Some evidence indicates that adding the anti-CD20 antibody rituximab to CHOP improves survival.
  - **High grade:** Very aggressive, rapidly growing cancers, but curable with chemotherapy in a high percentage of cases. Lymphoblastic lymphomas are treated like ALL. Burkitt's lymphoma is associated with EBV in Africa. There is a risk of tumor lysis syndrome with high-grade lymphomas.

Poor prognostic features in NHL include age > 60, LDH > 1× normal, poor performance status, and extranodal disease.

- **International Prognostic Index:** Predicts outcome based on pretreatment patient characteristics.
- **Rituximab:** An anti-CD20 antibody that targets B-cell lymphoma cells and leads to responses in roughly 50% of patients with low-grade lymphomas. Other anti-CD20 antibodies have been conjugated with radioisotopes (tositumomab and ibritumomab).
- **Important subtypes** are as follows:
  - **Mucosa-associated lymphoid tissue (MALT) lymphoma:** Gastric mucosa–associated lymphoma is linked to *H. pylori* infection; > 80% of MALT cases regress with antimicrobial therapy.
  - **Mantle cell lymphoma:** Acts like an intermediate-grade lymphoma in aggressiveness but is not curable with conventional chemotherapy (as with low-grade lymphoma). Median survival is three years.

IMPORTANT TRANSLOCATIONS

- **Burkitt's lymphoma:** t(8;14).
- **Follicular lymphoma:** t(14;18).
- **Philadelphia chromosome:** t(9;22) (CML and a subset of ALL).
- **Good-prognosis AML (M4-Eo):** inv16.
- **Acute promyelocytic leukemia:** t(15;17) retinoic acid receptor and promyelocytic leukemia gene.

HIV AND CANCER

- HIV is associated with an increased incidence of NHL, anal cancer, cervical cancer, Kaposi's sarcoma, and Hodgkin's disease.
- **Kaposi's sarcoma** is associated with HHV-8. Treated with α-interferon, topical retinoids, ABV or BV (Adriamycin, bleomycin, vincristine), liposomal doxorubicin, and paclitaxel.
- The optimal treatment of NHL in HIV is not clear, but NHL accounts for 15% of AIDS-related deaths.
- CNS NHL risk is also increased in HIV.
- Cervical cancer and anal cancer risks are increased by HPV and impaired cellular immunity.

SUPPORTIVE CARE/GROWTH FACTORS

Nausea and Vomiting

- **Types:**
  - **Acute emesis:** Occurs within 24 hours of receiving chemotherapy.
  - **Delayed emesis:** Begins after 24 hours (associated with cisplatin, carboplatin, or cyclophosphamide).
  - **Anticipatory emesis:** A conditioned response in patients who have had poor nausea control with previous treatments.
- **Treatment options:**
  - **Selective 5-HT3 receptor serotonin antagonists:** Ondansetron, granisetron, dolasetron.
  - **Prochlorperazine.**
  - **Dexamethasone.**
  - **Metoclopramide:** Must be given in high IV doses, but causes extrapyramidal side effects at those doses.
  - **Droperidol:** Dopaminergic blockade.

- **Lorazepam.**
- **Dronabinol and cannabinoids.**
- **NK1 receptor antagonists.**
- Combinations of agents are often necessary to achieve emetic control.

Myeloid Growth Factors (G-CSF, GM-CSF)

- **Prophylaxis of febrile neutropenia:** Indicated only in chemotherapy regimens with > 40% risk of neutropenic fever.
- Patients with neutropenia and sepsis, pneumonia, or fungal infection should get myeloid CSF in addition to antibiotics.
  - There is no indication for giving myeloid CSFs with uncomplicated neutropenic fever.
  - Safe to give in acute leukemia; reduces infectious complications.
  - Other uses for myeloid CSFs include mobilization of stem cells for transplant.
- GM-CSF side effects include constitutional symptoms and injection site reactions.
- Dosing begins at least 24–48 hours after chemotherapy administration and should always stop at least 24 hours before subsequent chemotherapy
- **Pegfilgrastim:** A long-acting, pegylated version of G-CSF.

The predominant side effect of G-CSF is bone pain.

Erythropoietin

- Anemia in cancer and/or chemotherapy impairs quality of life.
- The most commonly used dose is 40,000 U SQ weekly.
- The FDA-approved dose is 150 U/kg SQ TIW.
- Patients often need supplemental iron to respond to erythropoietin.
- Darbepoetin alfa is a new agent with a long half-life; may be given in less frequent dosing (q 2–3 weeks).

Anorexia

- Caused by cancer and/or chemotherapy.
- Interventions include the following:
  - Nutritional counseling.
  - **Appetite stimulants:** Dronabinol, cyproheptadine, corticosteroids, megestrol acetate.

Fatigue

- Usually multifactorial and include anorexia, anemia, depression, infection, hypoxia, deconditioning, and hypogonadism.
- Both causes and symptoms must be treated.
- Anemia is often a contributory factor; treat with transfusions or erythropoietic growth factors.
- Corticosteroids, megestrol acetate, counseling, physical therapy, and exercise may all help in selected patients.
- Stimulants may be used in selected terminally ill patients.

NOTES

ONCOLOGY

CHAPTER 15

Psychiatry

Amin Azzam, MD

PSYCHIATRY PEARLS

- All psychiatric illnesses can be divided into major illness categories (see Figure 15-1). As with medical illness, symptoms suggest major illness categories, which can then be further clarified. Unlike medical illness, there are no objective laboratory tests for psychiatric diagnostic clarification, so we must rely on further history, the specific time course of symptoms, and the clinician's subjective diagnostic impressions.
- Most psychiatric syndromes are diagnoses of exclusion—likely medical etiologies must be ruled out before you assume it is a psychiatric illness.
- Like medical illness, pharmacologic treatment follows from the diagnosis (see Figure 15-2). Psychotic disorders are treated with antipsychotics. Anxiety disorders are treated with anxiolytic agents. Mood disorders are treated with antidepressants or mood stabilizers.
- Some psychiatric syndromes have symptoms that transcend the major disease categories (e.g., schizoaffective disorder, which has both psychotic and mood disorder symptoms). For these syndromes, treatment generally involves medication with > 1 category, targeting each symptom separately.
- The choice of medication in each class should be based on several factors:
  - Proven efficacy for the illness being treated.
  - Patient demographics.
  - The likely side-effect profile and tolerability to the patient.
  - Patient preference (to maximize patient compliance).
  - Drug-drug interactions with other medications.
  - The choice of benzodiazepine to use should be based on the nature of the anxiety symptom being treated (see Figure 15-3).

ANXIETY DISORDERS

Panic Disorder

At least **two** untriggered panic attacks, **with fear of having another.** Diagnosis is by **exclusion.** Age of onset is in the 20s; the male-to-female ratio is 1:1. Prevalence is up to 4%.

Symptoms

Panic attacks must develop abruptly and peak within 10 minutes. They must also include at least four of the following: tachycardia, diaphoresis, shortness

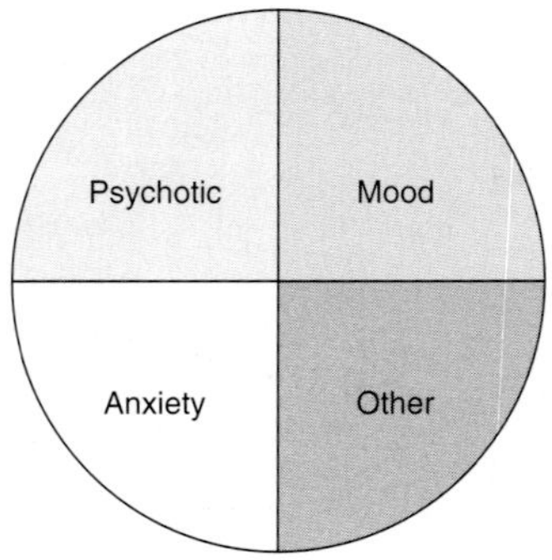

FIGURE 15-1. Major categories of psychiatric illness.

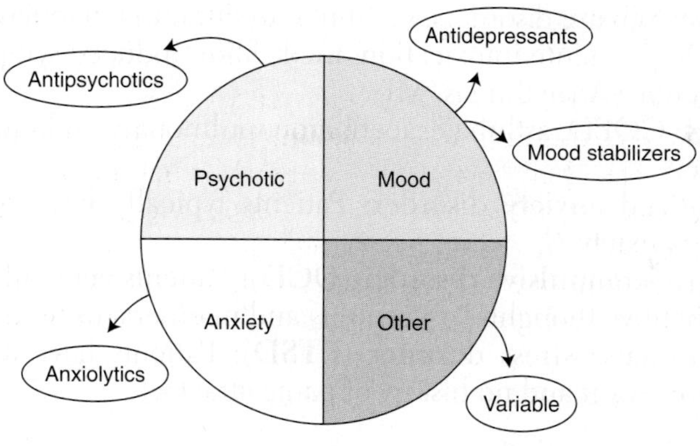

FIGURE 15-2. Pharmacologic management of psychiatric illness.

of breath, chest pain, nausea, dizziness, paresthesias, chills, derealization/depersonalization, and fear of losing control/going crazy/dying. A panic attack may be triggered or may occur spontaneously.

DIFFERENTIAL

- **Endocrine:** Hypoglycemia, hypothyroidism, hyperthyroidism, hyperparathyroidism, pheochromocytoma.

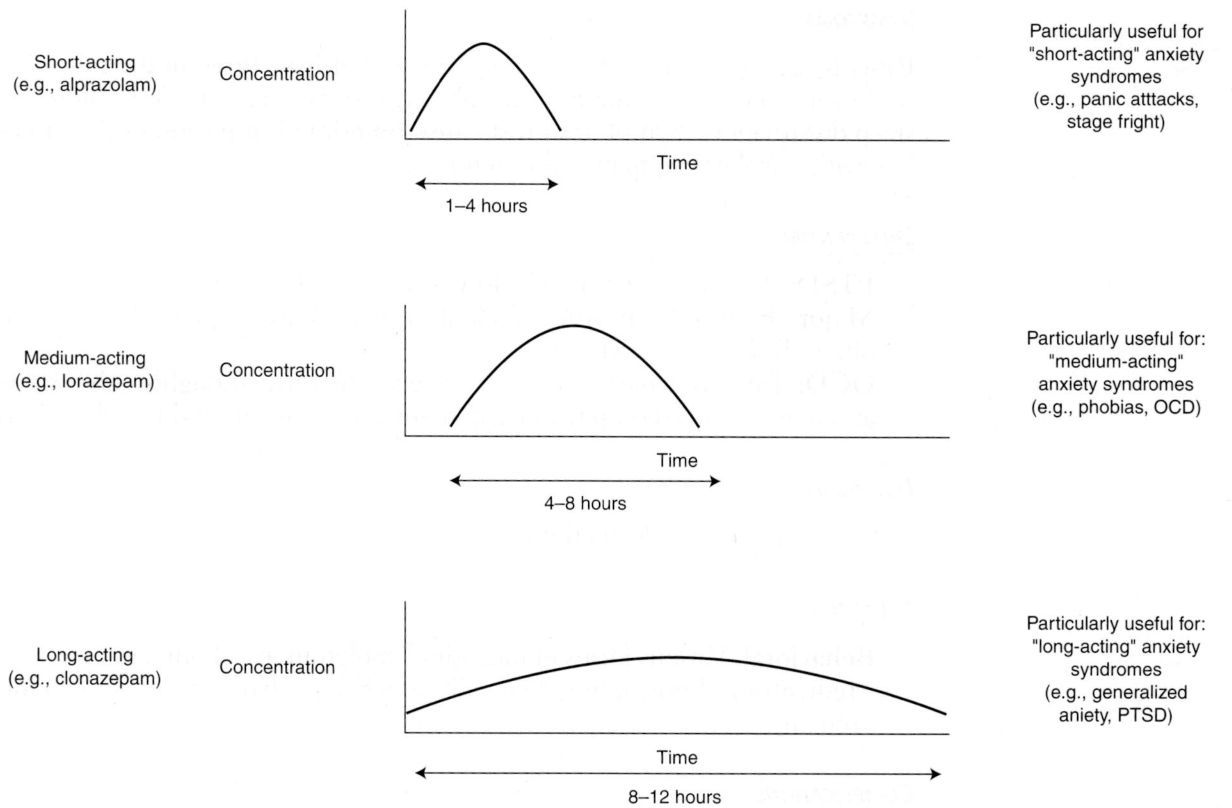

FIGURE 15-3. Length of action of benzodiazepines.

- **Neurologic:** Seizure disorders, vestibular dysfunction, neoplasms.
- **Pharmacologic:** Acute intoxication, medication-induced symptoms.
- **Cardiovascular:** Arrhythmias, MI.
- **Pulmonary:** COPD, asthma exacerbation, pulmonary embolus.
- **Psychiatric:**
  - **Generalized anxiety disorder:** Patients typically have more chronic baseline anxiety.
  - **Obsessive-compulsive disorder (OCD):** Patients generally have recurrent repetitive thoughts (obsessions) and mannerisms (compulsions).
  - **Post-traumatic stress disorder (PTSD):** Patients have a history of a traumatic event and no history of panic attacks.

DIAGNOSIS

Rule out all likely medical etiologies (e.g., ECG, electrolyte panel, CXR).

TREATMENT

- **Behavioral:** Various forms of individual and group psychotherapies.
- **Medication:** Benzodiazepine anxiolytic agents, β-blockers.

Panic disorder can occur with or without agoraphobia (fear of open spaces or of being alone in a crowd or leaving the home).

Generalized Anxiety Disorder

Uncontrollable worry about a **broad range of topics** (e.g., work/school, relationships, health) over time (i.e., more days than not for at least **six months**). Age of onset is variable; the male-to-female ratio is 1:2. Prevalence is up to 8%.

SYMPTOMS

Patients have poor control over the worry and at least **three** of the following: restlessness, poor concentration, irritability, easy fatigue, muscle tension, and sleep disturbances. Symptoms **must cause functional impairment** (i.e., interfere with social or occupational functioning).

DIFFERENTIAL

- **PTSD:** Patients must have a history of a traumatic event.
- **Major depressive disorder:** Patients usually have depressed mood and other physical symptoms.
- **OCD:** Patients typically have recurrent repetitive thoughts (obsessions) and mannerisms (compulsions), and anxiety is only around the obsessions.

DIAGNOSIS

Rule out all likely medical etiologies.

TREATMENT

- **Behavioral:** Various forms of individual and group psychotherapies.
- **Medication: Long-acting** benzodiazepine anxiolytic agents (e.g., clonazepam).

COMPLICATIONS

Often leads to **depression** if left untreated.

Specific Phobias

Fear of specific items. Age of onset is in **late childhood;** the male-to-female ratio is 1:2. Prevalence is up to 5%.

Symptoms

Excessive or unreasonable fear of a particular trigger; **patients realize that their response is excessive.** Must also cause **functional impairment** (i.e., must interfere with social or occupational functioning).

Differential

- **Panic disorder:** Panic attacks can be untriggered.
- **PTSD:** Patients avoid things only after having a traumatic event.
- **Generalized anxiety disorder:** Patients have chronic baseline anxiety about many things, not just when they are exposed to a trigger.

Treatment

- **Behavioral:** Exposure-response prevention therapy (exposes the patient to the stressful stimulus and prevents their usual fleeing response; will systematically desensitize the patient to the trigger).
- **Medication:** β-blockers; short-acting benzodiazepine anxiolytic agents (e.g., alprazolam).

Specific phobias are the most common anxiety disorder.

Obsessive-Compulsive Disorder (OCD)

Either obsessions or compulsions that cause significant impairment and that patients recognize as excessive or unreasonable. Age of onset is in childhood or early adulthood; the male-to-female ratio is 1:1. Prevalence is up to 3%.

Symptoms

- **Obsessions:** Recurrent or persistent thoughts that **cause** anxiety.
- **Compulsions:** Behaviors or rituals that temporarily **decrease** anxiety.
- **Patients must recognize that their symptoms are unreasonable** and that such symptoms are their own thoughts.

Differential

- **Delusional disorder:** Patients **do not realize** that the thoughts are their own.
- **Schizophrenia:** Patients usually have psychotic symptoms along with affective flattening, asociality, and avolition.
- **Generalized anxiety disorder:** Patients have anxiety in several different areas of their lives that are generally not relieved by compulsive acts.

Obsessions cause increased anxiety that is temporarily relieved by the compulsions.

Treatment

- **Behavioral:** Exposure-response prevention therapy; cognitive-behavioral therapy (teaches patients how to decrease their cognitive distortions of the stressor and how to change their behavioral response).
- **Medication:** Clomipramine, SSRIs (e.g., paroxetine, sertraline, fluvoxamine). **Higher doses than those used for depression are usually required.**

Complications

Often leads to depression if left untreated.

Post-Traumatic Stress Disorder (PTSD)

Reaction to a traumatic event characterized by reexperiencing, avoidance, and increased arousal. Age of onset is variable; the **male-to-female ratio is 1:2.** Prevalence is up to 3%, but 30% of Vietnam veterans are affected.

Symptoms

- Must have a perceived life-threatening trauma and all **three** of the following:
  1. Reexperiencing (flashbacks, nightmares, etc.).
  2. Avoidance (places, thoughts, feelings related to the trauma).
  3. Increased arousal (insomnia, hyperstartle, poor concentration, anger outbursts).
- Must have all symptoms for a **minimum of one month.**

Differential

- **Depression:** Patients do not have flashbacks to a traumatic event.
- **Generalized anxiety disorder:** Patients do not have a history of a traumatic event.
- **Adjustment disorder:** Patients have stress/anxiety/depression/behavioral changes that are related to a specific trigger but do not have all three primary symptoms: reexperiencing, avoidance, and increased arousal.

In acute stress disorder, symptoms last < 1 month. In PTSD, symptoms last > 1 month.

Treatment

- **Behavioral:** Various forms of individual therapy. **Group therapy is especially helpful.**
- **Medication:** SSRIs, sleep agents (e.g., trazodone), long-acting benzodiazepines (e.g., clonazepam).

Complications

- Long-term use of benzodiazepines can lead to psychological dependence. Prescribe with caution/selectivity.
- Avoidance of stimuli associated with the trauma can generalize to avoidance of wide-ranging things (which become secondarily associated with the trauma in the patient's mind). This leads to a far greater negative impact on the patient's life.

Prevention

Some research suggests that a **debriefing** shortly after the traumatic event may decrease the patient's likelihood of developing PTSD.

MOOD DISORDERS

Major Depressive Disorder

Age of onset is variable; the male-to-female ratio is 1:2. Lifetime prevalence in men is 10% and in women 20%. Risk is higher if there is a family history. **Untreated episodes usually last ≥ 4 months.**

Depression is the fourth largest cause of morbidity worldwide.

Symptoms

- Must have **depressed mood** *or* **loss of interest/pleasure** *and* **five** of the **SIG E CAPS** symptoms (see mnemonic).

- Must be a **change from baseline,** cause **functional impairment** (e.g., work, school, or social activities); and **last at least two weeks continuously.**

Differential

- **Adjustment disorder:** Patients have a known stressor that causes a reaction similar to a depressive episode, but the reaction is triggered specifically by that stressor.
- **Dysthymic disorder:** Patients have "low-level depression" (i.e., depression involving fewer than five **SIG E CAPS** symptoms) that **lasts at least two years.**
- **Anxiety disorders:** Generalized anxiety disorder, PTSD, OCD.
- **Medical "masqueraders":** Hypothyroidism, anemia, pancreatic cancer, Parkinson's.
- **Substance-induced mood disorder:** Illicit drugs, β-blockers, thiazide diuretics, digoxin, glucocorticoids, benzodiazepines, cimetidine, ranitidine, cyclosporine, sulfonamides, metoclopramide.

> ***Symptoms of major depressive disorder–***
>
> **SIG E CAPS**
>
> **S**leep (hypersomnia or insomnia)
> **I**nterest (loss of interest or pleasure in activities)
> **G**uilt (feelings of worthlessness or inappropriate guilt)
> **E**nergy (decreased)
> **C**oncentration (decreased)
> **A**ppetite (increased or decreased)
> **P**sychomotor agitation or retardation
> **S**uicidal ideation

Diagnosis

Eliminate potential medical etiologies (e.g., check TSH, CBC).

Treatment

- **Behavioral:** Various forms of individual and group psychotherapies.
- **Medication:** SSRIs; other classes of antidepressants. Choose medication on the basis of the symptom profile and anticipated side-effect tolerability.
- **Electroconvulsive therapy (ECT):** Often reserved for medication-resistant depression; **especially useful in the elderly.**

Psychotherapy and antidepressants together are more effective for depression than either treatment alone.

Complications

- Severely depressed patients can develop psychotic symptoms (e.g., auditory hallucinations, paranoid ideations, ideas of reference). These symptoms can be treated with a low dose of an antipsychotic agent.
- **Suicidality:** One of the major comorbidities of untreated depression is suicidality. Women generally have more attempts, but men's attempts are usually more lethal. Clinicians must assess the degree of risk (e.g., consider the number of prior attempts, degree of premeditation, lethality of method, and access to the proposed method) and hospitalize if necessary to ensure patient safety.

Bipolar Affective Disorder

Extreme mood swings between mania and depression. Age of onset is most commonly in the 20s and the 30s; the male-to-female ratio is 1:1. Prevalence is 1%. Risk is higher if there is a family history. There are two types: **type I,** which alternates between mania and depression; and **type II,** which alternates between depression and hypomania (i.e., fewer symptoms for a shorter duration).

Symptoms

- The symptoms of bipolar affective disorder are described by the mnemonic **DIG FAST.**
- Manic episodes **must last 4–7 days** in order to be called mania. Anything less is considered hypomania.

Symptoms of manic episodes—

DIG FAST

Distractibility
Insomnia (decreased need for sleep)
Grandiosity (increased self-esteem)
Flight of ideas (or racing thoughts)
Increased **A**ctivities/psychomotor **A**gitation
Pressured **S**peech
Thoughtlessness (poor judgment—e.g., spending sprees, unsafe sex)

- See the entry on depression for symptoms of the depressive episodes of bipolar disorder; remember the mnemonic **SIG E CAPS.**

DIFFERENTIAL

- **Major depressive disorder:** Patients have no history of a manic episode.
- **Schizoaffective disorder:** Patients have both **psychotic symptoms** and mood symptoms. Psychotic symptoms occur in the **absence** of mood symptoms.
- **Schizophrenia:** Patients do not have mood symptoms.

TREATMENT

- **Acute manic episode:** Hospitalize; consider antipsychotic agents (e.g., haloperidol, olanzapine, risperidone). Increase doses of mood stabilizers (lithium carbonate, valproic acid, carbamazepine [Tegretol]).
- **Maintenance treatment:** Mood stabilizers such as those listed above. Titrate to the lowest effective dose to maintain mood stability.
- **Depressive episodes:** Antidepressant agents; consider individual and group psychotherapies.

Treating a bipolar patient with antidepressant monotherapy can lead to a manic episode.

COMPLICATIONS

- In severe phases of mania or depression, patients can have psychotic symptoms.
- **Left untreated, many patients have progressively more rapid cycling** (more frequent and shorter-duration episodes).

PREVENTION

- Increase the mood stabilizer dose in the presence of imminent symptoms of mania.
- Educate patients to recognize the earliest signs of mania/depression (sleep changes are often the first sign), and encourage them to seek additional help early.

Psychotic = "break with reality."

PSYCHOTIC DISORDERS

Schizophrenia

A history of **severe** and **chronic** psychotic symptoms (> 6 months, or a lesser period if successfully treated; see below). There are several subtypes. **Age of onset is mostly in the 20s** for men and in the 20s–30s for women; the male-to-female ratio is 1:1. Prevalence is 1%; risk is higher if there is a family history. **Must cause functional impairment** (i.e., interfere with social or occupational functioning).

The 4 A's of schizophrenia:

Affective flattening
Asociality
Alogia (paucity of speech)
Auditory hallucinations

SYMPTOMS

Must have **two** or more of the following:

- **Delusions:** Fixed false beliefs.
- **Hallucinations:** Most often auditory but can be visual/gustatory/tactile as well.
- Disorganized speech.
- Grossly disorganized or catatonic behavior.
- **Negative symptoms:** Affective flattening, avolition, alogia (poverty of speech), asociality.

DIFFERENTIAL

- **Bipolar affective disorder:** Patients have psychotic symptoms only during extreme manic or depressive episodes.
- **Schizoaffective disorder:** Patients have psychotic symptoms **but also have prominent mood symptoms** (either depression or mania).
- **Delusional disorder:** Patients have **one** fixed false belief that is nonbizarre and that does not necessarily have an equally broad impact on their functioning.
- **Developmental delay (mental retardation):** Patients do not have overtly psychotic symptoms and **have not deteriorated from a higher-functioning baseline.**
- **OCD: Patients are aware** that their obsessions (recurring repetitive thoughts) are their own and do not stem from an external force.
- **Depression with psychotic features:** Patients have psychotic symptoms that occur only during depressive episodes, and the **depressive symptoms can occur without psychotic symptoms.**
- **Generalized anxiety disorder:** Patients have severe and chronic anxiety but no psychotic symptoms.
- **Substance-induced psychosis:** Especially associated with amphetamine or cocaine, both of which can cause paranoia and hallucinations. Patients have other signs/symptoms of substance use.
- **Medical "masqueraders":** Examples include neurosyphilis, herpes encephalitis, dementia, and delirium.
- **Neurologic "masqueraders":** Include complex partial seizures and Huntington's disease.

DIAGNOSIS

Diagnose by history. **Neuropsychological testing** can be helpful in clarifying the diagnosis but often is not indicated.

TREATMENT

There is often a prodromal phase of schizophrenia involving negative symptoms without the positive symptoms (delusions or hallucinations).

- Choose an antipsychotic agent that minimizes both symptoms and side-effect profile. **First-line agents are now atypical neuroleptics** (e.g., olanzapine, risperidone, quetiapine) because they **treat negative symptoms more effectively** than do typical neuroleptics (e.g., haloperidol). However, atypicals are much more expensive medications, so consider patients' financial resources when selecting medications.
- **Acute psychotic episode:** Hospitalize; increase the dose of antipsychotic agent and consider the use of anxiolytic agents (e.g., alprazolam, clonazepam). Group therapy can provide a forum for reality checks if patients can tolerate them.
- **Maintenance treatment: Titrate to the lowest effective dose of antipsychotic agent to maintain stability.** Group therapy and structured-day programs provide safety, socialization skills, and reality checks.

Patients newly diagnosed with schizophrenia ("first break") are at high risk for suicide attempts.

COMPLICATIONS

- Left untreated, will lead to a "**downward drift**" in socioeconomic class.
- Long-term use of typical neuroleptics (e.g., haloperidol) can lead to **tardive dyskinesias**—involuntary choreoathetoid movements of the face, lips, tongue, and trunk. Tardive dyskinesias should be treated by minimizing doses of neuroleptics or by switching to an atypical neuroleptic (e.g., olanzapine, risperidone, quetiapine). Can also be treated with a benzodiazepine (e.g., alprazolam, clonazepam) or a β-blocker (e.g., propranolol).

Delusional Disorder

Patients have a fixed false belief (delusion) that is nonbizarre. Prevalence is 0.025%. Age of onset is from the mid-20s to the 90s; the male-to-female ratio is roughly 1:1.

SYMPTOMS

- The delusion is often highly specific and organized into a system (i.e., patients can describe wide and varying evidence to support the delusion). This leads to hypervigilance and hypersensitivity.
- There is usually a relative lack of other symptoms, and patients often remain high functioning otherwise.

DIFFERENTIAL

- **Schizophrenia:** Patients often have a history of auditory hallucinations or other psychotic symptoms, such as prominent negative symptoms (affective flattening, avolition, alogia, asociality). Frequently there is greater functional impairment.
- **Substance-induced delusions:** Particularly associated with amphetamine and cannabis.
- **Medical conditions:** Hyper-/hypothyroidism, Parkinson's, Huntington's, Alzheimer's, CVAs, metabolic causes (hypercalcemia, uremia, hepatic encephalopathy), other causes of delirium.

TREATMENT

- Patients are often likely to refuse treatment and/or medications. Low-dose atypical neuroleptics (e.g., olanzapine, risperidone, quetiapine) may be helpful, but they must be balanced against patients' tendency to incorporate the medication into their delusional system.
- Do not pretend that the delusion is true, but do not argue with patients to prove it false. Instead, gently remind them of your goal of maximizing functionality.

Delusional disorder is far less common than schizophrenia and less responsive to medications, primarily owing to patients' lack of trust.

COMPLICATIONS

Many patients do not seek treatment, leading to progressive isolation and a decrease in productivity and/or functional status.

SUBSTANCE ABUSE DISORDERS

Chronic Abuse/Dependence

Substance abuse is a maladaptive pattern of use that occurs despite adverse consequences. Dependence is abuse and physiologic tolerance.

TREATMENT

For treatment of acute intoxication or withdrawal syndromes, see Chapter 10. All the dependencies are characterized by **relapsing and remitting** patterns. Optimal treatment varies from patient to patient but usually involves **combinations** of the following:

- **Pharmacologic substitutes:** Replace the substance of abuse with a longer-acting and less addictive pharmacologic equivalent. Examples include methadone for heroin, chlordiazepoxide (Librium) for alcohol, and clonazepam for short-acting benzodiazepines. Can be used either in a detoxification program (e.g., 21 days) or as a maintenance therapy (e.g., methadone maintenance).

- **Pharmacologic antagonists:** Decrease the pleasurable response associated with the substance of abuse. Examples include the following:
  - **Antabuse (disulfiram) for alcohol:** Blocks the efficacy of alcohol dehydrogenase, causing buildup of acetaldehyde.
  - **Naltrexone:** Thought to decrease alcohol craving.
- **Therapeutic communities:** Provide a safe, structured environment in which to boost attempts at maintaining early sobriety. Can be inpatient (residential) or outpatient, brief or long-term.
- **Self-help organizations:** Provide a regular and ongoing community of peers to maintain ongoing sobriety. Examples include Alcoholics Anonymous (AA) and Narcotics Anonymous (NA).
- **Family support/education:** Provide support to family members; offer an environment in which to learn from and commiserate with others. An example is Al-Anon.
- **Individual counseling/therapy:** Various techniques focus on the following:
  - Understanding and eliminating triggers for relapse.
  - **Harm reduction approach:** Minimizing use of the substance, which minimizes its functional impact on patients' lives.
  - **Abstinence model:** Getting patients to accept that they cannot minimize use but must abstain in order to improve their functional quality of life.
  - **Psychoeducation:** Educating patients regarding issues such as the cycle of relapses and remissions; the chronic nature of the illness; and available resources.

COMPLICATIONS

Chronic substance dependence leads to significant loss of productivity, functionality, and quality of life.

OTHER DISORDERS

Somatoform Disorders

A group of diseases in which patients complain of physical symptoms that have no clear medical etiologies. Affect 15% of all psychiatric patients and 20% of medical inpatients. Certain subtypes are more common in women (e.g., conversion disorder, pain disorder); others are more common in men (e.g., factitious disorder, malingering). All generally occur more often in those with lower socioeconomic status and education.

SYMPTOMS

Vary across the specific disorders, but all are insufficiently explained by medical causes alone. Demonstrate inconsistent findings and often lead to many unnecessary hospitalizations, procedures, and workups. Specific subtypes include the following:

- **Somatization disorder:** Complaints are in at least **two** organ systems. Caused by unconscious conflict.
- **Conversion disorder:** Complaints are in the **neurologic** system.
- **Pain disorder:** Complaints are of pain (predominantly).
- **Hypochondriasis:** Complaints and fear are of serious diseases.
- **Body dysmorphic disorder:** Complaints are about a perceived defective body or body part.

- **Factitious disorder:** Complaints are **consciously simulated by the patient** (vs. somatization disorder).
- **Malingering:** Complaints are **consciously simulated by the patient with specific secondary goals** as a primary motivator (vs. factitious disorder).

DIAGNOSIS

- Eliminate likely medical etiologies through standard medical workups. A balance must be struck between sufficient workup to rule out realistic causes and exhaustive workup to rule out extremely rare causes.
- Psychiatric consultation can help clarify specific diagnoses and therefore potential treatment options that could be most helpful.

Informal "curbside" consults of colleagues can be quite helpful and are preferable to the formal introduction of yet another medical provider.

TREATMENT

- **Minimize** the number of different providers involved in the care of the patient.
- Establish and maintain a **long-term, trusting doctor-patient relationship;** schedule regular outpatient visits and routinely inquire about psychosocial stressors.
- On each visit, perform at least a partial physical exam directed at the organ system of complaint, and gradually change the agenda to inquire about psychosocial issues in an empathic manner.
- **Refer patients to a mental health professional** to help them express their feelings, thereby minimizing physical symptoms as a proxy for those feelings.
- **Treat any secondary depression** (i.e., depression secondary to the sense of hopelessness associated with having the somatoform disorder).
- Some patients may benefit from the use of an anxiolytic agent (e.g., alprazolam).
- Be aware that some patients will develop psychological dependence on medications, so prescribe selectively.

Attention-Deficit Hyperactivity Disorder (ADHD)

Persistent (> 6 months) problems with **inattention** and/or **hyperactivity and impulsivity.** Prevalence is 3–5%; the male-to-female ratio is 3–5:1.

In order for an adult to be diagnosed with ADHD, symptoms must be present in childhood and must cause functional impairment.

SYMPTOMS

- Inattention, including at least **six** of the following:
    1. Poor attention to tasks, play activities, or schoolwork.
    2. Poor listening skills.
    3. Poor follow-through on instructions.
    4. Poor organizational skills.
    5. Avoidance of tasks requiring sustained mental effort.
    6. Frequent loss of things.
    7. Easy distractibility and forgetfulness.
    8. Frequent careless mistakes.
- Hyperactivity-impulsivity, including at least **six** of the following:
    1. Fidgetiness.
    2. Leaves rooms where sitting is expected.
    3. Excessive running/climbing.
    4. Subjective thoughts of restlessness.
    5. Difficulties with leisure activities.
    6. Acts as if "driven by a motor."
    7. Talks excessively.
    8. Interrupts others often.

Attention deficit can occur with or without hyperactivity.

DIFFERENTIAL

- **Med-seeking behavior:** Patients often present with a history of substance abuse (especially amphetamine abuse)
- **Bipolar affective disorder:** Inattention/racing thoughts occur only during manic episodes; are accompanied by a lack of need for sleep and by grandiosity/euphoria; and are cyclical in nature.
- **Substance-induced symptoms:** Especially amphetamine intoxication. Look for associated signs/symptoms of substance abuse.

Adults tend to have less hyperactivity than do children.

TREATMENT

- **Stimulants** (methylphenidate, others): Increase the dose as needed; use BID-TID dosing.
- **Antianxiolytics:** If there is a risk of abuse/dependence, bupropion (Wellbutrin) is a nonaddictive and reasonable first-line agent.
- **Behavioral therapy:** Focus on changing maladaptive behaviors and on learning more effective ones.

Patients with ADHD describe stimulants as slowing them down rather than making them "high."

Eating Disorders

Marked disturbances in eating behavior. **Two** major types:

- **Anorexia nervosa:** Patients have misperceptions of body weight, generally weigh < 85% of their ideal body weight, and self-impose severe dietary limitations. Affects 0.5–1.0% of adolescent girls; the male-to-female ratio is 1:10–20. More common in developed/Western societies and in more affluent socioeconomic strata.
- **Bulimia nervosa:** Episodic uncontrolled binges of food consumption followed by compensatory weight loss strategies (e.g., self-imposed vomiting, laxative and diuretic abuse, excessive exercise). Affects 1–3% of young women; the male-to-female ratio is 1:10.

SYMPTOMS

- Both anorexia and bulimia involve a marked misperception of body image and poor self-esteem.
- **Anorexia only:** Actual body weight must be < 85% of ideal body weight (for height and age). Also presents with **lanugo,** dry skin, lethargy, bradycardia, hypotension, cold intolerance, hypothermia, and hypocarotenemia.
- **Bulimia only:** Patients must have at least **three** months of binge-purging activity that occur at least **twice a week.** They must also have a sense of **loss of control** during food consumption binges. Patients often have signs of frequent vomiting (e.g., low chloride levels, pharyngeal lesions, **tooth enamel decay,** scratches on the dorsal surfaces of the fingers) and **enlarged parotid glands.**

Secondary amenorrhea may be a sign of an eating disorder in a young woman.

DIFFERENTIAL

Medical causes of weight loss and amenorrhea; failure to thrive.

DIAGNOSIS

Diagnose by history. A collateral history obtained from other family members is often helpful.

TREATMENT

- Correct electrolyte abnormalities.
- Psychotherapy.
- **Antidepressants:** SSRIs.

Personality Disorders

Persistent maladaptive characteristic patterns of behavior **that have been present since young childhood** and cause **significant impairment in patients' functioning in society.** All are coded on Axis II.

SYMPTOMS

There are several types, most often subdivided into clusters:

1. **Cluster A** (aka the "**weird**" personality disorders):
   a. Schizoid
   b. Schizotypal
   c. Paranoid
2. **Cluster B** (aka the "**wild**" personality disorders):
   a. Borderline
   b. Histrionic
   c. Narcissistic
   d. Antisocial
3. **Cluster C** (aka the "**wimpy**" personality disorders):
   a. Dependent
   b. Obsessive-compulsive personality
   c. Avoidant

DIFFERENTIAL

Mental retardation (will have below-normal intelligence).

DIAGNOSIS

Patients with personality disorders cannot be diagnosed on a single visit. Because there must be a persistent pattern of behavior, patients must be observed over time.

TREATMENT

- Personality disorders are both longstanding and pervasive and are thus **resistant to treatment.**
- **Dialectical behavioral therapy** has been shown to be an effective treatment of **borderline personality disorder.** Brief **cognitive-behavioral therapy** groups may also maximize effective coping strategies and minimize functional impact on patients' lives.
- **Mood stabilizers** (e.g., valproic acid, lithium, carbamazepine) may be of use in **antisocial** and **borderline personality disorders. SSRIs** (e.g., fluoxetine, sertraline, paroxetine) may be useful in treating **borderline, dependent,** and **avoidant personality disorders.**

PATIENT DECISION MAKING AND COMPETENCE

The fundamental question with regard to patient decision making is "Does the patient have the mental capacity to make decisions on his/her own behalf, or should you (or someone else) make decisions for him/her?" The answer depends on the **context** of care:

- **Patients with acute/emergent medical issues** (e.g., massive hemorrhage, delirium): In most states, doctors have the right to perform emergent medical care. Although not explicitly defined, "emergent" is generally thought of as "when there is an imminent loss of life or limb." Technically, without explicit patient or representative consent, you must confine your care to the treatment of emergent conditions.
- **Patients with acute psychiatric issues** (e.g., actively psychotic, floridly manic, dangerously suicidal): Again, laws vary from state to state, but most states allow for emergent psychiatric treatment. This may include medications (IM or IV if necessary), locked hospitalization, locked seclusion, or physical restraints.
- **Patients with subacute medical conditions** (e.g., nonemergent medical or surgical procedures): Patients have the right to refuse recommended treatment as long as they:
  - **Know and can repeat** the nature of the medical condition.
  - **Know and can repeat** the benefits/risks of and alternatives to the recommended treatment.
  - **Consistently** express their rationale for their decision.
- Patients with **subacute psychiatric conditions** (e.g., schizophrenia but not actively psychotic; depression but not currently actively suicidal; bipolar but not floridly manic): Recommended medical treatment should be offered just as if there were no psychiatric condition (see above). Laws regarding recommended psychiatric care vary significantly across states. Some states allow doctors significant power in forcing unwanted treatment, while others give patients significant rights to refuse, which can be overturned only in a court of law. Remember that if/when the condition becomes acute/emergent, most states allow psychiatric treatment.
- Patients with **advance directives:** By definition, patients may sign advance directives only when they have the mental capacity to do so. As long as the advance directive explicitly addresses the recommended/anticipated treatment, doctors must adhere to the patient's prestated wishes even if those wishes will lead to a worse outcome (including death). When the directive does not explicitly address an emergent or subacute medical condition (and the patient cannot respond), staff and/or the patient's family/friends must attempt to infer what the patient's wishes would be and treat accordingly.

THERAPEUTIC DRUGS IN PSYCHIATRY

Adverse Effects

Table 15-1 outlines both common and potentially serious adverse effects associated with psychiatric drugs.

Important Drug-Drug Interactions

- **Carbamazepine:**
  - Is an autoinducer of cytochrome P-450 isoenzyme, so the level needs to be rechecked and the dose often increased after several weeks of use.
  - Decreases serum level of OCPs.
  - Erythromycin, isoniazid, and H_2 blockers all increase carbamazepine levels.

TABLE 15-1. Adverse Effects of Commonly Administered Psychiatric Drugs

Class	Examples	Common Side Effects	Medically Serious Side Effects
SSRIs	Paroxetine (Paxil), fluoxetine (Prozac), sertraline (Zoloft), citalopram (Celexa), fluvoxamine (Luvox), others	Sedation, weight gain, GI discomfort, sexual dysfunction.	Serotonin syndrome (tachycardia, hypertension, fever, hyperthermia, myoclonus, convulsions, coma).
Antidepressants	Bupropion (Wellbutrin),	Insomnia, "jitteriness."	Lowered seizure threshold.
	venlafaxine (Effexor)	Constipation, dizziness.	Lowered seizure threshold, hypertension.
Mood stabilizers	Lithium	Cognitive dulling, tremor, sedation, nausea, diarrhea, T-wave flattening.	Lithium toxicity, **hypo**thyroidism (in long-term use), nephrogenic diabetes insipidus.
Mood stabilizers/ anticonvulsants	Valproic acid (Depakote),	Weight gain, sedation, cognitive dulling.	Thrombocytopenia.
	carbamazepine (Tegretol)	Same as above.	SIADH, agranulocytosis, Stevens-Johnson rash.
Typical high-potency antipsychotics	Haloperidol (Haldol), fluphenazine (Prolixin)	Sedation.	Acute dystonic reactions, neuroleptic malignant syndrome, tardive dyskinesia (in long-term use).
Typical midpotency antipsychotics	Thioridazine (Mellaril), chlorpromazine (Thorazine)	Sedation, anticholinergic side effects (dry mouth, constipation, urinary retention, tachycardia).	Acute dystonic reactions, neuroleptic malignant syndrome, tardive dyskinesia (in long-term use).
Typical low-potency antipsychotics	Thiothixene (Navane), perphenazine (Trilafon), trifluoperazine (Stelazine)	Orthostatic hypotension.	Acute dystonic reactions, neuroleptic malignant syndrome, tardive dyskinesia (in long-term use).
Atypical antipsychotics	Olanzapine (Zyprexa),	Weight gain, sedation.	Hypercholesterolemia, possible diabetes mellitus.
	Risperidone (Risperdal),	Weight gain.	Hyperprolactinemia; side effects of typical antipsychotics (when used in high doses).
	Quetiapine (Seroquel),		Cataracts.
	Clozapine (Clozaril)	Drooling.	Agranulocytosis.

- **Valproic acid:** Levels are increased by aspirin and anticoagulants.
- **Benzodiazepines:**
  - Levels are increased by disulfiram, ketoconazole, valproic acid, erythromycin, and cimetidine.
  - Diazepam (Valium) and alprazolam (Xanax) increase levels of digoxin and phenytoin.

NOTES

CHAPTER 16

Pulmonary Medicine

Christian Merlo, MD, MPH

COUGH

Healthy people rarely cough. Cough is one of the most common conditions for which patients seek medical attention. A systematic approach makes it possible to diagnose the cause in the majority of cases.

SYMPTOMS

Inquire about postnasal drip syndromes, asthma, GERD, treatment with ACEIs, and smoking. Productive cough usually represents an infectious or chronic process such as bronchiectasis. Cough productive of blood may represent malignancy, infection, or the first sign of connective tissue disease (e.g., Goodpasture's syndrome, Wegener's granulomatosis).

EXAM

Physical examination should focus on the nasal mucosa, lungs, heart, and extremities (for clubbing). Boggy nasal mucosa may be a sign of postnasal drip. Expiratory wheezing or crackles point to the need for further testing of the lower respiratory tract.

DIFFERENTIAL

Estimating the duration of cough is often the first step in focusing the differential diagnosis (see Figure 16-1).

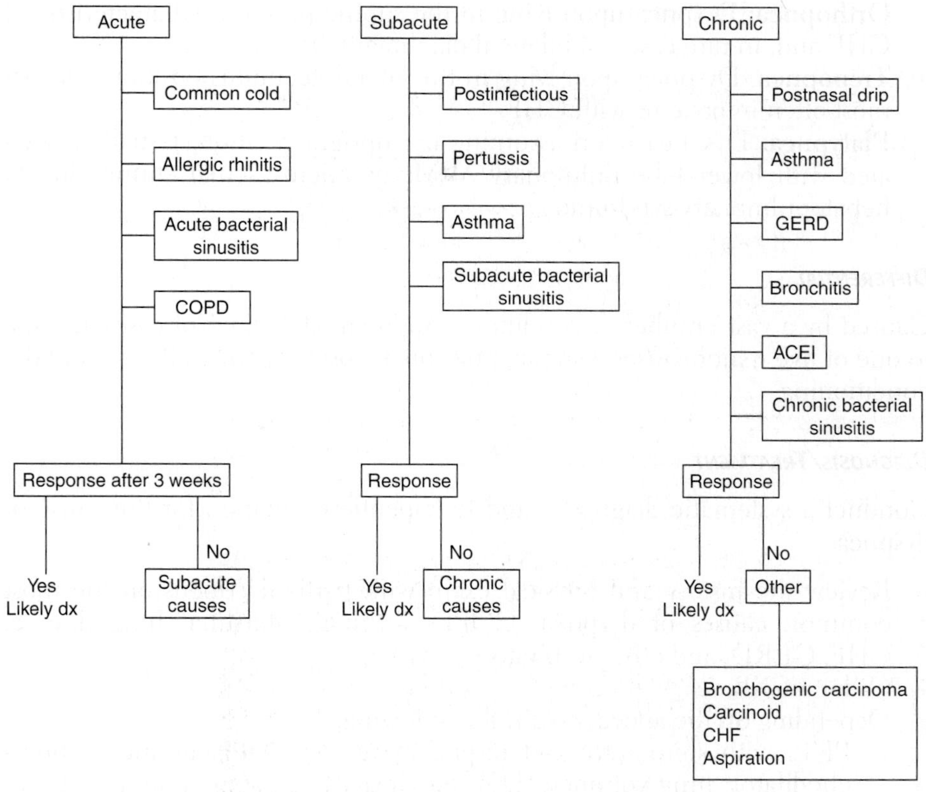

FIGURE 16-1. Algorithm for the differential diagnosis of cough.

- **Acute cough:** Of < 3 weeks' duration.
  - Viral infections are the most common cause.
  - Other causes include allergic rhinitis, acute bacterial sinusitis, COPD exacerbation, and infection with *Bordetella pertussis.*
  - May be the presenting symptom of left heart failure, asthma, or conditions that predispose patients to aspiration.
- **Subacute cough:** Of 3–8 weeks' duration.
  - Postinfectious cough is most common.
  - Subacute bacterial sinusitis, asthma, and infection with *B. pertussis* may all cause cough lasting between three and eight weeks.
- **Chronic cough:** Of > 8 weeks' duration.
  - Roughly 95% of cases are caused by postnasal drip, GERD, asthma, chronic bronchitis, bronchiectasis, or ACEI use.
  - It is important to remember that cough may have multiple etiologies.

The most common causes of chronic cough are postnasal drip, asthma, and GERD.

DIAGNOSIS/TREATMENT

Diagnosis and treatment depend on symptoms and response to treatment.

DYSPNEA

Dyspnea is the uncomfortable awareness of difficult, labored, or unpleasant breathing. Normal resting patients are unaware of the act of breathing.

SYMPTOMS/EXAM

It is important to quantify dyspnea on the basis of the amount of physical exertion that is required to produce the sensation.

- **Orthopnea:** Dyspnea upon lying in the supine position. Characteristic of CHF and, in rare cases, of bilateral diaphragmatic paralysis.
- **Trepopnea:** Dyspnea upon lying in the lateral decubitus position. Occurs most often in patients with CHF.
- **Platypnea:** Dyspnea upon assuming the upright position. Usually associated with lower lobe pulmonary AVMs or microvascular shunts due to hepatopulmonary syndrome.

DIFFERENTIAL

Caused by a vast number of conditions. Approximately 95% of cases are due to one of five major causes: cardiac, pulmonary, psychogenic, GERD, and deconditioning.

DIAGNOSIS/TREATMENT

Conduct a systematic diagnostic and therapeutic evaluation for the cause of dyspnea.

- Review the history and physical exam with particular focus on the most common causes of dyspnea: COPD, asthma, interstitial lung disease, CHF, GERD, and other respiratory disorders.
- Order a CXR.
- Depending on the above, obtain the following:
  - PFTs with spirometry and responsiveness to methacholine or bronchodilator; lung volumes, diffusion capacity, O_2 saturation at rest and with exercise, and flow volume loops (see Figure 16-2).

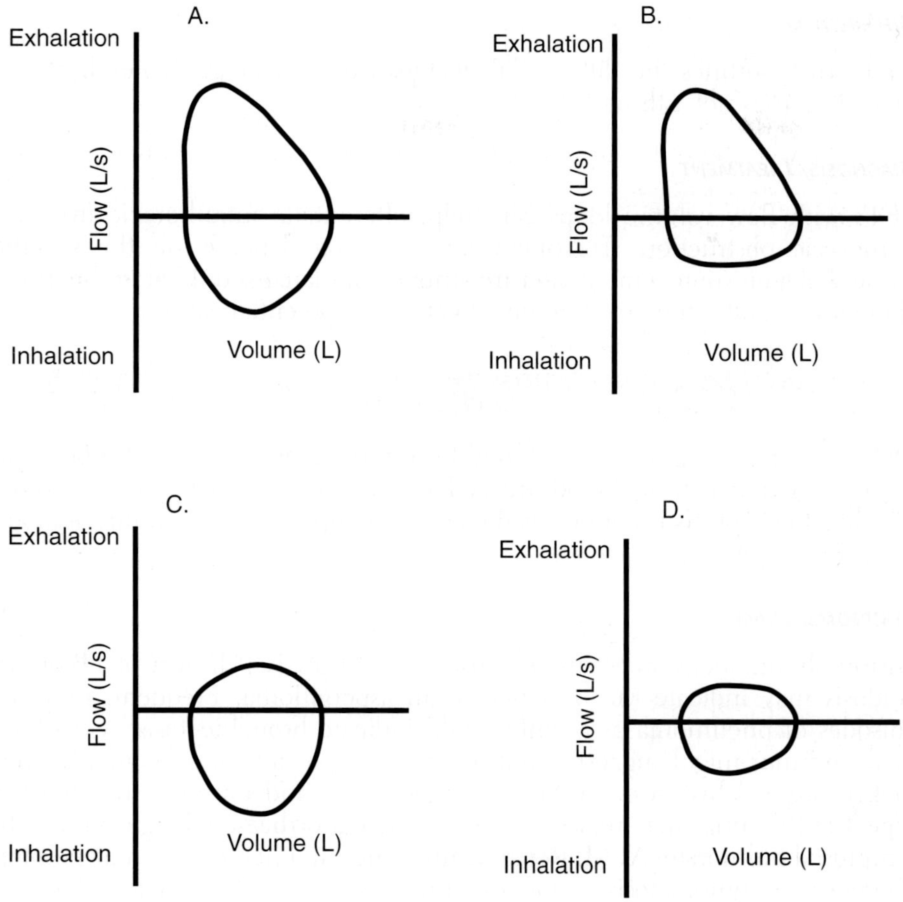

FIGURE 16-2. Flow volume loops.

A, normal pattern; *B*, variable extrathoracic obstruction; *C*,variable intrathoracic obstruction; *D*, fixed obstruction.

  - Noninvasive cardiac studies, including ECG and echocardiography +/– stress testing.
  - Chest CT; 24-hour esophageal pH monitoring.
- Final determination of the cause of dyspnea is made by observing which therapy relieves the symptoms.

WHEEZING

A wheeze is a continuous musical sound lasting > 100 msec. Wheezes can be high or low pitched, can consist of single or multiple tones, and can occur during inspiration or expiration.

SYMPTOMS/EXAM

Expiratory wheezes obtained by history or examination do **not** always point to a diagnosis of asthma. Inspiratory wheezes do **not** always suggest upper airway obstruction. When upper airway obstruction is present, however, patients typically develop dyspnea when the obstruction is < 8 mm in diameter and stridor when the diameter is < 5 mm. Polyphonic wheezes consisting of multiple notes suggest dynamic compression of the large, more central airways. Monophonic wheezes classically suggest disease of the smaller, lower airways.

DIFFERENTIAL

Table 16-1 outlines the differential diagnosis of wheezing. Remember, "All that wheezes is not asthma."

DIAGNOSIS/TREATMENT

PFTs with flow volume loops can help differentiate intrathoracic from extrathoracic obstruction. Treatment for wheezing depends on the specific cause. Lack of improvement after treatment is initiated should alert the physician either to alter therapy or to investigate other potential causes.

HEMOPTYSIS

Defined as the coughing up of blood from the trachea, bronchial tubes, and lungs. Can range from blood-streaked sputum to life-threatening bleeding. **Massive hemoptysis** is defined as the coughing up of > 100–600 mL of blood in a 24-hour period.

SYMPTOMS/EXAM

History should focus on common causes of hemoptysis. A history of TB or sarcoidosis may indicate the presence of an aspergilloma. Frequent, multiple episodes of pneumonia as a child could indicate bronchiectasis. A diastolic heart murmur might suggest mitral stenosis as a possible and frequently overlooked cause. A history of epistaxis, telangiectasias, and a bruit in the posterior aspect of the lungs may represent hereditary hemorrhagic telangiectasia with a ruptured pulmonary AVM. Renal insufficiency and hemoptysis may point to Wegener's granulomatosis or Goodpasture's syndrome. Weight loss, tobacco abuse, and cachexia may suggest malignancy.

DIFFERENTIAL

Blood expectorated from the upper respiratory tract and the upper GI tract can mimic blood coming from the trachea and below. Bronchitis, bronchogenic carcinoma, and bronchiectasis are the most common causes of he-

TABLE 16-1. Differential Diagnosis of Wheezing

Upper Airway Obstruction		Lower Airway Obstruction
Extrathoracic	**Intrathoracic**	
Vocal cord dysfunction	Tracheal stenosis	Allergic bronchopulmonary aspergillosis (ABPA)
Postnasal drip	Foreign body	Asthma
Laryngeal edema	Benign tumors	Aspiration
Malignancy	Tracheomalacia	Bronchiolitis
Relapsing polychondritis	Malignancy	Bronchiectasis
Wegener's granulomatosis		CF
		COPD
		CHF
		Parasitic infections
		PE

moptysis. Table 16-2 outlines the differential diagnosis of hemoptysis. Even after extensive evaluation, up to 30% of patients have no identifiable cause for hemoptysis.

DIAGNOSIS

- Routine evaluation for all patients with hemoptysis should include a history and physical exam, CBC with differential, UA, coagulation studies, ECG, and CXR. Bronchoscopy should also be strongly considered.
- Additional special studies (based on the history and physical) include expectorated sputum for acid-fast bacilli and cytology; thoracic CT scan; blood testing for BUN, creatinine, ANA, ANCA, and anti-GBM antibody; ABG analysis on room air; 100% O_2 to evaluate for shunt; and pulmonary arteriography.

TREATMENT

Treatment for hemoptysis is divided into two categories: supportive and definitive.

- **Supportive care:** Typically includes bed rest with supplemental O_2 and blood products if needed. In general, medications with antitussive effects should be avoided, as an effective cough is necessary to clear blood from the airways. If gas exchange becomes compromised, endotracheal intubation may become necessary. Generally, worsening of gas exchange precedes the need for transfusion.
- **Definitive treatment:**
  - **Nonmassive hemoptysis:** Treatment is directed at the specific cause (e.g., antibiotics for superinfected aspergilloma).
  - **Massive hemoptysis:** Treatment is directed toward bringing about abrupt cessation of bleeding. Urgent bronchoscopy may help localize the site of bleeding. Angiography of the bronchial arteries (a more common site of bleeding than the pulmonary arteries) has been shown to identify the bleeding site in > 90% of patients. When angiography is combined with embolization, bleeding can successfully be stopped in > 90% of patients. Emergency surgery for massive hemoptysis is controversial and is usually reserved for those who have failed embolization.

TABLE 16-2. Differential Diagnosis of Hemoptysis

MOST COMMON CAUSES	OTHER CAUSES
Bronchitis	Aspergilloma
Bronchogenic carcinoma	CHF
Bronchiectasis	CF
	Goodpasture's syndrome
	Lung abscess
	Mitral stenosis
	Pulmonary AVM
	PE/infarction
	Sarcoidosis
	TB
	Wegener's granulomatosis

HYPOXEMIA

Defined as a decrease in blood O_2 (in general, a PaO_2 of < 80 mmHg). An age adjustment given by the formula 80 – [(age – 20)/4] is used to define the lower limit of normal PaO_2.

Symptoms/Exam

Hypoxemia can lead to tissue hypoxia and cause impaired judgment and motor dysfunction. When hypoxia is long-standing, it leads to fatigue, drowsiness, and delayed reaction time. With severe hypoxia, the respiratory centers in the brain stem are affected, and death usually results from respiratory failure.

Differential

Calculation of the alveolar-arterial (A-a) oxygen gradient aids in narrowing the differential diagnosis. The A-a gradient is defined as $PiO_2 - (PaO_2 - PaCO_2/8)$. There are five general mechanisms of hypoxemia:

1. **Reduced inspired O_2** either from decreased total atmospheric pressure (P_{atm}) or from a decreased fraction of O_2 (FiO_2):
   - Transient exposure to low inspired O_2 is common on airline flights in which the cabin is pressurized to 5000–10,000 feet (PiO_2 = 100 mmHg).
     - FiO_2 is preserved (~21%), but total P_{atm} is decreased.
     - In patients with severe lung disease, PaO_2 may drop as low as 40 mmHg.
   - May also result from closed-space rescues (FiO_2 < 21%) or structure fires.
2. **Diffusion abnormality:**
   - A reduction in diffusion capacity **rarely** leads to abnormal pulmonary gas exchange.
   - It is estimated that DL_{CO} must fall to 10% of the individually predicted value to lead to hypoxemia.

Hypoxemia due to shunt does not correct with 100% O_2 therapy.

3. **Hypoventilation:**
   - Defined as decreased minute ventilation, resulting in an increase in $PaCO_2$ (as CO_2 increases, P_AO_2 decreases according to the alveolar gas equation).
   - Results in a **normal** A-a gradient.
4. **Ventilation-perfusion (V/Q) mismatch:**
   - Results when there is no perfusion to areas of ventilated lung.
   - The classic example is PE.
5. **Shunt:** Occurs when there is perfusion of nonventilated lung (pneumonia) or when there is a communication between the arterial and venous systems bypassing the lungs (intracardiac shunt or AVM).

Treatment

All patients with hypoxemia should be treated with supplemental O_2. Patients with a $PaO_2 \leq 55$ mmHg or with an O_2 saturation of ≤ 88% should be treated with long-term O_2 therapy. Patients with a $PaO_2 \leq 59$ mmHg or an O_2 saturation of ≤ 89% and evidence of cor pulmonale also qualify for long-term O_2 (to help reduce right heart failure).

PREOPERATIVE PULMONARY EVALUATION

Potential risk factors that are often thought to contribute to the risk of postoperative **pulmonary** complications include smoking, age, poor health status, obesity, COPD, asthma, and risk factors related to the specific surgical procedure to be performed.

- **Smoking:** Several studies have shown that smoking, even among those without chronic lung disease, is a risk factor for postoperative pulmonary complications. Among patients who smoke, stopping smoking at least eight weeks prior to surgery reduces risk. Smokers who stop smoking < 8 weeks prior to surgery may have a higher risk than do current smokers.
- **Age:** In general, advanced age is not thought to be a predictor of pulmonary complications.
- **Poor health status:** Inability to exercise is a strong predictor of postoperative pulmonary complications.
- **Obesity:** Although commonly thought of as a risk, obesity is not a significant risk factor for postoperative pulmonary complications.
- **COPD:** Patients with COPD are at increased risk for postoperative pulmonary complications. Prophylactic antibiotics do not reduce that risk.
- **Asthma:** It is controversial whether asthmatics are at increased risk for pulmonary complications in the postoperative period. In general, patients should not be wheezing and should have peak flow measures > 80% predicted prior to surgery. A course of steroids in the perioperative period does not increase the risk of pulmonary complications and should not increase the risk of wound-healing problems.
- **Procedure-related risk factors:** The surgical site is an important predictor of pulmonary complications. Risk increases with procedures closest to the diaphragm. General anesthesia and long-acting neuromuscular blockers also increase risk.

Smoking, COPD, poor exercise tolerance, surgical sites close to the diaphragm, and general anesthesia are important risk factors for postoperative pulmonary complications.

Preoperative Testing

- The history and physical exam are the most important aspects of the preoperative pulmonary assessment.
- PFTs should not be routinely performed, as spirometry has not been shown to identify high-risk patients who have not been recognized as such on clinical examination.
- Controversy exists as to whether an elevated $PaCO_2$ is a predictor of pulmonary complications.

Risk Reduction Strategies

- **Lung expansion exercises:** Incentive spirometry and other deep-breathing exercises reduce the risk of pulmonary complications by up to 50%.
- **Pain control:** Postoperative epidural analgesia reduces the risk of pulmonary complications and is recommended after high-risk thoracic, abdominal, and major vascular procedures. It also allows for early mobilization and better use of lung expansion exercises.

CHRONIC OBSTRUCTIVE PULMONARY DISEASE (COPD)

A disease state characterized by chronic airflow limitation that is no longer fully reversible, is usually progressive, and results from chronic bronchitis and emphysema. **Chronic bronchitis** is defined clinically as chronic productive cough for three consecutive months in two consecutive years. **Emphysema** is defined pathologically as abnormal enlargement of the airspaces distal to the terminal bronchioles with wall destruction. The most important risk factor for developing COPD is cigarette smoking. α_1-antitrypsin (AAT) deficiency is also a well-characterized genetic abnormality that predisposes individuals to the development of early-onset COPD.

SYMPTOMS/EXAM

Symptoms are usually not present until the individual has smoked > 1 pack per day for 20 years. Typically presents with chronic cough in the fourth or fifth decade of life. Dyspnea usually occurs only with moderate exercise, and not until the sixth or seventh decade of life. Chest wall hyperinflation, prolonged expiration, wheezing, and distant breath and heart sounds may be present. The patient may use accessory muscles and pursed lip breathing (**"pink puffer"**), and cyanosis may be present as well (**"blue bloater"**). Neck vein distention, tender liver, and lower extremity edema suggest cor pulmonale.

DIFFERENTIAL

Acute bronchitis, asthma, bronchiectasis, CF, CHF.

DIAGNOSIS

Along with a history and physical exam, testing modalities that are useful for diagnosing COPD and for evaluating the progression of disease include CXR, PFTs, ABG analysis, and AAT screening.

- **CXR:** Typically demonstrates decreased lung markings, increased retrosternal airspace, and flattened diaphragms.
- **PFTs:** Essential for diagnosis as well as for the evaluation of treatment and disease progression.
- **ABG analysis:** Acute exacerbations show hypoxemia and hypercarbia with acute respiratory acidosis.
- **AAT screening:** AAT deficiency accounts for < 1% of COPD cases. Low levels of AAT lead to basilar emphysema. CXR may show **decreased lung markings, predominantly in the bases** (usually in the apices with COPD from tobacco use).

TREATMENT

- **Acute exacerbations:** Where possible, the cause of the exacerbation should be treated.
  - **β_2-adrenergic** and **anticholinergic** agents are first-line therapy.
  - O_2 therapy is often necessary to treat hypoxemia. Hypercarbia can result from either a decreased respiratory drive with increased PaO_2 or increased V/Q mismatch with hyperoxia.
  - Systemic **corticosteroids** in either oral or IV form help decrease the length of exacerbation and improve FEV_1 in hospitalized patients.
  - **Antibiotics** are recommended by the American Thoracic Society for patients with an acute exacerbation who have a **change in sputum amount, consistency, or color.**
  - **Noninvasive positive pressure ventilation** is of benefit for patients with **severe** acute exacerbations of COPD, as it reduces in-hospital mortality, decreases the need for intubation, and diminishes hospital length of stay.

- **Stable chronic COPD:**
  - Smoking cessation.
  - **β_2-adrenergic** and **anticholinergic** agents help improve pulmonary function and reduce dyspnea. The long-acting β_2-adrenergic agent salmeterol is more effective than ipratropium at improving pulmonary function.
  - Long-term use of corticosteroids is controversial.
  - O_2 if indicated.
  - **Pulmonary rehabilitation** is associated with improved exercise tolerance and reduced pulmonary symptoms.
  - **Immunizations** for influenza and pneumococcus are recommended.
  - **Lung volume reduction surgery** initially benefits some patients, but lung function deteriorates to baseline within five years postsurgery.
  - Single- or double-**lung transplantation** is often indicated for willing patients with low FEV_1, hypercarbia, and cor pulmonale. Five-year survival following transplantation for COPD is approximately 40%.

Oxygen therapy is the only intervention known to increase life expectancy in hypoxemic COPD patients.

BRONCHIECTASIS

Defined as the irreversible dilatation and destruction of bronchi with inadequate clearance of mucus in the airways. Characterized by dilated airways and focal constrictive areas and, in some cases, by large, cystic, grapelike clusters resulting from progressive dilatation of the airways. Cycles of infection and inflammation lead to permanent remodeling and dilatation with viscous sputum production.

Symptoms/Exam

Patients often have cough productive of yellow or green sputum together with dyspnea and hemoptysis. May follow an episode or episodes of childhood pneumonia. Associated with postinfectious conditions (*Pseudomonas*, *Haemophilus*, TB, pertussis, measles, influenza, RSV, HIV), immunodeficiency (common variable immunodeficiency [CVID], IgA deficiency), congenital conditions (CF, Young's syndrome, primary ciliary dyskinesia, Kartagener's syndrome), autoimmune disease (SLE, RA, Sjögren's syndrome, relapsing polychondritis, IBD), or hypersensitivity (ABPA). Physical exam reveals crackles and wheezes. Acute exacerbations typically include changes in sputum production, increased dyspnea, increased cough and wheezing, fatigue, low-grade fever, decreased pulmonary function, changes in chest sounds, and radiographic changes.

Differential

COPD, interstitial fibrosis, pneumonia, asthma.

Diagnosis

Tests useful in making the diagnosis or in determining the underlying cause of bronchiectasis include the following:

- **CBC, including differential.**
- **Serum immunoglobulins** aid in screening for CVID, IgA/IgG deficiency, and ABPA.
- **High-resolution CT** has become the best tool for diagnosing bronchiectasis and aids in mapping airway abnormalities.

- **Spirometry** helps quantify the degree of airway obstruction.
- **Sputum sample** for bacterial and mycobacterial culture.
- **Sweat chloride test** for CF.
- **ANA, RF, anti-Ro/La.**

TREATMENT

- **Antibiotics** are the standard of care for acute exacerbations. A reasonable first-line choice would include a fluoroquinolone.
- **Bronchodilators** used routinely are helpful, as many patients have hyperresponsiveness that likely results from airway inflammation.
- **Inhaled corticosteroids** can reduce inflammation and improve dyspnea, cough, and pulmonary function in severe bronchiectasis.
- **Airway clearance techniques,** including chest physiotherapy, flutter devices, and percussive vests, aid in the clearance of secretions.
- Mucolytic agents such as **DNase** have been shown to be helpful in stable CF but are ineffective and potentially harmful in patients with stable idiopathic bronchiectasis.
- **Surgical resection** remains an option for patients with localized focal bronchiectasis.
- **Double-lung transplantation** has been performed among patients with severe bronchiectasis.

CYSTIC FIBROSIS (CF)

Cystic fibrosis is the most common lethal autosomal recessive disorder in Caucasians.

The most common lethal autosomal-recessive disorder in Caucasians, affecting 1 in every 3500 births. The disease is caused by mutations in the CF transmembrane conductance regulator (CFTR), leading to chloride channel dysfunction. Classically characterized by multisystem involvement of the sinuses, lungs, pancreas, liver, gallbladder, intestines, and bones and, in males, the vas deferens.

SYMPTOMS/EXAM

Most CF patients are diagnosed during childhood. A history of failure to thrive as a child, persistent respiratory infections (*Pseudomonas*), nasal polyposis, sinusitis, intestinal obstruction, malabsorption, recurrent pancreatitis, hepatobiliary disease, and male infertility are suggestive of CF. Exam may reveal increased chest AP diameter, upper lung field crackles, nasal polyps, hepatomegaly, and clubbing. Acute exacerbations are typically characterized by increased sputum production, dyspnea, fatigue, weight loss, and a decline in FEV_1.

DIFFERENTIAL

Immunodeficiency, asthma, ABPA.

DIAGNOSIS

Diagnosis requires both clinical and laboratory evidence of CFTR dysfunction.

- **Sweat chloride concentration:** The best screening test for CF for a patient with a suggestive clinical picture. Normal sweat chloride is < 40 mmol/L.
- **Genotyping:** Screening for the presence of two CFTR mutations known to cause CF. Newer tests screen for > 1000 different known mutations.
- **Nasal potential difference:** Directly evaluates CFTR function by measuring ion transport in the epithelial cells lining the interior of the nose.

- **CXR:** Shows hyperinflation, bronchiectasis, and upper lobe infiltrates. Nodules often represent mucoid impaction in the airways.

TREATMENT

- **Acute pulmonary exacerbations:** Treat with chest physical therapy, bronchodilators, DNase, and usually two antipseudomonal antibiotics.
- **Chronic stable CF:**
  - **Inhaled tobramycin** slows the decline in FEV_1 and is used for long-term therapy.
  - **Nebulized DNase** improves FEV_1 and should be offered to patients with daily cough, sputum production, and airflow obstruction.
  - **Aerobic exercise, flutter devices, and external percussive vests** help with regular airway clearance.
  - **Pancreatic enzymes** and the **fat-soluble vitamins A, D, E, and K** are given for malabsorption.
  - **Nutritional counseling** is essential for proper health maintenance to help prevent diabetic complications, osteoporosis, and weight loss.
  - **Double-lung transplantation** remains an option for severe progressive pulmonary disease.

PHYSIOLOGY PRIMER

Lung Physical Findings

Table 16-3 outlines physical findings typically associated with common lung conditions.

Lung Volumes

Common definitions are as follows (also see Figure 16-3):

- **Residual volume (RV):** Air in the lung at maximal expiration.
- **Expiratory reserve volume (ERV):** Air that can be exhaled after normal expiration.
- **Tidal volume (TV):** Air that enters and exits the lungs during normal respirations; generally 500 cc.
- **Inspiratory reserve volume (IRV):** Air in excess of TV that enters the lungs at full inspiration.

TABLE 16-3. Physical Findings Associated with Common Lung Conditions

	Tracheal Shift	Thoracic Expansion	Fremitus	Resonance	Breath Sounds	Egophony	Other
Consolidation (open bronchus)	–	↓	↑	↓	Tubular	Ipsilateral	Whispered pectoriloquy
Consolidation (atelectasis)	Ipsilateral	↓	↓	↓	↓	–	–
Pleural effusion	Contralateral	↓	↓	↓	↓	+ or –	–
Pneumothorax	Contralateral	–	↓	↑	↓	–	Coin test

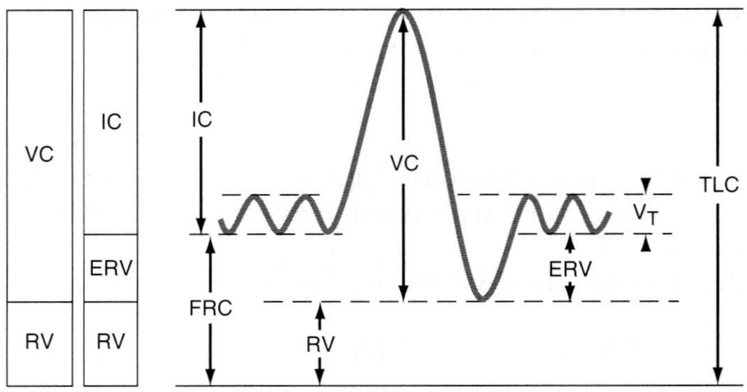

FIGURE 16-3. Lung volumes.

Lung volumes, shown by block diagram (left) and by spirogram tracing (right). VC, vital capacity; V_T, tidal volume. (Reproduced, with permission, from Weinberger SE. *Principles of Pulmonary Medicine*, 3rd ed. Philadelphia: W.B. Saunders, 1998.)

- **Functional reserve capacity (FRC):** RV + ERV.
- **Inspiratory capacity (IC):** TV + IRV.
- **Total lung capacity (TLC):** RV + ERV + TV + IRV.

Capacities are the sum of two or more volumes.

Alterations in Lung Function

Table 16-4 outlines changes in lung function associated with obstructive lung disease as well as those typically found with restrictive lung disease. Table 16-5 lists common pulmonary disorders by category.

DIAGNOSTICS IN PULMONARY MEDICINE

ABG Interpretation

Distinguishes respiratory acidosis from respiratory alkalosis.

- pH **decreases** by 0.08 for each 10-mmHg rise in P_{CO_2} in acute respiratory acidosis.

TABLE 16-4. Obstructive vs. Restrictive Lung Disease[a]

	FEV_1/FVC	TLC	RV	VC	MIP	MEP
Obstructive	↓	N to ↑	↑	↓	N	N
Restrictive						
Pulmonary parenchymal	N to ↑	↓	↓	↓	N	N
Extraparenchymal neuromuscular	N	↓	↑	↓	↓	↓
Extraparenchymal chest wall	N	↓	↑	↓	N	N

[a] MIP = maximum inspiratory pressure; MEP = maximum expiratory pressure.

TABLE 16-5. Diagnostic Categories of Common Pulmonary Disorders

OBSTRUCTIVE	RESTRICTIVE—PARENCHYMAL	RESTRICTIVE—EXTRAPARENCHYMAL
Asthma	Idiopathic pulmonary fibrosis	**Neuromuscular:**
COPD	Sarcoidosis	Diaphragmatic weakness/paralysis
Bronchiectasis	Drug- or radiation-related interstitial lung disease (ILD)	Myasthenia gravis
CF	Collagen vascular disease–related ILD	Guillain-Barré syndrome
		ALS
		Cervical spine injury
		Chest wall:
		Kyphoscoliosis
		Obesity
		Post-thoracoplasty

- pH **increases** by 0.08 for each 10-mmHg fall in $Paco_2$ in acute respiratory alkalosis.

CXR

- Often the first diagnostic test performed to evaluate pulmonary symptoms.
- Can reveal infiltrates, nodules, masses, effusion, and mediastinal and hilar abnormalities (see Tables 16-6 and 16-7).

CT Scan

- Offers several advantages over routine CXRs:
  - Cross-sectional images allow for comparison of different lesions that might be superimposed on CXR.
  - Better at characterizing lesions both by density and by size.
  - Particularly valuable in evaluating mediastinal and hilar disease.
- CT angiography (contrast injected and images rapidly acquired by helical scanning) can be used to detect PEs in segmental or larger vessels.
- High-resolution CT provides individual cross-sectional images of 1–2 mm and allows better recognition of bronchiectasis, emphysema, and ILD.

TABLE 16-6. Infiltrates Found on CXR

UPPER LOBE	LOWER LOBE
Ankylosing spondylitis	**B**ronchiectasis
Sarcoidosis	**A**spiration
Tuberculosis	**D**ermatomyositis/polymyositis
Eosinophilic granulomatosis	**A**sbestosis
Cystic fibrosis	**S**cleroderma
Silicosis	**SLE**, **S**jögren's syndrome
	Early Hamman-Rich syndrome
	Rheumatoid arthritis

TABLE 16-7. Masses Found on CXR

ANTERIOR MEDIASTINAL	POSTERIOR MEDIASTINAL
Teratoma	**B**ronchial cysts
Thymoma	**E**nterogenic cysts
Thymolipoma	**A**bscess
Thymic carcinoma/carcinoid	**N**on-Hodgkin's lymphoma
Thymic cyst	**N**eurogenic tumors
Thoracic thyroid	**P**ericardial cysts/**P**lasmacytoma
Terrible lymphoma	**H**odgkin's lymphoma

PET Scan

- A useful technique for the evaluation of solitary pulmonary nodules.
- Radiolabeled fluorodeoxyglucose is injected and rapidly transported into neoplastic cells, which then "light up" with PET imaging.

V/Q Scan

- Often used in the evaluation of PEs.
- Technetium-labeled albumin is injected into the vein and becomes trapped in the pulmonary capillaries following the distribution of blood flow.
- Radiolabeled xenon gas is inhaled to demonstrate the distribution of ventilation.
- Defects in perfusion that follow the distribution of a vessel and are not accompanied by defects in ventilation are called **mismatched defects** and may represent PEs.

Pulmonary Angiography

- Used to visualize the pulmonary arterial system.
- Contrast medium is injected through a catheter placed in the pulmonary artery.
- A **filling defect** or **cutoff** is often seen in cases of PE.
- Can also be used to investigate suspected pulmonary AVMs.

Bronchoscopy

- Allows for the direct visualization of the endobronchial tree.
- **Bronchoalveolar lavage** is a technique used to sample cells and organisms from the alveolar space using aliquots of sterile saline. It is most helpful for diagnosing infectious and neoplastic disease.
- **Transbronchial biopsy** is performed by passing a small forceps through the bronchoscope into the small airways to obtain parenchymal tissue. Transbronchial biopsy may be helpful in differentiating infection, neoplasm, ILD, granulomatous disease, and bronchiolitis obliterans with organizing pneumonia.
- **Transbronchial needle aspiration** involves the passing of a hollow-bore needle through the airway into a mass lesion or an enlarged lymph node. This is particularly useful in cases of mediastinal or hilar adenopathy, al-

lowing for the differentiation of neoplasm, sarcoidosis, fungal disease, and mycobacterial disease.

INTERSTITIAL LUNG DISEASE (ILD)

Represents a wide spectrum of diseases affecting the parenchyma of the lung. More than 200 known diseases are characterized by diffuse lung involvement. It is useful to separate such diseases into those of unknown and known etiology and then to distinguish them by the presence or absence of inflammation, fibrosis, or granulomas. Sarcoidosis, idiopathic pulmonary fibrosis (IPF), and fibrosis associated with connective tissue disease are most common.

SYMPTOMS/EXAM

Detailed history should focus on the onset of symptoms, family history, smoking history, and occupational and environmental exposures. Dyspnea is the most common presenting symptom. Gradual onset is consistent with IPF, whereas acute onset of dyspnea is more typical of Hamman-Rich syndrome or hypersensitivity pneumonitis (HP). A family history may help with cases of tuberous sclerosis and neurofibromatosis. Occupational and environmental exposures are critical, as they may help diagnose asbestosis or HP. Physical examination usually demonstrates **dry bibasilar crackles.** Inspiratory **squeaks** suggest a diagnosis of bronchiolitis obliterans with organizing pneumonia.

DIFFERENTIAL

The differential diagnosis of ILD is outlined in Tables 16-8 and 16-9.

DIAGNOSIS

- **Laboratory studies** to confirm the presence of a connective tissue disorder.
- **CXR** usually demonstrates a bibasilar interstitial pattern. May have upper lobe nodular pattern or honeycombing as well.
- **High-resolution CT:**
  - Helps **characterize** the disease, which may obviate the need for biopsy.
  - Helps **quantify** the extent of disease.
  - Helps **identify** the area to sample if biopsy is necessary.
- **PFTs** are useful for evaluating the extent of lung involvement. Commonly have a restrictive defect (low TLC), a normal or increased FEV_1/FVC ratio, and reduced DL_{CO}.
- **Lung biopsy** for disease confirmation and activity. Fiberoptic bronchoscopy with transbronchial biopsy is helpful in diagnosing sarcoidosis, eosinophilic granulomatosis, and HP. Open lung biopsy is preferred for making the diagnosis of IPF.

TREATMENT

Treatment is disease specific and usually supportive:

- **O_2** for hypoxemia ($PaO_2 < 55$ mmHg) at rest or with exercise.
- **Glucocorticoids** are usually recommended, but no placebo-controlled trials have yet been conducted, and there is no direct survival benefit.
- **Immunosuppressive** therapy with cyclophosphamide or azathioprine +/– steroids has been used with varying success.
- Lung transplantation is reserved for patients < 65 years of age with severe, refractory disease.

TABLE 16-8. Interstitial Lung Disease Characterized by Inflammation or Fibrosis

KNOWN ETIOLOGY	UNKNOWN ETIOLOGY
Asbestosis	Idiopathic interstitial pneumonias:
Drug reaction:	IPF[a]
Amiodarone	Acute interstitial pneumonia (Hamman-Rich)
Chemotherapeutic agents	Desquamative interstitial pneumonia
Radiation exposure	Respiratory bronchiolitis–associated
	Nonspecific interstitial pneumonia
	Bronchiolitis obliterans with organizing pneumonia
	Connective tissue disease:[a]
	SLE
	RA
	Scleroderma
	Dermatomyositis/polymyositis
	Sjögren's syndrome
	Crohn's disease/ulcerative colitis
	Amyloidosis
	Alveolar proteinosis
	Lymphangioleiomyomatosis
	Inheritable disease:
	Neurofibromatosis
	Tuberous sclerosis
	Hermansky-Pudlak syndrome

[a] The most common ILDs.

PLEURAL EFFUSION

Defined as the abnormal accumulation of fluid in the pleural space. Classified as **transudative** or **exudative.** In the United States, the most common causes are CHF, pneumonia, and cancer.

SYMPTOMS/EXAM

Patients often present with dyspnea and pleuritic chest pain. Examination of the chest typically demonstrates dullness to percussion, decreased or absent fremitus, and decreased breath sounds on the affected side. Elevated neck veins, an S3 gallop, and edema suggest CHF. Productive cough, fever, and

TABLE 16-9. Interstitial Lung Disease Characterized by Granulomas

KNOWN ETIOLOGY	UNKNOWN ETIOLOGY
Hypersensitivity pneumonitis	Sarcoidosis[a]
Berylliosis	Eosinophilic granulomatosis
	Wegener's granulomatosis
	Churg-Strauss syndrome

[a] The most common ILDs.

signs of consolidation suggest pneumonia. Lymphadenopathy may suggest malignancy, whereas ascites points to a hepatic cause.

DIFFERENTIAL

- A **transudative effusion** occurs because of an imbalance between hydrostatic and oncotic pressures. The main causes of transudative pleural effusion are CHF, cirrhosis, nephrotic syndrome, and PE.
- An **exudative effusion** occurs when inflammation leads to altered vascular permeability and protein-rich pleural fluid. Commons causes of exudative pleural effusions are malignancy, bacterial and viral pneumonia, TB, PE, pancreatitis, esophageal rupture, collagen vascular disease, chylothorax, and hemothorax.

DIAGNOSIS

- CXR may demonstrate blunting of the costophrenic angle. Decubitus films help determine if fluid is free flowing or loculated. The presence of > 1 cm of fluid on decubitus CXR suggests the presence of a significant amount of fluid.
- Diagnostic thoracentesis is performed on clinically significant effusions, and fluid is analyzed to distinguish transudate from exudate using Light's criteria (see Table 16-10) as well as to obtain pH, color, turbidity, cell count, glucose, Gram stain, bacterial/fungal/mycobacterial cultures, and cytology (see Table 16-11). Pleural fluid amylase, triglycerides, cholesterol, and hematocrit may also be analyzed given the appropriate clinical scenario (see Table 16-11).
- Pleural biopsy may aid in diagnosis of cancer or TB effusion.
- Evaluation for PE.

Drain pleural effusion if pH < 7.2, glucose < 40 mg/dL, or ⊕ Gram stain.

TREATMENT

- **Transudative pleural effusion:** Treatment is aimed at the underlying cause with therapeutic thoracentesis if the patient is symptomatic.
- **Exudative pleural effusion:**
  - **Malignant:** Consider pleurodesis in symptomatic patients who are unresponsive to chemotherapy or radiation.
  - **Parapneumonic:** Drainage of the pleural space is indicated if there is evidence of empyema (pH < 7.2, pus, glucose < 40 mg/dL, Gram stain positive).
  - **Hemothorax:** Requires drainage or fibrothorax will likely develop.
  - **Tuberculous:** Usually resolves with treatment of TB.

PNEUMOTHORAX

Defined as the presence of air in the pleural space. Traditionally classified as spontaneous, iatrogenic, or traumatic.

TABLE 16-10. Light's Criteria for Distinguishing Transudate from Exudate

	PLEURAL/SERUM PROTEIN	PLEURAL/SERUM LDH	PLEURAL FLUID LDH > 2/3 NORMAL
Transudate	< 0.6	< 0.5	No
Exudate	> 0.6	> 0.5	Yes

TABLE 16-11. Pleural Fluid Analysis and Interpretation

PLEURAL FLUID TEST	INTERPRETATION
pH	Pleural pH < 7.2 with parapneumonic effusion indicates the need for drainage.
Hematocrit	> 50% of peripheral hematocrit suggests hemothorax.
Glucose	< 60 mg/dL usually suggests a complicated parapneumonic effusion or malignancy. Can be seen with rheumatoid and lupus pleuritis, TB, and Churg-Strauss syndrome.
Triglycerides	> 110 mg/dL suggests chylothorax.
Cholesterol	> 250 mg/dL suggests pseudochlylothorax.
Lymphocytes	> 50% lymphocytes likely to be either tuberculous or malignant.
Eosinophils	> 10% most commonly due to pneumothorax. Less common causes include drug reaction, asbestos exposure, paragonimiasis, and Churg-Strauss syndrome.

- **Spontaneous** pneumothorax is not caused by any obvious precipitating factor. Classified as either **primary** (usually occurring in tall, thin males without clinically apparent lung disease) or **secondary** (occurring in patients with underlying lung disease or in women with a history of endometriosis around the time of menses)
- **Iatrogenic** pneumothorax is the result of diagnostic (thoracentesis) or therapeutic intervention (central venous catheter placement).
- **Traumatic** pneumothorax occurs with penetrating or blunt trauma that causes air to enter the pleural space as well as with acute compression of the chest that causes alveolar rupture.

SYMPTOMS/EXAM

Most patients present with unilateral chest pain (either sharp or steady pressure) and acute shortness of breath. The physical examination may be normal if the pneumothorax is small. If the pneumothorax is large, exam may reveal decreased chest movement, hyperresonance, decreased fremitus, and decreased breath sounds. Tachycardia, hypotension, and tracheal deviation should raise suspicion of tension pneumothorax.

DIFFERENTIAL

Acute PE, MI, pleural effusion, pneumonia, pericardial tamponade.

DIAGNOSIS

Confirmed through the identification of a thin visceral pleural line away from the chest wall on upright PA CXR. A CT scan of the thorax may help when the CXR is difficult to interpret because of severe underlying lung disease (e.g., CF).

TREATMENT

- Treatment involves both evacuating air from the pleural space and preventing recurrence. Small primary pneumothoraces usually resolve with simple observation and O_2 therapy. Supplemental O_2 accelerates the reabsorption of gas from the pleural space to about 8–9% per day. Larger, more symptomatic primary spontaneous pneumothoraces may be drained either with simple aspiration or with placement of a small-bore chest tube.

- Secondary spontaneous pneumothorax should be treated with a larger-bore chest tube attached to a water-seal device. Persistent air leaks and recurrences are more common with secondary than with primary spontaneous pneumothorax. For those with secondary spontaneous pneumothorax, recurrence is often prevented with instillation of sclerosing agents (e.g., talc) through the chest tube, video-assisted thoracoscopic surgery, or limited thoracotomy.
- Interventions to prevent recurrence in patients with primary spontaneous pneumothorax are usually recommended only after the second ipsilateral pneumothorax. Pilots and divers with primary spontaneous pneumothorax should be cautioned against such activity in the future because of the risk of contralateral pneumothorax.

Tension pneumothorax is a medical emergency requiring immediate decompression of the pleural space with a 14-gauge needle in the second intercostal space at the midclavicular line.

PULMONARY EMBOLISM (PE)

Defined as an obstruction of the pulmonary vasculature that is usually caused by venous thromboembolism (DVT). May also be the result of air, bone marrow, arthroplasty cement, tumor, infection, amniotic fluid, or talc. Ranges from clinically insignificant to massive embolus with sudden death. Risk factors are included in **Virchow's triad:**

- **Hypercoagulable state:** Associated with recent surgery, trauma, obesity, OCPs, pregnancy, cancer, immobilization, central venous catheters, and disorders of coagulation (antiphospholipid antibody, protein C/S deficiency, antithrombin III deficiency, factor V Leiden, and the prothrombin gene mutation).
- **Endothelial damage:** Associated with recent surgery or trauma or with previous DVT.
- **Stasis:** Associated with obesity, immobilization, CHF, and recent surgery.

SYMPTOMS/EXAM

Patients often present with acute-onset shortness of breath and pleuritic chest pain. Cough and hemoptysis may also be present. Physical examination may demonstrate low-grade fever, tachypnea, tachycardia, a loud P2, and JVD. Homans' sign and palpable cords on the calf may be present.

DIFFERENTIAL

MI, aortic dissection, pneumonia, pneumothorax, pericarditis, anxiety.

DIAGNOSIS

Accurate diagnosis remains difficult. Should be **suspected** when a patient presents with sudden-onset chest pain, dyspnea, tachycardia, and a normal CXR.

- **ABG:** May demonstrate **respiratory alkalosis,** hypoxemia, and an increased A-a gradient.
- **CXR:** Often normal, but may show **Hampton's hump** (wedge-shaped infarct) or **Westermark's sign** (relative oligemia in the region of the embolus), pleural effusion, or atelectasis.
- **ECG:** Sinus tachycardia is the most common finding. Less commonly seen is an S1Q3T3 pattern (S in lead I, Q in lead III, and an inverted T in lead III) suggesting right heart strain.

- **D-dimer:** some studies suggest a high negative predictive value with low pretest probability. However, the negative predictive value is much less in populations with a high prevalence of PE. Test characteristics vary by assay type, and assays also appear to be affected by embolus size and location. Currently not recommended as a single diagnostic test.
- **V/Q scan:** May demonstrate segmental regions of ventilation without perfusion (V/Q mismatch). Results are given as normal or low, indeterminate, or high probability for PE.
- **Lower extremity ultrasound:** May be used in conjunction with low or indeterminate V/Q scans to aid in the diagnosis of venous thromboembolism.
- **Spiral CT with IV contrast:** Sensitive for detecting proximal clots, but less sensitive with more distal emboli.
- **Pulmonary arteriogram:** The gold standard, but requires an invasive procedure with a skilled operator.

TREATMENT

- **Unfractionated heparin:** Bolus intravenously and continue using weight-based nomogram.
- **Low-molecular-weight heparin:** Can be given to low-risk patients with PE in place of IV unfractionated heparin.
- **Warfarin:** Long-term anticoagulation (six months) is usually recommended for those with no risk factors for future PEs.
- **Thrombolytics:** Generally recommended for patients with shock and no contraindications. Controversy exists for additional indications (e.g., right ventricular strain).

PULMONARY HYPERTENSION

Defined as a mean pulmonary artery pressure > 25 mmHg at rest or > 30 mmHg with exercise. Primary or idiopathic pulmonary hypertension (PPH) is a rare disease with an incidence of 1–2 per million with roughly a 3:1 female-to-male ratio. PPH may be familial or may occur sporadically. Secondary pulmonary hypertension is more common and is associated with disorders of the respiratory system (COPD, CF, pulmonary fibrosis); disorders of the heart (congenital heart disease, left ventricular dysfunction, mitral valve disease); chronic thromboembolic disease; pulmonary arterial hypertension related to collagen vascular disease (scleroderma, SLE, RA), HIV, or drugs (fenfluramine, phentermine, cocaine, methamphetamines); and miscellaneous causes (pulmonary veno-occlusive disease, pulmonary capillary hemangiomatosis, portopulmonary hypertension, sarcoidosis).

SYMPTOMS/EXAM

Patients with pulmonary hypertension typically complain of progressive dyspnea on exertion. In more advanced stages, patients may have exertional dizziness and even syncope. Raynaud's phenomenon is common in patients with PPH but may suggest an underlying collagen vascular disease. Cough and hemoptysis are rare in PPH but may be present in cases of pulmonary capillary hemangiomatosis. Hoarseness may also be present because of impingement of the left recurrent laryngeal nerve by a dilated pulmonary artery. Patients may have JVD, a right ventricular heave and right-sided S4, an increased P2, a murmur of tricuspid regurgitation, and the Graham Steell murmur of pulmonic insufficiency. In advanced disease, patients may present with hepatomegaly, pulsatile liver, and ascites.

DIFFERENTIAL

Left ventricular systolic failure, left ventricular diastolic dysfunction, causes of secondary pulmonary hypertension.

DIAGNOSIS

Treatment-based diagnostic evaluation to identify underlying disease is as follows:

- **Echocardiogram:** Provides an estimate of pulmonary artery pressure and helps identify left ventricular dysfunction, mitral valve disease, and congenital heart disease.
- **CXR:** Usually shows enlargement of the central pulmonary arteries with "pruning" of the peripheral vessels; may also show changes suggestive of COPD.
- **PFTs:** Help identify ILD, emphysema, and thoracic cage abnormalities as a cause of pulmonary hypertension.
- **V/Q scan:** All patients with pulmonary hypertension should have V/Q scanning to rule out chronic thromboembolic disease and should also have a subsequent pulmonary angiogram if subsegmental or segmental defects are present.
- **Sleep study:** For patients with loud snoring and daytime hypersomnolence; can identify obstructive sleep apnea as a potentially reversible cause of pulmonary hypertension.
- **Serologic testing:** For SLE, RA, scleroderma, and HIV. LFTs should also be performed as part of the workup.
- **Lung biopsy:** Rarely necessary and, in general, poorly tolerated.
- Patients should undergo **right heart catheterization** for the following purposes:
  - To confirm elevated pulmonary artery pressures and the absence of pulmonary venous hypertension.
  - To aid in determining prognosis, as those with high right atrial pressure and low cardiac index have the shortest survival rates.
  - To help determine the most appropriate therapy when used in conjunction with a vasodilator trial. An acute responder has reduced mean pulmonary arterial pressure with an increased or unchanged cardiac index.

TREATMENT

- In secondary pulmonary hypertension caused by disorders of the respiratory system (O_2, steroids, bronchodilators), chronic thromboembolic disease (anticoagulation, IVC filter, thromboendarterectomy), and pulmonary venous hypertension (afterload reduction, mitral valve repair/replacement), **treatment is aimed at disease.**
- In patients with PPH and other forms of pulmonary arterial hypertension, **treatment is based on response to vasodilators.**
  - **Acute responders** should be treated with anticoagulation and calcium channel blockers.
  - **Nonresponders** with New York Heart Association (NYHA) functional class III or IV should be treated with diuretics, anticoagulation, and bosentan, treprostinil, or epoprostenol. Bilateral lung transplantation remains a viable option for those who decline clinically despite maximal medical therapy.

SOLITARY PULMONARY NODULE

Defined as an isolated round lesion < 3 cm in diameter that is surrounded by pulmonary parenchyma. Abnormalities > 3 cm are termed masses and are usually malignant. Cancer affects 10–70% of those with solitary pulmonary nodules. Most benign lesions are infectious granulomas.

Lesions that increase in size or change in character are likely malignant and should be resected, assuming low surgical risk and no evidence of metastatic disease.

Symptoms/Exam

Patients are often asymptomatic but may present with cough, hemoptysis, and dyspnea. Older age and a history of cigarette smoking raise the suspicion of cancer. Patients should be questioned about prior TB and histoplasmosis. Physical examination of the lungs is frequently normal. However, examination of the lymphatic system may demonstrate lymphadenopathy.

Differential

Granuloma (old TB, histoplasmosis, foreign body reaction), bronchogenic carcinoma, metastatic disease (usually > 1), bronchial adenoma, round pneumonia.

Diagnosis

- Solitary pulmonary nodules are usually discovered incidentally.
- **Comparison of serial CXRs** is the **initial** step in determining the progression and extent of the nodule. Stability of findings on CXR for two years is considered a sign that the lesion is benign.
- **Chest CT** offers improved estimation of nodule size, characteristics (e.g., pattern of calcification), and interval growth (see Table 16-12). Contrast enhancement allows for the simultaneous evaluation of the mediastinum for lymphadenopathy.

TABLE 16-12. Chest CT Patterns and Associated Disease

Pattern	Disease
Calcification	
Laminated	Granulomatous disease
Popcorn	Hamartoma
Eggshell	Silicosis
Stippled	Malignancy
Eccentric	Malignancy
Margin contour	
Smooth	Likely benign
Scalloped	Intermediate risk of malignancy
Spiculated	Likely malignant
Corona radiata	Malignancy
Air-bronchus sign	Pneumonia; bronchoalveolar carcinoma

- **PET scan** may help provide staging information in the case of lung cancer. The diagnostic accuracy of detecting mediastinal involvement among patients with lung cancer is 65% by CT, 90% by PET, and > 95% using a combination of CT and PET.

TREATMENT

Currently, there are no evidence-based guidelines to address the approach to the solitary pulmonary nodule. When the probability of cancer is low (age < 35, nonsmoker, smooth nodule with diameter < 1.5 cm), the lesion should be monitored with serial HRCT at three-month intervals. When the probability of cancer is high (age > 35, smoker, spiculated nodule with diameter > 2 cm), the lesion should be resected if preoperative risk is acceptable and there are no other contraindications to surgery. When the probability of cancer is intermediate, additional testing (PET, transthoracic needle biopsy) may be warranted.

SARCOIDOSIS

A systemic disease of unknown etiology that primarily affects the lungs and lymphatics and is characterized by noncaseating granulomas. Commonly affects young and middle-age adults, often presenting with bilateral hilar adenopathy, pulmonary infiltrates, and skin lesions. The liver, lymphatics, salivary glands, heart, CNS, and bones may be involved as well.

SYMPTOMS/EXAM

Patients may present with nonspecific constitutional symptoms such as fever, fatigue, anorexia, weight loss, and arthralgias. Physical examination may reveal dry crackles, lymphadenopathy, parotid enlargement, splenomegaly, uveitis, or skin changes (erythema nodosum).

DIFFERENTIAL

Mycobacterial, fungal, bacterial (tularemia and brucellosis), and parasitic (toxoplasmosis) infection. Also includes berylliosis, lymphoma, hypersensitivity pneumonitis, Wegener's granulomatosis, and Churg-Strauss syndrome.

DIAGNOSIS

Diagnosis is made by a combination of clinical, radiographic, and histologic findings along with exclusion of other diseases that have a similar clinical picture. Workup should attempt to provide histologic evidence, evaluate the extent of disease, assess for disease progression, and determine whether therapy will benefit the patient.

The combination of bilateral hilar adenopathy, erythema nodosum, and joint symptoms (Löfgren's syndrome) usually resolves with corticosteroid treatment.

- **Baseline studies:**
  - **History:** Emphasis on occupational and environmental exposure.
  - **Physical examination:** Emphasis on the lung, skin, eye, liver, spleen, and heart.
  - Biopsy to obtain histologic confirmation of noncaseating granulomas.
  - CXR, PFTs, ECG.
  - Ophthalmologic evaluation.
  - LFTs, calcium, BUN/creatinine.
  - ACE level (not sensitive; value for monitoring disease is unclear).

- **Follow-up studies:**
  - Monitoring for resolution or progression of disease and for new-organ involvement.
  - Referral to subspecialists if there is evidence of disease progression or new-organ involvement.

TREATMENT

Systemic corticosteroids.

SLEEP-DISORDERED BREATHING

Sleep apnea is defined as intermittent cessation in airflow at the nose and mouth during sleep. It may be obstructive or central. Patients with **obstructive sleep apnea** (OSA) have episodic closure of the upper airway during sleep with continued respiratory efforts. Patients with **central sleep apnea** have cessation of both airflow and respiratory efforts. Central sleep apnea is often associated with CNS disorders, respiratory muscle weakness, cardiovascular disease, or pulmonary congestion, but it may also be idiopathic.

The key observation in making the diagnosis of central sleep apnea is that apneas are not accompanied by respiratory effort.

SYMPTOMS/EXAM

Daytime hypersomnolence, impaired cognition, snoring, witnessed gasping or choking at night, and witnessed apneic episodes while sleeping are common. Patients may have obesity and hypertension but may otherwise be normal. Patients with severe disease may have associated left ventricular failure, pulmonary hypertension, and right heart failure.

DIAGNOSIS

The overnight sleep study (polysomnogram) is used to identify onset of sleep and its various stages as well as to document apnea, hypopnea, and arousal. The polysomnogram can also help distinguish central sleep apnea from OSA. An overnight oximetry study may aid in the following:

- To **confirm** the diagnosis of sleep apnea when the pretest probability is high and the patient has recurrent episodes of O_2 desaturation.
- To **exclude** the diagnosis when the pretest probability is low and the patient has no O_2 desaturation.

TREATMENT

Options include weight loss, nasal continuous positive airway pressure (CPAP), and avoidance of alcohol and sedatives. Uvulopalatopharyngoplasty and mandibular advancement have had success in only a select group of patients. Tracheostomy provides instant relief but is often not first-line treatment.

LUNG TRANSPLANTATION

For patients with severe impairment due to lung disease and limited expected survival, lung transplantation offers the potential to improve quality of life as well as to prolong life. However, complications are frequent and may ultimately lead to graft dysfunction, which limits long-term survival. The limited number of acceptable donor lungs and increasing number of candidates have

Obs Sleep apnea - Hypoapnea :-

- Undiagnosed in 80% in US.
- prev. US - 2% ♀ 4% ♂
- Morbidity - HTN - 50-70% pt. OSA is risk factor for developing HTN indepen of obesity, age, alc intake & smoking.
  - may contribute to metabolic syn.
  - oxidative stress.
- large Study in progress - Sleep Heart health Study
  prelim findings ↑ risk CAD, CHF, Stroke.
- Race : Black, young < 25. M : F = 3:1, prev. ↑ c̄ age.
- Symp - Nocturnal - Snoring, apnea, freq arousal, tossing in bed
  Daytime - waking up s̄ being refreshed, morning headache, Excessive day time sleepiness (EDS)
- Epworth Sleepiness Score
  - > 10 ⇒ Sleepy.
  - 12 or more ⇒ greater propensity to fall asleep on Multiple Sleep Latency Test
  - Drawback - ↑ Score of ESS doesnot mean Shorter latencies on MSLT but ↑ Score means ↑ likelihood of falling asleep.
  - good thing - index for f/u.
- O/E Neck circumference 43 cm (17 in) ♂ / 37 cm (15 in) ♀ } ↑ risk of OSA
- Mallampati Score
  Class 1 - Full visibility of tonsils, Uvula & soft palate
  2 - Visibility of Hard & soft palate & upper part of tonsils & Uvula
  3 - Soft & hard palate & base of Uvula
  4 - Hard palate only.

  A 2006 study showed that each ↑ unit increase in Mallampati
  - odds of having OSA (i.e AHI > 5) increased by 2.5. } ← lead to.
  - AHI increased by 5 events per hour.

Obstructive - cessation of airflow c̄ respiratory effort.
Central - " " " with no " ".
Mixed - Begins as central & ends as an obs. apnea.
Hypoapnea - diff defn. But concensus (recent) is 30% reduction in flow associated c̄ 4% drop in oxygen saturation.

- polysomnography - (a) EEG, electrooculography, electromyography - sleep stage
  (b) ECG - single lead - Heart rhythm
  (c) ant. tibialis electromyography - Leg movmts
  (d) airflow at nose, mouth, effort, sat - Breathing.
- polysomnography is often followed by MSLT
- MSLT - consists of 4-5 naps of 20 min duration q 2 hrs during daytime & then latency to sleep onset - mean is calculated.
  - N latency is 10-15 min. In OSA it's < 10 min
  - Helpful to r/o narcolepsy. Narcoleptic have rapid eye movmt sleep on at least 2 of 4-5 naps during the day.
- PFT if evidence of cor pulmonale or if nocturnal symp s/o asthma eg SOB persists after waking or is asso c̄ wheezing
- Recent evidence OSA is not an indepen risk factor for dev. of Pulm HTN in absence of other lung disease.

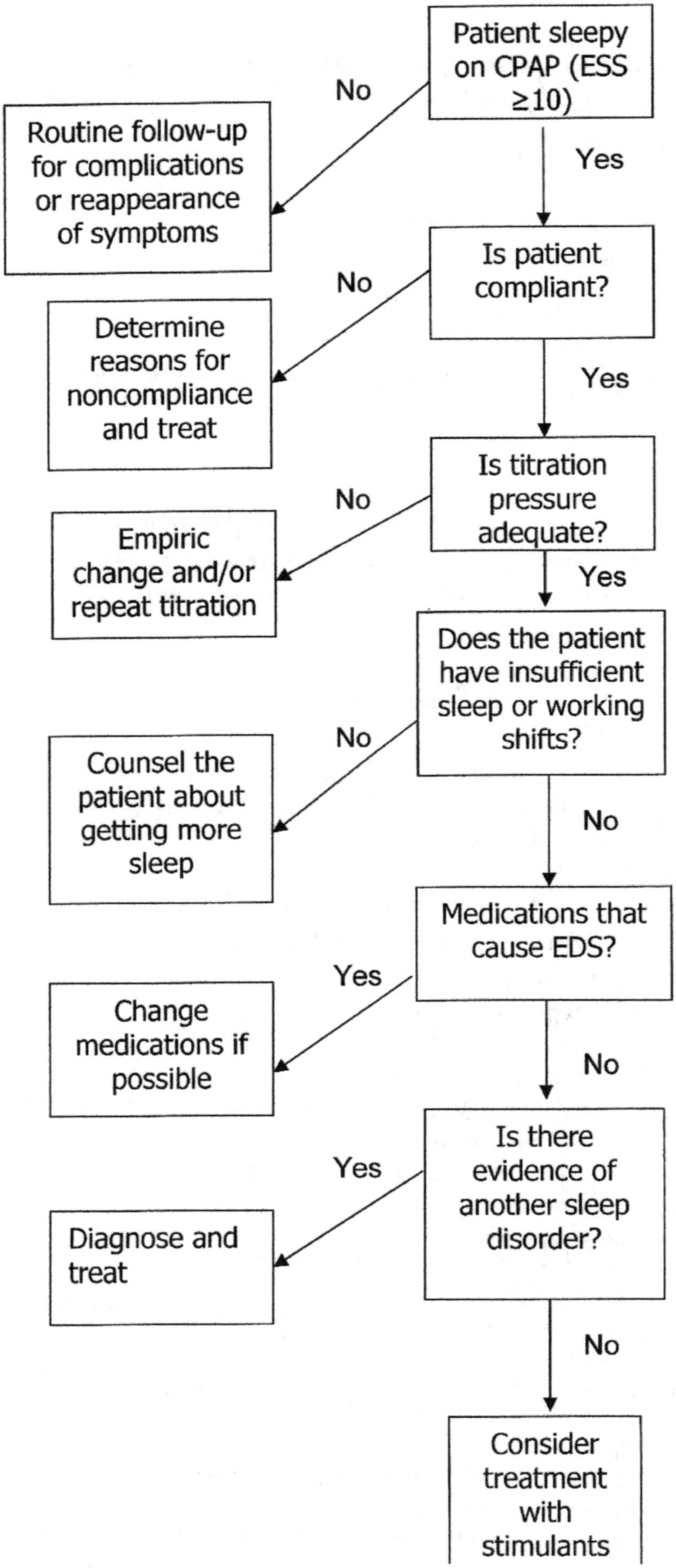

Management
(a) Mod - conservative (exclusive or very mild i.e. su... only.)
. wt loss
. avoid alc 4-6 hr prior to be...
- sleep on sides
(b) Nasal cpap -
• All pt c̄ AHI > 15 are elig... for CPAP regardless of s... (Medicare guidelines)
• 5-14.9 c̄ one of
- EDS
- HTN
- CV dz.
• ↓ HTN
improve LV EF. in CHF & ...

← Read flo on LHS.

Obesity-hypoventilation syn. or pickwickian syn:-
- OSA + hypoxemia & hypercarbia } whi... an...
- All pickwickian syn have ... but most pt c̄ OSA are not pickwickian.

led to long waiting times (e.g., 6–24 months) for lung transplantation. Currently, severe emphysema is the most common indication for lung transplantation in the United States. Other diseases for which it is indicated include CF, IPF, sarcoidosis, PPH, and pulmonary fibrosis related to collagen vascular disease.

Candidate Selection

Transplantation should be offered only to those with severe, advanced obstructive, fibrotic, or pulmonary vascular disease who have failed medical therapy and have a high likelihood of dying within the next 2–3 years. The following are recommended age limits for candidates:

- **Heart-lung transplantation:** ≤ 55 years of age.
- **Double-lung transplantation:** ≤ 60 years of age.
- **Single-lung transplantation:** ≤ 65 years of age.

Contraindications include severe extrapulmonary organ dysfunction, active or recent cigarette smoking, active cancer, drug dependence, severe malnutrition or obesity, and poor rehabilitation potential.

Organ Distribution

Allocation of lungs prior to 2005 was based solely on time accrued on the waiting list, regardless of severity of illness or medical emergency. In 2005, a lung allocation score was adapted to prioritize candidates based on wait list urgency and post-transplant survival.

Surgical Procedures

Single-lung transplantation is the most common procedure and is frequently performed for patients with emphysema or IPF. Double-lung transplantation is usually performed for patients with CF or bronchiectasis. Heart-lung transplantation is usually reserved for patients with Eisenmenger's syndrome and for those with severe lung disease and left ventricular dysfunction or advanced CAD.

Treatment Course and Outcomes

Immunosuppressive therapy is started in the perioperative period and is continued for life. Common long-term regimens include cyclosporine or tacrolimus in combination with azathioprine or mycophenolate mofetil and prednisone.

- **Quality of life:** Global improvement within the first three months after transplantation, but limited long-term data.
- **Complications:** Ischemia-reperfusion injury, bronchial anastomosis dehiscence or stenosis, infections (bacterial, CMV, aspergillosis), acute and chronic rejection are not infrequent and may limit survival.
- **Survival:** One-, three-, and five-year survival rates after lung transplantation are approximately 70%, 60%, and 50%, respectively.

NOTES

CHAPTER 17

Rheumatology

Jonathan Graf, MD

APPROACH TO ARTHRITIS

Tables 17-1 through 17-3 outline general approaches toward the differential diagnosis of arthritis and other rheumatic diseases. **Contraindications to arthrocentesis** include the following:

- Overlying soft tissue infection or cellulitis.
- Severe coagulopathy or bleeding disorder (INR > 3.0).

RHEUMATOID ARTHRITIS (RA)

Affects 1–2% of the U.S. population; exhibits a female-to-male predominance of 3:1. Its prevalence increases with age, with a typical age at onset of 20–40.

TABLE 17-1. Differential Diagnosis of Arthritis

Disease	Inflammation[a]	Joint Pattern	Peripheral Joint Involvement	Spinal Disease
RA	+	Symmetric/ polyarticular	Wrist/MCPs, PIPs/MTPs, ankles, knees	No (except C-spine)
SLE	+	Symmetric/ polyarticular	Wrist/MCPs/PIPs	No
Ankylosing spondylitis	+	Usually oligoarticular	Hips, shoulders, knees	Yes
Psoriatic arthritis	+	Asymmetric/ oligoarticular	Dactylitis, DIPs	Yes
Reactive arthritis	+	Asymmetric/ oligoarticular	Larger, weight-bearing joints; knees/ ankles	Yes
IBD-associated arthritis	+	Asymmetric/ oligoarticular	Larger joints	Yes
Gout (acute)	+	Monoarticular, polyarticular	First MTP, ankle, knee, MCPs/PIPs	No
Gout (chronic)	+	Monoarticular, polyarticular	Can mimic RA	No
Osteoarthritis	–	Monoarticular/ oligoarticular, polyarticular	DIPs, first carpal-metacarpal, knees, hips	Yes

[a] Symptoms and signs indicative of **inflammatory** joint disease include the following:

- Morning pain and/or stiffness > 30 minutes.
- Gelling phenomenon—worsening of symptoms with prolonged joint inactivity.
- Improvement in symptoms with use of the joint.
- Presence of erythema, warmth, and/or swelling in the joint.

TABLE 17-2. Characteristics of Synovial Fluid

Sign	Normal	Group 1: Noninflammatory (osteoarthritis, hypothyroidism)	Group 2: Inflammatory (RA, gout, spondyloarthropathy)	Group 3: Septic
Clarity	Transparent	Transparent	Slightly opaque	Opaque
Color	Clear	Yellow	Yellow-opalescent	Yellow-green
Viscosity	High	High	Low	Usually low
Culture	Negative	Negative	Negative	Often positive
WBCs/mm^3	< 200	200–2000	2000–50,000	> 50,000
PMNs (%)	< 25	< 25	> 50	> 75

TABLE 17-3. Laboratory Serologies in SLE and Other Rheumatic Diseases

	% Disease Association[a]							
	RA	SLE	SS	PSS	LS	P/DM	Wegener's	Other
ANA tests								
ANA	30–60	95–100	95	80–95	80–95	80–95	0–15	
Anti-dsDNA	0–5	60	N/A	N/A	N/A	N/A	N/A	
Anti-Sm	N/A	10–25	N/A	N/A	N/A	N/A	N/A	
Anti-SSA (Ro)	0–5	15–20	60–70	N/A	N/A	N/A	N/A	SCLE, neonatal lupus
Anti-SSB (La)	0–2	5–20	60–70	N/A	N/A	N/A	N/A	Neonatal lupus
Anticentromere	N/A	N/A	N/A	N/A	50	N/A	N/A	
Anti-SCL-70	N/A	N/A	N/A	33	20	N/A	N/A	
Non-ANA tests								
RF	70–80	20	75	25	25	33	50	
ANCA	N/A	1–5	N/A	N/A	N/A	N/A	93–96	
Anti-Jo-1	N/A	N/A	N/A	N/A	N/A	20–30	N/A	

[a] SS = Sjögren's syndrome; PSS = progressive systemic sclerosis; LS = limited scleroderma; P/DM = polymyositis/dermatomyositis; SCLE = subacute cutaneous lupus erythematosus.

Adapted, with permission, from Tierney LM et al (eds). *Current Medical Diagnosis & Treatment 2005,* 44th ed. New York: McGraw-Hill, 2005:809.

The most common joints affected are the hands, wrists, toes, ankles, and knees, although all joints with movable articulations can be involved.

SYMPTOMS/EXAM

Frequently associated with a prodrome of low-grade fever and malaise.

DIAGNOSIS

- **Diagnostic criteria (need four out of seven lasting > 6 weeks)** are as follows:
  - Morning stiffness
  - Arthritis involving three or more joint areas
  - Arthritis involving the hands
  - Symmetric arthritis
  - Serum RF
  - Radiographic changes consistent with disease
  - Rheumatoid nodules
- **Classic radiographic findings:** Periarticular osteopenia, joint space narrowing, juxta-articular erosions.
- **Common laboratory findings** include the following:
  - RF:
    - Usually an IgM antibody directed against an Fc fragment of IgG.
    - Present in 70–80% of patients with established disease.
    - Usually present in patients with extra-articular disease.
    - Not specific for RA; can be seen in other collagen vascular diseases and chronic infections (e.g., HCV).
  - ESR is frequently elevated but is neither sensitive nor specific.
  - Anemia of chronic disease.
  - Normal or elevated platelet count (vs. SLE).
  - Neutropenia can be seen with Felty's syndrome.
- **Extra-articular manifestations:**
  - Rheumatoid nodules, vasculitis, interstitial lung disease.
  - Serositis (pleuritis, pericarditis).
  - Ocular disease (episcleritis, uveitis, scleritis, keratitis).
  - Sjögren's syndrome.
  - Caplan's syndrome (large nodulosis of the lungs associated with anthracite coal exposure).
  - Amyloidosis.
  - Felty's syndrome (What is Felty's? The **ANS**wer = **A**rthritis, **N**eutropenia, and **S**plenomegaly).

Most extra-articular manifestations of RA are observed in patients who are RF positive and have long-standing erosive articular disease.

TREATMENT

Early use of disease-modifying antirheumatic drugs (DMARDs) is key. The "pyramid" is no longer board-eligible! NSAIDs are important for symptom flares, but the American College of Rheumatology recommends starting DMARD therapy within three months of diagnosis, either with single agents or as combination therapy.

- **Methotrexate:**
  - An antimetabolite used widely as a first-line DMARD.
  - **Dosage:** Weekly.
  - **Initial monitoring:** CXR, hepatitis serologies, CBC, LFTs, creatinine.
  - **Routine monitoring:** CBC, LFTs, creatinine.
  - **Contraindications:** Do not use in patients with known or suspected hepatic disease.
  - **Side effects:** Myelosuppression, hypersensitivity pneumonitis, pulmonary fibrosis, hepatic fibrosis, cirrhosis.

- **Sulfasalazine:**
  - An established first- or second-line DMARD.
  - **Initial monitoring:** CBC and G6PD level (if suspected); routine CBCs.
  - **Contraindications:** Can cause hemolysis in patients with G6PD deficiency and potential reactions in patients who are sulfonamide or aspirin sensitive.
  - **Other side effects:** GI intolerance, neutropenia, thrombocytopenia.
- **Leflunomide:**
  - An antimetabolite that is an effective first- or second-line DMARD.
  - **Dosage:** Daily (vs. weekly methotrexate), but half-life is > 2 weeks.
  - **Initial monitoring:** CBC, LFTs, hepatitis serologies, creatinine.
  - **Routine monitoring:** CBC, LFTs, creatinine.
  - **Side effects:** Myelosuppression, hepatotoxicity, diarrhea, rash.
- **Tumor necrosis factor (TNF) inhibitors:**
  - Usually added to the regimens of patients who are not responding well to other DMARDs.
  - Significantly retards the progression of erosive articular disease.
  - **Contraindications:** An increased incidence of opportunistic infections has been observed, particularly granulomatous infections such as TB and fungi.
  - **Other side effects:** Rare occurrence of leukopenias and demyelinating diseases.

TNF inhibitors can lead to activation of latent TB.

- **Antimalarials:**
  - Relatively weak DMARDs used in mild RA or in combination with other DMARDs.
  - **Monitoring:** Routine ophthalmologic exam.
  - **Side effects:** Can cause pigmented retinitis, visual loss, neuropathies, and myopathies.
- **Corticosteroids:**
  - Effective anti-inflammatory medications that may also retard bony erosions.
  - Use the lowest doses to prevent drug-induced complications.
  - **Initial monitoring:** BP, glucose, chemistry panel, lipid profile.
  - **Routine monitoring:** Bone densitometry in high-risk patients (length of treatment, higher dose, menopausal, etc.); monitoring of glucose and lipids as warranted.
  - **Side effects:** Glucose intolerance, hypertension, cataracts, avascular necrosis, osteoporosis.
- **Azathioprine:**
  - An antimetabolite used for severe or refractory RA.
  - **Initial monitoring:** CBC, LFTs, creatinine.
  - **Routine monitoring:** CBCs regularly or with change in dose.
  - **Contraindications:** Not to be used concomitantly with allopurinol.
  - **Side effects:** Myelosuppression, immunosuppression, hepatotoxicity, lymphoproliferative disorders.
- **Minocycline:**
  - Appears to show efficacy as a DMARD against RA, particularly in early disease.
  - **Monitoring:** No baseline or routine monitoring is required.
  - **Side effects:** Dizziness, skin hyperpigmentation, deposition into bone. Hyperpigmentation is sometimes reversible upon discontinuation of the drug.
- **Gold salts:**
  - Rarely used in modern practice, although some long-standing patients are maintained on therapy.

- Initial monitoring: CBC, creatinine, urine dipstick (protein).
- **Routine monitoring:** CBC and urine dipstick (protein) weekly for the first half year; then at a minimum before each injection.
- **Side effects:** Myelosuppression, proteinuria.

- **Penicillamine:**
  - Rarely used.
  - **Initial and routine monitoring:** CBC and urine dipstick (protein).
  - **Side effects:** Myelosuppression, proteinuria.

SYSTEMIC LUPUS ERYTHEMATOSUS (SLE) AND DRUG-INDUCED LUPUS

Systemic Lupus Erythematosus

Shows a female-to-male predominance of 9:1. Three times more common among African-Americans than among whites. Both genetic and environmental factors are involved. Nearly 90% of patients have joint symptoms.

DIFFERENTIAL

The differential diagnosis of SLE is outlined in Table 17-5.

DIAGNOSIS

- Four of the 11 clinical and laboratory criteria listed in Table 17-4 are needed for diagnosis.
- ANA testing is nearly 100% sensitive but is not specific for SLE (Table 17-5).
- Antibodies to dsDNA and Smith are specific (> 90% and > 95%, respectively) but not sensitive (50–60% and 30%, respectively).
- Antibody titers to dsDNA can correlate with disease activity, particularly renal disease.
- Antibodies to Smith and ANA titers do not correlate with disease activity.
- Depressed serum complement levels are frequently seen in SLE but can normalize in remission.

An elevated PTT in a patient with SLE suggests the presence of antiphospholipid antibodies.

TREATMENT

Nonpharmacologic treatment includes sun avoidance, sun protection, rest, and avoidance of stress. Pharmacologic treatment can be broken down according to disease severity:

- **Mild disease** (skin, joint, oral ulcers, serositis):
  - NSAIDs.
  - Topical corticosteroids for skin disease.
  - Low-dose systemic corticosteroids (< 10 mg/day).
  - Antimalarial medications (good for mild symptoms and skin disease).
- **Moderate disease** (cytopenias/hemolytic anemia, serositis, mild pneumonitis, mild myocarditis):
  - Moderately dosed systemic corticosteroids (approximately 0.5 mg/kg/day).
  - Steroid-sparing agents such as azathioprine, methotrexate (good for skin and arthritis), and mycophenolate mofetil.
- **Severe disease** (nephritis, severe CNS disease such as vasculitis, pulmonary hemorrhage):
  - High-dose corticosteroids (≥ 1 mg/kg/day).
  - IV cyclophosphamide (proven efficacy for nephritis; less established for other indications).
  - Azathioprine.
  - Mycophenolate mofetil.

TABLE 17-4. Diagnostic Criteria for SLE (4 of 11 Needed for Diagnosis)

Skin/**S**unlight:
1. Malar rash
2. Discoid rash
3. Photosensitivity

Serosa/mucous membranes:
4. Oral ulcers
5. Serositis (pleuritis/pericarditis)

Synovitis:
6. Arthritis

Seizures, "**S**"ychosis
7. Neurologic disease (seizures, psychosis)

"**S**"ellular casts, proteinuria:
8. Renal disease (any one of the following):
   a. > 0.5 g/day proteinuria
   b. ≥ 3+ dipstick protein
   c. Cellular casts

"**S**"ytopenias:
9. Hematologic disorders (any one of the following):
   a. Hemolytic anemia
   b. Leukopenia (< 4000/mL)
   c. Lymphopenia (< 1500/mL)
   d. Thrombocytopenia (< 100,000/mL)

Serologies:
10. Positive ANA
11. Immunologic abnormalities (any one of the following):
   a. Antibodies to native DNA
   b. Anti-Smith antibodies
   c. Antiphospholipid antibodies:
      1. False positive serologic test for syphilis
      2. Evidence of anticardiolipin antibodies
      3. Evidence of lupus anticoagulant

- IVIG (for antibody-mediated cytopenias).
- Plasmapheresis (extreme circumstances).

COMPLICATIONS

In addition to disease-related organ-specific damage, complications are as follows:

- Accelerated atherosclerosis; coronary heart disease.
- Transitional cell carcinoma and hematologic malignancies if the patient received cyclophosphamide.
- Opportunistic infections.

TABLE 17-5. Differential Diagnosis of SLE

DIFFERENTIAL	DISTINGUISHING FACTORS
Drug-induced lupus **(must be excluded)**	See below.
RA	Erosive arthritis.
Mixed connective tissue disease	Less severe renal disease; features of systemic sclerosis and/or inflammatory myopathy.
Vasculitis	Different serologies (see Table 17-3).
Acute drug reaction	Identification of offending agent.
Systemic sclerosis	Predominance of skin changes.

Drug-Induced Lupus

The most commonly associated drugs are hydralazine, procainamide, INH, quinidine, methyldopa, and chlorpromazine.

DIFFERENTIAL

Hallmarks that distinguish drug-induced lupus from SLE include the following:

- Equal prevalence among both sexes.
- Lack of severe renal and neurologic involvement.
- Lack of antibodies to DNA.
- Frequently normal levels of serum complement.
- Clinical and laboratory features remit upon discontinuation of the inciting agent.
- Presence of **antihistone antibodies** (sensitive but not specific for drug-induced lupus).

Neonatal lupus is classically associated with anti-Ro and anti-La antibodies.

Neonatal Lupus

Clinical features of neonatal lupus are as follows:

- Photosensitive rash, complete heart block, hepatitis, thrombocytopenia, hemolytic anemia.
- Passive transfer of maternal anti-Ro/SSA and anti-La/SSB antibodies in utero associated with disease.
- Most features remit when titers of antibodies wane in the neonate.
- Complete heart block is permanent.

SJÖGREN'S SYNDROME

Characterized by lymphocytic and plasma cell infiltration of affected exocrine glands throughout the entire body. Can be primary in etiology or secondary to another autoimmune disorder. Sjögren's exhibits a significant female-to-male predominance (9:1) and most commonly affects middle-aged individuals.

SYMPTOMS/EXAM

The clinical characteristics of Sjögren's syndrome are as follows (common ABIM-tested associations are in boldface):

- **Dry mouth (xerostomia), dental caries,** impaired taste and/or smell, dysphagia.
- **Keratoconjunctivitis sicca: Burning, itching eyes;** diminished lacrimation; thickened/sticky tears; photophobia.
- Parotid enlargement.
- Dryness of the skin and vaginal mucosa.
- **Pancreatitis.**
- Interstitial lung disease, **lymphocytic interstitial pneumonitis,** tracheobronchitis sicca.
- **Type 1 RTA,** interstitial nephritis.
- Neuropsychiatric diseases of various etiologies.
- Vasculitis.

DIFFERENTIAL

Drugs (e.g., anticholinergic medications), HCV, HIV, and sarcoidosis may present with dry eyes and dry mouth. HIV and sarcoidosis may also present with glandular infiltration.

DIAGNOSIS

- **Biopsy** of minor lip/salivary gland reveals lymphocytic foci in glands.
- **Labs:** Frequently positive ANA, RF, and anti-SSA/anti-SSB (see Table 17-3); hypergammaglobulinemia.
- Ancillary testing can demonstrate decreased tear production, low salivary flow, and sicca.

TREATMENT

Seek symptom relief with the following:

- Artificial tears and saliva.
- Sugarless candies and frequent water sipping.
- Aggressive oral hygiene.
- Avoidance of anticholinergic and decongestant medications.
- Cholinergic agonist medications to stimulate saliva production.

COMPLICATIONS

Lymphoproliferative disorders, including lymphomas; Waldenström's macroglobulinemia.

SERONEGATIVE SPONDYLOARTHROPATHIES

The four diseases are grouped because:

- *"Seronegative" = serologies negative for ANA and RF.*
- *"Spondylo-" = spinal arthritis.*

Include four disorders: ankylosing spondylitis, psoriatic arthritis, IBD-associated arthritis, and reactive arthritis (Reiter's syndrome) (see Table 17-6).

Ankylosing Spondylitis

Shows a predominance of **males over females;** characterized by an early age of onset (generally < 35 years). Prevalence is 0.2–0.5% among whites in the United States (higher prevalence among Scandinavians).

TABLE 17-6. Features of Seronegative Spondyloarthropathies

Disease	Sacroiliitis	Percentage with Positive HLA-B27	Other Manifestations
Ankylosing spondylitis	Symmetric	90	Uveitis, aortitis.
Psoriatic arthritis	Asymmetric	75	Skin disease in 80% of cases; DIP arthritis is common.
Reactive arthritis	Asymmetric	50 (when sacroiliitis is present)	Classic triad: conjunctivitis, urethritis, and arthritis (more commonly of larger peripheral joints than of the spine); keratoderma blennorrhagicum (pustular rash on soles of feet).
IBD-associated arthritis	Symmetric	50 (when sacroiliitis is present)	GI disease is usually present, more commonly Crohn's than ulcerative colitis.

Symptoms

- Inflammatory low back pain that worsens in the morning and with inactivity but improves with exercise.
- Progressive pain and stiffening of the spine.
- Transient acute arthritis (pain and swelling) of the larger peripheral joints.

Exam

- Tenderness of the sacroiliac joints to palpation.
- Reduced lumbar lordosis.
- Reduced chest expansion diameter.
- Limited range of motion of the neck.

Differential

- RA (affects numerous symmetric, small peripheral joints of the hands and feet).
- Noninflammatory, mechanical low back pain (vs. the characteristics detailed above).
- Diffuse idiopathic skeletal hyperostosis (DISH).
- Osteitis condensans ilei (sclerosis of the iliac bone in childbearing women).
- Infectious sacroiliitis.

Diagnosis

- Consistent history.
- Radiographic evidence of sacroiliitis and/or spinal involvement (see Figure 17-1):
  - Bilateral sclerosis of the sacroiliac joints.
  - Squared-off vertebral bodies.
  - "Shiny" corners of vertebral bodies.
  - Symmetric, bamboo-like syndesmophytes between vertebral bodies.
- HLA-B27 positive in the majority of cases (**not diagnostic;** seen in 8% of the normal population).
- Elevated ESR and negative RF.

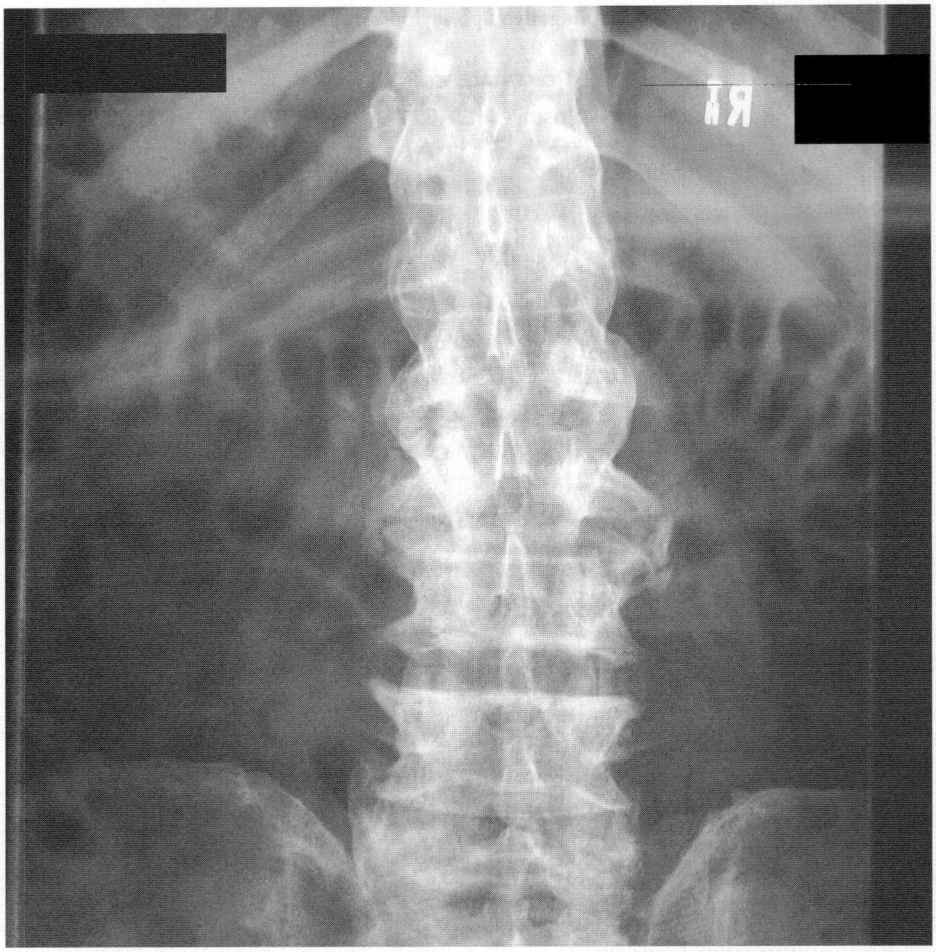

FIGURE 17-1. Spinal x-ray showing changes associated with a spondyloarthropathy.

(Courtesy of Jonathan Graf, MD, 2004.)

Treatment

- NSAIDs.
- Sulfasalazine or methotrexate for peripheral arthritis.
- TNF-α antagonists for significant disease.
- Aggressive **physical therapy** to enable spinal fusion in an advantageous position.

Complications

All of the following are board-eligible classic associations:

- Anterior uveitis.
- Aortitis and aortic regurgitation (more rarely, cardiac conduction system involvement).
- Apical pulmonary fibrosis (mimics TB—be careful!).
- Pseudoarthroses can occur when a fused spine is severed in a traumatic accident, which can cause spinal cord compromise.

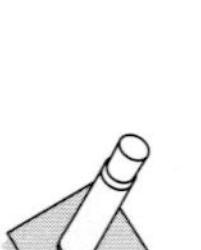

Apical pulmonary fibrosis can look like TB.

Psoriatic Arthritis

Peripheral arthritis, dactylitis, and enthesitis (inflammation of the tendinous insertions of the joints; seen with other HLA-B27-related diseases as well). Found in 15–20% of patients with psoriatic skin disease. Skin disease precedes arthritis in 80% of cases.

Symptoms/Exam

The clinical presentation of psoriatic arthritis is further outlined in Table 17-7.

Diagnosis

- Characteristic presentation.
- Radiographic findings include the following:
  - Marginal erosions of bone.
  - Characteristic "pencil-in-cup" deformities of distal digits.
  - Periosteal bone formations and calcifications of entheses.
  - Sacroiliitis and spondylitic changes of the spine (frequently asymmetric).

Treatment

- NSAIDs.
- Methotrexate, sulfasalazine, and other DMARDs for peripheral arthritis.
- TNF-α inhibitors.
- **Avoid corticosteroids if possible** (tapering can cause skin disease to flare).

Psoriasis precedes most cases of psoriatic arthritis.

Reactive Arthritis

Males (particularly young men) are affected more often than females. Eighty percent of white and 50–60% of African-American patients are HLA-B27 positive. Develops within days to weeks of antecedent infection:

- **GI disease:** *Salmonella, Shigella, Campylobacter, Yersinia.*
- **GU disease (urethritis):** *Chlamydia.*
- Idiopathic.

Symptoms/Exam

- Frequently asymmetric involvement of larger, weight-bearing joints.
- Spinal involvement is seen in 20% of patients.

TABLE 17-7. Five Major Patterns in Psoriatic Arthritis

Pattern	Joint Involvement
DIP involvement	Can be monoarticular or asymmetric; **nail pitting and onycholysis** (see Figure 17-2).
Pseudo-rheumatoid	Symmetric, smaller joint polyarthritis.
Oligoarticular	Erosive arthritis, dactylitis **("sausage digit")**.
Arthritis mutilans	Severe, osteolytic, deforming (telescoping digits).
Spondylitis	Sacroiliitis and/or ankylosing spondylitis.

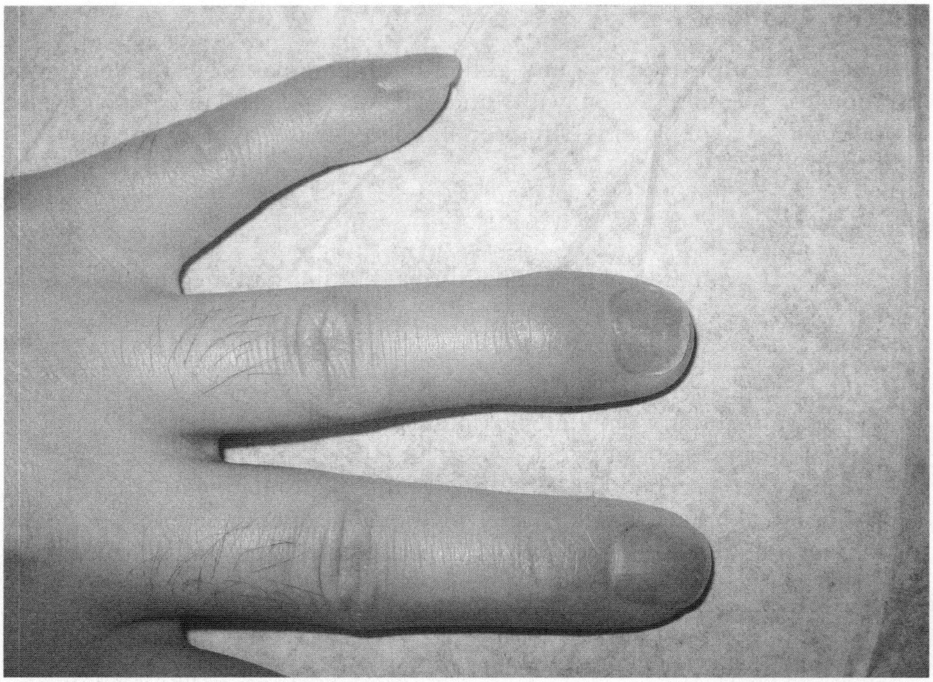

FIGURE 17-2. Onycholysis in a psoriatic arthritis patient.

(Courtesy of Jonathan Graf, MD, 2004.) (Also see Color Insert.)

- Conjunctivitis, urethritis, mucocutaneous ulcerations.
- Keratoderma blennorrhagicum (pustular eruptions on the soles of the feet).
- Systemic signs (fever, weight loss) are not unusual.

Differential

Septic and gonococcal arthritis, crystal-induced arthritis, seronegative RA, other seronegative spondyloarthropathies.

Diagnosis

- Inflammatory pattern on arthrocentesis.
- Culture of affected joints is sterile.
- Test for chlamydia if history or exam suggest this.

Treatment

- NSAIDs.
- Antibiotics for chlamydia-related reactive arthritis.
- Sulfasalazine, methotrexate, and other DMARDs for recalcitrant peripheral arthritis.

Complications

Aortitis and aortic regurgitation (rare).

Inflammatory Bowel Disease (IBD)–Associated Arthritis

Twenty percent of patients with IBD have associated arthritis. Associated more often with Crohn's disease than with ulcerative colitis. Arthritis usually appears after the onset of GI disease.

SYMPTOMS/EXAM

- Peripheral arthritis, enthesitis, and dactylitis:
  - Asymmetric, oligoarticular.
  - Large joint involvement.
  - Frequently nonerosive.
  - Flares in concert with intestinal disease.
- Spinal arthritis:
  - Symmetric inflammatory sacroiliitis and spondylitis.
  - Mimics ankylosing spondylitis.
  - The course of the disease is independent of intestinal disease.

DIFFERENTIAL

Ankylosing spondylitis, enteropathic reactive arthritis, Whipple's disease, seronegative RA.

TREATMENT

NSAIDs; treatment of intestinal disease (controls peripheral arthritis).

Hyperuricemia increases the risk of gout, but most patients with hyperuricemia will not get gout.

CRYSTALLINE-INDUCED ARTHROPATHIES

Include gout, pseudogout, and calcium pyrophosphate dihydrate deposition disease.

Hyperuricemia

The causes of hyperuricemia and its relation to gout are outlined in Table 17-8.

TABLE 17-8. Causes of Hyperuricemia

Overproduction of uric acid:

- Genetic metabolic defects:
  - Lesch-Nyhan syndrome
  - Glycogen storage diseases
  - Psoriasis
- Myeloproliferative disorders/large tumor burden malignancies
- Idiopathic

Underexcretion of uric acid:

- Idiopathic
- Chronic renal disease
- Medication induced:
  - Thiazide diuretics
  - Loop diuretics
  - Cyclosporine
- Metabolic:
  - Lactic acidosis
  - Alcoholism
  - Ketoacidosis
  - Lead nephropathy (saturnine gout)

Gout

Usually associated with abnormal uric acid metabolism and hyperuricemia; can be associated with uric acid stones and urate nephropathy (renal toxicity). Males are affected more often than females (9:1). Onset is generally after age 30; almost always **postmenopausal** in women.

Symptoms

- Sudden-onset, self-limited, recurrent, acute mono- or oligoarticular arthritis.
- Can progress to chronic deforming polyarthritis after multiple attacks.
- **Tophi:** Deposits of uric acid crystals in joints, bone, tendon, cartilage, and subcutaneous tissues.
- **Podagra:** The most commonly affected joint is the first MTP.
- Other affected joints include the knees, ankles, feet, elbows, and hands.
- **Intercritical periods:** Asymptomatic periods can last months or years.

Exam

- Erythema, swelling, warmth, and tenderness to palpation of affected joints.
- Cellulitis-like erythema of overlying skin and soft tissue.
- Classically exhibits a monoarticular presentation, but can be oligoarticular or polyarticular in long-standing disease.
- Presence of tophi on external ears, elbows, hands, and feet.
- Fever is common but rarely exceeds 39°C.

Differential

Cellulitis, septic arthritis, pseudogout, reactive arthritis, RA, lead poisoning.

Diagnosis

- Uric acid is abnormally elevated at some point in 95% of cases, but **this is not diagnostic and is not needed to make a diagnosis.**
- Synovial fluid aspiration reveals the following:
  - An inflammatory pattern.
  - Sterile cultures.
  - Negatively birefringent, needle-like crystals (the crystals are yellow under polarized light, when the red compensator is pointed in parallel to the crystals (think **yeLLow = paraLLel**) (see Figure 17-3).
- Radiographs of chronic tophi show "rat-bite" erosions adjacent to affected joints.
- Measure urinary uric acid excretion to distinguish underexcreters from overproducers of uric acid (< 600–800 mg/day = underexcreter).

Treatment

Guidelines for the treatment of gout are outlined in Table 17-9.

Complications

Complications associated with treatment are as follows:

- **Allopurinol:**
  - An acute gouty attack may occur if allopurinol used without a concomitant NSAID, colchicine, or corticosteroid agent.
  - Hypersensitivity syndrome (increased in renal disease and elevated serum metabolite levels).
  - Fever, desquamating rash, hepatitis, vasculitis.

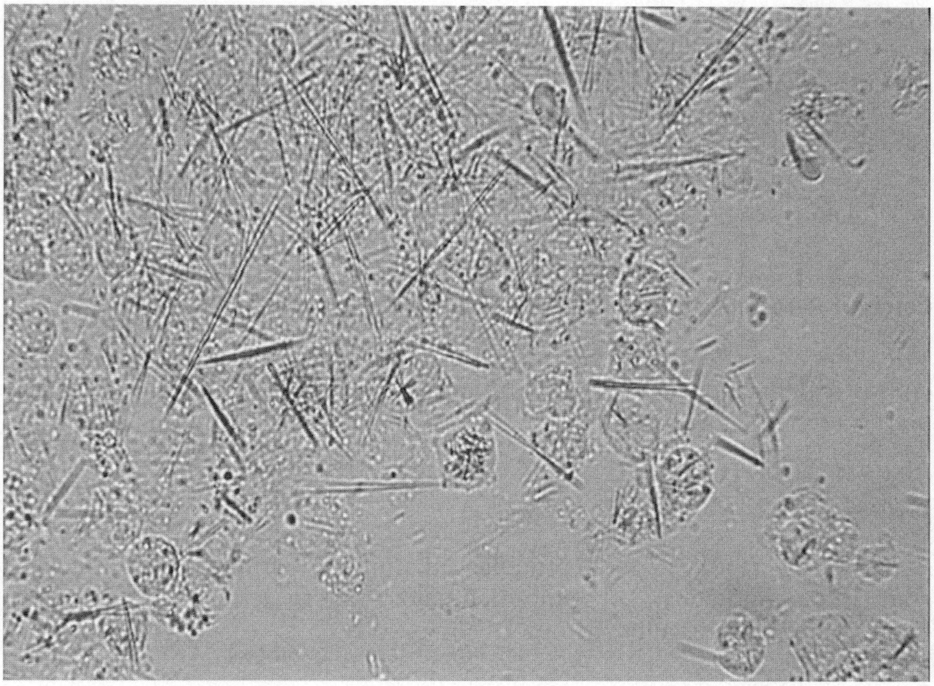

FIGURE 17-3. Gout crystals.

(Courtesy of Jonathan Graf, MD, 2004.) (Also see Color Insert.)

TABLE 17-9. Treatment of Gout

DRUG	USAGE
Acute attack	
NSAID (indomethacin)	Until symptoms resolve (1–2 weeks, 50–75 mg TID).
Colchicine	Within 48 hours of onset of attack (0.6 mg/hour until resolution of toxicity).
Corticosteroids	Oral in NSAID-intolerant patients; intra-articular injections for monoarticular disease.
After	
Nothing	Many patients will experience few if any future attacks and choose no further uric acid therapy.
Diet	Low purine (at best, can lower uric acid 1 mg/dL); alcohol avoidance.
Medication management	Discontinue precipitating medications.
Colchicine	0.6 mg QD BID to prevent future attacks; 0.6/day × 1–2 weeks while initiating uric acid–lowering therapies.
Allopurinol (xanthine oxidase inhibitor)	Best for uric acid overproducers, tophaceous gout, and urate nephropathy. Give 100 mg (starting) to 300 mg/day.
Probenecid	Best for uric acid underexcretors (uricosuric). Give 500 mg/day (starting) to 2 g/day.

- Increases the effect and toxicity of azathioprine (blocks its metabolism).

- **Probenecid:**
  - Hypersensitivity.
  - Loss of efficacy in patients with advanced renal disease.
  - Precipitates urate nephropathy and nephrolithiasis if used in tophaceous gout or in patients with a history of urate calculi.

Calcium Pyrophosphate Dihydrate Deposition Disease (CPPD)

Accelerated or unusual distribution of degenerative joint disease should raise your suspicion for CPPD.

The clinical spectrum ranges from pseudogout to asymptomatic chondrocalcinosis (calcification of articular cartilage surface). CPPD may also occur as part of a systemic disease.

Pseudogout

Acute and/or recurrent monoarticular inflammatory arthropathy mimicking gout (including podagra). Pseudo-rheumatoid-pattern acute arthritis is more uncommon. Onset is after age 60.

Diagnosis

- Normal serum urate level.
- **Chondrocalcinosis** is visualized on x-rays of the knees and wrists.
- Synovial fluid aspiration reveals the following:
  - Inflammatory fluid profile in acute attacks.
  - Weakly **positive** birefringent **rhomboid-shaped crystals** (opposite of urate).

Treatment

NSAIDs, intra-articular injection of corticosteroid, colchicine for chronic chemoprevention.

CPPD as part of underlying metabolic disorders—

HOT PAW

Hemochromatosis
Ochronosis
Thyroid (hypothyroidism)
Parathyroid (hypoparathyroidism)
Acromegaly
Wilson's disease

Chondrocalcinosis

An accelerated degenerative joint disease characterized by osteoarthritis of unusual joints (e.g., the shoulders, ankles, elbows, MCPs). Characterized by a frequently asymptomatic deposition of CPPD crystals along articular surfaces. Aggressive disease or unusual age at presentation should prompt evaluation and treatment of an underlying metabolic disorder (see the mnemonic **HOT PAW**).

INFLAMMATORY MYOPATHIES

Table 17-10 outlines the clinical characteristics of various inflammatory myopathies.

Polymyositis

A systemic inflammatory disorder that specifically targets the proximal musculature. Women are affected more often than men by a ratio of 2:1; the average age of onset is 40–60 years. May have a mild association with malignancy.

TABLE 17-10. Characteristics of Inflammatory Myopathies

	PAIN	MUSCLE WEAKNESS	SKIN INVOLVEMENT	RESPONSE TO STEROIDS
Polymyositis	–	Proximal	–	+
Dermatomyositis	–	Proximal	+	+
Inclusion body myositis	–	Distal	–	–
Polymyalgia rheumatica	++	None	–	++

SYMPTOMS/EXAM

- Progressive muscle weakness of the neck and upper and lower extremities.
- **Weakness** is more common than **pain.**
- **Proximal muscles are affected more than distal muscles.**
- Difficulty swallowing.

DIFFERENTIAL

- Inclusion body myositis (**distal muscles are affected more than proximal muscles).**
- Polymyalgia rheumatica (**pain** is more common than weakness).
- Myositis secondary to other autoimmune diseases.
- Myositis secondary to malignancy.
- Medication-related myopathies (steroid, statin, colchicine).
- Toxin- or endocrine/metabolic-related myopathy.
- Myasthenia gravis.
- Genetic myopathies.

DIAGNOSIS

- Elevated markers of muscle enzymes (CK and/or aldolase) for both diagnosis and follow-up of disease.
- EMG is nonspecific and shows abnormal polyphasic potentials, fibrillations, and high-frequency action potentials.
- Biopsy of affected muscle shows endomysial lymphocytic inflammatory infiltrate.

TREATMENT

- Corticosteroids (0.5–1.0 mg/kg/day).
- DMARDs (methotrexate, azathioprine) for steroid sparing or recalcitrant disease.

COMPLICATIONS

- **Antisynthetase syndrome:** Interstitial lung disease, Raynaud's phenomenon, arthritis (associated with **anti-Jo-1 antibodies**).
- Myocarditis.
- Respiratory muscle failure.
- Swallowing difficulties and aspiration.

Dermatomyositis

Often associated with occult malignancy. Amyopathic dermatomyositis is a variant with a characteristic skin disease.

SYMPTOMS/EXAM

- Similar to polymyositis.
- Characteristic skin rashes.
- **Gottron's papules:** A scaly rash over the extensor surfaces.
- **Shawl sign:** Erythema in a sun-exposed V-neck or shoulder distribution.
- **Heliotrope rash:** A violaceous rash over the eyelids, sometimes with periorbital edema.
- **Facial erythema:** A diffuse, dusky rash.
- Periungual erythema and dilated periungual capillaries.

Once dermatomyositis is diagnosed, serious investigation of underlying occult malignancy should be sought, especially age-appropriate cancer screening.

DIAGNOSIS

- Similar to polymyositis.
- **Muscle biopsy:** Perivascular and perifascicular lymphocytic inflammatory infiltrate with destruction of microvasculature.

TREATMENT

- Similar to polymyositis.
- IVIG for refractory cases.
- Treatment of underlying malignancy (if present).

Inclusion Body Myositis

Characterized by distal more than proximal muscle weakness; weakness is more frequently asymmetric than symmetric. More insidious in onset than polymyositis or dermatomyositis. "Treatment resistant" compared to other inflammatory myopathies. Characteristic inclusion bodies are seen on muscle biopsy. Older white males are more frequently affected.

SYSTEMIC SCLEROSIS (SCLERODERMA)

The clinical characteristics of systemic sclerosis are outlined in Table 17-11.

Limited Scleroderma

SYMPTOMS/EXAM

- Characterized primarily by the **CREST** syndrome: **C**alcinosis, **R**aynaud's phenomenon, **E**sophageal dysmotility, **S**clerodactyly (distal to wrist), and **T**elangiectasias.

TABLE 17-11. Characteristics of Systemic Sclerosis

DISEASE TYPE	FREQUENCY OF CASES (%)	ORGANS INVOLVED	ANTIBODIES
Limited scleroderma	80	CREST, pulmonary hypertension	ANA, anticentromere
Progressive systemic sclerosis	20	Proximal skin, kidney, heart, lung, GI tract	ANA, anti-SCL-70

- Also presents with arthralgia and arthritis, fever and malaise, abnormal periungual capillary dropout or dilatation, digital ulcerations, and tapering of distal digits.

TREATMENT

Treatment is outlined in Table 17-12.

COMPLICATIONS

The prognosis is generally more favorable than that of diffuse scleroderma, but later-onset pulmonary hypertension and other vasculopathic processes affect mortality.

Progressive (Diffuse) Systemic Sclerosis

SYMPTOMS/EXAM

- Skin involvement **proximal to the wrists,** including the arms, chest, and face.
- Tendon friction rubs.
- Early **scleredema** (soft tissue swelling of affected joints).
- Features of CREST.

DIFFERENTIAL

Morphea and linear scleroderma (characteristic localized skin disease), limited scleroderma, scleromyxedema, eosinophilic fasciitis, eosinophilia-myalgia syndrome.

TREATMENT

Treatment is outlined in Table 17-13.

VASCULITIS

Approach to Vasculitis

Vasculitis can be classified as either primary or secondary. Figure 17-4 categorizes primary vasculitis according to vessel size. Secondary causes of vasculitis are as follows:

- Infections (particularly indolent, chronic infections such as subacute bacterial endocarditis and HCV).

TABLE 17-12. Symptomatic Treatment of Limited Scleroderma

DISORDER	TREATMENT
Raynaud's	Body-warming techniques, calcium channel–blocking agents.
Digital ulcerations	Raynaud's therapies as above; aspirin, topical nitrates, prostacyclin analogs.
Esophageal dysmotility	Elevate the head of the bed and avoid late-night meals; H_2 blocker or PPI.
Pulmonary hypertension	O_2, calcium channel blocker, prostacyclin analogs, bosentan.

TABLE 17-13. Symptomatic Treatment of Diffuse Scleroderma

Organ	Complication	Treatment
Kidney	Renal crisis (malignant hypertension, renal failure, and micrangiopathic hemolytic anemia).	ACEIs.
Lung	Interstitial pneumonitis, interstitial fibrosis.	Corticosteroids,[a] immunosuppressants.
Heart	Myocarditis, myocardial fibrosis, heart failure, pericardial effusions, conduction system disease.	Corticosteroids,[a] immunosuppressants, CHF therapy, pacemakers.
GI	Delayed gastric emptying, intestinal malabsorption, bacterial overgrowth.	Frequent small meals, promotility agents, antibiotics.

[a] Corticosteroids are usually avoided in scleroderma (unless severe organ-related disease leaves little other choice) because they may precipitate renal crisis.

- Medications (hypersensitivity vasculitis, leukocytoclastic vasculitis, ANCA-associated vasculitis).
- Collagen vascular disease.
- Malignancy.

Primary Vasculitis Syndromes

WEGENER'S GRANULOMATOSIS

Necrotizing **granulomatous** arteritis of the small arteries, arterioles, and capillaries. Characterized by cavitating **nodules of the upper and lower respiratory tract (lungs and sinuses)** and by **glomerulonephritis.** Organs and systems affected include the upper and lower respiratory tract, kidney, eye, ear, nerve, skin, gingiva, and joints.

SYMPTOMS/EXAM

- Fever, malaise, weight loss.
- Sinusitis, epistaxis, otitis media, gingivitis, stridor, mastoiditis.

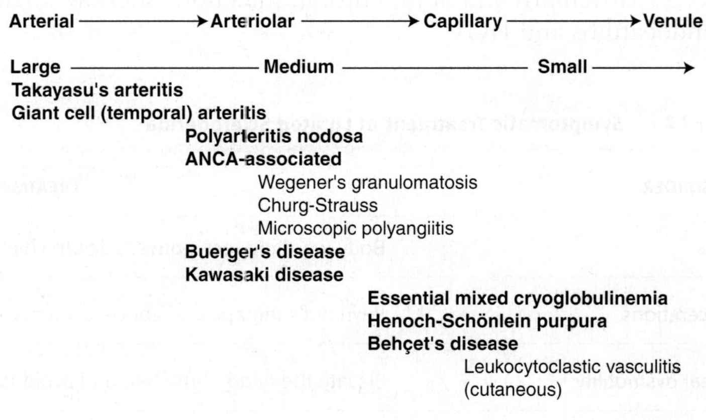

FIGURE 17-4. Classification of primary vasculitis according to size of vessel involved.

- Cough, hemoptysis, dyspnea.
- Arthritis, scleritis, neuropathy, skin rashes, hematuria.

Diagnosis

- Elevated ESR; normal serum complement levels.
- **ANCA positive: c-ANCA** (anti-proteinase 3) more than **p-ANCA.**
- CXR and chest CT show fixed pulmonary nodules, cavities, and/or infiltrates.
- UA with active sediment.
- Characteristic biopsy.

Treatment

- **Induction:** Cyclophosphamide and corticosteroids.
- **Remission:** Methotrexate, TMP-SMX.

Churg-Strauss Angiitis

Males are affected more often than females. Organs and systems affected include the lung, heart, nerve, and kidney.

Symptoms/Exam

- **Asthma,** nasal polyps, allergic rhinitis.
- Mono- and peripheral neuropathy.
- Fever, rash, myalgias, arthralgias, weight loss.
- Cough, dyspnea, angina pectoris.
- Glomerulonephritis is less common than in other ANCA-associated diseases.

The triad of asthma, eosinophilia, and a positive p-ANCA strongly suggests Churg-Strauss.

Diagnosis

- **Peripheral eosinophilia.**
- Normal serum complement levels.
- **Positive p-ANCA.**
- CXR shows fleeting pulmonary infiltrates.
- Biopsy of affected tissue demonstrates extravascular eosinophils.

Treatment

- High-dose corticosteroids,
- Immunosuppressants for steroid-unresponsive disease.

Microscopic Polyangiitis (MPA)

Medium- or, more commonly, small-vessel vasculitis and capillaritis. Characterized by pulmonary hemorrhage and by glomerulonephritis and renal failure. Organs and systems affected include the lung, kidney, nerve, and skin. Often confused with polyarteritis nodosa (see Table 17-14).

Symptoms/Exam

- Fever, malaise, myalgias, arthralgias, weight loss.
- Hemoptysis, dyspnea.
- Hematuria/active sediment.
- Mono-/polyneuropathy, skin rashes (palpable purpura).

TABLE 17-14. Polyarteritis Nodosa vs. Microscopic Polyangiitis

	PAN	MPA
Vessel size	Medium	Medium and small
Skin	Ulcer/nodule/livedo reticularis	Palpable purpura
Lung	Rare	Capillaritis/alveolar hemorrhage
Renal	Renal artery aneurysms/renal infarction	Glomerulonephritis

Diagnosis

- Elevated ESR, normal serum complement levels.
- **p-ANCA (anti-MPO) positive.**
- Tissue biopsy demonstrates alveolar hemorrhage/necrotizing capillaritis/glomerulonephritis.

Treatment

Corticosteroids; cytotoxic agents.

Polyarteritis Nodosa (PAN)

Necrotizing arteritis of medium-sized vessels. Active infection with **HBV** predisposes to the development of disease. Organs affected include the kidney, nerves, GI/mesentery, brain, skin, heart, testes, and joints. Often confused with MPA (see Table 17-14).

*Primary vasculitides involving the lungs and kidneys ("pulmonary-renal" pattern) include Wegener's, Goodpasture's, microscopic polyangiitis, and Churg-Strauss but **not PAN,** which rarely affects the lungs.*

Symptoms/Exam

- Fever, malaise, weight loss, hypertension, **abdominal pain.**
- Arthritis or arthralgias, myalgias.
- **Neuropathies** (mono- or polyneuritis).
- **Skin rash** (livedo reticularis, nodules, ulcerations).

Diagnosis

- Elevated ESR.
- The majority of cases are **ANCA negative.**
- Normal serum complement levels.
- HBV serologies.
- Angiography shows aneurysmal dilations of affected arteries (see Figure 17-5).
- Site-directed biopsy.

Treatment

- High-dose corticosteroids.
- Cytotoxic immunosuppressive agents (e.g., cyclophosphamide).

Polymyalgia Rheumatica (PMR)

Associated with proximal/axial skeletal pain and stiffness; fever, malaise, and weight loss; and elevated ESR. Rare before age 50; usually affects **older female patients.** Associated with giant cell (temporal) arteritis.

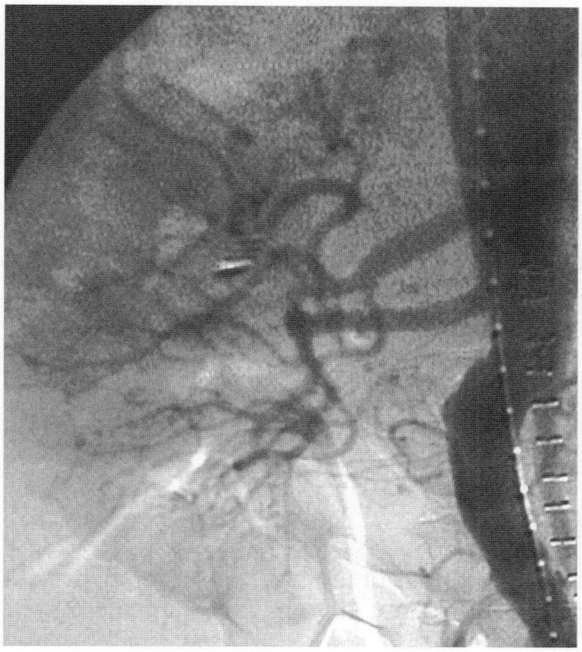

FIGURE 17-5. PAN of the right kidney (note the aneurysms in the superior pole of the kidney).

(Courtesy of Jonathan Graf, MD, 2004.)

SYMPTOMS/EXAM

- Joints affected include the shoulders, hip girdles, and low back and, less commonly, the peripheral joints.
- **No muscular weakness** (vs. polymyositis).
- Fever, malaise, and weight loss can be profound.

The CK is normal in PMR, and there is no weakness. Remember that PMR is an "-algia," not an "-itis."

DIAGNOSIS

- Characteristic joint involvement (shoulders, hips).
- Elevated ESR (> 40).
- Constitutional features.
- Prompt response to corticosteroids.

TREATMENT

Small to moderate doses of corticosteroids.

GIANT CELL ARTERITIS

Up to 20% of PMR patients have giant cell arteritis, whereas up to 60% of giant cell patients have PMR.

Arteritis of large and medium-sized vessels. The most common vasculitis in North America and Europe; affects patients > 50 years of age. Blindness results from involvement of posterior ciliary arteries/ischemic optic neuritis. Strong association with PMR.

SYMPTOMS/EXAM

- Severe headache.
- Scalp/temporal artery tenderness.

- Jaw claudication, sore throat, amaurosis fugax.
- Fever, malaise, and weight loss.

Failure to consider giant cell arteritis as a cause of new fever, headache, or vision loss in the elderly can result in permanent vision loss if biopsy and high-dose steroids are delayed

DIAGNOSIS

- Age > 50.
- Elevated ESR (> 50).
- New-onset headache.
- Tender, nodular, or pulseless temporal artery.
- Characteristic angiographic findings.
- Characteristic temporal artery biopsy.

TREATMENT

High-dose corticosteroids.

TAKAYASU'S ARTERITIS

Pulseless aortitis and vasculitis of the large vessels/branches of the aorta. Most prevalent in East Asia; **women < 40 years of age** are most commonly affected.

Because giant cell arteritis is a patchy process, biopsies should be taken at several sites and from both temporal arteries.

SYMPTOMS/EXAM

- Fever, malaise, myalgia, arthralgia, weight loss, progressive claudication.
- Evidence of limb and/or organ ischemia.
- Hypertension, bruits, abnormal pulses, **systolic BP discrepancies measured between limbs,** aortic valvular regurgitation murmur.

DIAGNOSIS

- Elevated ESR is common but not universal.
- CXR may suggest aortic abnormalities.
- Angiography of aorta/branches shows stenoses/aneurysms.
- Biopsy reveals granulomatous arteritis +/– variable numbers of giant cells.

Takayasu's is also known as "pulseless disease" because the arteries it involves–the aorta and its branches–can narrow and result in reduced radial and femoral pulses and BP.

TREATMENT

- Corticosteroids.
- Aggressive BP control.
- Surgical bypass of ischemic vessels once systemic disease is controlled.

Other Vasculitides

CRYOGLOBULINEMIA

All cryoglobulins are immune complexes that precipitate at ≤ 4°C. Cryoglobulinemias are divided into three types:

HCV infection is the most common cause of cryoglobulinemia in the United States.

- **Type 1:** Monoclonal (seen in multiple myeloma and Waldenström's macroglobulinemia). Acrocyanosis (blue digits) and hyperviscosity complications are more common than vasculitis.
- **Type 2:** Monoclonal antibodies (RF) against polyclonal immune targets.
- **Type 3:** Polyclonal antibodies (RF) against polyclonal immune targets.
- Types 2 and 3 can both be **idiopathic** or caused by **HCV** or other chronic infections, malignancies, or collagen vascular diseases (especially Sjögren's syndrome).
- Clinically, signs of vasculitis are seen—e.g., glomerulonephritis, palpable purpura, and neuropathy.

BUERGER'S DISEASE (THROMBOANGIITIS OBLITERANS)

Thromboses of medium-sized arteries and veins, usually of the hands or feet. Most commonly affects **males who smoke** heavily. Treat by discontinuing smoking.

BEHÇET'S DISEASE

Recurrent **oral and genital ulcerations,** skin ulcerations, pathergy (worsening of ulcerations with provocation), and erythema nodosum. Other characteristics are as follows:

- **Ocular disease:** Keratitis, hypopyon, uveitis, retinal vasculitis, blindness.
- Seronegative arthritis.
- Thrombophlebitis.
- **CNS abnormalities:** Cerebral vasculitis, meningoencephalitis, myelitis, cranial neuropathies.

Treat with corticosteroids and/or immunosuppressants.

Three rheumatic diseases associated with oral ulcers are Behçet's, SLE, and reactive arthritis.

RELAPSING POLYCHONDRITIS

Episodic inflammatory attacks involving the **cartilage of the ears, nose, larynx, and trachea.**

- May be idiopathic or secondary to another autoimmune, collagen vascular, or malignant disease.
- Noncartilaginous involvement includes fever, polyarthritis, scleritis, uveitis, middle/inner ear inflammation, and vasculitis.
- Treat with corticosteroids, dapsone, colchicine, and immunosuppressants (for refractory disease).
- Complications include chronic deformities of the ear (cauliflower ear), nasal septum collapse **(saddlenose)**, laryngotracheal chondritis and stenoses, hearing loss, vertigo, tinnitus, and valvular heart disease.

INFECTIOUS ARTHRITIS

Nongonococcal Arthritis

Acute-onset, **monoarticular** joint pain, swelling, warmth, and erythema. Gram-positive species (***S. aureus, Streptococcus***) are common causative organisms. Gram-negative species (*E. coli, Pseudomonas*) are less commonly involved. Patients with previous joint damage (traumatic or inflammatory), IV drug use, endocarditis, and prosthetic joints are at highest risk.

Prosthetic infections: Think S. epidermidis.

SYMPTOMS/EXAM

Fevers, chills, inability to bear weight or pain with joint motion, large joint effusions, very hot and tender joint.

DIAGNOSIS

- Blood cultures are positive in 50% of cases.
- Arthrocentesis reveals leukocytosis (usually > 50,000, > 90% PMN predominance), culture positive, Gram stain positive in only 75% (*S. aureus*).
- X-rays reveal demineralization, joint erosions, narrowing, osteomyelitis, and periostitis.

Treatment

- IV antibiotics (often needed for up to six weeks).
- Serial arthrocentesis if effusion reaccumulates, or surgical drainage if the patient fails medical therapy or the disease involves inaccessible sites (e.g., the hip).

Complications

Articular destruction, septicemia.

Gonococcal Arthritis (Disseminated Infection)

Most common in patients < 40 years of age; women are more frequently affected than men.

Symptoms/Exam

- **Migratory** polyarthralgias and tenosynovitis.
- A papulopustular skin rash that may involve the palms and soles.
- Fever.

Diagnosis

- Arthrocentesis reveals leukocytosis (commonly > 50,000), 25% Gram stain positive, < 50% culture positive.
- Blood cultures, rectal and throat swab cultures, urethral cultures (70–86% sensitive).

Recurrent bouts of disseminated gonococcal infection should prompt evaluation for complement deficiency (C5–C9).

Treatment

- IV antibiotics (third-generation cephalosporin) until clinical improvement is seen, followed by the oral equivalent or a quinolone antibiotic for a 7- to 10-day total course.
- Empiric therapy or testing for chlamydia is recommended.

Tuberculous Arthritis

Most common in children, immunosuppressed patients, and the elderly. Can occur shortly after primary infection or as a reactivation phenomenon. Fewer than 50% of patients with tuberculous arthritis will have an abnormal CXR. Patients with spinal disease (Pott's) rarely have extraspinal involvement.

Symptoms/Exam

- Insidious-onset, subacute or chronic monoarticular joint swelling, pain, and warmth followed by destructive arthritis, contractures, and abscess/sinus drainage.
- **Pott's disease** presents as insidious onset of back pain with involvement of the thoracic and lumbar spine.

Diagnosis

Isolation of acid-fast bacilli from joint fluid or synovial biopsy.

Treatment

As for pulmonary TB, although a longer treatment course may be necessary.

COMPLICATIONS

Joint destruction, invasion of adjacent soft tissues and bone, paraplegia (Pott's disease).

Lyme Arthritis

Early Lyme disease (stages 1 and 2) may have migratory arthralgias and myalgias along with flulike symptoms and erythema migrans rash. **Advanced Lyme** (stage 3) presents as an **acute monoarthritis of the knee;** less common is oligo- or polyarthritis.

The most common joint involved in Lyme arthritis (stage 3) is the knee.

DIAGNOSIS

- **Arthrocentesis:** PMN-predominant leukocytosis (average ~25,000); cultures for *Borrelia burgdorferi* is typically negative.
- **American College of Physicians recommendations for diagnosis:** Objective arthritis with both ELISA and Western blot confirmatory tests to *B. burgdorferi.*

TREATMENT

Treat advanced Lyme arthritis (stage 3) with doxycycline (4 weeks) or ceftriaxone (2–4 weeks).

MISCELLANEOUS DISEASES

Adult Still's Disease

Presents with high-spiking **fevers,** diaphoresis, chills, sore throat, an evanescent salmon-colored **rash** coincident with fevers, erosive arthritis, serositis, and lymphadenopathy. Laboratory findings reveal **leukocytosis,** anemia, seronegativity, transaminitis, and **hyperferritinemia.** Treat with NSAIDs and corticosteroids.

Consider Still's in a young adult with fever of unknown origin and markedly elevated ferritin (usually > 1000) whose workup for infection and malignancy is negative.

Sarcoidosis

Arthritis associated with sarcoidosis is either acute or chronic. See Chapter 16 for nonarticular manifestations of sarcoidosis.

- **Acute sarcoid arthritis = Löfgren's syndrome,** which presents with **periarthritis** (ankle/knee most common), **erythema nodosum,** and **hilar adenopathy** on CXR. Resolution of acute disease occurs in 2–16 weeks with minimal therapy, NSAIDs, and colchicine.
- **Chronic sarcoid arthritis** usually involves minimally inflamed joints with synovial swelling/granulomata. Treat with NSAIDs, corticosteroids, and immunosuppressants.

Cholesterol Emboli Syndrome

Precipitated by invasive arterial procedures in patients with atherosclerotic disease. Features include fever, livedo reticularis, cyanosis/gangrene of the digits, vasculitic/ischemic ulcerations, **eosinophilia, renal failure,** and other end-organ damage.

NOTES

CHAPTER 18

Women's Health

Linda Shiue, MD

BREAST CANCER SCREENING AND PREVENTION

The second deadliest cancer in women. Risk factors include include the following:

- A family history, particularly of premenopausal breast cancer.
- Positive mutations of BRCA1 or BRCA2.
- Age > 40.
- Estrogen exposure, HRT.
- Age at menarche < 12; age at first birth > 30; age at menopause > 55.
- OCP use is probably not a risk factor in average-risk women but may be in those with a positive family history.
- Alcohol use.
- A history of benign breast biopsy.
- A history of atypical hyperplasia on breast biopsy.

DIAGNOSIS

Types of screening are as follows:

- **Breast self-examination (BSE):** Not standardized, and **not shown to have benefit.**
- **Clinical breast examination (CBE):** Not standardized; has a sensitivity of approximately 50%.
- **Mammography:** Screening should start at age 40 or 50 and should continue until age 70 (controversial for those < 50 and > 70 years of age). Sensitivity is 90% and is higher in older than in younger women. Screen patients in their 40s every year (cancer can be more aggressive even though it is less prevalent) and every 1–2 years for patients ≥ 50 years of age (no organization takes a definitive position).
- BRCA1/BRCA2 mutation testing for those with the following risk factors:
  - A family history of premenopausal breast cancer.
  - Known breast cancer.
  - Breast and ovarian cancer in the same patient.
  - A family history of male breast cancer.

PREVENTION

Women with positive mutations of BRCA1 and BRCA2 should undergo intensive surveillance and may consider prophylactic mastectomy and/or oophorectomy as well as tamoxifen therapy.

BREAST MASSES

SYMPTOMS

May be found on exam or on mammography. An abnormality found on mammography may not correlate with the actual mass.

EXAM

Bilateral breast examination should include palpation of the axillae and nipples. Malignant lesions are associated with the following traits:

- Single
- Hard
- Immovable
- Irregular borders

- Size ≥ 2 cm
- Possible nipple discharge
- Skin changes, axillary adenopathy

DIAGNOSIS/TREATMENT

Diagnostic modalities available are triaged on the basis of age and clinical suspicion using the above characteristics.

- **Imaging:**
  - Ultrasound if age < 35
  - Mammography if age > 35
- **Biopsy:**
  - Fine-needle aspiration (FNA)
  - Large-needle (core) biopsy
  - Open biopsy/excision
- **Treatment:**
  - **Benign masses:** Clinical follow-up and routine screening as described above.
  - **Malignant masses:** Treatment is based on pathology and clinical staging and may include a combination of surgery, chemotherapy, and/or radiation.

Up to 80% of breast biopsies are benign. If the patient has a mass and a normal mammogram, further diagnosis is needed.

CERVICAL CANCER SCREENING

Cervical cancer screening through use of the Pap smear was introduced in the 1960s, leading to a significant decline in the incidence of cervical cancer in the United States. Nonetheless, cervical cancer is the second most common cancer among women worldwide and the sixth most common cancer in the United States. It is caused by the human papillomavirus, a common STD (HPV-16 and -18 are considered high-risk types). Risk factors include multiple sexual partners, early onset of intercourse, other STDs, smoking, low socioeconomic status (SES), and HIV/immunosuppression.

SYMPTOMS

Usually asymptomatic or may present with irregular bleeding, postcoital bleeding, pelvic pain, or abnormal vaginal discharge.

EXAM

Abnormal findings on pelvic exam include cervical discharge, ulceration, and a pelvic mass or fistula. All visible lesions should be biopsied even if the Pap smear is normal.

DIFFERENTIAL

Cervicitis, vaginitis, STD, actinomycosis.

DIAGNOSIS

- Guidelines for Pap screening are as follows:
  - The American College of Physicians (**ACP**) and the United States Preventive Services Task Force (**USPSTF**) recommend that sexually active women between the ages of 20 and 65 be screened every three years. Those with known risk factors or a history of abnormal Pap smears should be screened annually.

- The American Cancer Society (**ACS**) recommends that screening begin within three years of initiation of intercourse.
- Screening may be stopped at approximately age 70. **Older women who have not had a recent Pap test merit screening.**
- No further screening is indicated for those who have undergone a TAH for benign reasons.

- Abnormalities are diagnosed with colposcopy and biopsy.

Treatment

- Table 18-1 outlines treatment options associated with specific cytologic abnormalities found on Pap smear.
- For **invasive cancer:**
  - Treat early-stage disease with radical hysterectomy and lymph node dissection.
  - Adjuvant radiation and chemotherapy for advanced disease.

CHLAMYDIA SCREENING

Chlamydia is a common infection. Up to 25% of men are asymptomatic carriers, and as many as 70% of infected women are asymptomatic. Chlamydia is a major cause of infertility, PID, and ectopic pregnancy. Risk factors include the following:

All sexually active women through age 25 (or older in the presence of risk factors) should be screened for chlamydia infection once a year.

- **Young age** (prevalence among sexually active adolescents is 5–10%).
- Multiple sexual partners over the last three months (or a partner with a similar history).
- Inconsistent use of barrier methods.
- Low SES, single marital status, or a history of prior STDs.

Symptoms

Often asymptomatic, but may present with urethritis/cervicitis, PID (endometritis or salpingitis), acute epididymitis, neonatal infection (ophthalmia neonatorum, pneumonia), trachoma, or lymphogranuloma venereum. Screening is recommended for the following:

- **All pregnant women** at the first prenatal visit (CDC); women < 25 years of age and other high-risk patients should also be screened in the third trimester.

TABLE 18-1. Management of Cervical Cytologic Abnormalities

Abnormality	Management
Atypical squamous cells of uncertain significance (ASCUS)	Serial Pap smears; triage with HPV testing or immediate colposcopy.
Atypical glandular cells	Colposcopy and/or endometrial sampling.
Low-grade squamous intraepithelial lesion (LSIL)	Colposcopy (or triage in adolescents or postmenopausal patients).
High-grade squamous intraepithelial lesion (HSIL)	Colposcopy; possibly diagnostic excisional procedure (laser conization, cold-knife conization, loop electrosurgical excision procedure [LEEP], loop electrosurgical conization).

- Nonpregnant women with the risk factors noted above.
- Sexually active women through age 25 (or older if risk factors are present at the annual exam).

EXAM

Conduct a pelvic exam for evidence of vaginitis, cervicitis, and cervical motion tenderness.

DIFFERENTIAL

Vaginitis, other STDs.

DIAGNOSIS

Screening methods include ligase chain reaction (LCR) on urine or cervical swab, cell culture, and direct fluorescent antibody/enzyme immunoassay (DFA/EIA).

TREATMENT

Azithromycin 1 g PO × 1, or doxycycline 100 mg PO BID × 7 days.

COMPLICATIONS

Infertility and ectopic pregnancy due to PID, perihepatitis (Fitz-Hugh–Curtis syndrome), Reiter's syndrome.

CONTRACEPTION

Table 18-2 describes common contraceptive methods and outlines their contraindications and side effects.

DOMESTIC VIOLENCE

The leading cause of injuries in women. Abuse may be physical, mental (including denial of financial or health care access), or sexual. Affects individuals from all socioeconomic groups. May also occur in same-sex partners. Pregnancy may initiate or exacerbate abuse.

SYMPTOMS

All patients should be screened. Patients may present with no symptoms or with multiple somatic complaints, depression, or injuries unexplained by their history. There may also be a delay in seeking care.

EXAM

Conduct mental status exam; look for signs of new, old, or chronic trauma.

DIFFERENTIAL

Psychological illness, physical illness, somatization.

TREATMENT

- Conduct a risk assessment (frequency, weapons, substance abuse, threats of suicide, homicide).

Warning signs of OCP complications–

ACHES

Abdominal pain
Chest pain
Headache (severe)
Eye (blurred vision)
Sharp leg pain

IUD side effects–

PAINS

Period that is late
Abdominal cramps
Increase in body temperature
Noticeable vaginal discharge
Spotting

Domestic violence questions–

SAFE

Stress and **S**afety:
Do you feel safe in your relationship?
What happens when you and your partner disagree?
Afraid or **A**bused:
Have you or your children ever been physically threatened or abused?
Have you ever been forced to have sexual intercourse?
Friend or **F**amily Awareness:
Are your friends or family aware of what is happening?
Would they support and help you?
Emergency **E**scape Plan:
Are you in danger now, and would you like to go to a shelter or talk with someone?
Do you have a place where you and your children could go in an emergency?

TABLE 18-2. Contraceptive Methods

METHOD	DESCRIPTION	SIDE EFFECTS
Behavioral methods		**High failure rate.**
Rhythm	Uses **body temperature** and **cervical mucus consistency** to predict fertile periods.	
Coitus interruptus	Withdrawal of the penis before ejaculation.	
Barrier methods		
Diaphragm, cervical cap	Domed sheet of rubber or latex placed over the cervix. Must be fitted by a physician and remain in the vagina **6–8 hours** after intercourse.	Possible allergy to latex or spermicides; risk of UTI and TSS.
Condom	Latex sheath placed over the penis during intercourse.	Possible allergy to latex or spermicides.
IUD	Plastic and/or metal device placed in the uterus. Causes a local sterile inflammatory reaction within the uterine wall so that sperm are engulfed and destroyed. Mirena is an IUD that is impregnated with a progestin.	Increased vaginal bleeding, uterine perforation, IUD migration, infection, increased risk of PID, ectopic.
Hormonal methods		
OCPs	Suppress ovulation by inhibiting FSH/LH; change the consistency of cervical mucus, making the endometrium unsuitable for implantation.	Nausea, breast tenderness, acne, mood changes, hypertension, hepatic adenoma, weight gain, increased risk of venous thromboembolism (VTE).
Levonorgestrel (Norplant) (discontinued in 2002)	**Progestin-only** subdermal implant. Suppresses ovulation and changes the consistency of cervical mucus, making the endometrium unsuitable for implantation. **Lasts for five years.**	Irregular vaginal bleeding, weight gain, galactorrhea, acne, breast tenderness, headache. Difficult removal.
Postcoital "morning after pill"	Progesterone +/– estrogen taken within 72 hours of intercourse to suppress ovulation or discourage implantation.	Nausea, vomiting, fatigue, headache, dizziness, breast tenderness.
Depot medroxyprogesterone (Depo-Provera)	IM injection **given every three months.** Suppresses ovulation and changes the consistency of cervical mucus, making the endometrium unsuitable for implantation.	Irregular vaginal bleeding, depression, weight gain, breast tenderness, **delayed restoration of ovulation after discontinuation** (6–18 months).
Medroxyprogesterone/ estradiol cypionate (Lunelle) (recalled 2002)	Monthly IM injection. Suppresses ovulation by inhibiting FSH/LH; changes the consistency of cervical mucus, making the endometrium unsuitable for implantation.	Nausea, breast tenderness, acne, mood changes, hypertension, hepatic adenoma, weight gain, increased risk of VTE.
Transdermal contraceptive patch (Ortho Evra)	Combination estrogen/progesterone transdermal patch that is **changed once a week.**	Local dermal reaction, nausea, breast tenderness, acne, mood changes, hypertension, hepatic adenoma, weight gain, increased risk of VTE.

TABLE 18-2. Contraceptive Methods (continued)

METHOD	DESCRIPTION	SIDE EFFECTS
Hormonal methods (continued)		
Contraceptive vaginal ring (NuvaRing)	Intravaginal ring that is **worn for three weeks of each four-week cycle.** Suppresses ovulation by inhibiting FSH/LH; changes the consistency of cervical mucus, making the endometrium unsuitable for implantation.	Nausea, breast tenderness, acne, mood changes, hypertension, hepatic adenoma, weight gain, increased risk of VTE.
Surgical sterilization (tubal ligation, vasectomy)	Tubes are ligated, cauterized, or mechanically occluded, and the vas deferens is cut.	Tubal ligation may result in bleeding, infection, failure, or ectopic pregnancy and is essentially irreversible. By contrast, > **50% of men with reversed vasectomies are fertile.**
Natural family planning/ periodic abstinence		
Rhythm/calendar method	Determining the fertile period on the basis of the last menstrual period (LMP).	High failure rate (especially the rhythm method).
Ovulation method	Determining the fertile period on the basis of changes in cervical mucus or basal body temperature, or using home ovulation testing to detect LH surge.	Cannot be used in women with irregular cycle lengths.

Adapted, with permission, from Le T et al. *First Aid for the USMLE Step 2,* 4th ed. New York: McGraw-Hill, 2003.

- Determine if the patient has a safety plan (see the mnemonic **SAFE**).
- Report to law enforcement.

All women should be screened for domestic violence, including during the preconception visit.

DYSURIA

Symptom of burning during urination.

SYMPTOMS

Pain, tingling, and/or burning in the perineum during or just after urination. UTIs have an abrupt onset of symptoms, whereas other causes have a more stuttering course.

EXAM

Determine temperature; conduct an abdominal exam. Consider a pelvic exam if vaginitis or STDs are a concern.

DIFFERENTIAL

UTI, STDs (gonorrhea, chlamydia, HSV, trichomoniasis), vaginitis, interstitial cystitis (sterile urine, normal UA, significant frequency and dysuria), atrophic vaginitis, irritants (spermicide, douching).

Diagnosis

- UA; possible STD testing (DNA amplification for gonorrhea and chlamydia).
- Obtain a urine culture only for suspected pyelonephritis or complicated UTI (see the section on UTIs below).

Suspect chlamydia urethritis or other sexually transmitted disease when the patient presents with a stuttering course as opposed to sudden onset of symptoms.

Treatment

- Treat the underlying cause.
- Consider symptomatic treatment with **phenazopyridine** for no longer than two days (tell the patient that her urine may appear orange while she is on the drug).

HIRSUTISM

Increased male-pattern hair growth. A clinical manifestation of increased androgen levels.

Symptoms

- Increased hair growth, often of facial or chest hair.
- May present with associated amenorrhea and signs of virilization (e.g., deepening voice, male-pattern baldness, clitoromegaly, male body habitus).

Exam

- Note body habitus (obesity).
- Look for male-pattern hair growth, acne, signs of Cushing's (acanthosis nigricans, thin skin, bruising), galactorrhea.
- Abdominal and ovarian exam for mass lesions.

Virilization and/or abrupt onset of hirsutism may indicate an androgen-secreting tumor.

Differential

- PCOS is by far the most common cause. May also be idiopathic. Other etiologies include the following:
  - Congenital adrenal hyperplasia
  - Medications (androgenic progestins in OCPs, danazol)
  - Cushing's syndrome
  - Sertoli-Leydig cell ovarian tumor
  - Luteoma of pregnancy
  - Adrenal neoplasm
  - Hyperprolactinemia
- Non-PCOS or idiopathic causes of hirsutism are distinguished by:
  - Abrupt, short duration (< 1 year) or sudden progressive worsening.
  - Onset in the third decade of life or later (not peripubertal).
  - Virilization.

Diagnosis

- **No labs** are indicated for patients with **long-standing hirsutism,** regular menses, and familial factors.
- **All others:** Testosterone, prolactin, DHEAS (if there is associated virilization or if symptoms are of rapid onset).
- **Ultrasound** in the presence of elevated androgens and if a tumor is suspected.

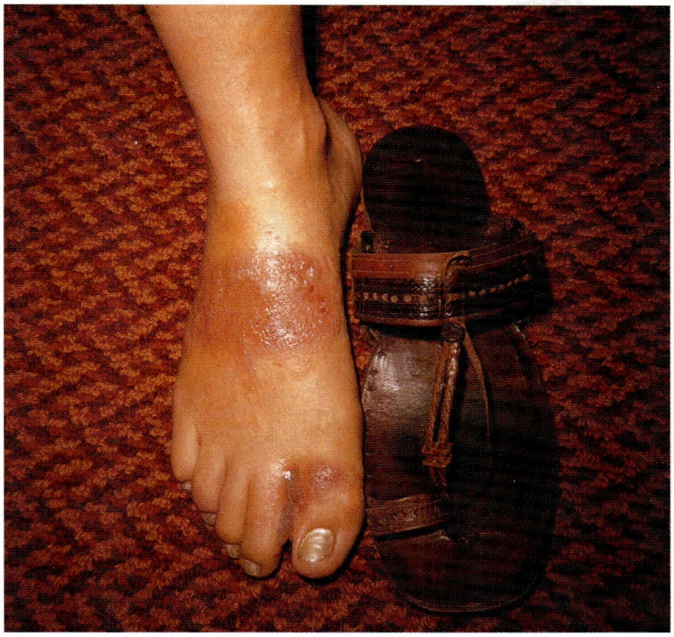

FIGURE 1-2. Contact dermatitis.

Erythematous papules, vesicles, and serous weeping localized to areas of contact with the offending agent are characteristic. (Reproduced, with permission, from Hurwitz RM. *Pathology of the Skin: Atlas of Clinical-Pathological Correlation.* Stamford, CT: Appleton & Lange, 1991:3.)

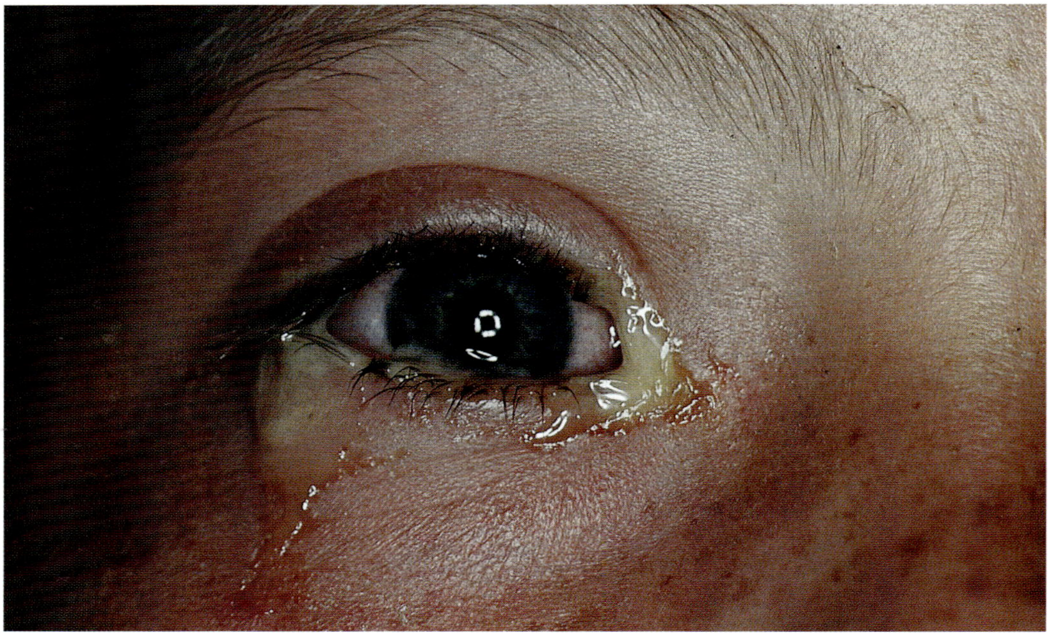

FIGURE 2-1. Bacterial conjunctivitis.

(Reproduced, with permission, from Knoop KJ, Stack LB, Storrow AB. *Atlas of Emergency Medicine*, 2nd ed. New York: McGraw-Hill, 2002:30.)

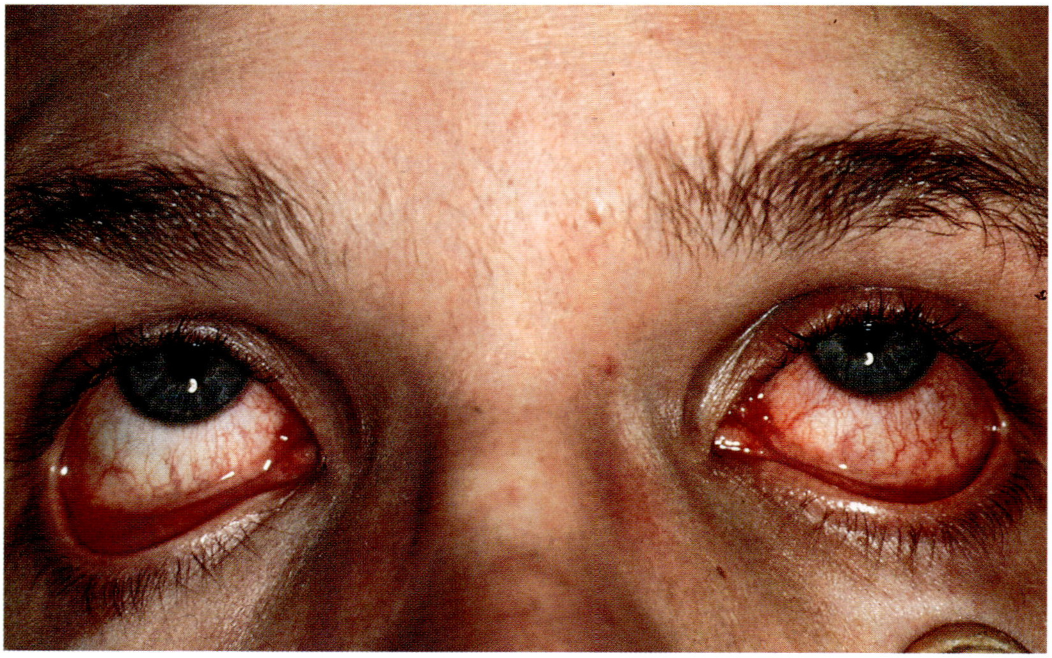

FIGURE 2-2. Viral conjunctivitis.

(Reproduced, with permission, from Knoop KJ, Stack LB, Storrow AB. *Atlas of Emergency Medicine*, 2nd ed. New York: McGraw-Hill, 2002:31.)

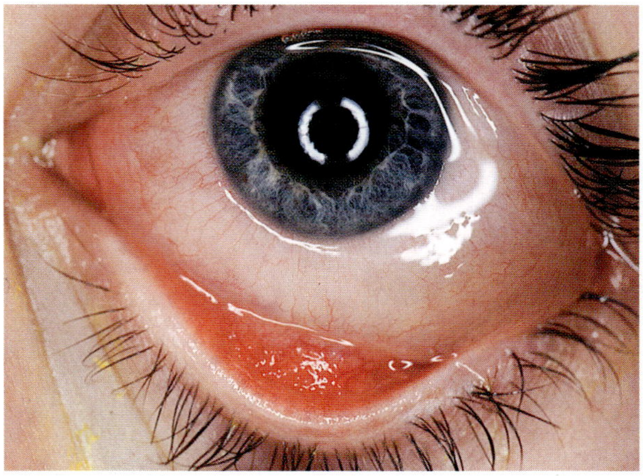

FIGURE 2-3. Allergic conjunctivitis.

(Courtesy of Timothy D. McGuirk, DO. Reproduced, with permission, from Knoop KJ, Stack LB, Storrow AB. *Atlas of Emergency Medicine*, 2nd ed. New York: McGraw-Hill, 2002:36.)

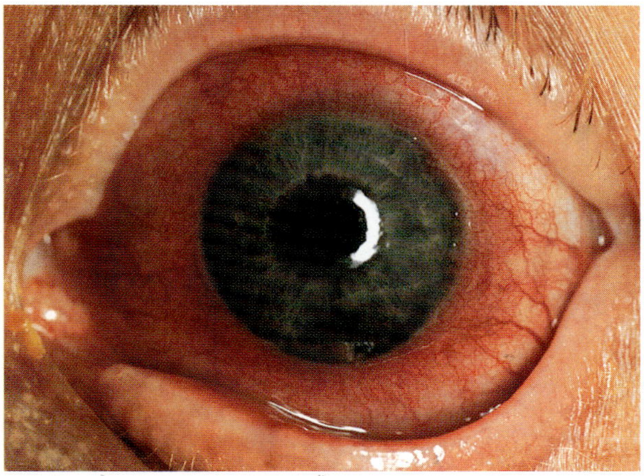

FIGURE 2-4. Anterior uveitis.

(Reproduced, with permission, from Knoop KJ, Stack LB, Storrow AB. *Atlas of Emergency Medicine*, 2nd ed. New York: McGraw-Hill, 2002:52.)

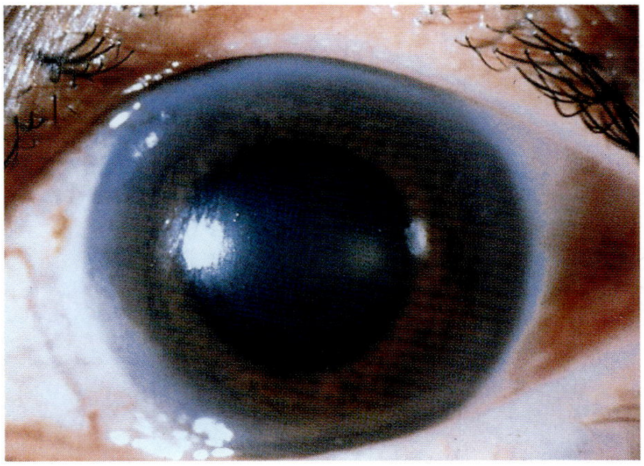

FIGURE 2-5. Acute angle-closure glaucoma.

(Courtesy of Gary Tanner, MD. Reproduced, with permission, from Knoop KJ, Stack LB, Storrow AB. *Atlas of Emergency Medicine*, 2nd ed. New York: McGraw-Hill, 2002:49.)

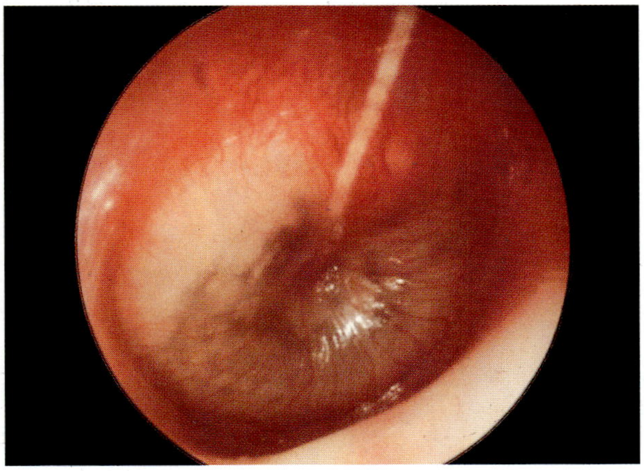

FIGURE 2-6. Acute otitis media.

(Courtesy of Richard A. Chole, MD, PhD. Reproduced, with permission, from Knoop KJ, Stack LB, Storrow AB. *Atlas of Emergency Medicine*, 2nd ed. New York: McGraw-Hill, 2002:118.)

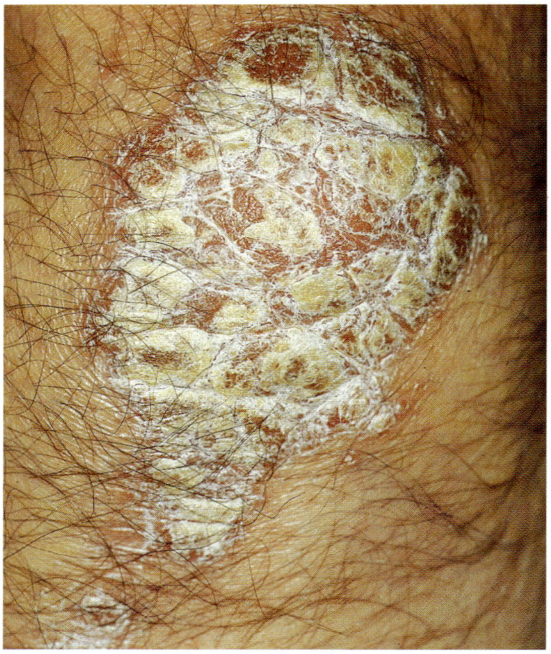

FIGURE 5-2. Psoriasis vulgaris (elbow).

A well-demarcated erythematous plaque is seen with a thick white scale. (Reproduced, with permission, from Wolff K, Johnson RA, Suurmond D. *Fitzpatrick's Color Atlas and Synopsis of Clinical Dermatology*, 5th ed. New York: McGraw-Hill, 2005:57.)

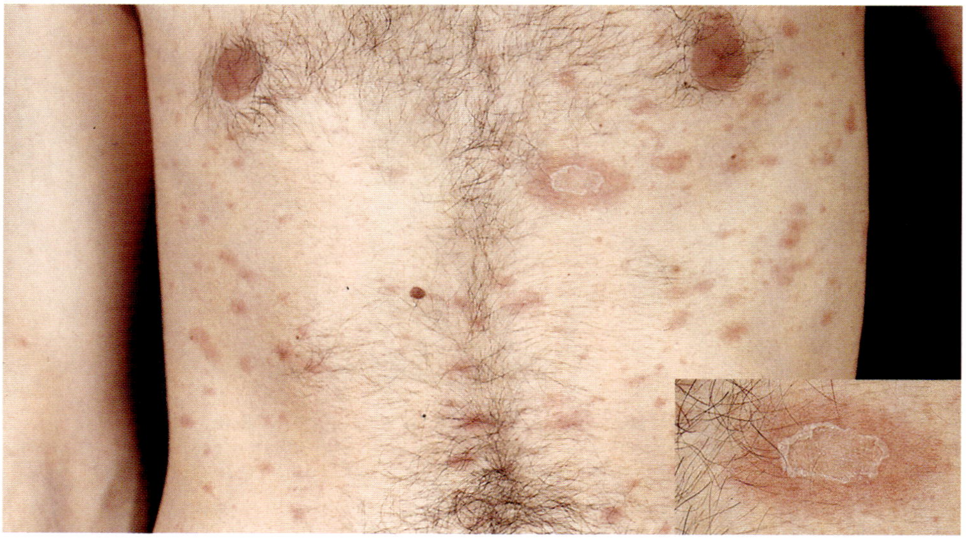

FIGURE 5-3. Pityriasis rosea.

Pink plaques with an oval configuration are seen that follow the lines of cleavage. Inset: Herald patch. The collarette of scale is more obvious on this magnification. (Reproduced, with permission, from Wolff K, Johnson RA, Suurmond D. *Fitzpatrick's Color Atlas and Synopsis of Clinical Dermatology*, 5th ed. New York: McGraw-Hill, 2005:119.)

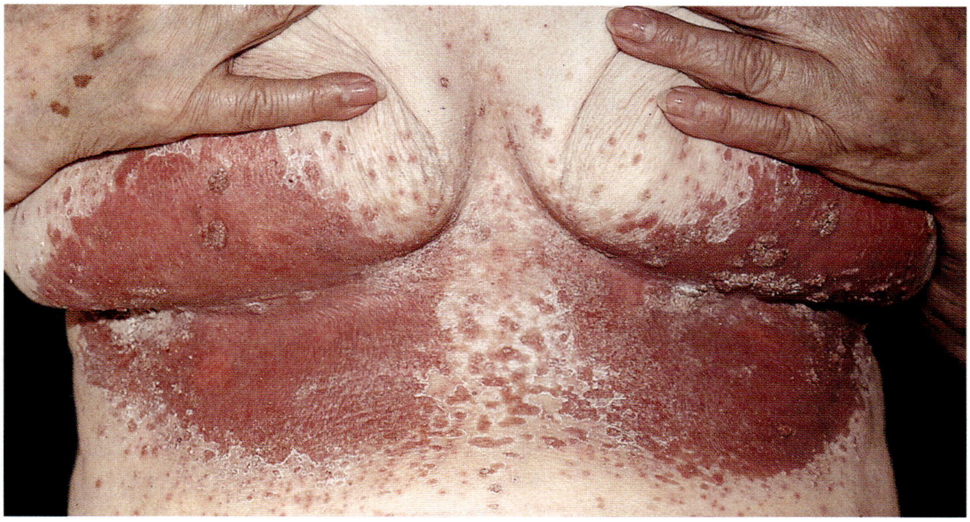

FIGURE 5-4. Cutaneous candidiasis—intertrigo.

Small peripheral satellite papules and pustules coalesce to create a large eroded area in the submammary region. (Reproduced, with permission, from Wolff K, Johnson RA, Suurmond D. *Fitzpatrick's Color Atlas and Synopsis of Clinical Dermatology*, 5th ed. New York: McGraw-Hill, 2005:719.)

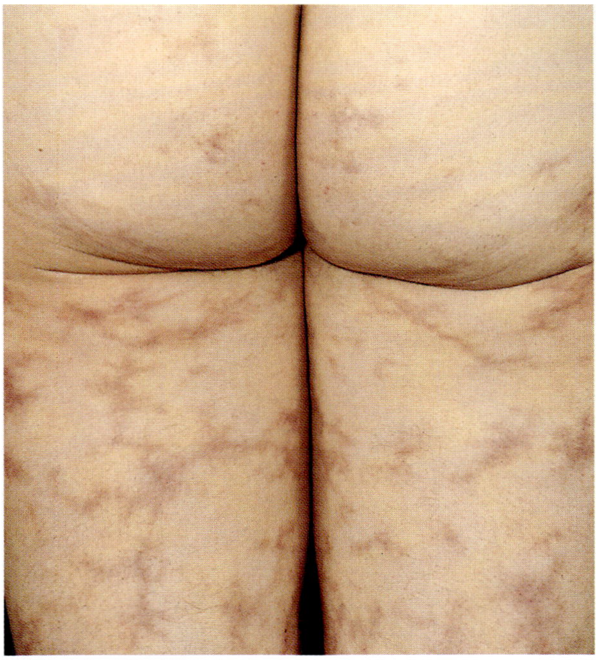

FIGURE 5-6. Symptomatic livedo reticularis.

A bluish, netlike, arborizing pattern is seen on the posterior thighs and buttocks and is defined by violaceous, erythematous streaks resembling lightning. (Reproduced, with permission, from Wolff K, Johnson RA, Suurmond D. *Fitzpatrick's Color Atlas and Synopsis of Clinical Dermatology*, 5th ed. New York: McGraw-Hill, 2005:381.)

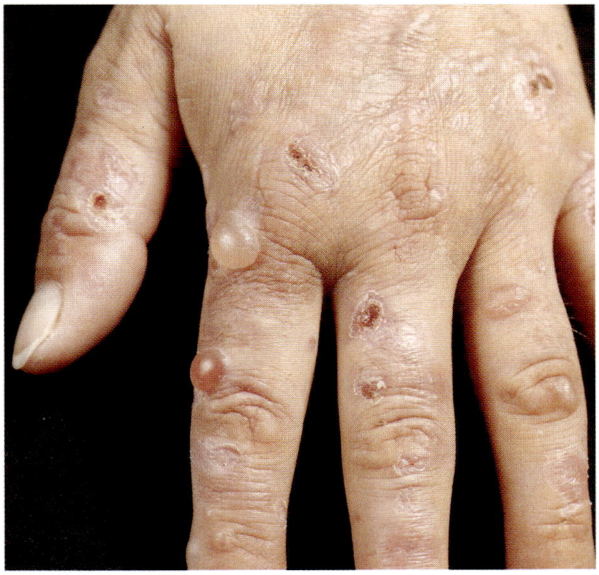

FIGURE 5-7. Porphyria cutanea tarda.

Bullae on the dorsum of the hand. (Reproduced, with permission, from Wolff K, Johnson RA, Suurmond D. *Fitzpatrick's Color Atlas and Synopsis of Clinical Dermatology*, 5th ed. New York: McGraw-Hill, 2005:247.)

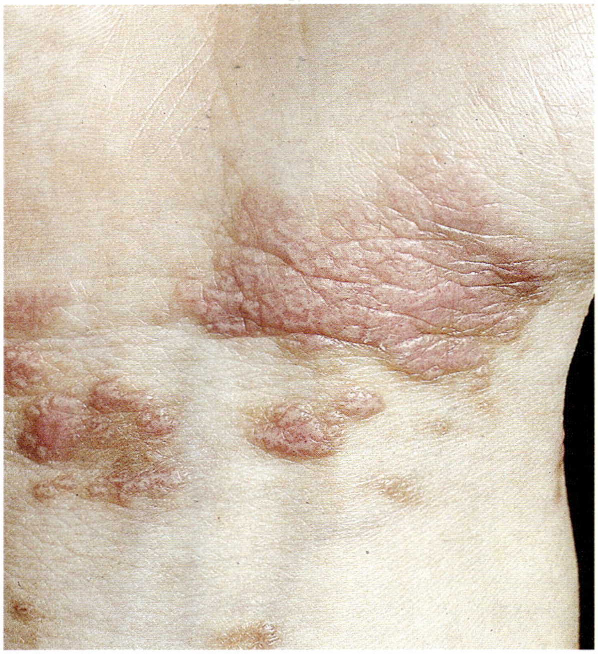

FIGURE 5-8. Lichen planus.

Flat-topped, polygonal, sharply defined, shiny violaceous papules. (Reproduced, with permission, from Wolff K, Johnson RA, Suurmond D. *Fitzpatrick's Color Atlas and Synopsis of Clinical Dermatology*, 5th ed. New York: McGraw-Hill, 2005:125.)

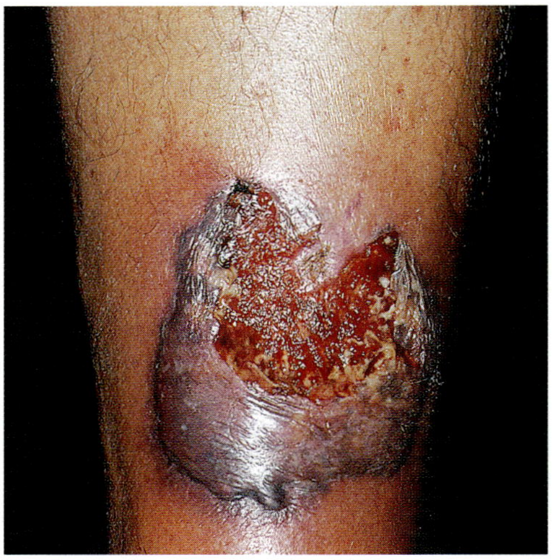

FIGURE 5-10. Pyoderma gangrenosum.

A painful ulcer with a dusky-red peripheral rim and an undermined border. (Reproduced, with permission, from Wolff K, Johnson RA, Suurmond D. *Fitzpatrick's Color Atlas and Synopsis of Clinical Dermatology*, 5th ed. New York: McGraw-Hill, 2005:153.)

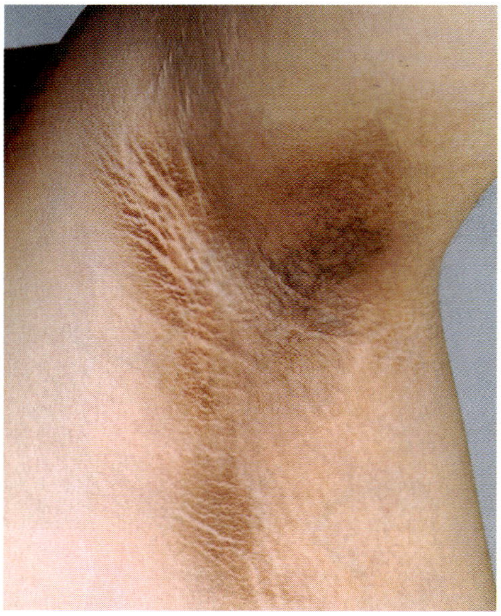

FIGURE 5-11. Acanthosis nigricans.

Velvety, dark-brown epidermal thickening of the neck. (Reproduced, with permission, from Wolff K, Johnson RA, Suurmond D. *Fitzpatrick's Color Atlas and Synopsis of Clinical Dermatology*, 5th ed. New York: McGraw-Hill, 2005:87.)

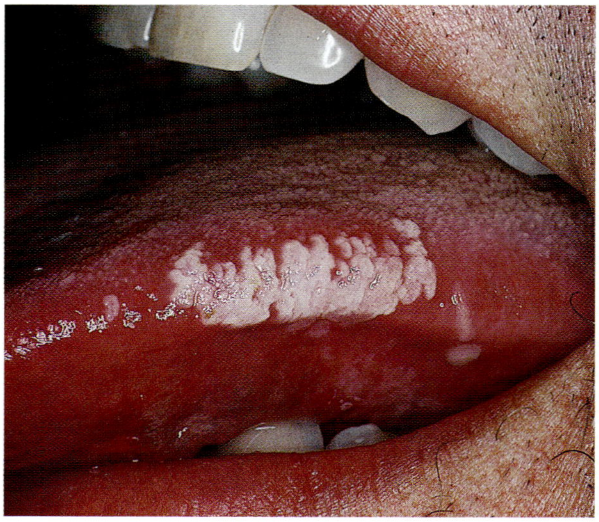

FIGURE 5-12. Oral hairy leukoplakia.

Corrugated white plaque on the lateral tongue. Essentially pathognomonic for HIV infection. (Reproduced, with permission, from Wolff K, Johnson RA, Suurmond D. *Fitzpatrick's Color Atlas and Synopsis of Clinical Dermatology*, 5th ed. New York: McGraw-Hill, 2005:943.)

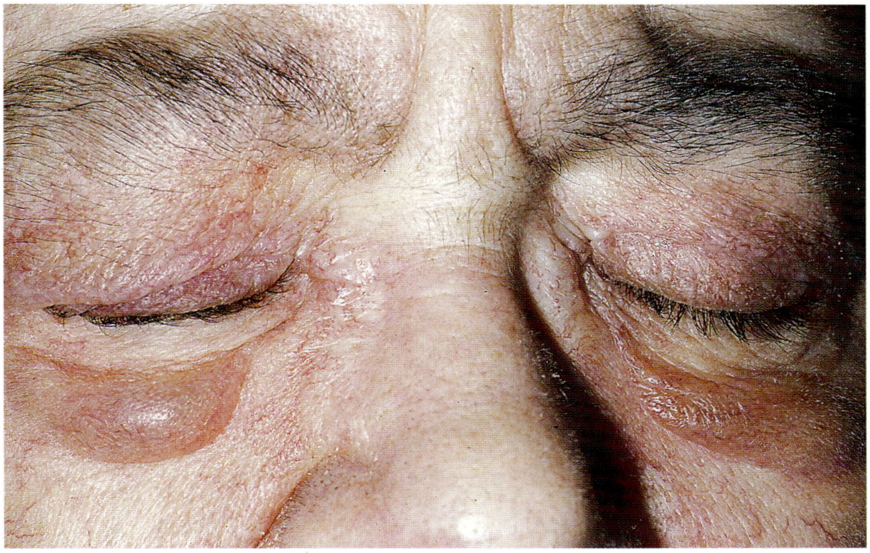

FIGURE 5-15. Dermatomyositis—heliotrope.

Violaceous (reddish-purple) rash and edema of the eyelids. (Reproduced, with permission, from Wolff K, Johnson RA, Suurmond D. *Fitzpatrick's Color Atlas and Synopsis of Clinical Dermatology*, 5th ed. New York: McGraw-Hill, 2005:373.)

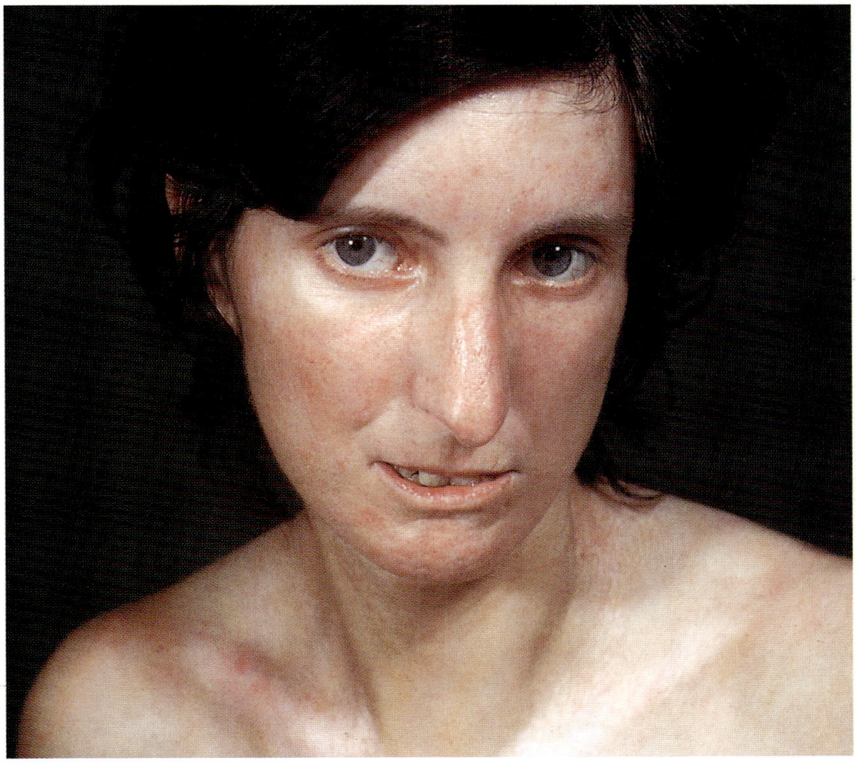

FIGURE 5-17. Scleroderma—masklike facies.

Stretched, shiny skin with loss of normal facial lines. (Reproduced, with permission, from Wolff K, Johnson RA, Suurmond D. *Fitzpatrick's Color Atlas and Synopsis of Clinical Dermatology*, 5th ed. New York: McGraw-Hill, 2005:400.)

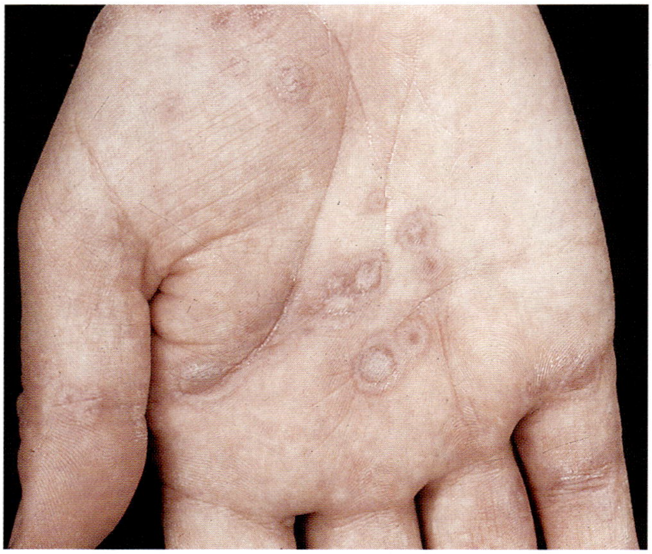

FIGURE 5-18. Erythema multiforme.

Targetoid lesions on the palms. (Reproduced, with permission, from Wolff K, Johnson RA, Suurmond D. *Fitzpatrick's Color Atlas and Synopsis of Clinical Dermatology*, 5th ed. New York: McGraw-Hill, 2005:141.)

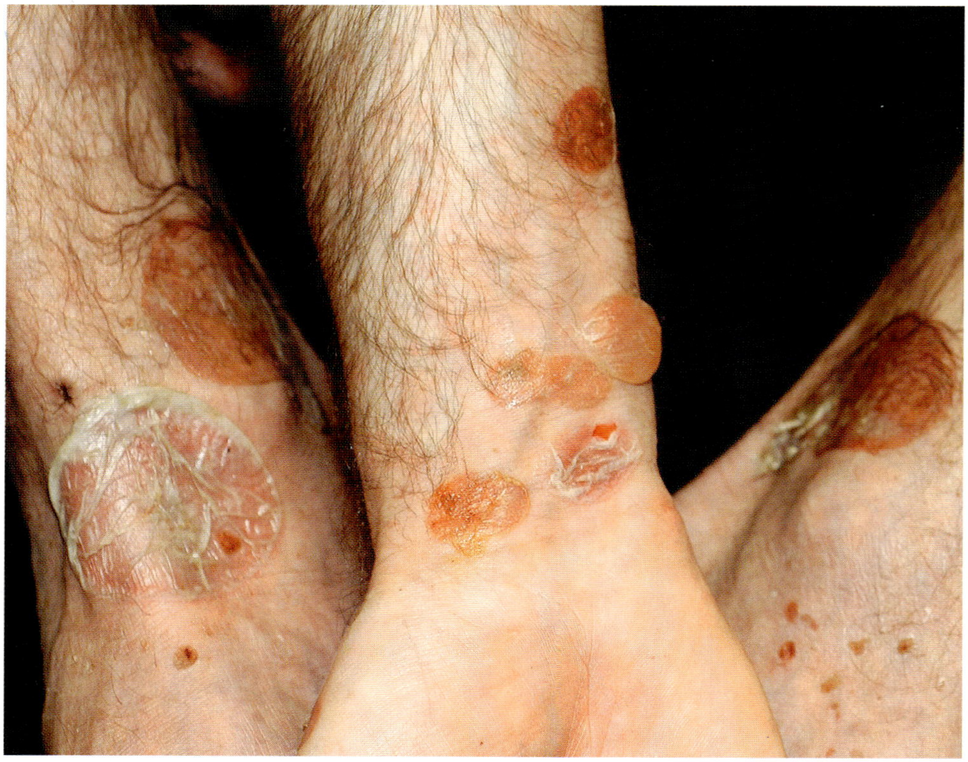

FIGURE 5-19. Bullous pemphigoid.

Tense bullae with serous fluid are seen in a patient with HIV infection. Postinflammatory pigmentary alteration is present at sites of prior lesions. (Reproduced, with permission, from Wolff K, Johnson RA, Suurmond D. *Fitzpatrick's Color Atlas and Synopsis of Clinical Dermatology*, 5th ed. New York: McGraw-Hill, 2005:103.)

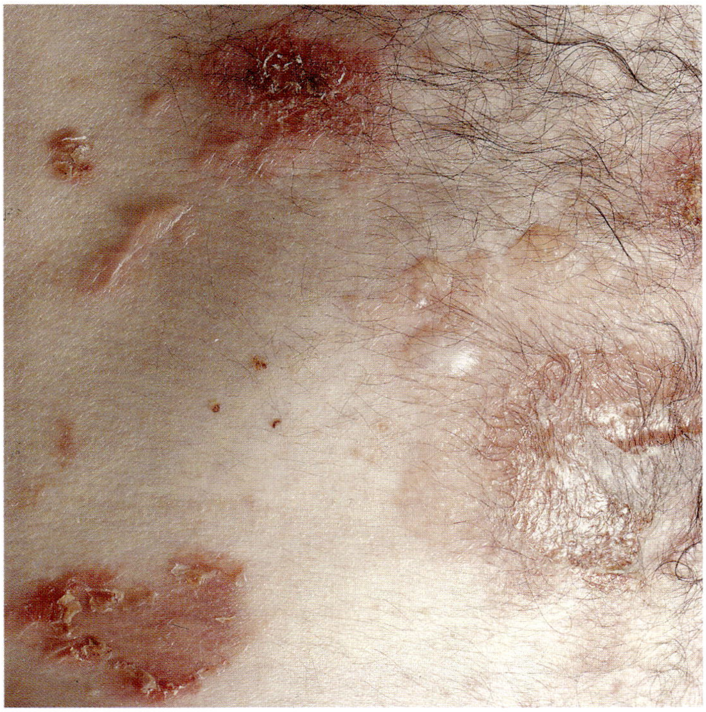

FIGURE 5-20. Pemphigus vulgaris.

Owing to the fragility of the blisters, pemphigus vulgaris presents as erosions. (Reproduced, with permission, from Wolff K, Johnson RA, Suurmond D. *Fitzpatrick's Color Atlas and Synopsis of Clinical Dermatology*, 5th ed. New York: McGraw-Hill, 2005:104.)

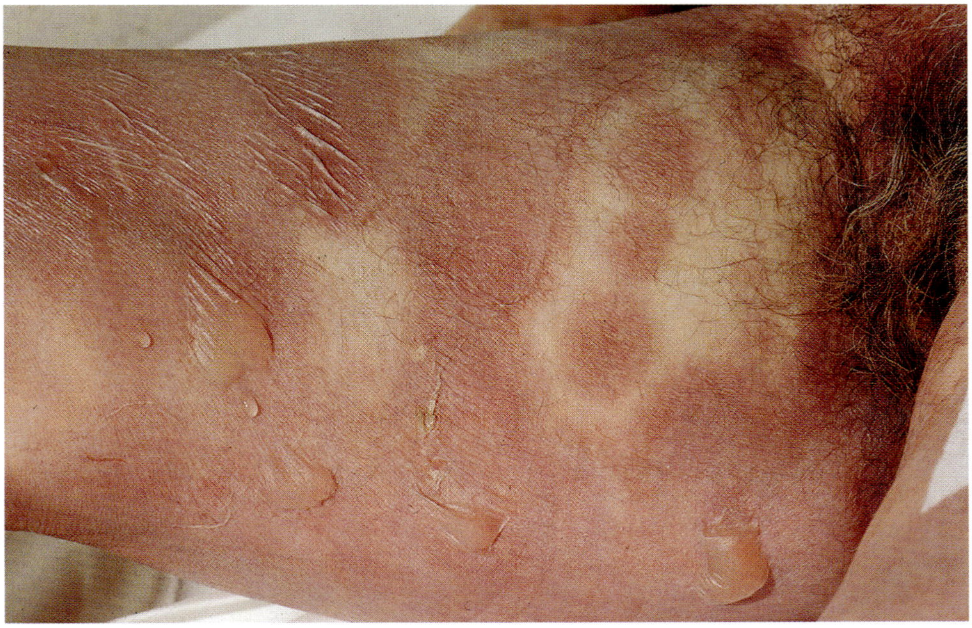

FIGURE 5-21. Stevens-Johnson syndrome.

Generalized eruption of initially targetlike lesions that become confluent, brightly erythematous, and bullous. (Reproduced, with permission, from Wolff K, Johnson RA, Suurmond D. *Fitzpatrick's Color Atlas and Synopsis of Clinical Dermatology*, 5th ed. New York: McGraw-Hill, 2005:145.)

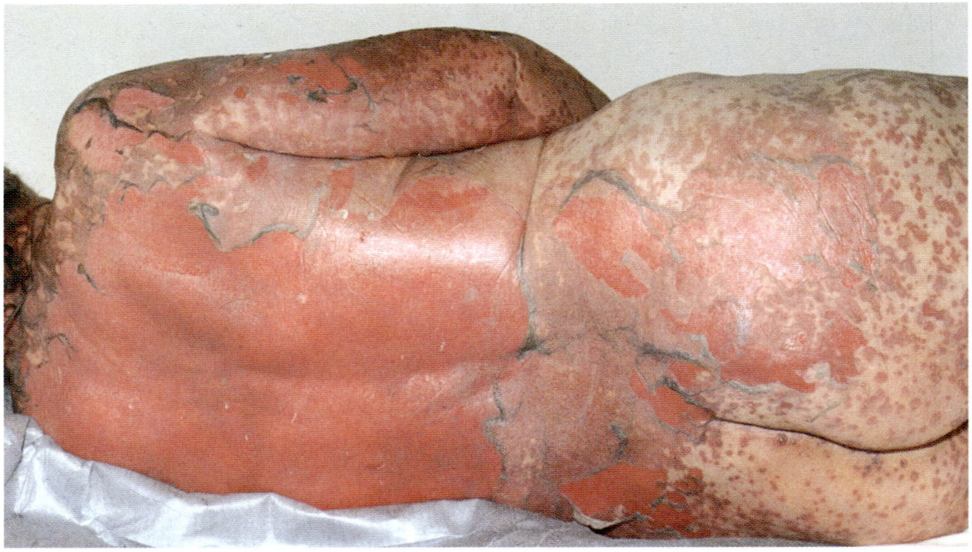

FIGURE 5-22. Toxic epidermal necrolysis.

Bulla formation with rapid desquamation revealing denuded, erosive areas. (Reproduced, with permission, from Wolff K, Johnson RA, Suurmond D. *Fitzpatrick's Color Atlas and Synopsis of Clinical Dermatology*, 5th ed. New York: McGraw-Hill, 2005:147.)

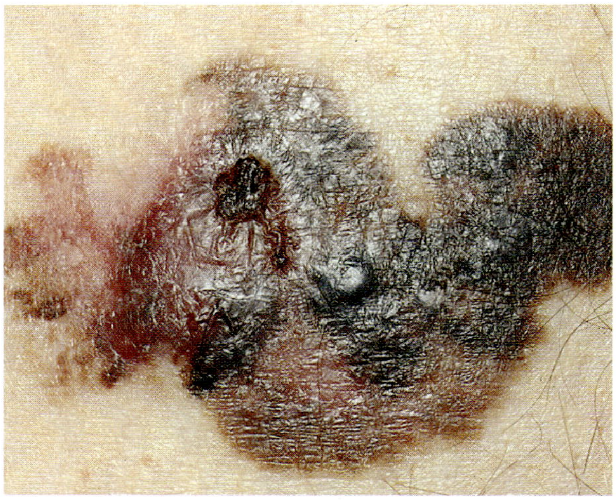

FIGURE 5-23. Superficial spreading melanoma.

A highly characteristic lesion with an irregular pigmentary pattern and scalloped borders. (Reproduced, with permission, from Wolff K, Johnson RA, Suurmond D. *Fitzpatrick's Color Atlas and Synopsis of Clinical Dermatology*, 5th ed. New York: McGraw-Hill, 2005:318.)

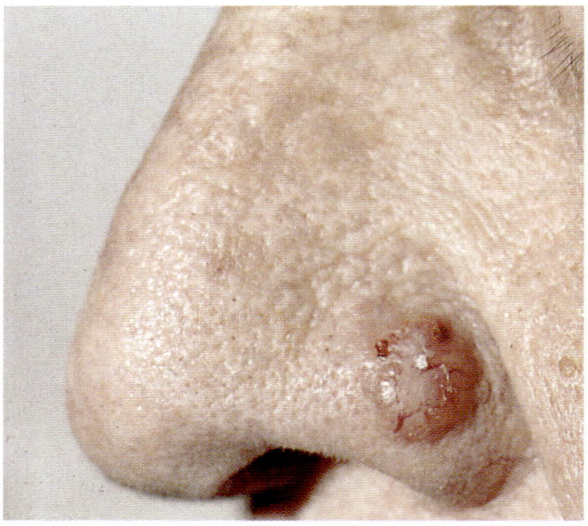

FIGURE 5-24. Nodular basal cell carcinoma.

A smooth, pearly nodule with telangiectasias. (Reproduced, with permission, from Wolff K, Johnson RA, Suurmond D. *Fitzpatrick's Color Atlas and Synopsis of Clinical Dermatology*, 5th ed. New York: McGraw-Hill, 2005:283.)

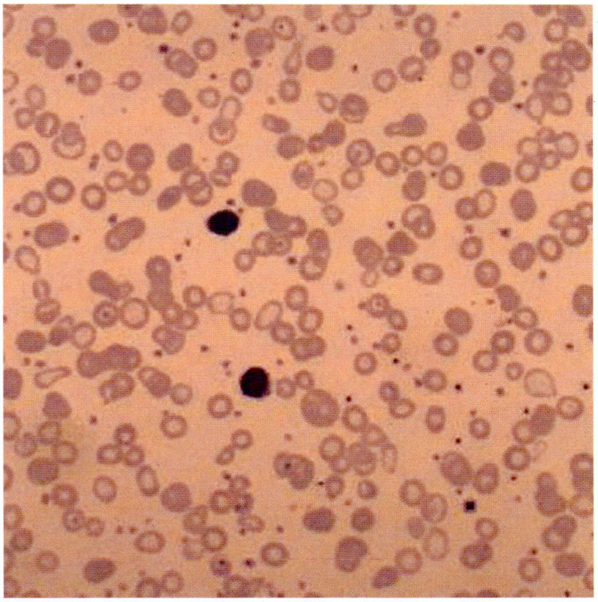

FIGURE 9-2. Iron deficiency anemia.

Note hypochromic cells (prominent central pallor) and microcytosis (RBCs smaller than the nucleus of the lymphocyte). There is also prominent thrombocytosis, a common associated finding with iron deficiency.

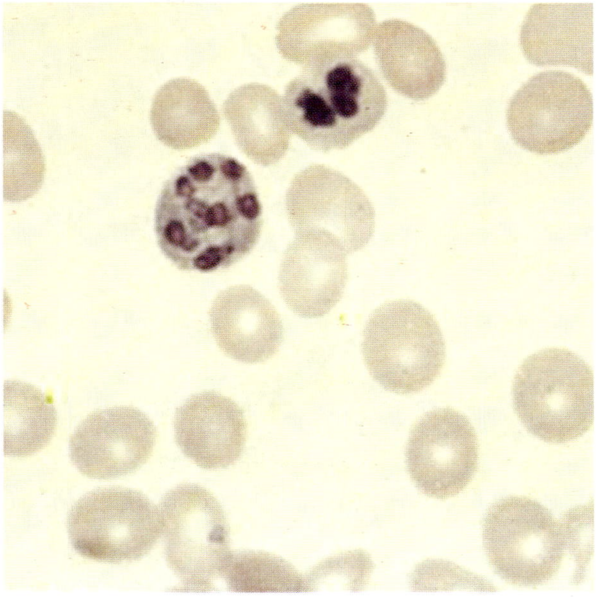

FIGURE 9-3. Megaloblastic anemia.

Note macro-ovalocytes and prominent hypersegmented neutrophil. (Reproduced, with permission, from Babior BM, Bunn HF. Megaloblastic anemias. In Kasper DL et al [eds]. *Harrison's Principles of Internal Medicine,* 16th ed. New York: McGraw-Hill, 2005.)

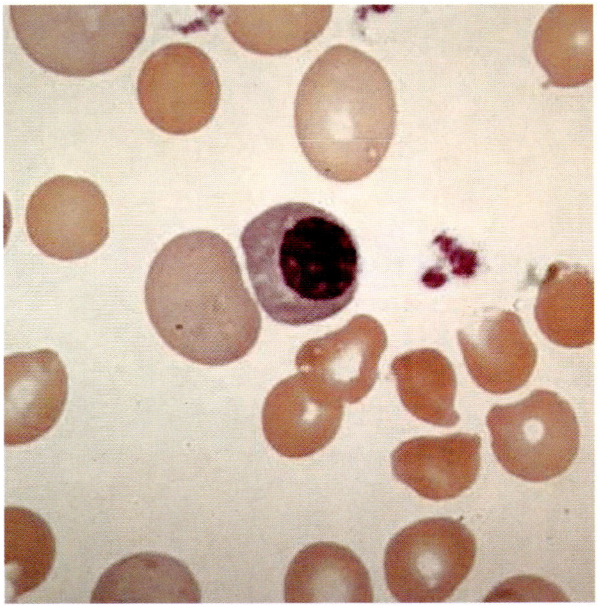

FIGURE 9-5. Bite cells.

Several characteristic bite cells are present in this patient with G6PD deficiency with acute oxidative hemolysis. (Courtesy of L Damon. Reproduced, with permission, from Linker CA. Hematology. In Tierney LM et al [eds]. *Current Medical Diagnosis & Treatment 2005,* 44th ed. New York: McGraw-Hill, 2005.)

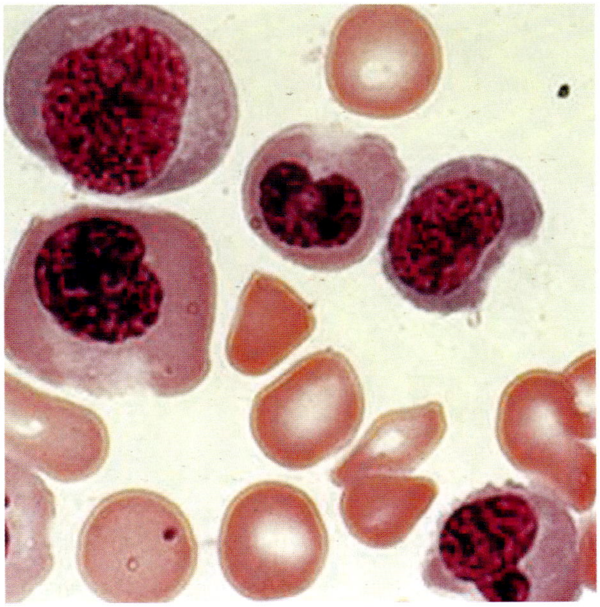

FIGURE 9-6. Spherocytes.

Characteristic spherocytes (small, round RBCs without central pallor) are present in addition to signs of markedly increased RBC synthesis (polychromasia, nucleated RBCs) in a patient with extravascular immune hemolysis. (Reproduced, with permission, from RS Hillman, MD, and KA Ault, MD, courtesy of the American Society of Hematology Slide Bank.)

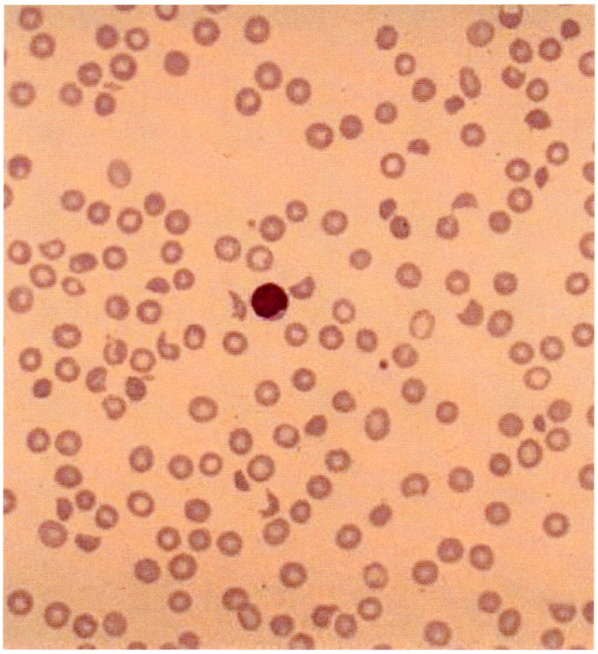

FIGURE 9-7. Schistocytes.

A large number of fragmented RBCs is characteristic of microangiopathic or intravascular hemolysis. In this case, the patient had HUS. (Courtesy of L Damon. Reproduced, with permission, from Linker CA. Hematology. In Tierney LM et al [eds]. *Current Medical Diagnosis & Treatment 2005*, 44th ed. New York: McGraw-Hill, 2005.)

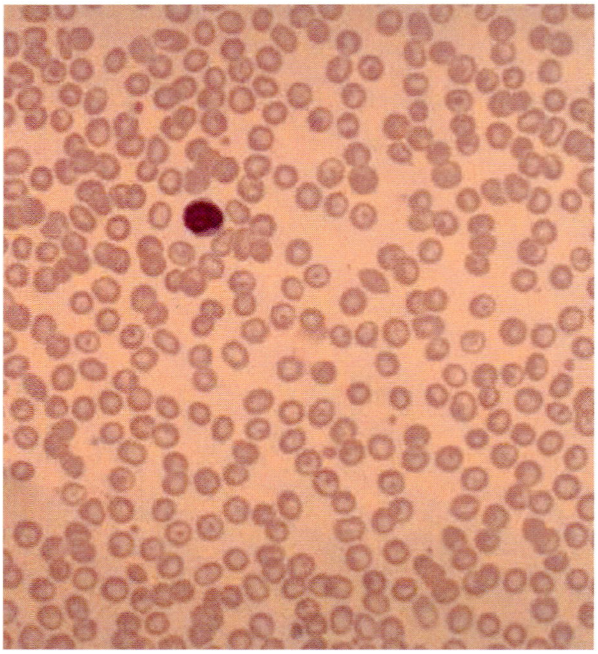

FIGURE 9-8. β-thalassemia major.

Note microcytic, hypochromic cells, target cells, and nucleated RBCs. (Courtesy of L Damon. Reproduced, with permission, from Linker CA. Hematology. In Tierney LM et al [eds]. *Current Medical Diagnosis & Treatment 2005*, 44th ed. New York: McGraw-Hill, 2005.)

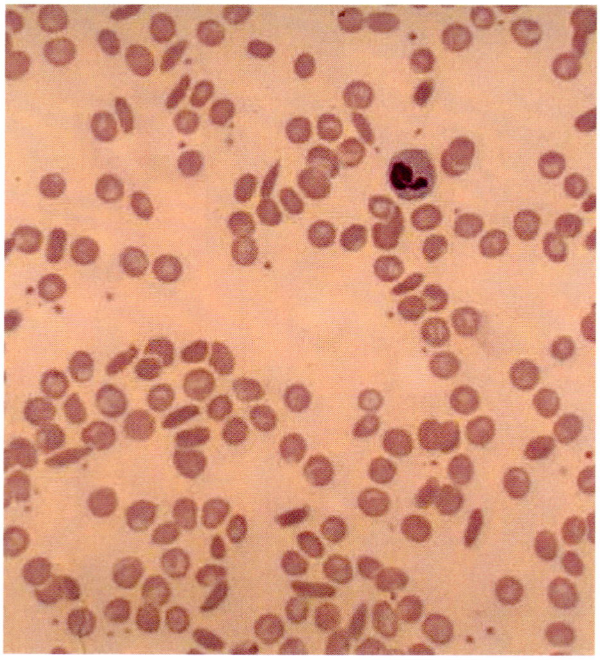

FIGURE 9-9. Sickle cell anemia.

Multiple sickle forms are characteristic. (Courtesy of L Damon. Reproduced, with permission, from Linker CA. Hematology. In Tierney LM et al [eds]. *Current Medical Diagnosis & Treatment 2005*, 44th ed. New York: McGraw-Hill, 2005.)

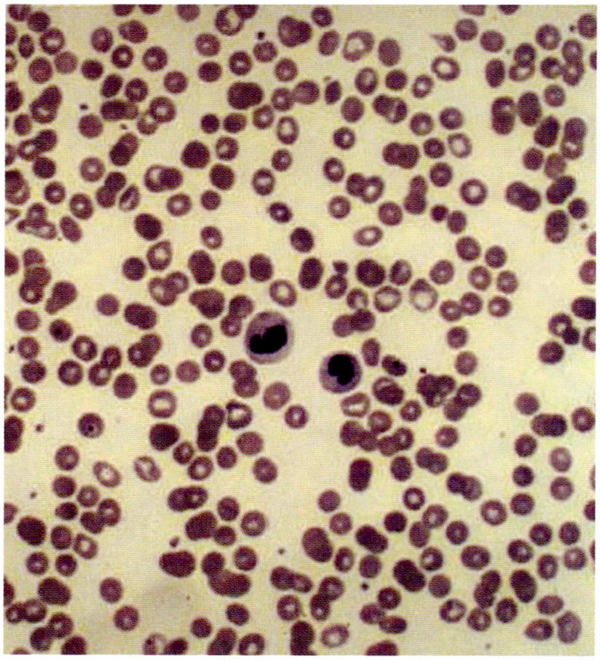

FIGURE 9-10. Myelodysplasia.

Both neutrophils in this slide demonstrate hypogranulation and hypolobation (pseudo–Pelger-Huët anomaly), suggesting myelodysplasia. (Courtesy of L Damon. Reproduced, with permission, from Linker CA. Hematology. In Tierney LM et al [eds]. *Current Medical Diagnosis & Treatment 2005*, 44th ed. New York: McGraw-Hill, 2005.)

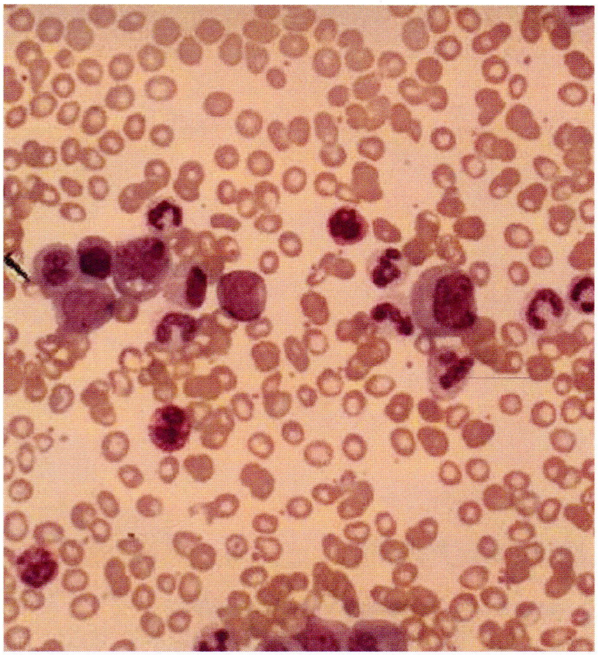

FIGURE 9-11. Chronic myelogenous leukemia.

Note the large number of immature myeloid forms in the peripheral blood, including metamyelocytes, myelocytes, and promyelocytes, as well as a large number of eosinophils and basophils. (Courtesy of L Damon. Reproduced, with permission, from Linker CA. Hematology. In Tierney LM et al [eds]. *Current Medical Diagnosis & Treatment 2005*, 44th ed. New York: McGraw-Hill, 2005.)

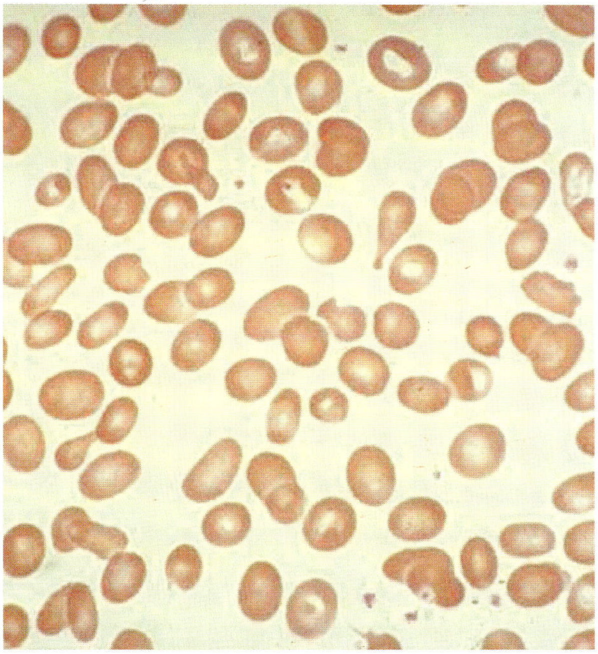

FIGURE 9-12. Myelofibrosis.

Note the large number of teardrop cells suggestive of bone marrow infiltrative disease.(Courtesy of L Damon. Reproduced, with permission, from Linker CA. Hematology. In Tierney LM et al [eds]. *Current Medical Diagnosis & Treatment 2005*, 44th ed. New York: McGraw-Hill, 2005.)

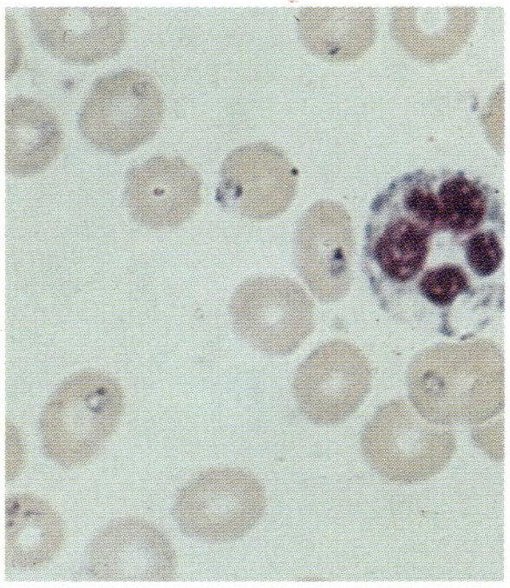

FIGURE 11-1. Babesiosis on a blood smear.

Note parasites within RBCs resembling malaria. Tetrads and classic "Maltese crosses" are rare but diagnostic of babesiosis. (Reproduced, with permission, from *Bench Aids for the Diagnosis of Malaria Infections,* 2nd ed. Geneva: World Health Organization, 2000.)

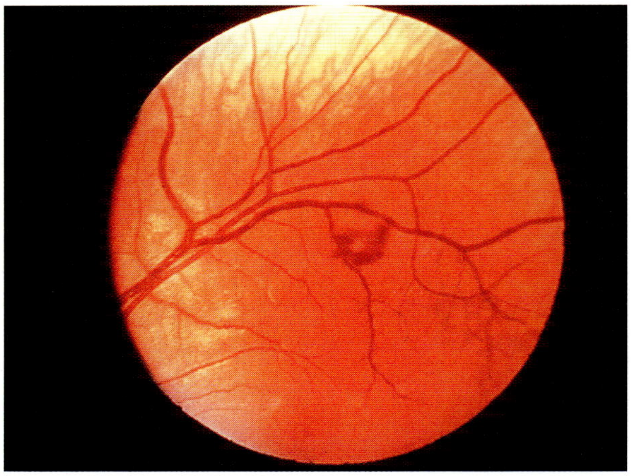

FIGURE 11-2. Roth's spot in endocarditis.

This retinal image shows a lesion with central clear areas surrounded by hemorrhage. (Courtesy of William E. Cappaert, MD. Reproduced, with permission, from Knoop KJ, Stack LB, Storrow AB. *Atlas of Emergency Medicine,* 2nd ed. New York: McGraw-Hill, 2002:80.)

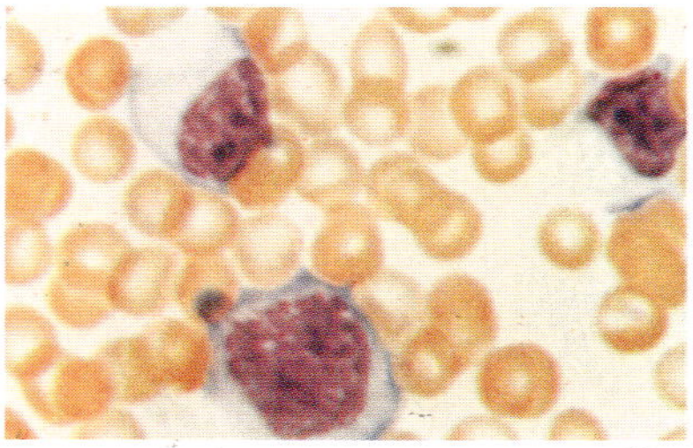

FIGURE 11-5. Atypical lymphocytosis seen in infectious mononucleosis and other infections.

These reactive T lymphocytes are large with eccentric nuclei and bluish-staining RNA in the cytoplasm. (Reproduced, with permission, from Braunwald E et al [eds]. *Harrison's Principles of Internal Medicine,* 15th ed. New York: McGraw-Hill, 2001.)

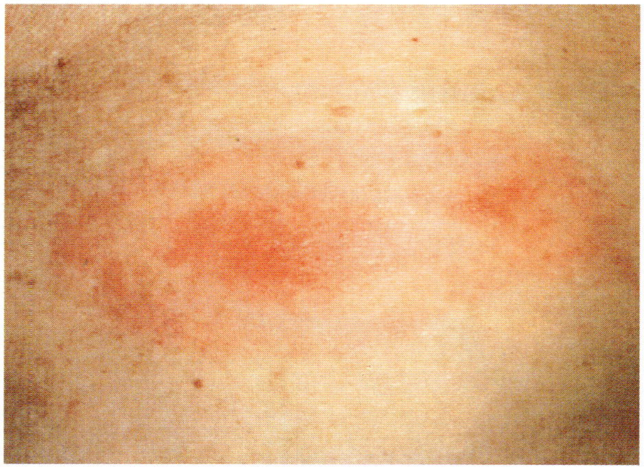

FIGURE 11-6. Erythema chronicum migrans seen in Lyme disease.

The classic "bull's eye" lesion consists of an outer ring where the spirochetes are found, an inner ring of clearing, and central erythema due to an allergic response at the site of the tick bite. Note that some lesions may consist of just the outer annular erythema wth central clearing. (Reproduced, with permission, from Braunwald E et al [eds]. *Harrison's Principles of Internal Medicine,* 15th ed. New York: McGraw-Hill, 2001.)

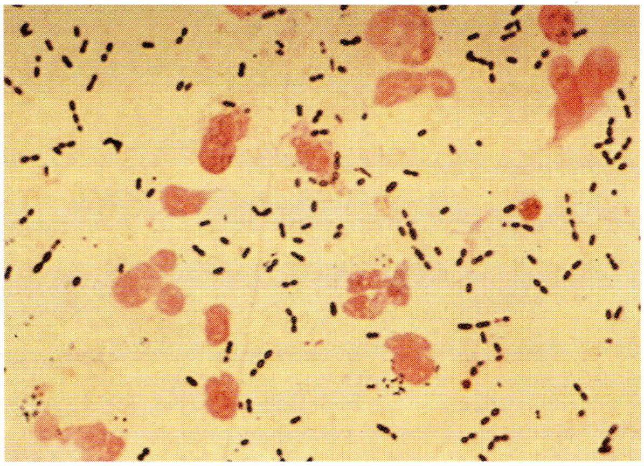

FIGURE 11-7. Pneumococcal pneumonia.

This Gram-stained sputum sample shows many neutrophils and lancet-shaped gram-positive cocci in pairs and chains, indicating infection with *S. pneumoniae*. (Courtesy of Roche Laboratories, Division of Hoffman-LaRoche Inc., Nutley, NJ.)

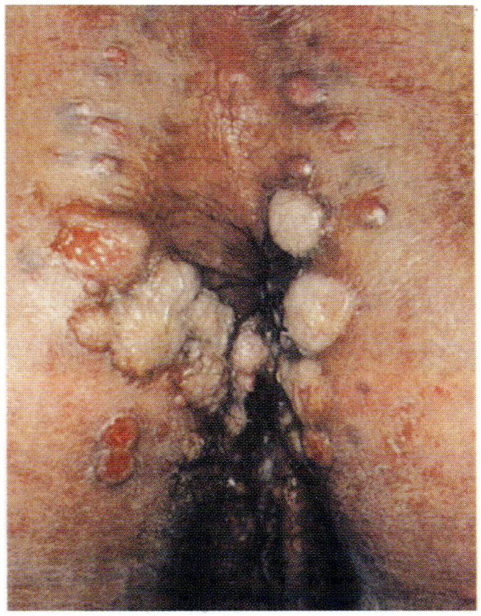

FIGURE 11-8. Condylomata lata in secondary syphilis.

(Reproduced, with permission, from Kasper DL et al [eds]. *Harrison's Principles of Internal Medicine*, 16th ed. New York: McGraw-Hill, 2005:979.)

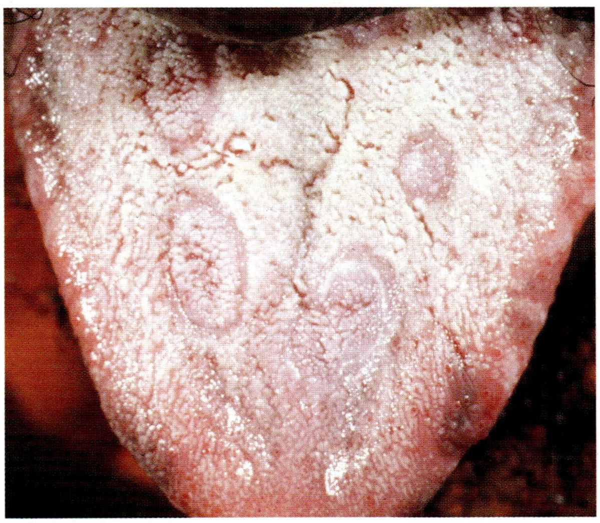

FIGURE 11-9. Mucous patches in secondary syphilis.

Note the multiple painless grayish-white erosions with a red periphery on the dorsal and lateral tongue. These highly infectious mucosal lesions contain large numbers of treponemes. (Courtesy of Ron Roddy. Reproduced, with permission, from Kasper DL et al [eds]. *Harrison's Principles of Internal Medicine*, 16th ed. New York: McGraw-Hill, 2005:980.)

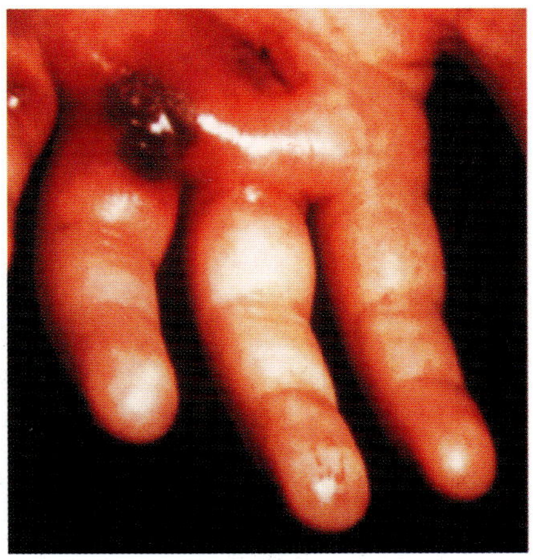

FIGURE 11-10. Ecthyma gangrenosum with *Pseudomonas* in a neutropenic patient.

Note the red papule with a necrotic center. (Reproduced, with permission, from Kasper DL et al [eds]. *Harrison's Principles of Internal Medicine*, 16th ed. New York: McGraw-Hill, 2005:890.)

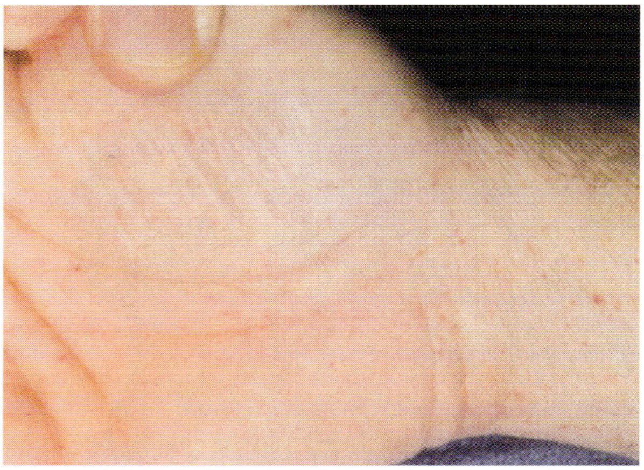

FIGURE 11-11. Rocky Mountain spotted fever.

(Reproduced, with permission, from Braunwald E et al [eds]. *Harrison's Principles of Internal Medicine,* 15th ed. New York: McGraw-Hill, 2001: Color Plate IID-45.)

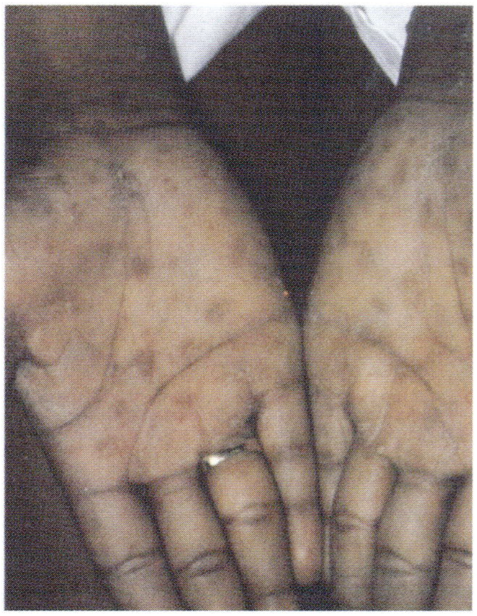

FIGURE 11-12. Secondary syphilis.

(Reproduced, with permission, from Kasper DL et al [eds]. *Harrison's Principles of Internal Medicine,* 16th ed. New York: McGraw-Hill, 2005:979.)

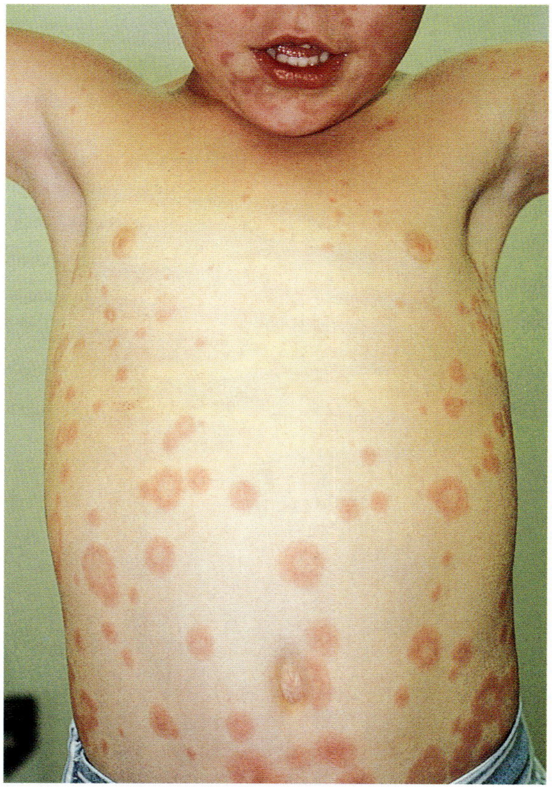

FIGURE 11-13. Erythema multiforme.

(Courtesy of Michael Redman, PA-C. Reproduced, with permission, from Knoop KJ, Stack LB, Storrow AB. *Atlas of Emergency Medicine,* 2nd ed. New York: McGraw-Hill, 2002:378.)

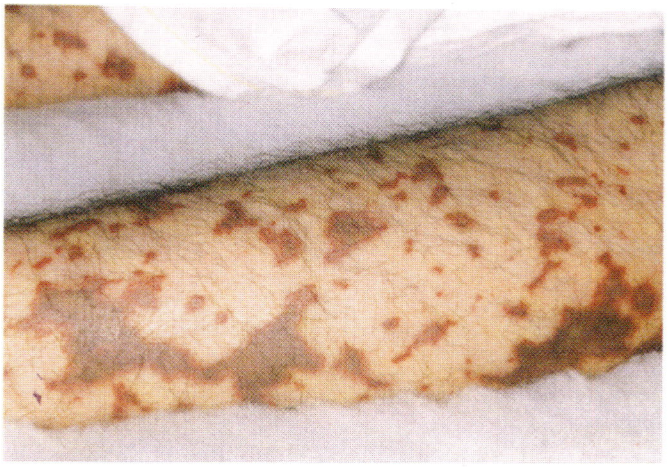

FIGURE 11-14. Acute meningococcemia.

(Courtesy of Stephen E. Gellis, MD. Reproduced, with permission, from Kasper DL et al [eds]. *Harrison's Principles of Internal Medicine*, 16th ed. New York: McGraw-Hill, 2005:284.)

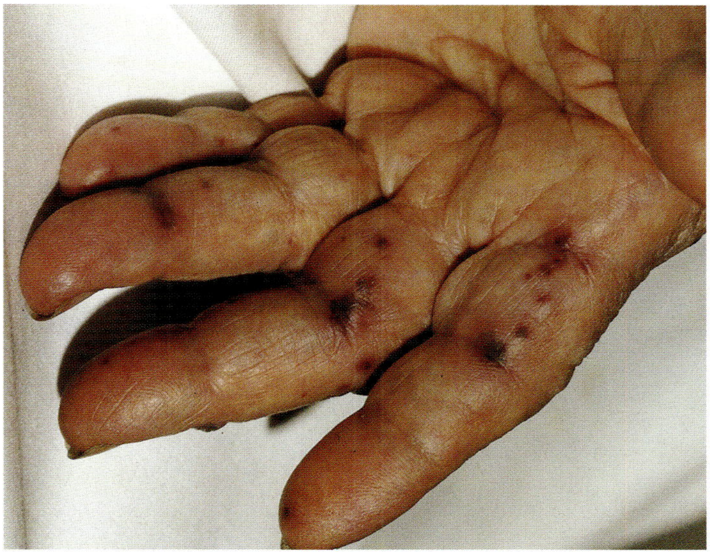

FIGURE 11-15. Janeway lesions in endocarditis.

(Reproduced, with permission, from Wolff K, Johnson RA, Suurmond D. *Fitzpatrick's Color Atlas and Synopsis of Clinical Dermatology*, 5th ed. New York: McGraw-Hill, 2005:636.)

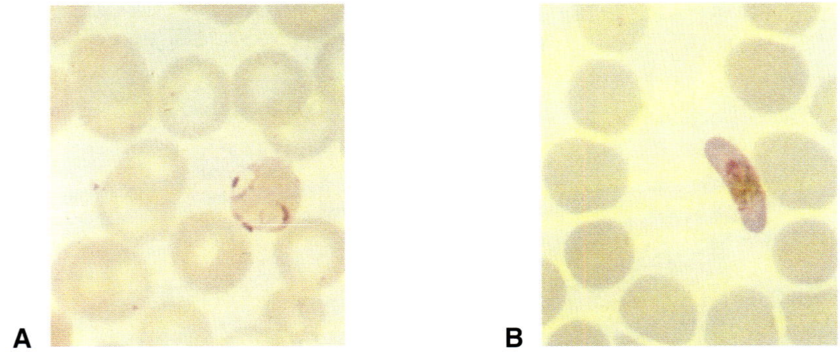

FIGURE 11-16. Falciparum malaria on a thin blood smear.

(**A**) Young signet-ring-shaped parasites are seen for all species of *Plasmodium*, but only *P. falciparum* shows multiple parasites within a single RBC. (**B**) Banana-shaped gametocytes are diagnostic for *P. falciparum*. (Reproduced, with permission, from *Bench Aids for the Diagnosis of Malaria Infections*, 2nd ed. Geneva: World Health Organization, 2000.) (Also see Color Insert.)

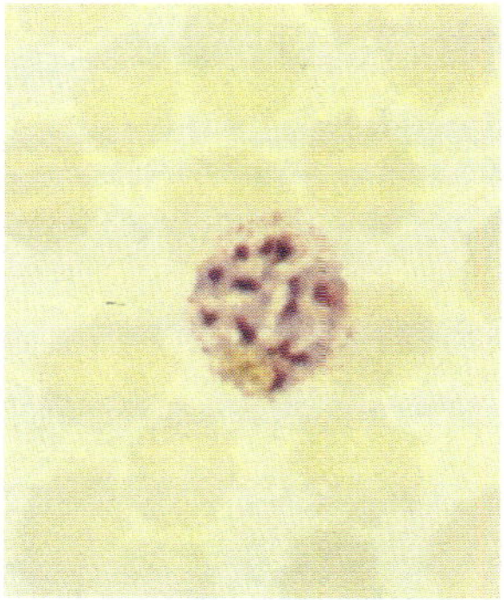

FIGURE 11-17. Vivax malaria on a thin blood smear.

Mature schizonts ready to burst and release many daughter parasites are seen in *P. vivax*, *P. ovale*, and *P. malariae* infections. They are not seen in the blood with *P. falciparum*. (Banana-shaped gametocytes are diagnostic for *P. falciparum*. (Reproduced, with permission, from *Bench Aids for the Diagnosis of Malaria Infections*, 2nd ed. Geneva: World Health Organization, 2000.) (Also see Color Insert.)

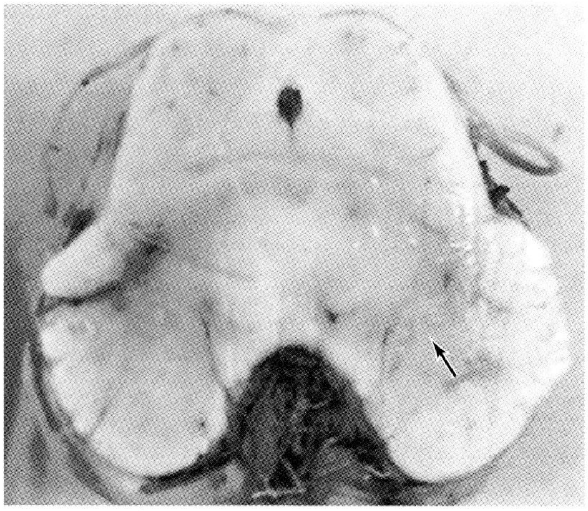

FIGURE 13-1. Midbrain of a 45-year-old woman with Parkinson's disease, showing depigmentation of the substantia nigra (arrow).

(Reproduced, with permission, from Waxman S. *Clinical Neuroanatomy*, 25th ed. New York: McGraw-Hill, 2003: Figure 13-9.)

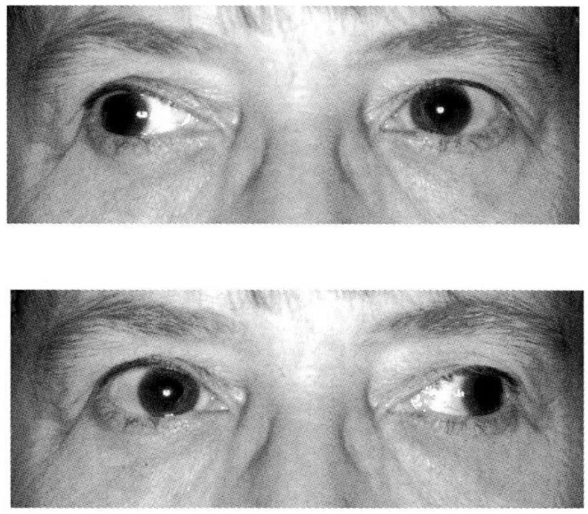

FIGURE 13-3. Bilateral internuclear ophthalmoplegia due to multiple sclerosis.

(Reproduced, with permission, from Riordan-Eva P. *Vaughan & Asbury's General Ophthalmology*, 16th ed. New York: McGraw-Hill, 2004: Figure 14-12.)

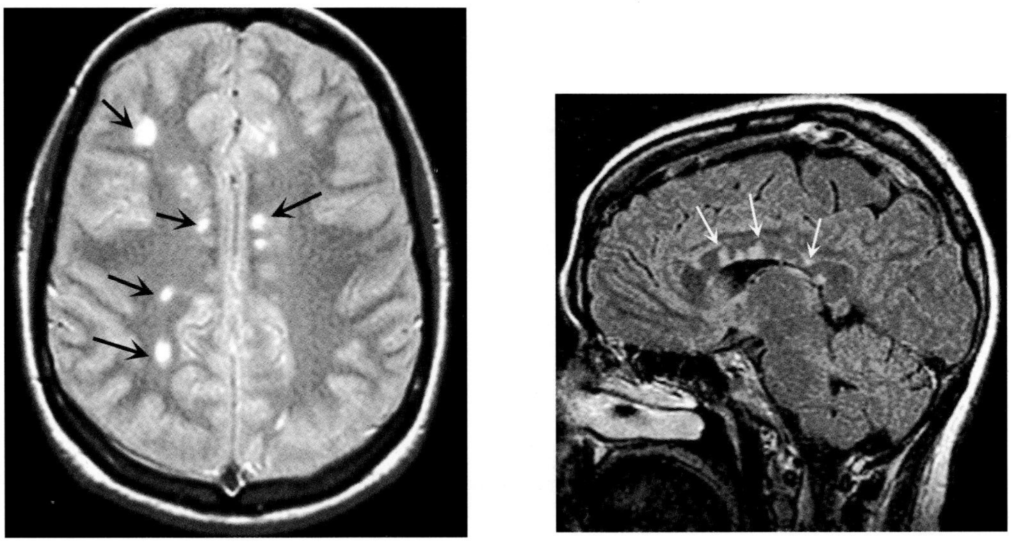

A *B*

FIGURE 13-4. MRI findings in MS.

(A) Axial image from T2-weighted sequence demonstrates multiple bright signal abnormalities in white matter, typical for MS. (B) Sagittal T2-weighted FLAIR (fluid-attenuated inversion recovery) image in which the high signal of CSF has been suppressed. CSF appears dark, while areas of brain edema or demyelination appear high in signal, as shown here in the corpus callosum (*arrows*). Lesions in the anterior corpus callosum are frequent in MS and rare in vascular disease. (Reproduced, with permission, from Kasper DL et al [eds]. *Harrison's Principles of Internal Medicine*, 16th ed. New York: McGraw-Hill, 2005:2464.)

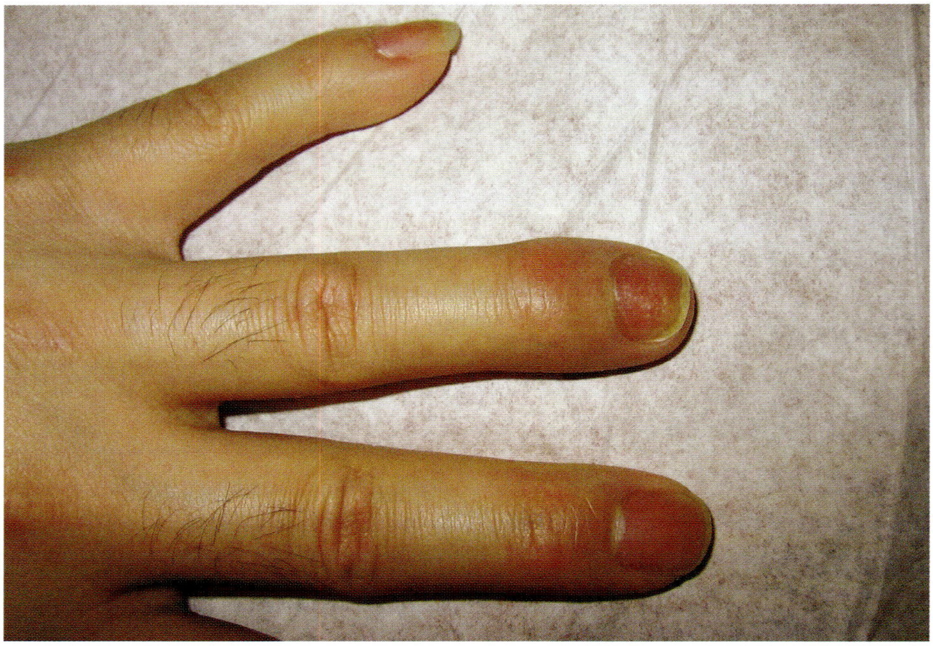

FIGURE 17-2. Onycholysis in psoriatic arthritis patient.

(Courtesy of Jonathan Graf, MD, 2004.)

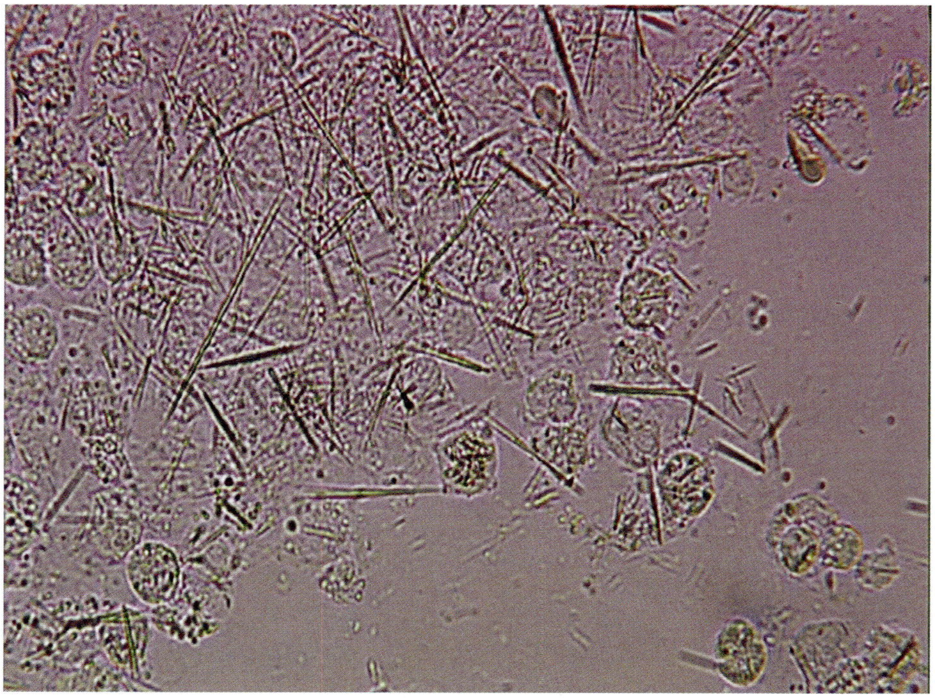

FIGURE 17-3. Gout crystals.

(Courtesy of Jonathan Graf, MD, 2004.)

TREATMENT

- Treat the underlying cause.
- **Nonpharmacologic treatment:** Shaving, depilatories, electrolysis, laser treatment, eflornithine hydrochloride cream (Vaniqa), weight loss.
- **Antiandrogen therapy:** OCPs, spironolactone.

INFERTILITY

Inability to conceive after **one year** of unprotected intercourse.

EXAM

Exam is often unremarkable. Look for hirsutism, goiter, galactorrhea, and an abnormal pelvic exam.

DIFFERENTIAL

Etiologies include the following:

- Factors related to the male partner (e.g., quantity and quality of sperm).
- Ovulatory dysfunction (failure, prolactinoma, thyroid disease, PCOS, other causes of anovulation).
- Luteal-phase defects (implantation).
- Uterine abnormalities (congenital [e.g., septum], DES exposure, fibroids, polyps, synechiae from prior manipulation).
- Tubal and peritoneal abnormalities (PID, severe endometriosis, adhesions).
- Cervical abnormalities.

DIAGNOSIS

- Semen analysis.
- Serum FSH, LH, TSH, prolactin.
- Postcoital (ferning) test.
- Possibly endometrial biopsy, hysterosalpingography and/or laparoscopy.

It is important to rule out male infertility first, as it is the source of the problem in 40% of cases and is easy to evaluate.

TREATMENT

Treat the underlying cause:

- Sperm or egg donation.
- Ovulation induction (clomiphene, menotropins [e.g., Pergonal]).
- Laparoscopy (e.g., to remove endometriosis implants).
- Advanced reproductive technologies (IVF).

MEDICAL ISSUES IN PREGNANCY

Teratogenic Drugs

Table 18-3 lists common teratogens and their effects.

Chronic Hypertension

Hypertension that is present before conception or at < 20 weeks' gestation, or that persists > 6 weeks postpartum.

WOMEN'S HEALTH

TABLE 18-3. Teratogenic Drugs

TERATOGEN	EFFECT
Alcohol	Fetal alcohol syndrome, intrauterine growth retardation (IUGR), cardiac defects.
Cocaine	Bowel atresias, IUGR, microcephaly.
Streptomycin	CN VIII damage/ototoxicity.
Tetracycline	Tooth discoloration, inhibition of bone growth, small limbs, syndactyly.
Sulfonamides	Kernicterus.
Quinolones	Cartilage damage.
Isotretinoin	Heart and great vessel defects, craniofacial dysmorphism, deafness.
Iodide	Congenital goiter, hypothyroidism, mental retardation.
Methotrexate	CNS malformations, craniofacial dysmorphism, IUGR.
DES	Clear cell adenocarcinoma of the vagina/cervix, genital tract abnormalities (cervical hood, T-shaped uterus, hypoplastic uterus), cervical incompetence.
Thalidomide	Limb reduction (phocomelia), ear and nasal anomalies, cardiac and lung defects, pyloric or duodenal stenosis, GI atresia.
Coumadin	Stippling of bone epiphyses, IUGR, nasal hypoplasia, mental retardation.
ACEIs	Oligohydramnios, fetal renal damage.
Lithium	Ebstein's anomaly, other cardiac disease.
Carbamazepine	Fingernail hypoplasia, IUGR, microcephaly, neural tube defects.
Phenytoin	Nail hypoplasia, IUGR, mental retardation, craniofacial dysmorphism, microcephaly.
Valproic acid	Neural tube defects, craniofacial and skeletal defects.

Adapted, with permission, from Le T et al. *First Aid for the USMLE Step 2,* 4th ed. New York: McGraw-Hill, 2003.

SYMPTOMS

Asymptomatic. Ask about headaches and edema.

EXAM

Cardiovascular exam.

DIFFERENTIAL

Chronic hypertension, pregnancy-induced hypertension, preeclampsia, eclampsia.

Diagnosis

BP monitoring, possibly CBC, liver panel, UA, 24-hour urine collection, ECG.

Treatment

May need to change preconception antihypertensive medication based on the risk of teratogenicity. Commonly used antihypertensives include β-blockers, methyldopa, and hydralazine. **ACEIs and diuretics are contraindicated.**

It is important to reevaluate the antihypertensive regimen in women contemplating pregnancy.

Complications

Increased risk of preeclampsia (1 in 3).

Pregestational Diabetes

Diabetes prior to conception.

Symptoms

Hyperglycemia.

Exam

Retinal exam; cardiovascular exam, including BP; podiatric exam.

Differential

Gestational diabetes.

Diagnosis

Glycohemoglobin, creatinine, 24-hour urine for protein and creatinine. Early ultrasound and AFP.

The goal in the mother with preexisting diabetes is good control before conception.

Treatment

Tight control with insulin (see Table 18-4). **Sulfonylureas are contraindicated.** Metformin has recently been used. Close fetal surveillance.

Complications

Common complications associated with pregestational diabetes are outlined in Table 18-5. Outcomes are improved with good control before conception as well as with tight control during pregnancy.

TABLE 18-4. Blood Sugar Goals During Pregnancy

Time of Fingerstick Glucose Measurement	Glucose
Fasting	60–90
1 hour postprandial	130–140
2 hours postprandial	< 120

TABLE 18-5. Complications of Pregestational Diabetes Mellitus

MATERNAL COMPLICATIONS	FETAL COMPLICATIONS
DKA or HHNK	Macrosomia
Preeclampsia/eclampsia	Cardiac and renal defects
Cephalopelvic disproportion (from macrosomia) and need for C-section	Neural tube defects
	Hypocalcemia
Preterm labor	Polycythemia
Infection	Hyperbilirubinemia
Polyhydramnios	IUGR
Postpartum hemorrhage	Hypoglycemia from hyperinsulinemia
Maternal mortality	Respiratory distress syndrome
	Birth injury (shoulder dystocia)
	Perinatal mortality

Adapted, with permission, from Le T et al. *First Aid for the USMLE Step 2,* 4th ed. New York: McGraw-Hill, 2003.

MENOPAUSE

Permanent cessation of menstruation (one year without menses). The median age of onset in the United States is 51. Premature menopause/ovarian failure is cessation of menses in patients ≤ 40 years of age.

Symptoms

Vasomotor instability (hot flashes, nocturnal awakening), mood changes, and symptoms of urogenital atrophy. Urogenital atrophy can lead to dyspareunia, urinary frequency, and an increased incidence of vaginal infections and dysuria.

> ***Menopause wreaks HAVOC–***
>
> **H**ot flashes
> **A**trophy of
> **V**agina
> **O**steoporosis
> **C**oronary artery disease

Exam

Decreased breast size, vaginal dryness, genital tract atrophy.

Differential

Premature ovarian failure, infections (e.g., TB if night sweats predominate and there are TB risk factors), malignancy.

Diagnosis

Take an appropriate history; determine serum FSH.

Treatment

Estrogen works best for the symptoms of menopause, but the risks associated with its use need to be carefully considered.

Nonhormonal treatment of the symptoms of menopause is preferred:

- Treat osteoporosis.
- Treat vaginal symptoms—intravaginal estrogen (low-dose), moisturizers (Replens), lubricants.
- Treat vasomotor instability—clonidine, venlafaxine and SSRIs, gabapentin, herbal medications (black cohosh, soy).
- Hormone replacement therapy (HRT) should be considered only for intractable vasomotor and urogenital symptoms, or inability to tolerate other

treatments for osteoporosis. Recent data from the Women's Health Initiative show increased risk of thromboembolic disease, stroke, CAD, and breast cancer in women taking combination HRT.

MENSTRUAL DISORDERS

Irregular Menses

Abnormalities in the frequency, duration, volume, and/or timing of menses.

- **Menorrhagia:** Prolonged and/or excessive uterine bleeding that is cyclic.
- **Metrorrhagia:** Bleeding at irregular and frequent intervals.
- **Menometrorrhagia:** Prolonged and/or excessive bleeding at irregular intervals.
- **Polymenorrhea:** Cycles < 21 days.
- **Oligomenorrhea:** Cycles > 35 days.
- **Amenorrhea:** Absence of menses for ≥ **6 months.**
- **Hypomenorrhea:** Cyclic light flow.

SYMPTOMS

Patients complain of abnormal vaginal bleeding.

EXAM

Pelvic exam, Pap smear.

DIFFERENTIAL

Table 18-6 outlines the differential diagnosis of abnormal uterine bleeding.

TABLE 18-6. Causes of Abnormal Uterine Bleeding

MENSTRUAL ABNORMALITY	DIFFERENTIAL
Menorrhagia	Leiomyoma, adenomyosis, endometrial hyperplasia or polyps, endometrial or cervical cancer, primary bleeding disorders, pregnancy complications.
Metrorrhagia	Endometrial polyps, endometrial or cervical cancer, pregnancy complications, exogenous estrogen.
Menometrorrhagia	Same as above.
Polymenorrhea	Anovulation.
Oligomenorrhea	**Pregnancy** (most common), hypothalamic-pituitary-gonadal axis disruption, systemic disease.
Hypomenorrhea	Hypogonadotropic hypogonadism, OCPs, Asherman's syndrome, outlet obstruction.

Adapted, with permission, from Le T et al. *First Aid for the USMLE Step 2,* 4th ed. New York: McGraw-Hill, 2003.

DIAGNOSIS

- **Ovulatory bleeding:** Transvaginal ultrasound, D&C (gold standard), hysteroscopy, sonohysterogram.
- **Anovulatory bleeding:** β-hCG, CBC, coagulation factors, endocrine tests (FSH, LH, TSH, prolactin, testosterone, DHEAS).
- **Postmenopausal or chronic:** Requires endometrial biopsy.

TREATMENT

Treat the underlying cause:

- **Ovulatory:** NSAIDs, OCPs.
- **Anovulatory:** OCPs or cyclic progestin.
- **Profuse bleeding:** High-dose estrogen, D&C, endometrial ablation, hysterectomy.

Amenorrhea

Primary or secondary absence of menses. Distinguished as follows:

- **Primary:** Absence of menses and secondary sexual characteristics by age 14, or absence of menses with or without secondary sexual characteristics by age 16.
- **Secondary:** Previously normal menses; absence for **six months.**

SYMPTOMS

Ask about pregnancy symptoms, galactorrhea, headaches, visual changes, hirsutism, acne, stress, medications, and menopausal symptoms. There may also be weight loss (e.g., in eating disorders, exercise).

EXAM

Look for secondary sexual characteristics, virilization (male-pattern hair loss/growth, acne, clitoromegaly), galactorrhea, and abnormalities on pelvic exam.

DIAGNOSIS

Primary amenorrhea is diagnosed as defined above. Secondary amenorrhea is diagnosed as follows:

- Rule out pregnancy.
- Check **TSH** and **prolactin.**
  - If TSH is abnormal, suspect a thyroid disorder.
  - If prolactin is elevated, suspect a **prolactinoma.** Check CT or MRI to visualize the pituitary.
- If TSH and prolactin are normal, **give progestin challenge** (in low estrogen state, no withdrawal bleed).

TREATMENT

Treat the underlying cause.

OSTEOPOROSIS

Bone loss leading to an increased risk of fractures, particularly of the vertebrae, hip, and long bones (proximal femur and distal radius). The mortality from complications of hip fractures is equal to that from breast cancer in women > 50 years of age. Risk factors include the following:

- White or Asian ethnicity
- Low weight
- Menopause
- Glucocorticoid use
- Anovulation
- Tobacco, alcohol use
- A family history of osteoporosis
- Older age
- Falls
- Poor eyesight
- Low calcium intake (e.g., secondary to anticonvulsant use, excess vitamin A, hyperparathyroidism, overreplacement of thyroid hormone).

Symptoms

Asymptomatic or may present with back pain or fractures.

Exam

May be normal. Patients may be thin and have a "dowager's hump" (kyphosis).

Diagnosis

DEXA imaging measures bone mineral density (BMD) at the spine and hip. **Osteoporosis is diagnosed if BMD (T-score) is ≥ 2.5 SDs below that of a young, normal woman.**

Treatment

- Calcium 1500 mg QD, vitamin D 800 IU QD, weight-bearing exercises.
- Smoking cessation.
- Bisphosphonates (alendronate, risedronate) are first-line agents. Selective estrogen receptor modulators, or SERMs (raloxifene, tamoxifen), are currently being evaluated.
- Estrogen.
- Calcitonin (helpful for pain after an acute fracture; not as effective as others in the long term).
- Vertebroplasty for symptoms.
- PTH IM.

PELVIC INFLAMMATORY DISEASE (PID)

Infection of the ascending genital tract, including the endometrium, oviducts, ovaries, uterine wall, and peritoneum. May be acute, subacute, or chronic. Risk factors include multiple sexual partners, unprotected intercourse, young age at first intercourse, mucopurulent cervicitis, IUD use, and prior PID.

Symptoms

One to three days of lower abdominal pain, possibly accompanied by fever, nausea, and vomiting. May occur after recent menses; may present with abnormal discharge.

Exam

Pelvic exam to look for cervical motion tenderness, discharge, other pelvic tenderness, **"chandelier sign."**

DIFFERENTIAL

Ectopic pregnancy, endometriosis, ovarian tumors or hemorrhagic cysts, adnexal torsion, UTI/pyelonephritis, appendicitis, diverticulitis, regional ileitis, IBD.

DIAGNOSIS

- **Minimal** diagnostic criteria are as follows:
  - Lower abdominal, adnexal, and cervical motion tenderness.
  - Fever > 38°C.
  - Elevated ESR; WBC > 10K.
  - Presence of gonorrhea or chlamydia infection.
  - Pelvic abscess on ultrasound.
- **Definitive diagnosis:** Laparoscopy (pus in peritoneum).

TREATMENT

Treat for gonorrhea, chlamydia, and anaerobes with ceftriaxone, doxycycline, clindamycin, or metronidazole for 14 days. Always treat gonorrhea and chlamydia even if only one pathogen has been identified given the high prevalence of coinfection. Hospitalization is advised if patients:

- Present with tubo-ovarian abscess, peritonitis, high fever, or a high WBC count.
- Are noncompliant, unable to tolerate PO medications, or nulliparous.
- Are adolescent.
- Show no improvement after 48–72 hours of oral therapy.

> ***Complications of PID–***
>
> **I FACE PID**
>
> **I**nfertility
> **F**itz-Hugh–Curtis syndrome (perihepatitis or inflammation of the liver capsule and adjacent peritoneal surfaces)
> **A**bscess
> **C**hronic pelvic pain
> **E**ctopic pregnancy
> **P**eritonitis
> **I**ntestinal obstruction
> **D**isseminated: sepsis, endocarditis, arthritis, meningitis

COMPLICATIONS

The complications of PID are outlined in the mnemonic **I FACE PID.**

CHRONIC PELVIC PAIN

Roughly 90% of cases have a gynecologic etiology; GI diseases are the second most common cause. Endometriosis is the most common etiology in populations with a low incidence of STDs, whereas chronic PID is most common in the presence of a high incidence of STDs. Etiologies can be further broken down as follows:

- **Gynecologic:** Endometriosis, chronic PID, adenomyosis, uterine leiomyomata (see above).
- **GI:** IBS, diverticulitis.
- **GU:** Interstitial cystitis.
- **Musculoskeletal:** Fibromyalgia.
- **Psychiatric:** Depression, somatization, domestic violence, narcotic and other substance abuse.

SYMPTOMS

- Pain below the umbilicus lasting > 6 months.
- May be consistent or intermittent, cyclic or acyclic.
- Includes disorders with laparoscopically evident pathology and those without (40%).

EXAM

Abdominal and pelvic exam.

DIAGNOSIS

- Conduct a careful history and physical and review previous workup results to determine the following:
  - The character of the pain.
  - The patient's social and sexual history.
  - Psychiatric evaluation.
- **Labs:** CBC, cultures, ultrasound, laparoscopy, UA, pregnancy test.

The treatment of chronic pelvic pain requires a multidisciplinary approach.

TREATMENT

- Requires a multidisciplinary approach involving a psychologist.
- Trust is a key issue.
- **Sequential drug treatment:** NSAIDs, OCPs, GnRH agonist analogs, antibiotics (doxycycline).
- Surgery (TAH-BSO, adhesiolysis) is a last resort.

PRECONCEPTION CARE

Patients contemplating pregnancy should undergo preventive counseling in order to optimize maternal and fetal health.

SYMPTOMS

Ask about preexisting illness and risk factors (e.g., domestic violence, substance use, alcohol use and smoking, medications, environmental hazards, seat belt use, use of smoke detectors, family history of genetic defects).

Preconception counseling optimizes the health of the mother and fetus before pregnancy.

EXAM

BP, weight, general physical exam.

DIAGNOSIS

- Rubella, STD screen.
- Screen for other infections (HBV, HIV, TB) if the patient is high risk.

TREATMENT

- Nutrition (folate, iron, multivitamins with folate **before** the patient gets pregnant).
- Immunizations.
- Genetic counseling if indicated by family history or risk factors.

POLYCYSTIC OVARIAN SYNDROME (PCOS)

A syndrome characterized by menstrual irregularity and hyperandrogenism. Onset is typically **peripubertal.**

SYMPTOMS

Patients seek treatment for **hirsutism, amenorrhea,** or infertility.

EXAM

Virilization, obesity, acne, hypertension, and acanthosis nigricans may be present. Enlarged cystic ovaries may be found on bimanual exam.

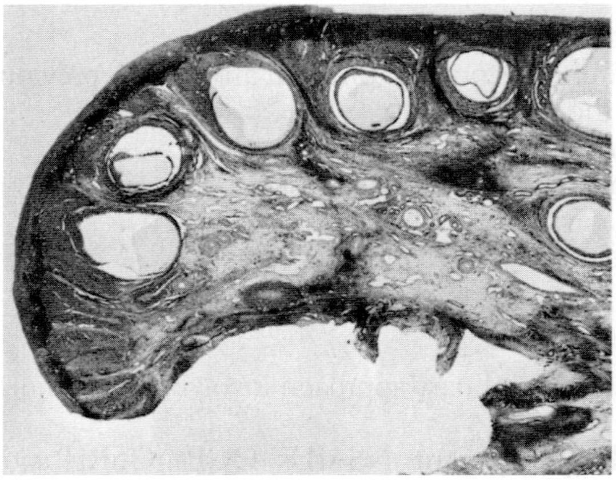

FIGURE 18-1. Polycystic ovaries.

(Reproduced, with permission, from DeCherney AH, Nathan L. *Current Obstetric & Gynecologic Diagnosis & Treatment*, 9th ed. New York: McGraw-Hill, 2003:709.)

Differential

- **Irregular menses:** See the section on menstrual disorders.
- **Androgen excess:** Adrenal or ovarian tumor, congenital adrenal hyperplasia, Cushing's syndrome.

The presence of polycystic ovaries is neither necessary nor sufficient to make the diagnosis of PCOS.

Diagnosis

- **Minimal criteria:** Menstrual irregularity (amenorrhea or oligomenorrhea), hyperandrogenism (clinical or biochemical).
- Other characteristics may include infertility and insulin resistance.
- **Labs: Serum LH-to-FSH ratio > 3:1;** increased serum androstenedione and DHEA.
- Ultrasound may reveal enlarged ovaries with numerous large subcapsular cysts (see Figure 18-1).

Treatment

- Treatment depends on the target symptom, but **weight loss and OCPs are best overall.**
- **Surgery** (ovarian) can be used as a last resort.
- Symptom-specific treatment is as follows:
  - **Insulin resistance:** Weight reduction, possibly metformin.
  - **Infertility:** Clomiphene, metformin.
  - **Hirsutism, acne:** Hair removal methods, OCPs, spironolactone, other acne treatment.
  - **Endometrial protection:** OCPs or intermittent progestin therapy.
  - **Cardiovascular protection:** Control of cardiac risk factors.

POSTMENOPAUSAL BLEEDING

Any vaginal bleeding that occurs after menopause. Always considered abnormal. Etiologies include vaginal atrophy (most common), exogenous hormones, nongynecologic sources, endometrial hyperplasia, polyps, submucosal fibroids, endometrial cancer, and cervical cancer.

Symptoms

Patients may complain of "**spotting**" or heavier, menses-like bleeding.

Exam

- Conduct a pelvic exam to look for anatomic abnormalities, including vaginal atrophy, vaginal lesions, or cervical polyps, and to palpate for fibroids.
- A Pap smear must be obtained to look for cervical cancer.

Any vaginal bleeding that occurs after menopause merits investigation.

Diagnosis

Endometrial biopsy; transvaginal ultrasound to assess endometrial thickness.

Treatment

Treat the underlying cause. Endometrial cancer requires a hysterectomy.

SEXUALLY TRANSMITTED DISEASES (STDs)

More than 15 million cases of STD are diagnosed in the United States each year.

Symptoms

None (asymptomatic screening), or may present with dysuria or discharge.

Exam

- Obtain appropriate labs.
- Conduct dermatologic and pelvic exams.
- Anyone who presents for STD screening should be offered **HBV vaccine** as well as **HAV vaccine** if high risk (IV drug users, MSM).
- Women with chlamydia should be rescreened at 3–4 months and no later than 12 months to check for reinfection.

Diagnosis/Treatment

Table 18-7 outlines the diagnosis and treatment of common STDs.

URINARY TRACT INFECTION (UTI)

Infection of the bladder and/or kidneys. May be complicated or uncomplicated:

- **Uncomplicated:** UTI in a young, healthy, nonpregnant woman. Species most commonly involved are *E. coli* and *Staphylococcus saprophyticus.* Less common are *Proteus mirabilis, Klebsiella* spp., *Enterococcus,* and *Chlamydia.*
- **Complicated:** UTI in anyone else (male, elderly, hospital acquired, pregnant, indwelling catheter, recent catheterization, anatomic abnormalities, recent antibiotics, symptoms > 1 week at presentation, immunosuppression, diabetes, recurrent UTI, history of resistant UTI).

Symptoms

- Presents with dysuria, frequency, and urgency.
- There may also be **gross hematuria,** fever, flank pain, or suprapubic pain.

TABLE 18-7. Diagnosis and Treatment of Sexually Transmitted Infections

INFECTION	DIAGNOSTIC TEST	TREATMENT
Gonorrhea	LCR, culture.	Cefixime 400 mg PO × 1; ceftriaxone 125 mg IM × 1.
Chlamydia/NGU	LCR, culture.	Azithromycin 1 g PO × 1; doxycycline 100 mg BID PO × 7 days.
Genital HSV	Clinical exam; HSV culture and HSV-1/HSV-2 serotypes.	**First episode:** ■ Acyclovir 400 mg PO TID × 7–10 days or 200 mg PO 5×/day. ■ Famciclovir 250 mg PO TID. ■ Valacyclovir 1 g PO BID. **Recurrences:** ■ Acyclovir 400 mg PO TID × 5 days, 200 mg PO 5×/day, or 800 mg PO BID. ■ Famciclovir 125 mg PO BID × 5 days. ■ Valacyclovir 500 mg PO BID × 3–5 days or 1 g QD for 5 days. **Suppression:** ■ Acyclovir 400 mg PO BID. ■ Famciclovir 25 mg PO BID. ■ Valacyclovir 500 mg QD or 1 g QD.
PID	See PID section.	**Outpatient:** ■ Ofloxacin 400 mg PO BID × 14 days. ■ Levofloxacin 500 mg PO QD × 14 days. **Parenteral:** ■ Cefotetan 2 g IV QD × 12 days plus doxycycline 100 mg PO or IV QD × 12 days.
HIV	HIV antibodies.	Multiple antiretroviral regimens.
Syphilis	RPR, VDRL, darkfield microscopy.	Penicillins.

EXAM

Temperature, abdominal exam, flank tenderness. Conduct a pelvic exam if other etiologies are suspected.

DIFFERENTIAL

See the section on dysuria.

DIAGNOSIS

UA and urine culture if complicated infection is suspected.

TREATMENT

- For **uncomplicated** infections, give a **three-day** course of oral TMP-SMX or ciprofloxacin or a **seven-day course of nitrofurantoin.**
- For **complicated** infections, a **longer course** of broad-spectrum antibiotics, typically a fluoroquinolone, should be used.

TABLE 18-8. Wet Mount Criteria in Diagnosing Vaginitis

Diagnosis	Discharge	Cells	pH	Whiff
Bacterial vaginosis	Grayish-white, fishy odor	Clue cells	> 4.5	Positive with KOH
Yeast	Thick, white, like cottage cheese	Pseudohyphae with KOH (see Figure 18-2)	3.5–4.5	Negative
Trichomoniasis	Profuse, yellow-green, frothy, malodorous	Motile trichomonads	3.5–4.5	Negative

VAGINITIS

The normal environment of the vagina is acidic (pH 3.5–4.5) and contains mixed bacterial flora (lactobacilli, diphtheroids, and S. *epidermidis*). A change in this environment due to medications, illness, or frequent intercourse can lead to bacterial overgrowth.

The triad of pruritus, malodor, and/or burning are characteristics of abnormal vaginal discharge.

Symptoms

Patients complain of abnormal discharge (odor, color, quantity) and symptoms such as itching, burning, soreness, dysuria, and dyspareunia.

Exam

Conduct a pelvic exam, particularly for:

- Vulvar edema/erythema.
- Discharge.
- **Cervicitis:** Friability, purulent discharge, **"strawberry cervix"** (petechiae in trichomonal infection).

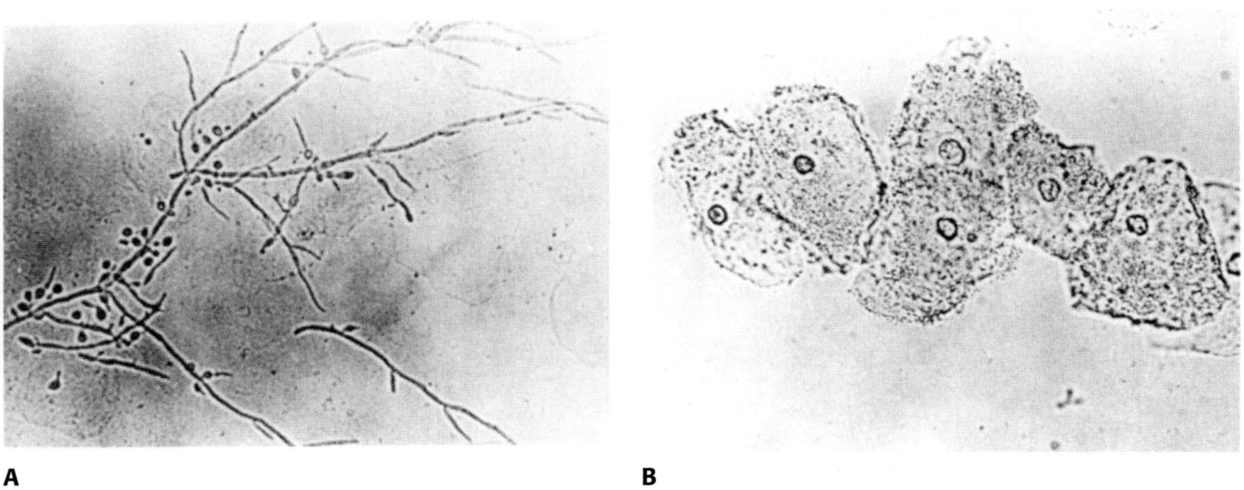

FIGURE 18-2. Causes of vaginitis.

(A) Pseudohyphae in candidal vaginitis. (B) Clue cells in *Gardnerella vaginalis.* (Reproduced, with permission, from DeCherney AH, Nathan L. *Current Obstetric & Gynecologic Diagnosis & Treatment*, 9th ed. New York: McGraw-Hill, 2003:651, 653.)

Differential

UTI, normal (physiologic), cancer, noninfectious/irritants (spermicide, douching).

Diagnosis

- Wet mount (pH and microscopy in saline and KOH) (see Table 18-8 and Figure 18-2).
- Consider UA and/or STD testing.

Treatment

Treat the underlying cause:

- **UTI:** See the UTI section above.
- **Bacterial vaginosis:** Metronidazole (500 mg PO BID × 7 days or 2 g × 1, or topical) or clindamycin (PO or topical). May resolve spontaneously; recurrence is common.
- **Candida:** Fluconazole 150 mg × 1, or various topicals.
- **Trichomoniasis:** Metronidazole at the same doses as for bacterial vaginosis.

APPENDIX

Abbreviations and Symbols

Abbreviation	Meaning
A-a	alveolar-arterial (oxygen gradient)
AASK	African-American Study of Kidney Disease and Hypertension
AAT	α_1-antitrypsin
ABG	arterial blood gas
ABI	ankle-brachial index
ABPA	allergic bronchopulmonary aspergillosis
ABPA-CB	allergic bronchopulmonary aspergillosis with central bronchiectasis
ABPA-S	allergic bronchopulmonary aspergillosis—seropositive
ABV	Adriamycin, bleomycin, and vincristine
ABVD	Adriamycin, bleomycin, vincristine, and dacarbazine
ACA	anterior cerebral artery
ACC	American College of Cardiology
ACD	anemia of chronic disease
ACEI	angiotensin-converting enzyme inhibitor
ACh	acetylcholine
AChE	acetylcholinesterase
AChR	acetylcholine receptor
ACL	anterior cruciate ligament
ACLS	advanced cardiac life support
ACP	American College of Physicians
ACS	American Cancer Society
ACTH	adrenocorticotropic hormone
AD	autosomal dominant, Addison's disease
ADA	American Diabetes Association
ADH	antidiuretic hormone
ADHD	attention-deficit hyperactivity disorder
ADP	adenosine diphosphate
ADPKD	adult dominant polycystic kidney disease
AF	atrial fibrillation
AFB	acid-fast bacillus
AFFIRM	Atrial Fibrillation Follow-up Investigation of Rhythm Management
AFP	α-fetoprotein
AFS	allergic fungal sinusitis
AG	anion gap
AHA	American Heart Association
AICA	anterior inferior cerebellar artery
AICD	automatic implantable cardioverter defibrillator
AIDS	acquired immunodeficiency syndrome
AIN	acute interstitial nephritis
ALL	acute lymphoblastic leukemia
ALS	amyotrophic lateral sclerosis
ALT	alanine aminotransferase
AMA	antimitochondrial antibody
AML	acute myeloid leukemia
ANA	antinuclear antibody
ANC	absolute neutrophil count
ANCA	antineutrophil cytoplasmic antibody
AP	anteroposterior
APL	acute promyelocytic leukemia
APLAS	antiphospholipid antibody syndrome
APO E2	apolipoprotein E2
APS	autoimmune polyglandular syndrome
APUD	amine precursor uptake and decarboxylation
AR	autosomal recessive
ARB	angiotensin receptor blocker
ARDS	acute respiratory distress syndrome
ARF	acute respiratory failure
5-ASA	5-aminosalicylic acid
ASA	acetylsalicylic acid
ASCA	Anti-*Saccharomyces cerevisiae* antibody
ASCUS	atypical squamous cells of uncertain significance
ASD	atrial septal defect
AST	aspartate aminotransferase
AT	angiotensin, atrial tachycardia

Abbreviation	Meaning
ATN	acute tubular necrosis
ATPase	adenosine triphosphatase
ATRA	*all*-trans retinoic acid
AV	arteriovenous, atrioventricular
AVF	arteriovenous fistula
AVM	arteriovenous malformation
AVN	avascular necrosis
AVNRT	atrioventricular nodal reentrant tachycardia
AVRT	atrioventricular reentrant tachycardia
AXR	abdominal x-ray
AZT	azidothymidine (zidovudine)
BCC	basal cell carcinoma
BCG	bacille Calmette-Guérin
BEP	bleomycin, etoposide, and Platinol (cisplatin)
BID	twice daily
BIW	twice weekly
BM	bowel movement
BMD	bone mineral density
BMI	body mass index
BMT	bone marrow transplant
BNP	B-natriuretic peptide
BOOP	bronchiolitis obliterans with organizing pneumonia
BP	blood pressure
BPH	benign prostatic hypertrophy
bpm	beat per minute
BPV	benign positional vertigo
BRAT	bran, rice, applesauce, toast (diet)
BSE	breast self-examination
BUN	blood urea nitrogen
BV	bleomycin and vincristine
CABG	coronary artery bypass graft
$CaCO_3$	calcium carbonate
CAD	coronary artery disease
c-ANCA	cytoplasmic antineutrophil cytoplasmic antibody
CBC	complete blood count
CBE	clinical breast examination
CBW	current body weight
CCK	cholecystokinin
CD	cluster of differentiation
CDC	Centers for Disease Control and Prevention
CF	cystic fibrosis
CFTR	cystic fibrosis transmembrane regulator
CHF	congestive heart failure
CHOP	cyclophosphamide, doxorubicin hydrochloride, Oncovin (vincristine), and prednisone
CIDP	chronic inflammatory demyelinating polyneuropathy
CIWA	Clinical Institute Withdrawal Assessment
CK	creatine kinase
CKD	chronic kidney disease
CK-MB	creatine kinase, MB fraction
CLL	chronic lymphocytic leukemia
CMC	carpometacarpal (joint)
CML	chronic myelogenous leukemia
CMML	chronic myelomonocytic leukemia
CMT	Charcot-Marie-Tooth (disease)
CMV	cytomegalovirus
CN	cranial nerve
CNS	central nervous system
COMT	catechol-O-methyltransferase
COPD	chronic obstructive pulmonary disease
COX	cyclooxygenase
CP	ceruloplasmin
CPAP	continuous positive airway pressure
CPK	creatine phosphokinase
CPPD	calcium pyrophosphate dihydrate
CPR	cardiopulmonary resuscitation
CrAg	cryptococcal antigen
CRBSI	catheter-related bloodstream infection
CREST	calcinosis, Raynaud's phenomenon, esophageal dysmotility, sclerodactyly, and telangiectasia (syndrome)
CRF	corticotropin-releasing factor
CRH	corticotropin-releasing hormone
CRP	C-reactive protein
CSF	cerebrospinal fluid
CSS	Churg-Strauss syndrome
CT	computed tomography
CTA	computed tomographic angiography
CTCL	cutaneous T-cell lymphoma
CTP	Child-Turcotte-Pugh (scoring)
CVA	cerebrovascular accident
CVID	common variable immunodeficiency
CXR	chest x-ray
D&C	dilation and curettage
D_2	ergocalciferol
D_3	cholecalciferol
d4T	didehydrodeoxythymidine (stavudine)
DAP	3,4-diaminopyridine
DASH	Dietary Approach to Stop Hypertension (study)
DBP	diastolic blood pressure
DC	direct current
DCCT	Diabetes Control and Complication Trial
DCIS	ductal carcinoma in situ
DDAVP	1-deamino (8-D-arginine) vasopressin
ddC	dideoxycytosine

Abbreviation	Meaning
ddI	dideoxyinosine
DEET	diethyltoluamide
DES	diethylstilbestrol
DEXA	dual-energy x-ray absorptiometry
DF	discriminant factor
DFA	direct fluorescent antibody
DGI	disseminated gonococcal infection
DH	dermatitis herpetiformis
1,25-DHD	1,25-dihydroxycholecalciferol
DHEA	dehydroepiandrosterone
DHEAS	dehydroepiandrosterone sulfate
DHIC	detrusor hyperactivity with impaired contractility
DI	diabetes insipidus
DIC	disseminated intravascular coagulation
DIG	Digitalis Investigation Group (trial)
DIP	distal interphalangeal (joint)
DISH	diffuse idiopathic skeletal hyperostosis
DJD	degenerative joint disease
DKA	diabetic ketoacidosis
DLB	dementia with Lewy bodies
DL_{CO}	diffusing capacity of carbon monoxide
DM	diabetes mellitus
DMARD	disease-modifying antirheumatic drug
DNA	deoxyribonucleic acid
DNase	deoxyribonuclease
DNR	do not resuscitate
DOC	deoxycorticosterone
2,3-DPG	2,3-diphosphoglycerate
DPOA-HC	durable power of attorney for health care
DRE	digital rectal examination
dsDNA	double-stranded DNA
DTIC	dacarbazine
DTRs	deep tendon reflexes
DTs	delirium tremens
DVT	deep venous thrombosis
DWI	diffusion-weighted imaging
EBNA	Epstein-Barr nuclear antigen
EBV	Epstein-Barr virus
ECG	electrocardiography
ECT	electroconvulsive therapy
ED	erectile dysfunction
EECP	enhanced external counterpulsation
EEG	electroencephalography
EF	ejection fraction
EGD	esophagogastroduodenoscopy
EHEC	enterohemorrhagic *E. coli*
EIA	enzyme immunoassay
ELISA	enzyme-linked immunosorbent assay

Abbreviation	Meaning
EM	electron microscopy, erythema multiforme
EMG	electromyography
EMS	emergency medical services
EN	erythema nodosum
ENT	ears, nose, and throat
EOM	extraocular muscle
EP	etoposide and Platinol (cisplatin), evoked potential
EPHESUS	Eplerenone Post-AMI Heart Failure Efficacy and Survival Study
EPO	erythropoietin
ER	emergency room, estrogen receptor
ERCP	endoscopic retrograde cholangiopancreatography
ERV	expiratory reserve volume
ESR	erythrocyte sedimentation rate
ESRD	end-stage renal disease
ETEC	enterotoxigenic *E. coli*
EtOH	ethanol
ETT	exercise treadmill test
EVH	esophageal variceal hemorrhage
FAP	familial adenomatous polyposis
FBHH	familial benign hypocalciuric hypercalcemia
FDA	Food and Drug Administration
FDG	fluorodeoxyglucose
F-dUMP	5-fluorodeoxyuridine monophosphate
Fe_{Na}	fractional excretion of sodium
FEV_1	forced expiratory volume in one second
FFP	fresh frozen plasma
FiO_2	fraction of inspired oxygen
FN	false negative
FNA	fine needle aspiration
FOBT	fecal occult blood test
FRC	functional reserve capacity
FSH	follicle-stimulating hormone
FT_3	free triiodothyronine
FT_4	free thyroxine
FTA	fluorescent treponemal antibody
5-FU	5-fluorouracil
FUO	fever of unknown origin
FVC	forced vital capacity
GABA	γ-aminobutyric acid
GABHS	group A β-hemolytic streptococcus
GAD	generalized anxiety disorder
GBM	glomerular basement membrane
GBS	Guillain-Barré syndrome
G-CSF	granulocyte colony-stimulating factor
GDM	gestational diabetes mellitus
GERD	gastroesophageal reflux disease
GFR	glomerular filtration rate
GGT	γ-glutamyltransferase
GH	growth hormone

Abbreviation	Meaning
GHB	γ-hydroxybutyrate
GHRH	growth hormone–releasing hormone
GI	gastrointestinal
GIST	gastrointestinal stromal tumor
GM-CSF	granulocyte-macrophage colony-stimulating factor
GnRH	gonadotropin-releasing hormone
G6PD	glucose-6-phosphate dehydrogenase
GU	genitourinary
HAART	highly active antiretroviral therapy
HACEK	*Haemophilus, Actinobacillus, Cardiobacterium, Eikenella, Kingella*
HAV	hepatitis A virus
HbA_{1c}	hemoglobin A_{1c}
HBeAg	hepatitis B early antigen
HBIG	hepatitis B immune globulin
HBsAg	hepatitis B surface antigen
HBV	hepatitis B virus
hCG	human chorionic gonadotropin
HCO_3	bicarbonate
HCTZ	hydrochlorothiazide
HCV	hepatitis C virus
1,25-HD	1,25-hydroxycholecalciferol
HDL	high-density lipoprotein
HDV	hepatitis D virus
HEENT	head, eyes, ears, nose, and throat
HELLP	hemolysis, elevated LFTs, low platelets (syndrome)
HEV	hepatitis E virus
HF	heart failure
HGE	human granulocytic ehrlichiosis
HGH	human growth hormone
HHV	human herpesvirus
HIAA	hydroxyindole acetic acid
HIDA	hepato-iminodiacetic acid (scan)
HIPA	heparin-induced platelet activation
HIT	heparin-induced thrombocytopenia
HIV	human immunodeficiency virus
HIVAN	human immunodeficiency virus–associated nephropathy
HL	hearing loss
HLA	human leukocyte antigen
HME	human monocytic ehrlichiosis
HNPCC	hereditary nonpolyposis colorectal cancer
HOCM	hypertrophic obstructive cardiomyopathy
HOPE	Heart Outcomes Prevention Evaluation (study)
HOT	Hypertension Optimal Treatment (trial)
HP	hypersensitivity pneumonitis
hpf	high-power field
HPV	human papillomavirus

Abbreviation	Meaning
HR	heart rate
HRCT	high-resolution computed tomography
HRS	hepatorenal syndrome
HRT	hormone replacement therapy
11β-HSD	11β-hydroxysteroid dehydrogenase
HSIL	high-grade squamous intraepithelial lesion
HSV	herpes simplex virus
5-HT	5-hydroxytryptamine
HTLV	human T-cell leukemia virus
HUS	hemolytic-uremic syndrome
IABP	intraaortic balloon pump
IBD	inflammatory bowel disease
IBS	irritable bowel syndrome
IC	inspiratory capacity
ICA	internal carotid artery
ICD	implantable cardiac defibrillator
ICP	intracranial pressure
ICS	inhaled corticosteroid
ICU	intensive care unit
IFE	immunofixation electrophoresis
Ig	immunoglobulin
IGF	insulin-like growth factor
IHSS	idiopathic hypertrophic subaortic stenosis
IL	interleukin
ILD	interstitial lung disease
IM	intramuscular
IMRT	intensity-modulated radiation therapy
INH	isoniazid
INO	internuclear ophthalmoplegia
INR	International Normalized Ratio
IPF	idiopathic pulmonary fibrosis
IPSS	inferior petrosal sinus sampling
ITP	idiopathic thrombocytopenic purpura
IUD	intrauterine device
IUGR	intrauterine growth retardation
IV	intravenous
IVC	inferior vena cava
IVDU	intravenous drug user
IVF	in vitro fertilization
IVIG	intravenous immunoglobulin
IVP	intravenous pyelography
JAMA	*Journal of the American Medical Association*
J-I	jejunoileal
JNC 7	Joint National Committee on the Prevention, Detection, Evaluation, and Treatment of High Blood Pressure, Seventh Report
JVD	jugular venous distention
JVP	jugular venous pressure
KCl	potassium chloride
KOH	potassium hydroxide

Abbreviation	Meaning
KS	Kaposi's sarcoma
LA	left atrial
LAD	left anterior descending (artery)
LAP	leukocyte alkaline phosphatase
LBBB	left bundle branch block
LBP	lower back pain
LCIS	lobular carcinoma in situ
LCR	ligase chain reaction
LCV	leukocytoclastic vasculitis
LDH	lactate dehydrogenase
LDL	low-density lipoprotein
LEEP	loop electrosurgical excision procedure
LEMS	Lambert-Eaton myasthenic syndrome
LES	lower esophageal sphincter
LFTs	liver function tests
LGIB	lower GI bleeding
LH	luteinizing hormone
LLQ	left lower quadrant
LMN	lower motor neuron
LMP	last menstrual period
LMWH	low-molecular-weight heparin
LP	lumbar puncture
LR	likelihood ratio
LS	limited scleroderma
LSIL	low-grade squamous intraepithelial lesion
LT_4	levothyroxine
LTBI	latent tuberculosis infection
LTOT	long-term oxygen therapy
LUQ	left upper quadrant
LV	left ventricular
LVH	left ventricular hypertrophy
LVRS	lung volume reduction surgery
MAC	*Mycobacterium avium* complex
MAHA	microangiopathic hemolytic anemia
MAID	mesna, Adriamycin, ifosfamide, and dacarbazine
MALT	mucosa-associated lymphoid tissue
MAOI	monoamine oxidase inhibitor
MCA	middle cerebral artery
MCI	mild cognitive impairment
MCL	medial collateral ligament
MCP	metacarpophalangeal (joint)
MCV	mean corpuscular volume
MDD	major depressive disorder
MDI	metered-dose inhaler
MDMA	3,4-methylene-dioxymethamphetamine ("Ecstasy")
MDR	multidrug resistance
MDS	myelodysplastic syndrome
MELAS	mitochondrial myopathy, encephalopathy, lactic acidosis, and strokelike episodes (syndrome)
MELD	Model for End-Stage Liver Disease

Abbreviation	Meaning
MEN	multiple endocrine neoplasia
MEP	maximum expiratory pressure
MERRF	myoclonic epilepsy and ragged red fibers
MET	metabolic equivalent
MF	mycosis fungoides
MFH	malignant fibrous histiocytoma
MG	myasthenia gravis
MGUS	monoclonal gammopathy of undetermined significance
MHATP	microhemagglutination assay—*Treponema pallidum*
MI	myocardial infarction
MIBG	metaiodobenzylguanidine
MIBI	methoxyisobutyl isonitrile (stress test)
MIP	maximum inspiratory pressure
MMA	middle meningeal artery
MMI	methimazole
MMR	measles, mumps, rubella (vaccine)
MMSE	mini-mental status examination
6-MP	6-mercaptopurine
MPA	microscopic polyangiitis
MPGN	membranoproliferative glomerulonephritis
MPO	myeloperoxidase
MR	magnetic resonance
MRA	magnetic resonance angiography
MRC	magnetic resonance cholangiography
MRCP	magnetic resonance cholangiopancreatography
MRI	magnetic resonance imaging
MRSA	methicillin-resistant S. *aureus*
MS	multiple sclerosis
MSA	multisystem atrophy
MSM	men who have sex with men
MTP	metatarsophalangeal (joint)
NA	Narcotics Anonymous
nAChR	nicotinic acetylcholine receptor
NAEPP	National Asthma Education and Prevention Program
$NaHCO_3$	sodium bicarbonate
NASPE	National Association for Sport and Physical Education
NBW	normal body weight
NCEP-ATPIII	National Cholesterol Education Program Adult Treatment Panel III
NCS	nerve conduction study
NF	neurofibromatosis
NGU	nongonococcal urethritis
NHANES	National Health and Examination Survey
NHL	non-Hodgkin's lymphoma
NHLBI	National Heart, Lung, and Blood Institute
NIH	National Institutes of Health

Abbreviation	Meaning
NIPPV	noninvasive positive pressure ventilation
NPO	nil per os (nothing by mouth)
NPV	negative predictive value
NREM	non–rapid eye movement
NS	normal saline
NSAID	nonsteroidal anti-inflammatory drug
NSCLC	non–small cell lung cancer
NSTEMI	non-ST-elevation myocardial infarction
NVE	native-valve endocarditis
NYHA	New York Heart Association
O&P	ova and parasites
OCD	obsessive-compulsive disorder
OCP	oral contraceptive pill
OR	operating room
OSA	obstructive sleep apnea
OTC	over the counter
PA	primary aldosteronism, pernicious anemia
PAC	plasma aldosterone concentration, premature atrial contraction
$PaCO_2$	partial pressure of carbon dioxide in arterial blood
PAN	polyarteritis nodosa
p-ANCA	perinuclear antineutrophil cytoplasmic antibody
PaO_2	partial pressure of oxygen in arterial blood
PAOP	pulmonary artery occlusion pressure
PASP	pulmonary artery systolic pressure
P_{atm}	atmospheric pressure
PBC	primary biliary cirrhosis
PCA	patient-controlled anesthesia
PCI	percutaneous coronary intervention
PCO_2	partial pressure of carbon dioxide
PCOP	pulmonary capillary occlusion pressure
PCOS	polycystic ovarian syndrome
PCP	*Pneumocystis jiroveci* cystic pneumonia
P_{Cr}	plasma creatinine
PCR	polymerase chain reaction
PCV	procarbazine, CCNU (lomustine), and vincristine
PCW	pulmonary capillary wedge (pressure)
PDA	patent ductus arteriosus
P/DM	polymyositis/dermatomyositis
PE	pulmonary embolism
PEEP	positive end-expiratory pressure
PEF	peak expiratory flow
PET	positron emission tomography
PFTs	pulmonary function tests
PHN	postherpetic neuralgia
PICA	posterior inferior cerebellar artery
PID	pelvic inflammatory disease
PiO_2	partial pressure of inspired oxygen
PIOPED	Prospective Investigation of Pulmonary Embolism Diagnosis
PIP	proximal interphalangeal (joint)
P_{K+}	plasma potassium
PLED	period lateralizing epileptiform discharge
PLMD	period limb-movement disorder
PLMS	periodic limb movements in sleep
PMI	point of maximal insertion
PMN	polymorphonuclear (leukocyte)
PMR	polymyalgia rheumatica
P_{Na}	plasma sodium
PNH	paroxysmal nocturnal hemoglobinuria
PO	per os (by mouth)
PO_2	partial pressure of oxygen
PORT	Patient Outcomes Research Team
P_{osm}	plasma osmolality
PPD	purified protein derivative
PPH	primary pulmonary hypertension
PPI	proton pump inhibitor
PPN	peripheral parenteral nutrition
PPV	positive predictive value
PR	progesterone receptor
PRA	plasma renin activity
PRBC	packed red blood cells
PRCA	pure red cell aplasia
PRN	as needed
PSA	prostate-specific antigen
PSC	primary sclerosing cholangitis
PSI	Pneumonia Severity Index
PSP	progressive supranuclear palsy
PSS	progressive systemic sclerosis
PSVT	paroxysmal supraventricular tachycardia
PT	prothrombin time
PTCA	percutaneous transluminal coronary angioplasty
PTH	parathyroid hormone
PTHC	percutaneous transhepatic cholangiography
PTHrP	parathyroid hormone–related protein
PTSD	post-traumatic stress disorder
PTT	partial thromboplastin time
PTU	propylthiouracil
PUD	peptic ulcer disease
PV	polycythemia vera
PVC	premature ventricular contraction
PVE	prosthetic-valve endocarditis
$P\bar{v}mO_2$	mixed venous arterial saturation
PVX	Pneumovax (vaccine)
QD	once daily
QHS	at bedtime

Abbreviation	Meaning
QID	four times daily
QOD	every other day
RA	rheumatoid arthritis, right atrial, refractory anemia
RAEB	refractory anemia with excess blasts
RAEB-T	refractory anemia with excess blasts in transformation
RAI	radioactive iodine
RAIU	radioactive iodine uptake
RALES	Randomized Spironolactone Evaluation Study
RAPD	relative afferent pupillary defect
RARS	refractory anemia with ringed sideroblasts
RAST	radioallergosorbent test
RBBB	right bundle branch block
RBC	red blood cell
RDW	red-cell distribution width
REM	rapid eye movement
RF	rheumatoid factor
RICE	rest, ice, compression, and elevation
RLQ	right lower quadrant
RLS	restless leg syndrome
RNA	ribonucleic acid
RPGN	rapidly progressive glomerulonephritis
RPR	rapid plasma reagin
RR	respiratory rate
RSV	respiratory syncytial virus
RTA	renal tubular acidosis
RUQ	right upper quadrant
RV	residual volume, right ventricular
RVH	right ventricular hypertrophy
SAAG	serum-ascites albumin gradient
SADNI	selective antibody deficiency with normal immunoglobulins
SAH	subarachnoid hemorrhage
SAMe	S-adenosyl-L-methionine
SARS	severe acute respiratory syndrome
SBE	subacute bacterial endocarditis
SBP	spontaneous bacterial peritonitis, systolic blood pressure
SCA	superior cerebellar artery
SCC	squamous cell carcinoma
SCD	sequential compression device
SCLC	small cell lung cancer
SCLE	subacute cutaneous lupus erythematosus
SD	standard deviation
SERM	selective estrogen receptor modulator
SES	socioeconomic status
SGA	small for gestational age
SHEP	Systolic Hypertension in Elderly Patients (study)
SIADH	syndrome of inappropriate secretion of antidiuretic hormone
SIRS	systemic inflammatory response syndrome
SJS	Stevens-Johnson syndrome
SLE	systemic lupus erythematosus
SMA	smooth muscle antibody
SOD	superoxide dismutase
SPEP	serum protein electrophoresis
SQ	subcutaneous
SS	Sjögren's syndrome
SSA	sulfosalicylic acid
SSKI	saturated solution of potassium iodide
SSPE	subacute sclerosing panencephalitis
SSRI	selective serotonin reuptake inhibitor
STD	sexually transmitted disease
STEMI	ST-elevation myocardial infarction
SVC	superior vena cava
SVR	systemic vascular resistance
$T_{1/2}$	half-life
T_3	triiodothyronine
T_4	thyroxine
TAH	total abdominal hysterectomy
TAH-BSO	total abdominal hysterectomy and bilateral salpingo-oophorectomy
TB	tuberculosis
TBG	thyroid-binding globulin
TBNA	transbronchial needle aspiration
3TC	dideoxythiacytidine (lamivudine)
TCA	tricyclic antidepressant
TD	tetanus and diphtheria (vaccine)
TEDS	thromboembolic disease stockings
TEE	transesophageal echocardiography
TFTs	thyroid function tests
Tg	thyroglobulin
TG	triglyceride
TIA	transient ischemic attack
TID	three times daily
TIPS	transjugular intrahepatic portosystemic shunt
TIW	three times per week
TLC	total lung capacity
TLS	tumor lysis syndrome
TMP-SMX	trimethoprim-sulfamethoxazole
TN	true negative
TNF	tumor necrosis factor
TNM	tumor, node, metastasis (staging)
tPA	tissue plasminogen activator
TPN	total parenteral nutrition
TPO	thyroid peroxidase
TRALI	transfusion-related acute lung injury
TRH	thyrotropin-releasing hormone
TS	transferrin saturation
TSH	thyroid-stimulating hormone

Abbreviation	Meaning
TSHR	thyroid-stimulating hormone receptor
TSI	thyroid-stimulating immunoglobulin
TSS	toxic shock syndrome
TSST	toxic shock syndrome toxin
TTE	transthoracic echocardiography
TTKG	transtubular K^+ gradient
TTP	thrombotic thrombocytopenic purpura
TUIP	transurethral incision of the prostate
TURP	transurethral resection of the prostate
TV	tidal volume
UA	urinalysis
UAG	urine anion gap
UC	ulcerative colitis
U_{Cr}	urine creatinine
UDCA	ursodeoxycholic acid
UFH	unfractionated heparin
UGIB	upper GI bleeding
U_{K+}	urine potassium
UKPDS	United Kingdom Prospective Diabetes Study
UMN	upper motor neuron
U_{Na}	urine sodium
U_{osm}	urine osmolality
UPEP	urinary protein electrophoresis
URI	upper respiratory infection
USPSTF	United States Preventive Services Task Force
UTI	urinary tract infection
UV	ultraviolet
V/Q	ventilation-perfusion (ratio)
Val-HeFT	Valsartan Heart Failure Trial
VAP	ventilator-assisted pneumonia
VATS	video-assisted thoracoscopy
VBI	vertebrobasilar insufficiency
VC	vital capacity
VDRL	Venereal Disease Research Laboratory
VF	ventricular fibrillation
VLDL	very low density lipoprotein
VMA	vanillylmandelic acid
VSD	ventricular septal defect
V_T	tidal volume
VT	ventricular tachycardia
VTE	venous thromboembolism
vWD	von Willebrand's disease
vWF	von Willebrand's factor
VZIG	varicella-zoster immune globulin
VZV	varicella-zoster virus
WBC	white blood cell
WHI	Women's Health Initiative
WHO	World Health Organization
WNL	within normal limits
WPW	Wolff-Parkinson-White (syndrome)
Z-E	Zollinger-Ellison syndrome

Index

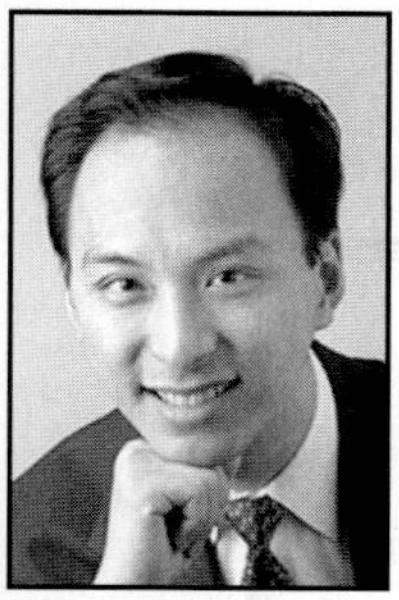

Tao Le, MD

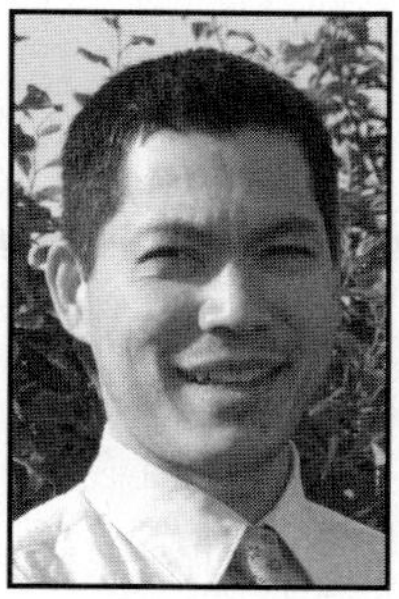

Peter Chin-Hong, MD

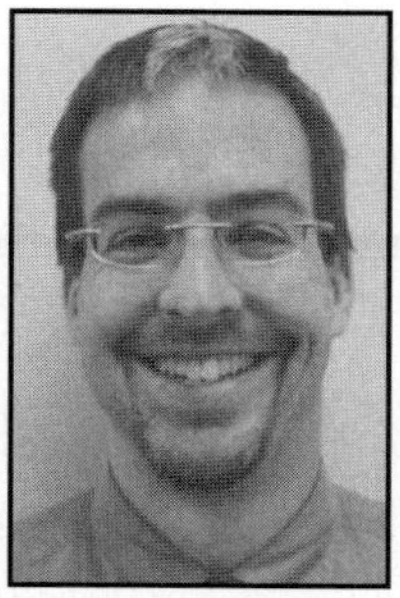

Thomas E. Baudendistel, MD, FACP

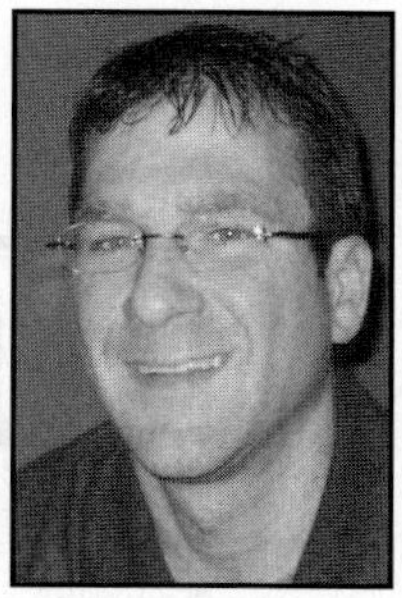

Lewis Rubinson, MD, PhD

Tao Le, MD

Tao has led multiple medical education projects over the past 14 years. As a medical student, he was editor-in-chief of the University of California, San Francisco *Synapse,* a university newspaper with a weekly circulation of 9000. Subsequently, he authored *First Aid for the Step 2 CK, First Aid for the USMLE Step 2 CS,* and *First Aid for the USMLE Step 3,* and led the most recent revision of *First Aid for the USMLE Step 1.* At Yale, he was a regular guest lecturer on the USMLE review courses and an adviser to the Yale University School of Medicine curriculum committee. Tao earned his medical degree from the University of California, San Francisco in 1996 and completed his residency training and board certification in internal medicine at Yale–New Haven Hospital. Tao subsequently went on to co-found Medsn and served as its Chief Medical Officer. He is also founder and Editor-in-Chief of the USMLERx test bank series. He is currently pursuing research in asthma education as a fellow in allergy and clinical immunology at the Johns Hopkins Asthma and Allergy Center.

Peter Chin-Hong, MD

Peter is Assistant Professor in the division of Infectious Diseases at UCSF and site co-leader of the Doris Duke Clinical Research Fellowship Program for medical students. He was born and raised in Trinidad, West Indies, and received his undergraduate and medical degrees at Brown University in Providence, Rhode Island. Seeking a more balmy clime, he completed Internal Medicine residency training and a fellowship in Infectious Diseases at UCSF, and joined the faculty there in 2002. He is board certified in internal medicine and infectious diseases. He is actively involved in teaching nurses, medical students, residents and fellows and is a frequent speaker for UCSF continuing medical education courses, including the annual Internal Medicine Board Certification and Recertification Review. He has authored chapters in various medical texts (including *Current Diagnosis and Treatment in Otolaryngology, Current Diagnosis and Treatment in Sexually Transmitted Infections,* and the *Encyclopedia of Gastroenterology*) and penned several original scientific articles based on an active research program in infectious diseases of immunocompromised hosts. He sees patients at the UCSF Medical Center as well as at the Positive Health Practice, Ward 86, San Francisco General Hospital.

Thomas E. Baudendistel, MD, FACP

Tom is the chair of the Society of Hospital Medicine's national ethics committee and is the Associate Program Director of the Internal Medicine Residency at California Pacific Medical Center in San Francisco. Prior to join ing CPMC in 2002, he graduated magna cum laude from Duke University with a B.S. in zoology and psychology and was the Dean's Award recipient at the University of Missouri-Columbia where he received his M.D. in 1995. He completed his Internal Medicine residency and chief residency at UCSF and then joined the Hospitalist faculty at UCSF in 1999. He is board certified in Internal Medicine, has lectured nationally on numerous clinical and bioethical topics, and currently edits the clinical vignette series for *The Hospitalist.* He has been a contributor on *Current Consult Medicine, The Patient History: Evidence-based Approach, Hospital Medicine for the pda, The Saint-Frances Guide to Inpatient Medicine,* the *UCSF Housestaff Handbook,* and edited the *Companion Web Page* for *Current Medical Diagnosis and Treatment.*

Lewis Rubinson, MD, PhD

Lewis is a nationally recognized expert on mass casualty critical care responses for disasters, particularly those due to outbreaks. Recently, he completed a fellowship in Pulmonary and Critical Care Medicine at Johns Hopkins and joined the clinical staff of the Bend Memorial Clinic in Bend, Oregon. Lewis has published a number of peer-reviewed manuscripts on central venous catheter-related bloodstream infections and more recently on the delivery of medical care in the wake of large-scale outbreaks. He is the Vice-Chair and Chair-elect of the Society of Critical Care Medicine's (SCCM) subcommittee for Fundamentals of Disaster Medicine, is a core developer of SCCM's Hospital Mass Casualty Disaster Management course, and has chaired a number of expert committees regarding mass casualty critical care. Dr. Rubinson has lectured internationally on topics related to bioterrorism and mass casualty critical care. He was a member of Phi Beta Kappa and graduated summa cum laude with a BS in Chemistry from the University of Michigan. Lewis received his medical degree from Northwestern University Medical School, where he was elected to the Alpha Omega Alpha honor society. He completed his Internal Medicine residency at UCSF, and also received a Doctor of Philosophy in Clinical Investigation from Johns Hopkins University, where he was elected to the Delta Omega honor society.

ABOUT THE AUTHORS